Veterinary Neuroanatomy and Clinical Neurology

Second Edition

ALEXANDER DE LAHUNTA, D.V.M., Ph.D.

Professor of Anatomy
Chairman, Department of Clinical Sciences
Director, Veterinary Medical Teaching Hospital
New York State College of Veterinary Medicine
Cornell University, Ithaca, New York

Illustrated by
Lewis L. Sadler, William P. Hamilton IV and Grant S. Lashbrook

W. B. SAUNDERS COMPANY
Philadelphia/London/Toronto/Mexico City/Rio de Janeiro/Sydney/Tokyo

W. B. Saunders Company: West Washington Square
Philadelphia, PA   19105

1 St. Anne's Road
Eastbourne, East Sussex BN21 3UN, England

1 Goldthorne Avenue
Toronto, Ontario M8Z 5T9, Canada

Apartado 26370—Cedro 512
Mexico 4, D.F., Mexico

Rua Coronel Cabrita, 8
Sao Cristovao Caixa Postal 21176
Rio de Janeiro, Brazil

9 Waltham Street
Artarmon, N.S.W. 2064, Australia

Ichibancho, Central Bldg., 22-1 Ichibancho
Chiyoda-Ku, Tokyo 102, Japan

Library of Congress Cataloging in Publication Data

DeLahunta, Alexander, 1932–

Veterinary neuroanatomy and clinical neurology.

Includes index.

1. Veterinary neurology.   2. Veterinary anatomy.   3. Neuroanatomy.   I. Title.

SF895.D44 1983   636.089′68   82–42607

ISBN 0–7216–3029–4

Veterinary Neuroanatomy and Clinical Neurology   ISBN   0-7216-3029-4

Last digit is the print number: 9   8   7   6   5   4   3

FOREWORD

This book has been made possible by the willingness of my original department head, Dr. Robert E. Habel, and present chairman, Dr. Howard E. Evans, to allow me to spend my research time and energy outside the Department of Anatomy in the areas of clinical neurology and neuropathology. The cooperation received from the clinical departments and the Department of Pathology also has made possible the studies that are the basis for this book.

To follow neuroanatomy to its logical conclusion is to explore its function. For a veterinarian, the knowledge of normal function is the basis for understanding the pathophysiology of abnormal function. In the nervous system, this is the study of clinical neurology. Neuroanatomy, neurophysiology, neuropathology, and clinical neurology are a logical sequence of studies that are integrated readily into a single course.

With some modification, this is the subject matter that is taught to first-year veterinary students at the New York State College of Veterinary Medicine. The academic year consists of two semesters. During the first semester the students study the gross anatomy of the dog, including the various components of the peripheral nervous system, followed by a dissection of the brain and spinal cord. This anatomy and the dissection procedure are described in *Miller's Guide to the Dissection of the Dog,* by H. E. Evans and A. de Lahunta. A complete preserved dog brain is provided for each pair of students. Following the dissection each pair of students sections another preserved dog brain transversely, and relates the gross features of the transverse sections to their dissection to obtain a three-dimensional orientation.

In the second semester, the neuroanatomy course is taught in a vertically integrated manner according to functional systems. For each functional system the anatomy of the major components is described, along with its normal function. This is followed by a consideration of the clinical signs that occur if the function of the system is disturbed, and a description and differential diagnosis of the diseases that typically affect this system. Films of clinical patients are used to demonstrate the clinical signs produced by the various diseases. Slides of gross and microscopic lesions are shown to emphasize the clinical-neuroanatomic relationships and to stress characteristic features of some of the diseases.

Clinical diagnoses of disease of the nervous system probably depend more on the understanding of the anatomy of the system than any other diagnoses. The first-year student is in a unique position to study both simultaneously. The direct application of the anatomic study to the disease process and clinical diagnosis not only is logical for this system but also permits the first-year veterinary student the opportunity to work with the clinical patient. Not only does this approach stimulate the student to learn, but it is equally exciting for the professor to teach in this manner.

This book has been written primarily to complement this method of teaching at the New York State College of Veterinary Medicine. It is not intended to be a complete treatise on all aspects of veterinary neuroanatomy, clinical neurology, and neuropathology. It is hoped that its organization will permit the book to be of special use to the practitioner in arriving at a clinical diagnosis. Some of the specialized ancillary diagnostic procedures and therapeutic techniques that are not considered in this book in any depth are described amply in *Canine Neurology*, by B. F. Hoerlein. Similarly, a more detailed account of canine neuroanatomy may be found in *Miller's Anatomy of the Dog,* by

H. E. Evans and G. C. Christensen, and in *Functional Mammalian Neuroanatomy*, by
T. W. Jenkins.

If errors or omissions are found, or the reader has a strong difference of opinion,
the author would like to be informed. This book is the result of the cooperation of
knowledgeable individuals. Its improvement depends on continued cooperation, so that
the information presented is as accurate as possible.

Many thanks are extended to my former students, whose enthusiasm and expertise
kept urging me to learn more about each clinical patient and disease process. Special
thanks go to Dr. John Cummings, whose excellence in neuroanatomy and neuropathology continually contributed to my better understanding of the nervous system. There
are many others throughout the veterinary college who could be singled out for
mention, but all are part of this institution's cooperative academic environment that
provides the stimulus to pursue knowledge.

Special thanks are given to Karen Allaben-Confer and Muriel G. Keller for their
secretarial expertise, and to Esther Wilcox for her excellent histologic preparation of
neuropathologic specimens.

The outstanding artistic work of the first five chapters was done by Lewis L. Sadler,
who was medical illustrator for the Department of Anatomy at the New York State
College of Veterinary Medicine. The remaining chapters were illustrated by Grant
Lashbrook, formerly Art Director for the Health Sciences at W. B. Saunders Co.
William P. Hamilton IV, medical illustrator for the Department of Anatomy at the
New York State College of Veterinary Medicine, contributed to the second edition.
This excellent work is greatly appreciated.

ALEXANDER DE LAHUNTA

CONTENTS

INTRODUCTION

PURPOSE

This textbook was written primarily for the veterinary student and secondarily for the veterinary practitioner. It is organized to provide the veterinary student with a concept of the development, organization, and function of the nervous system as a basis for understanding disorders of the nervous system.

For the experienced clinician, descriptions of the more common neurologic diseases are found in chapters for the system primarily affected by that disease (e.g., polyneuritis or coonhound paralysis is in Chapter 4, Lower Motor Neuron—General Somatic Efferent System), or in the chapters devoted to a compilation of neurologic diseases by species (Chapters 21, 22). In these chapters, each disease will be described or located in the textbook for the reader. The index should provide ready access to descriptions of specific clinical signs and diseases.

ACCURATE DIAGNOSIS

The primary objective of this textbook is to teach the morphologic and physiologic features of the nervous system in order to provide a basis for the student to diagnose the location of lesions that occur in this system. This is the anatomic diagnosis. An additional goal is to teach the student some of the features and causes of the different kinds of diseases that affect the nervous system. An intelligent diagnosis of disease of the nervous system is entirely dependent upon a firm knowledge of the anatomy, physiology, and pathology of this system. Rational prognosis and treatment can be based only on accurate diagnosis. To perform an accurate neurologic diagnosis, it is necessary to be able to answer the following questions: Where is the disease process located, and what is its nature? The answer to the first question is dependent on the examiner's knowledge of the anatomy and physiology of the nervous system. The answer to the question on the pathogenesis of the lesion depends on a knowledge of pathology and the various basic sciences concerned with the causes of disease, such as microbiology and virology.

Although mortality is high in diseases of the nervous system in which regenerative capabilities are limited, it is the obligation of the diagnostician to diagnose the disease accurately so that transient neurologic disturbances can be recognized and appropriate therapy can be offered when it is applicable. The medical and surgical equipment for the treatment of neurologic disease is improving continually. A firm basis in the interpretation of neurologic examinations increases the confidence of the practitioner.

Proper application and interpretation of the neurologic examination should show the diagnostician where the lesion is located. In considering the various kinds of lesions that occur in the nervous system, the following general list should be reviewed to avoid overlooking a disease.

Inflammation. Inflammation is a pathologic process involving a reaction of blood vessels and tissues to physical, chemical, and biologic agents—the reaction of tissues to an irritant. In the consideration of neurologic disease, it usually refers to the tissue reaction to a microorganism.

SUPPURATIVE INFLAMMATION. This is an inflammation characterized by a neutrophilic

1

response and the products of necrosis of tissue and inflammatory cells, usually caused by bacteria, protozoa, or fungi.

NONSUPPURATIVE INFLAMMATION. This type of inflammation is characterized by a lymphocytic or monocytic response and usually is caused by a viral agent.

Degeneration. Degeneration is the deterioration of cells from lack of blood supply (ischemia), from abnormal cellular metabolism caused by an inherited cellular defect, by abnormalities of other systems (nephritis-uremia, hepatitis, hypoxia), or by intoxicants. Abiotrophy is cell degeneration due to an intrinsic defect in essential metabolism necessary for survival and function.

Trauma. Trauma is physical injury to the nervous system.

Malformation. Malformation is developmental abnormality of the nervous system.

Neoplasia. Primary neoplasia is the uncontrolled, continuous proliferation of a cell belonging to the nervous system, while a metastatic neoplasm is the uncontrolled growth of a malignant neoplastic cell which spreads to the nervous system from a primary neoplasm in another organ by metastasis. Such growths have no orderly structure or useful function.

THE NEURON

In this book the neuron is defined as consisting of a dendritic zone, axon, cell body, and telodendron. The dendritic zone is the "receptor" portion in which the stimulus of the internal or external environment becomes converted into an impulse in the neuron. The axon is the cell process that courses from the dendritic zone to the telodendron. The telodendron is the ending of the neuron at which the impulse leaves the neuron; it is often referred to as the synapse. The cell body consists of the nucleus and major organelles, and may be located anywhere along the axon.

For example, a sensory neuron in the peripheral nervous system for proprioception may have its dendritic zone in a neuromuscular spindle in a skeletal muscle of the limb. The axon courses toward the spinal cord through a specific peripheral nerve, a branch of one spinal nerve, its dorsal root, and into the dorsal grey column of that spinal cord segment to synapse in a nucleus within that column. The telodendron is the end of the neuron at the synapse in that nucleus. The cell body is located in the spinal ganglion associated with the

dorsal root that the axon courses through. It is actually intercalated in the axon at this point.

The dendritic zone and cell body of a motor neuron of the peripheral nervous system are closely associated in the ventral grey column of one segment of the spinal cord. The axon leaves the cell body, and courses through the white matter to leave the spinal cord in a ventral root. It continues into that segment's spinal nerve, then travels to a branch of the spinal nerve, and by way of a specific peripheral nerve it reaches the skeletal muscle to be innervated. It ends in a telodendron at the neuromuscular ending in a motor end-plate.

Within the central nervous system, a neuron of the dorsal spinocerebellar tract is an example of a sensory or afferent neuron to the cerebellum. Its dendritic zone and cell body are closely associated in a nucleus in the dorsal grey column of the spinal cord. The impulse is initiated here by synapse with a sensory proprioceptive neuron of the peripheral nervous system. The axon passes across the grey and white matter to join a tract on the dorsal superficial surface of the lateral funiculus. The axon continues rostrally in this dorsal spinocerebellar tract, traversing the length of the spinal cord and caudal medulla; at the caudal medulla it enters the cerebellum through the caudal cerebellar peduncle. It courses through the cerebellar medulla and white matter of a folium, and ends in a telodendron in the granular layer of the cerebellum; here it synapses with the dendritic zone of a granular cell neuron.

Within the central nervous system, the Purkinje cell of the cerebellum is an example of an efferent neuron in the cerebellar cortex. Its dendritic zone is located in the molecular layer of the cerebellar cortex. Telodendria of granular cell neurons synapse on these processes to initiate the impulse in the Purkinje cell. The cell body is located in the Purkinje cell layer of the cerebellar cortex. The axon travels from the cell body through the granular layer, into and through the white matter of that cerebellar folium, and into the white matter of the cerebellar medulla. Here it ends in a telodendron on the dendritic zone of another efferent neuron located in a nucleus in the cerebellar medulla.

FUNCTIONAL SYSTEMS

This book is primarily organized along the lines of functional systems rather than by re-

TABLE 1–1. FUNCTIONAL CLASSIFICATION OF THE NERVOUS SYSTEM

System	Innervation
I. Afferent (A) – sensory	
Somatic (S)	
General (GSA)	"Pain," temperature, touch – spinal nerves, CN V
Special (SSA)	Vision – CN II; hearing – CN VIII
Visceral (V)	
General (GVA)	Organ content and distention, chemical changes; splanchnic — spinal nerves, CN VII, IX, X
Special (SVA)	Taste – CN VII, IX, X; smell – CN I
Proprioception (P)	
General (GP)	Muscle and joint movement – spinal nerves, CN V
Special (SP)	Vestibular system, balance – CN VIII
II. Efferent (E) – motor	
Somatic (S)	
General (GSE)	Striated skeletal muscle associated with somite and somatic mesoderm origin – spinal nerves, CN III, IV, VI, XII
Visceral (V)	
General (GVE)	Smooth muscle, cardiac muscle, glands, sympathetic – spinal and splanchnic nerves, parasympathetic – CN III, VII, IX, X, XI
Special (SVE)	Striated muscle from branchial arch mesoderm — CN V, VII, IX, X, XI

gions of the nervous system. It is my opinion that for teaching purposes this is the best way to conceptualize the organization of the nervous system, which will provide a basis for understanding the disorders that affect the various portions of the nervous system. Some of these functional systems are derived from a classification of the peripheral nervous system based on its functional components. The sensory portion has components that continue in the central nervous system. The classification is outlined in Table 1–1.

SENSORY (AFFERENT)

The afferent or sensory portion of the peripheral nervous system is classified on the basis of the location of the dendritic zone (the origin of the impulse) in the body.

Somatic Afferent. The somatic afferent system has its dendritic zone on or near the surface of the body, derived from the somatopleure where it receives the various stimuli from the external environment.

GENERAL SOMATIC AFFERENT (GSA). The general somatic afferent system comprises the neurons distributed by the fifth cranial nerve and all the spinal nerves to the surface of the head, body, and limbs, respectively, that are sensitive to touch, temperature, and noxious stimuli.

SPECIAL SOMATIC AFFERENT (SSA). The special somatic afferent system involves specialized receptor organs limited to one area deep within the body surface, but stimulated by changes in the external environment. These include light to the eyeball (cranial nerve II) and air waves indirectly to the membranous labyrinth of the inner ear (cranial nerve VIII, cochlear division).

Visceral Afferent. The visceral afferent system has its dendritic zone in the wall of the various viscera of the body. This is tissue derived mostly from splanchnopleure and stimulated by changes in the internal environment.

GENERAL VISCERAL AFFERENT (GVA). The general visceral afferent system is composed of neurons distributed by the seventh, ninth, and tenth cranial nerves to visceral structures of the head, and by the tenth cranial nerve and the spinal nerves to the viscera of the body cavities and blood vessels throughout the trunk and limbs. This widely distributed system is stimulated primarily by the distention of visceral walls and chemical changes.

SPECIAL VISCERAL AFFERENT (SVA). The special visceral afferent system contains the neurons in the seventh, ninth, and tenth cranial nerves whose dendritic zones are limited to the specialized receptors for taste. The specialized receptor neuron for olfaction or cranial nerve I is also a component of this system.

Proprioception. The modality of proprioception is sometimes included in the general somatic afferent system. Here it will be considered as a separate functional system because of its clinical significance. It is the system responsible for detecting changes in the position of the trunk, limbs, and head.

GENERAL PROPRIOCEPTION (GP). The general proprioceptive system is distributed widely throughout all the spinal nerves and the fifth cranial nerve, with receptors located in muscles, tendons, and joints deep to the surface of the body. The receptors respond to changes in length and position of the structures at points where they are located.

SPECIAL PROPRIOCEPTION (SP). The special proprioceptive system is composed of the receptors specialized to respond to movements of the head located in the membranous labyrinth of the inner ear. These neurons, concerned with the orientation of the head in space, are in the vestibular division of the vestibulocochlear nerve (cranial nerve VIII).

MOTOR (EFFERENT)

The efferent or motor portion of the peripheral nervous system is classified on the basis of where the neuron terminates, or the site of its telodendron. This peripheral motor system also is referred to as the lower motor neuron, because it is the final neuron that innervates the muscle cell. Its cell body and dendritic zone are in the spinal cord grey matter (brain stem), and its axon is in the ventral root, spinal (cranial) nerve, and peripheral nerve. It terminates in a muscle cell at the neuromuscular ending.

Somatic Efferent. The somatic efferent system has its telodendria in voluntary striated muscles derived from somites and somatic mesoderm (skeletal), and head myotomes.

GENERAL SOMATIC EFFERENT (GSE). The general somatic efferent system is made up of neurons in the third, fourth, sixth, and twelfth cranial nerves and all the spinal nerves that innervate the extraocular and tongue muscles, and the muscles of the axial and appendicular skeletons.

Visceral Efferent. The visceral efferent system has its telodendria in involuntary smooth muscle of viscera (splanchnic mesoderm), in blood vessels, cardiac muscle, and glands, and in voluntary muscles in the head associated with visceral function.

GENERAL VISCERAL EFFERENT (GVE). The general visceral efferent system is the lower motor neuron of the autonomic nervous system. It is a two neuron-lower motor neuron system that includes neurons in the third, seventh, ninth, tenth and eleventh cranial nerves and all of the spinal nerves. It is distributed widely throughout the head and body, and has both sympathetic and parasympathetic divisions.

SPECIAL VISCERAL EFFERENT (SVE). The special visceral efferent system is composed of efferent neurons in the fifth, seventh, ninth, tenth, and eleventh cranial nerves that innervate the striated muscle derived from the branchial arch mesoderm. These muscles are associated with visceral structures and functions in the head: jaw, face, palate, pharynx, larynx, and the esophagus in the neck and thorax.

A prerequisite for the use of this textbook is the knowledge and understanding of the gross anatomy of the peripheral and central nervous systems of domestic animals. This can be obtained by dissection of a dog as described in *Miller's Guide to the Dissection of the Dog,* by H. E. Evans and A. de Lahunta. The last section of this book, entitled the nervous system, specifically describes a dissection of the dog brain and spinal cord that should provide the student with the basic knowledge needed for the successful use of this textbook.

The following references may be useful adjuncts to the study of neuroanatomy, clinical neurology, and neuropathology. For neuroanatomy the textbook by T. W Jenkins on *Functional Mammalian Neuroanatomy* is especially recommended. It is based on the dog and provides some clinical application of the functional anatomy. *Miller's Anatomy of the Dog* by H. E. Evans and G. C. Christensen is an excellent source for canine neuroanatomy. For clinical neurology and especially therapy, the textbook by B. F. Hoerlein, *Canine Neurology, Diagnosis and Treatment,* is recommended.

Throughout this text the anatomic descriptions are based on the dog unless otherwise stated. Major species differences of clinical importance are described.

REFERENCES

1. Adams, R. D., and Sidman, R. L.: Introduction to Neuropathology. New York, McGraw-Hill, 1968.
2. Blackwood, W., McMenemey, W. H., Meyer, A., Norman, R. M., and Russell, D. S.: Greenfield's Neuropathology. Baltimore, Williams & Wilkins, 1963.
3. Brain, Walter R.: Diseases of the Nervous System. 6th ed., London, Oxford University Press, 1962.
4. Crosby, E. C., Humphrey, T., and Lauer, E. W.: Correlative Anatomy of the Nervous System. New York, Macmillan, 1962.
5. Curtis, B. A., Jacobson, S., and Marcus, E. M.: An Introduction to the Neurosciences. Philadelphia, W. B. Saunders Co., 1972.
6. Evans, H. E., and Christensen, G. C.: Miller's Anatomy of the Dog. 2nd ed., Philadelphia, W. B. Saunders Co., 1979.
7. Evans, H. E., and de Lahunta, A.: Miller's Guide to the Dissection of the Dog. 2nd ed., Philadelphia, W. B. Saunders Co., 1980.
8. Fankhauser, R., and Luginbühl, H.: Pathologische Anatomie des zentralen und peripheren Nervensystems der Haustiere. Berlin, Verlag Paul Parey, 1968.
9. Frauchiger, E., and Fankhauser, R.: Vergleichende Neuropathologie des Menschen und der Tiere. Berlin, Springer-Verlag, 1957.
10. Gilroy, J., and Meyer, J. S.: Medical Neurology. London, The Macmillan Co., 1969.
11. Hoerlein, B. F.: Canine Neurology. Diagnosis and Treatment. 3rd ed., Philadelphia, W. B. Saunders Co., 1978.
12. House, E. L., and Pansky, B.: A Functional Approach to Neuroanatomy. New York, McGraw-Hill, 1960.
13. Innes, J. R. M., and Saunders, L. Z.: Comparative Neuropathology. New York, Academic Press, 1962.
14. Jenkins, T. W.: Functional Mammalian Neuroanatomy. 2nd ed., Philadelphia, Lea & Febiger, 1978.
15. McGrath, J. T.: Neurologic Examination of the Dog with Clinicopathologic Observations. 2nd ed., Philadelphia, Lea & Febiger, 1960.
16. Merritt, H. H.: A Textbook of Neurology. 4th ed., Philadelphia, Lea & Febiger, 1967.
17. Minckler, J.: Pathology of the Nervous System. New York, McGraw-Hill, 1968.
18. Nickel, R., Schummer, A., and Seiferle, E.: Lehrbuch der Anatomie der Haustiere. Band IV Nervensystem, Sinnesorgane, Endokrine Drüsen. Berlin, Verlag Paul Parey, 1975.
19. Palmer, A. C.: Introduction to Animal Neurology. 2nd ed., Philadelphia, F. A. Davis, 1976.
20. Papez, J. W.: Comparative Neurology. New York, T. Y. Crowell Co., 1929.
21. Peele, T. L.: The Neuroanatomic Basis of Clinical Neurology. 2nd ed., New York, McGraw-Hill, 1961.
22. Ranson, S. W., and Clark, S. L.: The Anatomy of the Nervous System. 10th ed., Philadelphia, W. B. Saunders Co., 1959.
23. Singer, M.: The Brain of the Dog in Section. Philadelphia, W. B. Saunders Co., 1962.

2

THE DEVELOPMENT OF THE NERVOUS SYSTEM

THE NEURAL TUBE

The central nervous system is a tubular structure originating from a proliferation of ectoderm referred to as neuroectoderm, which is situated dorsal to the notochord along the axis of the embryo. The thickened ectoderm, known as the neural plate, invaginates along this axis until the lateral extremities of the original plate, the neural folds, meet centrally and fuse over the neural groove to form a neural tube and canal. The margins of the nonneural ectoderm fuse dorsal to the neural tube and the two layers of ectoderm separate. As this fusion and separation of ectodermal layers occurs, a longitudinal column of cells arises from the junction of nonneural and neural ectoderm and separates from these two structures when the neural tube is formed. These two bilateral columns, situated dorso-lateral to the neural tube throughout its length, are the columns of neural crest cells (Fig. 2–1).

Closure of the neural tube progresses rostrally and caudally from the level of the site of development of the rhombencephalon, the most caudal division of the brain. The rostral opening, or rostral neuropore, closes as the brain vesicles develop. The caudal opening at the caudal extremity of the spinal cord closes later or not at all. In some animals it communicates with the subarachnoid space of the leptomeninges at the conus medullaris (Fig. 2–2).

The rostral end of the neural tube develops rapidly and produces three vesicles: the prosencephalon, mesencephalon, and rhombencephalon, moving from rostral to caudal (Fig. 2–3). Early in its development the prosencephalon has a lateral enlargement, the optic vesicle, which grows out to contact the adjacent ectoderm. The further development of this primordial eyeball is considered in the section on the visual system. Two additional swellings from the rostral prosencephalon grow laterally and dorsally out of the neural tube. These telencephalic vesicles completely overgrow the original vesicular system and form the cerebral hemispheres. The portion of the prosencephalon that remains at the rostral end of the neural tube is the diencephalon. The optic vesicles remain associated with the diencephalon. The lumen of the diencephalon, the third ventricle, communicates rostrolaterally with the lumen of each telencephalon by the interventricular foramina. The latter lumina are the lateral ventricles of the cerebral hemispheres. The nuclei of the thalamus and hypothalamus develop in the diencephalon. The neurohypophysis is a ventral outgrowth of the diencephalon.

The lumen of the mesencephalon is reduced to a narrow tubular structure, called the mesencephalic aqueduct.

From the rostral rhombencephalon, the cerebellum or dorsal metencephalon develops dorsally. Concomitant developmental changes in the neural tube form the ventral metencephalon or pons. The caudal rhombencephalon forms the myelencephalon or medulla oblongata. The fourth ventricle is the lumen of the neural canal in the rhombencephalon. It communicates with the meningeal spaces that

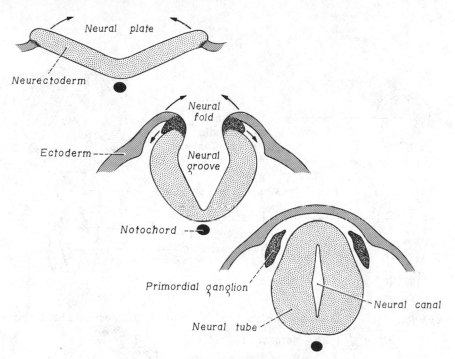

Figure 2–1. Development of the neural tube.

develop around the neural tube by way of openings that arise in the wall of the neural tube. These openings are called lateral apertures and are located caudal to the cerebellum (see Fig. 3–2).

Cell Differentiation. In the first stage of development within the wall of the neural tube, the cells commonly referred to as neuroepithelial or neuroectodermal cells are organized in a pseudostratified arrangement (Fig. 2–4). The cell membrane of each cell connects to both sides of the wall of the neural tube, but the nuclei are at different levels. These cells are all actively mitotic, increasing the size and thickness of the tube. The nuclei migrate within the wall of the tube, and their position depends upon the cell's stage of mitosis.

During interphase the nuclei are located on the external surface of the tube. DNA or chromosomal duplication occurs in that position. As the nucleus enters mitosis it migrates through its cytoplasm to the luminal surface. The cytoplasm and peripheral cell membrane also retract to that position where cell division is completed. The two new daughter cells extend their cell membrane to the periphery, and the nucleus migrates to the external surface again. Since the nucleus is at the outer

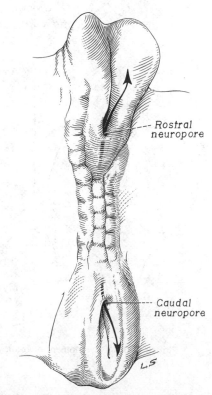

Figure 2–2. Dorsal view of neural tube closure.

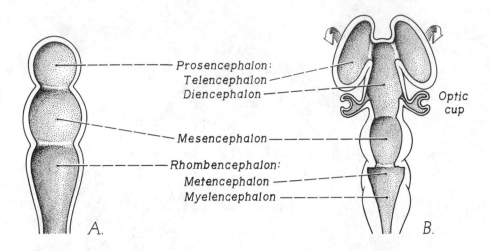

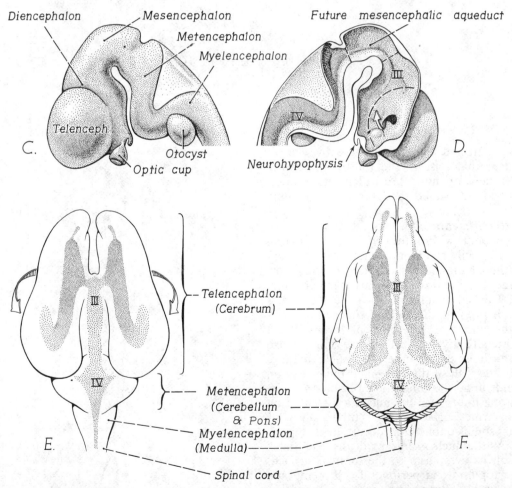

Figure 2–3. Development of brain vesicles. *A:* three-vesicle stage; *B–F:* five-vesicle stages.

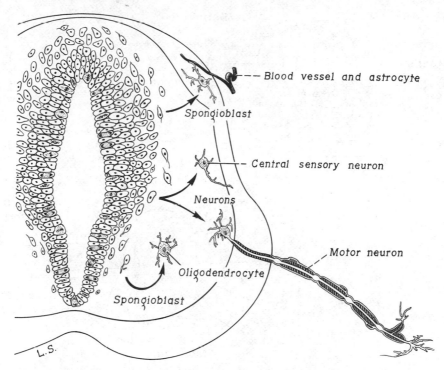

Figure 2–4. Mitosis and differentiation of neuroepithelial cells.

surface during interphase, when cell division ceases in any one neuroepithelial cell and differentiation begins, it occurs on the surface of the neural tube. Thus in a short time a new layer of differentiated cells appears on the external surface of the actively mitotic layer.[28]

The cells that are differentiated are of two types. Immature neurons, the parenchymal cells, usually are referred to as neuroblasts, but this is misleading because once a neuron is formed it will not divide again, as is inferred in the term neuroblast. The differentiated neuron grows extensively to become a mature, functioning cell, but it does not divide further. Spongioblasts are the second type of cell. These are the progenitors of the neuroectodermal supporting cell for the nervous system, the neuroglia (glue). Two of the three forms of glial cells are derived from these spongioblasts: astrocytes and oligodendrocytes (see Fig. 2–4).

As more primitive neurons and spongioblasts are differentiated and grow and produce processes, the neural tube is arranged into three concentric layers (Fig. 2–5). Adjacent to the neural tube is the germinal layer of proliferating neurocpithclial cclls. This proliferative function ultimately is exhausted and the multicellular layer is reduced to a single layer of cells, ranging from squamous to columnar, called ependymal cells. The ependymal cells line the entire lumen of the neural tube, which includes the ventricular system in the brain and the central canal of the spinal cord. Peripheral to the germinal layer in the embryonic neural tube is the thick layer of differentiated cell bodies, mostly composed of primitive neurons and spongioblasts. This is the mantle layer that becomes the grey matter of the definitive spinal cord and nuclei of the brain stem. After migration to the external surface of the neural tube, this layer becomes the cerebral cortex of the telencephalon. The external layer in the neural tube is the marginal layer composed mostly of the growing processes of the cell bodies in the mantle layer. These are the tracts of the white matter.

From the mesencephalon caudally, a longitudinal groove, the sulcus limitans, is apparent in the lateral wall of the neural canal. The neural canal can be divided into dorsal and ventral portions by a dorsal plane at the level of this sulcus. The dorsal portion is called the alar plate, and the ventral portion the basal plate. Functionally, the alar-plate mantle layer is concerned predominantly with sensory systems and the basal-plate mantle layer with motor systems (see Fig. 2–5).

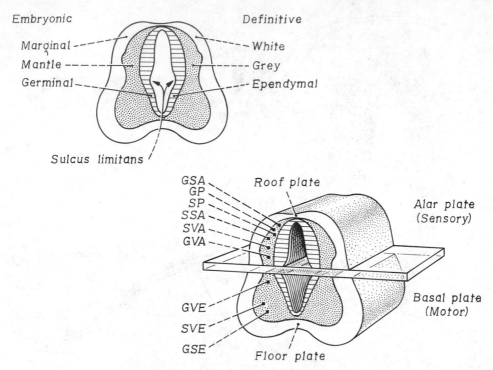

Figure 2–5. Functional organization of neural tube.

SPINAL CORD

The spinal cord provides the best example of the symmetric development of the neural tube by layers. Ventral growth of the two basal plates and associated marginal zones leaves a separation between the two sides—the ventral median fissure. The mantle and marginal layers of the alar plates grow dorsally. The dorsal marginal layers fuse medially to form the dorsal median septum. The mantle layer of the alar plate becomes the dorsal grey column, and that of the basal plate the ventral grey column. The mantle zone at the plane of the sulcus limitans is the intermediate grey column (Fig. 2–6).

Not only is there a gross topographic differentiation of function of primitive neurons between the alar and basal plates, but within the mantle layer of each plate neurons are arranged in functional columns. The general visceral afferent and general visceral efferent columns are located adjacent to each other on either side of the dorsal plane through the sulcus limitans. The general somatic afferent and general proprioception columns are located dorsally in the alar plate of the mantle layer, and the general somatic efferent column is located ventrally in the basal plate of the mantle layer. Because the relative size of the components of each spinal cord segment depends on the volume of tissue to be innervated, at the levels of the limbs the spinal cord segments responsible for their innervation are enlarged, forming the cervical and lumbosacral intumescences. Studies have shown that the ultimate growth to maturity of a neuron in the peripheral nervous system depends on its appropriate innervation of a muscle cell or formation of a peripheral receptor.[21] The lack of such innervation results in degeneration of the neuron. In the cervical and thoracolumbar regions where appendages are not innervated, the immature primitive neurons in the basal-plate mantle layer and the spinal ganglion that fail to innervate structures will degenerate. The shape of the ventral grey column depicts this phenomenon and shows further anatomic subdivision of the mantle layer.

In the basal-plate mantle layer the general somatic efferent neurons located medially innervate axial skeletal musculature. Those located laterally innervate appendicular skeletal muscles. Within these areas neuronal cell bodies can be grouped further according to the specific peripheral nerve that contains the axon of these cell bodies, and specific muscle innervation.[1]

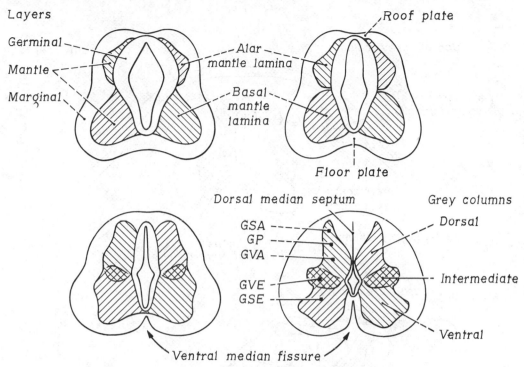

Figure 2–6. Development and functional organization of the spinal cord.

The growth of axons of the basal-plate neurons through the adjacent marginal layers and outside the neural tube forms the ventral root and part of the spinal and peripheral nerves. This includes the general somatic efferent neurons located in the ventral grey column and the general visceral efferent neurons (preganglionic neurons of the autonomic nervous system lower motor neuron) located in the intermediate grey column adjacent to the sulcus limitans. This intermediate grey column is evident only in the thoracic, part of the lumbar, and the sacral spinal cord segments. In the other segments it was present in the embryo but subsequently degenerated. These general visceral efferent neurons terminate in ganglia in the peripheral nervous system that contain the cell bodies of the postganglionic axons in this two neuron–lower motor neuron system (see Fig. 2–8).

Neural Crest. The neural crest cells are the cell bodies in the longitudinal column of cells dorsolateral to the neural tube. Along the spinal cord, these provide the neurons that form the spinal ganglia at each segment. Neural crest cells migrate adjacent to the somites and proliferate into a collection of cell bodies that will become spinal ganglia (Fig. 2–7). The axon that grows centrally into the alar-

plate dorsal grey column forms the dorsal root. Distally it forms the sensory component of the spinal and peripheral nerves. The point of penetration of the marginal layer of white matter by axons of the dorsal and ventral roots divides the spinal cord white matter into three regions called funiculi. These are dorsal, lateral, and ventral on each side of the spinal cord. The formation of spinal ganglia is only one of the many outcomes of the neural crest cells. Prior to its segregation into ganglia, an early migration of cells from this column provides melanoblasts to the epidermis and the cell bodies of postganglionic axons in the two neuron-general visceral efferent system. These cell bodies form the ganglia of the sympathetic trunk and the abdominal plexus autonomic ganglia, as well as the cells of the adrenal medulla (Fig. 2–8). These adrenal medullary cells do not grow processes but synthesize and elaborate into the blood stream the same endocrine substance—norepinephrine—that is the neurotransmitter at the telodendron of the postganglionic axon derived from the neural crest cells. The general visceral efferent neurons located in the wall of the viscera also may be derived from the neural crest. Although melanoblasts and these general visceral efferent neurons seem to be unrelated, their com-

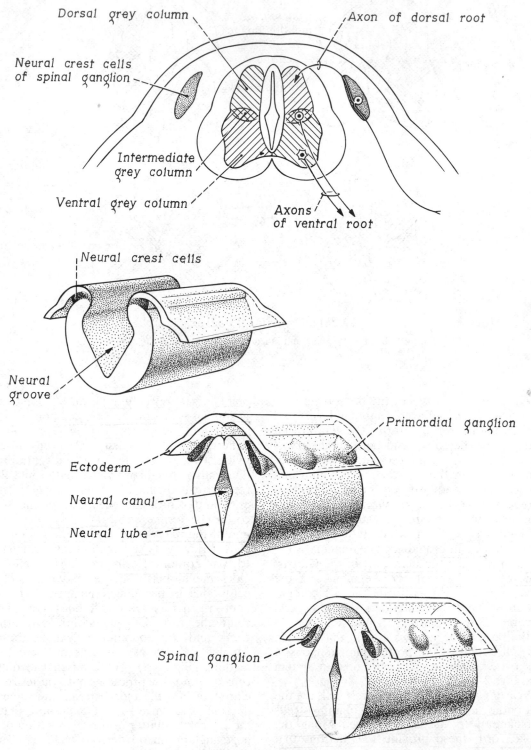

Figure 2–7. Spinal ganglia development from neural crest.

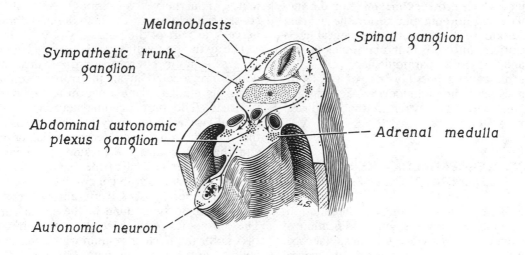

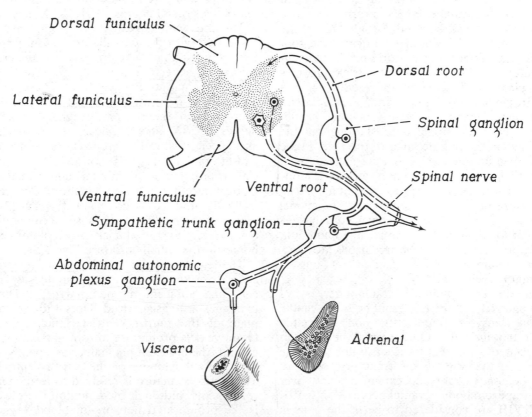

Figure 2–8. Neural crest contribution to development of general visceral efferent neuron.

mon denominator is the unique metabolism of tyrosine, which provides melanin for the melanoblast and norepinephrine for the neuron. In addition to these cells, the neural crest differentiates into cells found in branchial arch cartilage, thyroid parafollicular (C) cells, odontoblasts, and possibly part of the leptomeninges and the lemmocytes, or Schwann cells, that form the myelin of the peripheral nervous system.

MYELENCEPHALON—MEDULLA OBLONGATA (Plates 3–7)

The basic formation of the medulla oblongata involves only a slight modification of the development described for the spinal cord. The potential roof-plate region in the neural tube is expanded extensively instead of being displaced by proliferating alar-plate and marginal-layer tissue as it is in the spinal cord. This relegates the entire alar and basal plates of the neural tube to a lateral and ventral position. The region of the ventral median fissure is filled in by neural tissue. The lumen of the central canal enlarges to form the fourth ventricle, which is covered dorsally only by the thin, single cell layer of ependyma, the roof plate. The sulcus limitans present on the ventrolateral wall of the fourth ventricle provides the plane of division of the medulla into a ventromedial basal plate and a dorsolateral alar plate having the same functional significance as in the spinal cord. Throughout the brain stem the mantle layer of the neural tube is broken up into nuclei that are collections of cell bodies with a common purpose, interspersed with neuronal processes. Some nuclei are more distinct than others. The functional columns described in the spinal cord have a similar location in the brain stem. In addition, there are added neurons organized into functional columns that have components only in cranial nerves (Fig. 2–9).

In domestic animals cranial nerves VI through XII and the trapezoid body are caudal to the transverse fibers of the pons associated with the medulla. Only cranial nerve V is associated with the transverse fibers of the pons. In the primate the transverse fibers of the pons are larger and extend caudally over the trapezoid body. Cranial nerves V, VI, VII, and VIII are considered to be in the pons in these species. Some veterinary neuroanatomists have also included cranial nerves VI through VIII in the pons, leaving cranial

nerves IX through XII in the medulla. In this text, cranial nerves VI through XII will be considered as part of the medulla and cranial nerve V as part of the pons.

The sixth and twelfth cranial nerves contain general somatic efferent neurons whose cell bodies are located in an interrupted column along the median plane adjacent to the fourth ventricle. The preganglionic neurons of the general visceral efferent system have axons in the seventh, ninth, and tenth cranial nerves and the cell bodies are located in an interrupted column medial to the sulcus limitans. This relationship of the general somatic efferent and general visceral efferent columns is comparable to that found in the spinal cord. The cell bodies of the special visceral efferent system form a nuclear column which was originally located between the GSE and GVE columns, but migrated to a ventrolateral position closer to the source of their stimulus from sensory neurons in the trigeminal nerve. This phenomenon of migration is called neurobiotaxis. As a result of this migration, the axons from this nucleus course toward the ventricle before coursing ventrolaterally and into their respective cranial nerves—VII, IX, X, and XI.

The sensory components of cranial nerves associated with the medulla arise from primitive neurons that develop from neural crest cells and from ectodermal cells that proliferate from branchial groove ectoderm. These latter are referred to as cranial placodes. These two sources form the sensory ganglia of cranial nerves VII, IX, and X concerned with general and special visceral afferent (taste) function, and of cranial nerve VIII concerned with special proprioception (vestibular) and special somatic afferent (auditory) function. The centrally situated axons grow into the alar-plate region of the medulla to synapse on cell bodies comparable to the dorsal grey column cell bodies in the spinal cord (see Fig. 2–9).

The leptomeninges that surround the entire central nervous system form from neural crest cells and adjacent mesodermal cells. These meninges are vascularized. Dorsal to the roof plate of the fourth ventricle, the capillary blood vessels proliferate to form a plexus that extends the adjacent pia mater and ependymal layer into the lumen of the fourth ventricle. This entire structure is referred to as the choroid plexus, although by definition the plexus is the proliferated network of blood vessels. This proliferation occurs in two symmetric sagittal lines parallel to the median plane, from the caudal part of the fourth ventricle rostrally

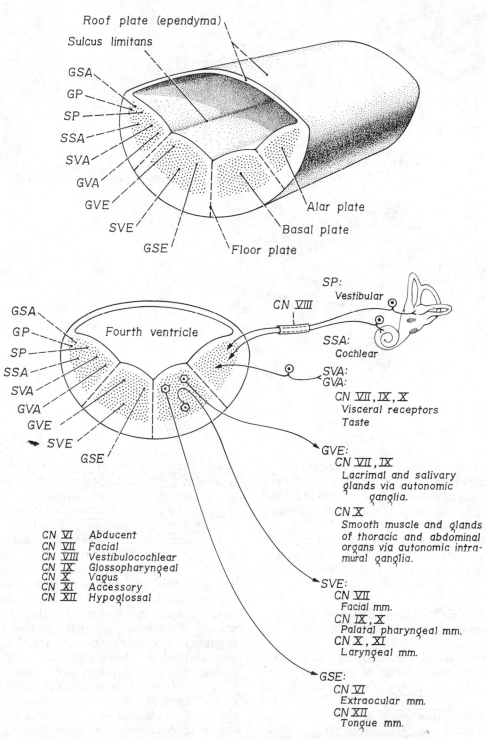

Figure 2–9. Functional organization of cranial nerves VI to XII in the myelencephalon.

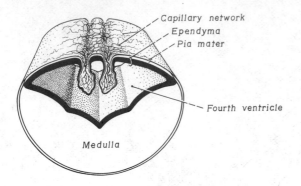

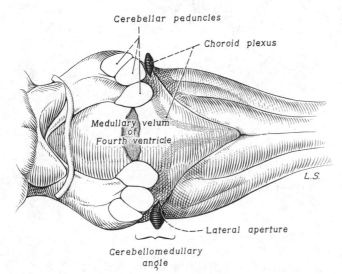

Figure 2–10. Development of roof plate and choroid plexus of fourth ventricle.

to the level of the cerebellar peduncles, where the plexuses turn laterally. At this point there is an opening in the roof plate called the lateral aperture. At the level of the lateral aperture these choroid plexuses protrude from the lumen of the fourth ventricle out through the lateral aperture, where they are visible at the cerebellomedullary angle (Fig. 2–10).

METENCEPHALON—CEREBELLUM
(Plates 3–9) **AND PONS** (Plates 8–9)

The initial development of the metencephalon is comparable to that of the myelencephalon. Cranial nerve V is associated with this division of the brain stem (Fig. 2–11). Its motor neurons function in the special visceral efferent system. Its sensory neurons, whose cell bodies are situated in the trigeminal ganglion, function predominantly in the general somatic afferent system, with some in the general proprioceptive system. The central axons of these neurons grow into the alar-plate region of the metencephalon and course rostrally into the mesencephalon and caudally through the entire myelencephalon to synapse on alar-plate neurons (see Fig. 2–11).

The cerebellum, or dorsal metencephalon, is formed from the proliferation of the germinal neuroepithelial cells of the alar plate. This growth dorsolaterally from each side overgrows the roof plate of the fourth ventricle so that the cerebellum forms the dorsal boundary of the fourth ventricle in the metencephalon. The cerebellum is thus the dorsal metencephalon. The development of the cerebellar cortex and nuclei are considered in Chapter 13. The ventral metencephalon is the pons. Migration of alar-plate neurons forms the pontine nucleus on the ventral aspect of the metencephalon. The axons of these neurons course dorsally into the cerebellum, producing the transverse fibers of the pons, which demarcate the ventral surface of the pons (Fig. 2–12).

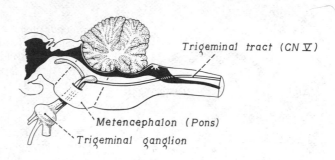

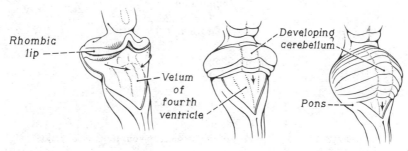

Figure 2–11. Development of the metencephalon: surface view, afferent portion of cranial nerve V.

MESENCEPHALON—MIDBRAIN
(Plates 9–12)

Symmetric proliferation of the walls of the neural tube in the mesencephalon reduces the size of the neural canal to a narrow tube, the mesencephalic aqueduct. This is smaller rostrally at the point where it joins the third ventricle, and larger caudally where it is continuous with the fourth ventricle beneath the rostral medullary velum.

Cranial nerves III and IV are associated with the midbrain. These contain general somatic efferent axons that innervate extraocular muscles. The cell bodies are in the same topographic nuclear column as those for cranial nerves VI and XII, adjacent to the median plane ventral to the aqueduct. The alar plate

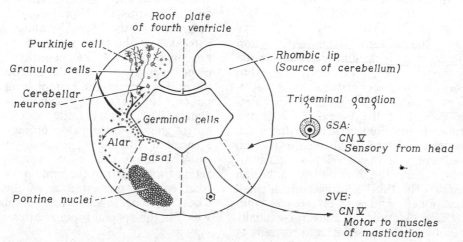

Figure 2–12. Development of the metencephalon: transverse section, pontine nucleus.

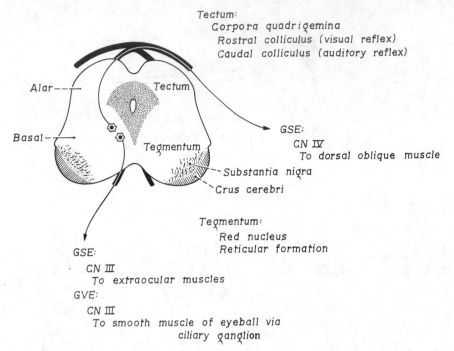

Figure 2–13. Development of the mesencephalon: transverse section.

proliferates dorsally to form the tectum of the midbrain, which is divided into paired rostral and caudal colliculi. These are associated with visual and auditory reflex functions, respectively. The crus cerebri on the ventral aspect of the midbrain results from the caudal growth of descending telencephalic projection neurons. These are in the internal capsule rostral to the midbrain (Fig. 2–13).

DIENCEPHALON—INTERBRAIN
(Plates 12–15)

Rostral to the region of the mesencephalon the sulcus limitans is no longer evident in the primitive neural tube, and the diencephalon and telencephalon are considered to be developments of the alar-plate tissue. The symmetric development of the lateral walls of the neural tube in the diencephalon reduces the neural canal to a vertical slit on the median plane. Adhesion of the developing thalamus in the center forms the interthalamic adhesion and separates the third ventricle into a small dorsal component and a larger ventral component. These two portions converge caudally at the mesencephalic aqueduct and rostrally at

the level of the interventricular foramina. There is only roof plate along the median plane over the small dorsal portion of the third ventricle, and a small choroid plexus is developed along this roof plate on both sides of the median plane. At the interventricular foramina these are continuous with the choroid plexuses of the lateral ventricles (Fig. 2–14).

The dorsal portion of the diencephalon forms the thalamus, which is a complex of numerous nuclei and tracts of neuronal processes. The nervous tissue constituting the walls and floor of the ventral portion of the third ventricle forms the hypothalamus. A ventral outgrowth of the hypothalamus, including an extension of the third ventricle, produces the neurohypophysis. The neurohypophysis becomes associated with the contribution from the oral ectoderm, the hypophyseal (Rathke's) pouch, to form the hypophysis (pituitary gland). The original optic vesicles that grew out of the prosencephalon ultimately become associated with the diencephalon (see Fig. 2–3). The axons that grow caudally from the retina (optic cup) in the optic nerve and optic tract enter a nuclear area of the thalamus. These optic nerve axons form cranial nerve II, which is the special somatic afferent or visual system.

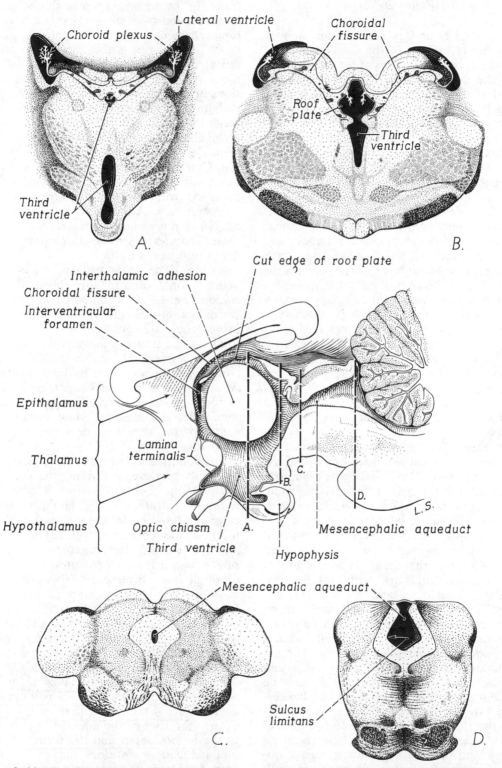

Figure 2–14. Relationship of the diencephalon and mesencephalon. *A:* Transverse section of middiencephalon; *B:* transverse section of caudal diencephalon; *C:* transverse section of rostral mesencephalon; *D:* transverse section of caudal mesencephalon.

TELENCEPHALON—CEREBRUM
(Plates 9–16)

The rostral boundary of the brain stem is the lamina terminalis of the diencephalon. It forms the rostral boundary of the third ventricle of the diencephalon. The optic chiasm is located at the ventral portion of this lamina. At this level the telencephalic vesicle grew out of the original prosencephalon, a short distance rostrally and in a large curve caudally and ventrally. The lumen of this vesicle is the lateral ventricle, which communicates with the diencephalic third ventricle by means of the interventricular foramen on either side, at the level of the lamina terminalis (Fig. 2–15).

At one aspect of the medial wall the telencephalic vesicle development is retarded, and at that point the entire wall of the neural tube is reduced to a single layer of ependymal cells comparable to the roof plate of the rhombencephalon (fourth ventricle) and diencephalon (third ventricle), with which it is continuous. This layer of cuboidal ependymal cells is attached to the crus and body of the fornix on one side and the stria terminalis which is on the opposite side located in the groove between the caudate nucleus and the thalamus. In this area of limited development a choroid plexus is formed and protrudes into the lateral ventricle.

The extensive development of projection processes from brain stem neurons to the telencephalon, and from telencephalic neurons to the brain stem, creates a thick layer of white matter between the diencephalon and telencephalon. This is the internal capsule.

Cell Bodies. The telencephalic neuronal cell bodies are located in one of two general locations. One of these is the subcortical-basal nuclei (caudate nucleus, lentiform nucleus, amygdala, claustrum) and the other is the cerebral cortex. The cerebral cortex can be divided into three regions on an evolutionary and anatomic basis. The archipallium includes the hippocampus and fornix system. The paleopallium includes the olfactory bulbs and peduncles, and the pyriform lobe cortex. The neopallium includes the remainder of the cerebrum, which contains the numerous gyri dorsal to the rhinal sulcus (Fig. 2–16). Comparative evolutionary studies show the continual development of the neopallium in higher animals relegating the archipallium and paleopallium to a lesser portion anatomically. The surface of the amphibian cerebrum is smooth and comprises the archipallium dorsally, the paleopallium laterally, and basal nuclei ventrally. In the advanced reptile the basal nuclei have receded from the surface and have been replaced ventrally by the paleopallium. A small lateral area is the neopallium and the dorsal area is the archipallium. In mammals the neopallium has overgrown the other divisions of the cerebral cortex so that the paleopallium is entirely on the ventral surface of the cerebrum ventral to the rhinal sulcus, and the archipallium is rolled medially into the lateral ventricle as an internal gyrus—the hippocampus. Continual development of the neopallium has resulted in the characteristic gyri and sulci observed over most of the exposed surface of the cerebrum. Although at birth the puppy brain has the primary gyri and sulci present, these undergo extensive development in the first 3 to 6 weeks of life.

Axons. The axons of telencephalic cortical neurons form tracts that are classified as association fibers if they course between areas of cortex within one cerebral hemisphere. If the axons leave the cerebrum to enter the brain stem via the internal capsule, they are called projection fibers. Those that cross the cerebral cortex of one hemisphere to the opposite hemisphere are commissural fibers (Fig. 2–17). All of these axons are intermixed in the centrum semiovale, the mass of white matter in the center of the cerebrum dorsal to the lateral ventricle.

The commissural fibers of the telencephalon originally all develop through the lamina terminalis (Fig. 2–18). The rostral commissure located ventrally in the lamina terminalis courses primarily between paleopallial structures and basal nuclei (amygdala) on each side. Another small group of commissural fibers runs between the archipallium (hippocampus) of either side, forming the hippocampal commissure. The largest group of commissural fibers forms the corpus callosum. This primarily connects the neopallial areas of each hemisphere. Beginning in the lamina terminalis, it extends caudally over the diencephalon as the telencephalic vesicle expands caudally in its development. The corpus callosum forms between the archipallium and neopallium on the medial side of the hemisphere, and thus constitutes the roof of the lateral ventricle dorsal to the hippocampus and the fornix. The septum pellucidum develops out of the rostral part of the lamina terminalis, between the genu of corpus callosum and the body of the fornix (see Fig. 2–18).

In the telencephalon the germinal layer ul-

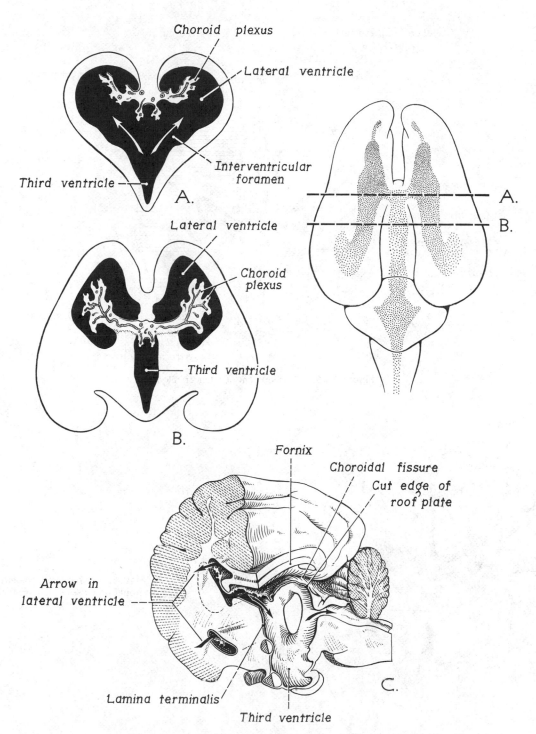

Figure 2–15. Development of choroid plexus and ventricular system of diencephalon and telencephalon.

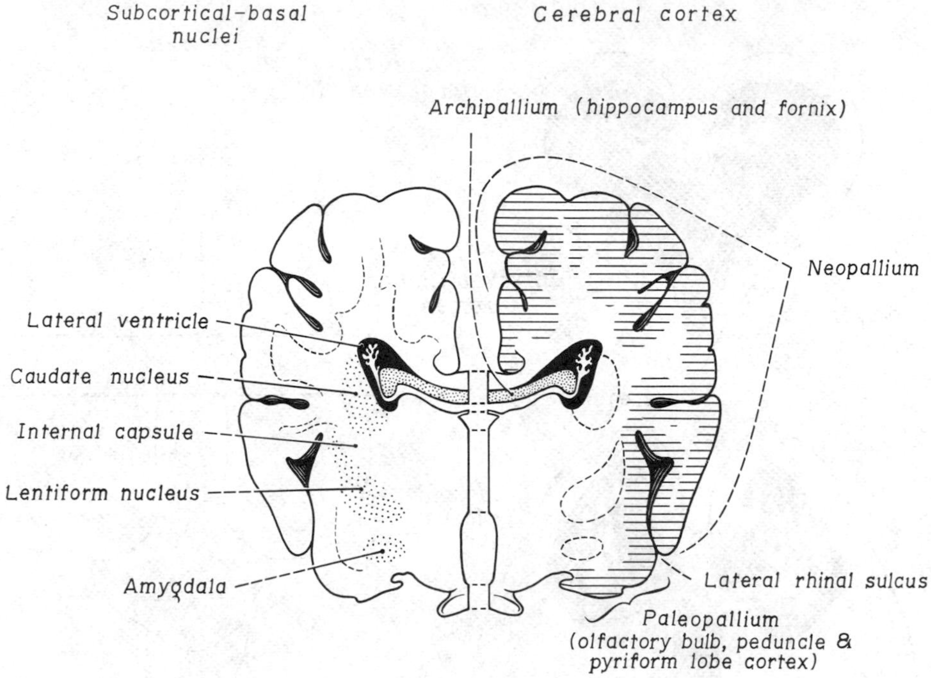

Subcortical–basal
nuclei   *Cerebral cortex*

Archipallium (hippocampus and fornix)

Neopallium

Lateral ventricle

Caudate nucleus

Internal capsule

Lentiform nucleus

Amygdala

Lateral rhinal sulcus

Paleopallium
(olfactory bulb, peduncle &
pyriform lobe cortex)

Figure 2–16. Development of telencephalon.

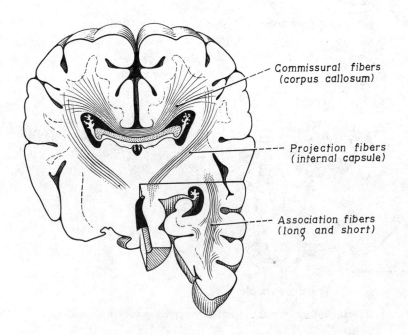

Commissural fibers
(corpus callosum)

Projection fibers
(internal capsule)

Figure 2–17. Development of
neuronal processes in telencephalon.

Association fibers
(long and short)

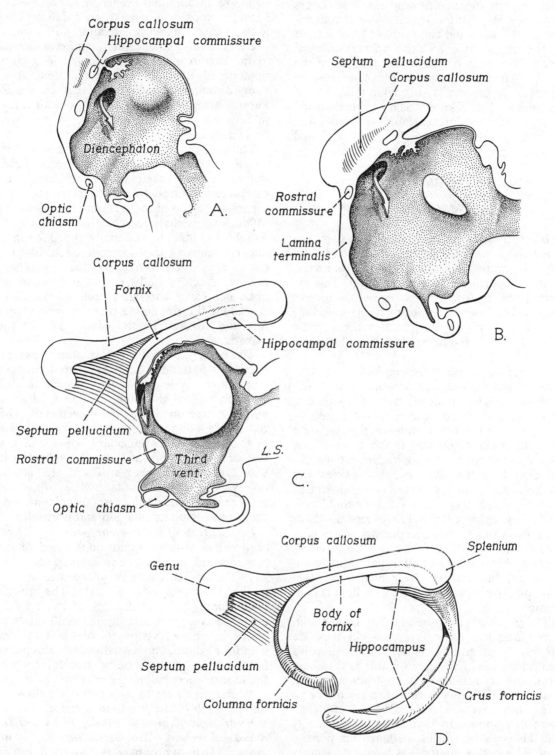

Figure 2–18. Development of telencephalic commissural pathways.

timately is replaced by the ependyma of the lateral ventricle. Except for the area of the basal nuclei, the mantle and marginal layers reverse their positions by means of the migration of the neuronal cell bodies to the surface of the neural tube and the primary internal (medial) growth of the axons that leave the cerebral cortex. Remnants of this telencephalic germinal layer persist throughout the life of the animal. This is known as the subependymal zone, and consists of a variable-sized collection of small cells that are thought to be a continual source of glia and small neurons.

MALFORMATIONS[25]

BRAIN MALFORMATIONS

Hydrocephalus. Many circumstances can cause the ventricular cerebrospinal fluid pressure to elevate and dilate the lateral ventricles, at the expense of the telencephalon. This hypertensive hydrocephalus causes extensive degeneration of the telencephalon, especially its neopallium. The subject of hydrocephalus is considered in the discussion of cerebrospinal fluid in Chapter 3.

Hypoplasia of the Prosencephalon. Calves have been observed with a failure of the telencephalic vesicles to develop, along with cranioschisis and encephalocele. If the neurectoderm of the prosencephalon failed to separate from the skin ectoderm at the level of the rostral neuropore, this could prevent the development of the telencephalic vesicles and create a defect in the calvaria—cranioschisis, through which the nervous tissue would protrude—encephalocele.[44] These animals have hypoplasia of the prosencephalon, which consists of a complete lack of cerebral hemispheres (telencephalic aplasia) and a malformed diencephalon. In addition, the caudal brain stem is relatively normal but the cerebellum is malformed.

These animals have been observed to stand, nurse, and live for a few days but they are obtunded and have no vision. They do perceive painful stimuli. Evidence for this is voluntary struggling to remove a limb from a painful stimulus and throwing the head from side to side. They have also reacted by sudden movement in response to loud noises. Presumably the diencephalic nuclei mediate this perception. This malformation has been erroneously referred to as anencephaly, which would be a complete failure of brain development.[11]

Cerebral meningocele and meningoenceph-

alocele have been reported in pigs, with a variety of associated brain malformations.[50] Cranium bifidum and exencephaly occurred in a kitten exposed in utero to griseofulvin being used to treat ringworm infection in its dam.[47]

Exencephaly. Exencephaly and craniofacial malformation have been observed in a large number of newborn Burmese kittens from many different locations in the United States. Parents are normal, and usually one or a few in any one litter are affected. A recessive hereditary cause is suspected.

The exencephaly consists of a mass of skin-covered meninges and cerebral hemispheres that project from the cranial cavity through an extensive opening—cranioschisis—in the frontoparietal region of the calvaria. The ventricles of the exencephalic cerebral hemisphere are variably dilated. Occasionally the dilation is massive, causing the skin-covered saclike exencephalic vesicle to fold over the face. There are no olfactory bulbs or peduncles and no optic nerves or chiasm. Caudal to the diencephalon, the remaining brain is grossly normal and covered by the caudal part of the calvaria.

The upper jaw and the nose area are shortened and flattened. No nares, nasal cavities, or planum nasale is evident. There is a cleft on each side of the center of the nose area, with vibrissae on either side of each cleft. This represents a duplication which is also apparent in the two pairs of maxillary bones and two sets of canine teeth and may be reflected in the cerebral hemispheres. There are usually no eyeballs grossly evident. The orbits are present. The mandibles are prominent, and the tongue is often enlarged and protrudes.

Duplication of the Prosencephalon. Newborn calves with complete duplication of the prosencephalon have been observed sporadically. The cranial cavity is enlarged to accommodate the increased brain tissue. The calvaria is complete. Varying degrees of facial duplication accompany the brain malformation. There are usually two sets of nasal cavities with four ethmoid bones with cribriform plates for the four olfactory bulbs, one for each of the four telencephalons. Four orbits, eyes, and optic nerves correlate with two optic chiasms, one for each of the two diencephalons.

Hydranencephaly—A Model for Viral-Induced Cerebral Malformation in Animals. Hydranencephaly is the condition in which each cerebral hemisphere has been reduced to a cerebrospinal fluid-filled membranous sac within a relatively normal sized cra-

nial cavity. The wall of the sac consists of leptomeninges, a glial membrane, and ependymal remnants with no remains of cortical parenchyma.[16] This predominantly affects the neopallium, with relative sparing of the archipallium and paleopallium.

In some instances the cause of the malformation is a viral agent that destroys the developing telencephalon.[23, 24] The malformation is the result of necrosis of already differentiated nervous tissue, and aplasia caused by the necrosis of still actively mitotic germinal neuroectodermal tissue. Cells from the latter usually migrate outward from the mantle layer to form the glia and neurons of the cerebral cortex. Interference with the blood supply of this germinal layer, causing ischemic necrosis of these precursor cells, also produces this lesion.

The bluetongue virus has been shown to produce this lesion in both clinical and experimental studies.[8, 38, 39, 46] This virus causes systemic disease in sheep that is characterized by fever, lameness, and erosions and ulcerations of the oral and nasal mucosae. The live-virus vaccine produced to establish immunity in sheep was found to cause brain malformations, including hydranencephaly in lambs born from ewes immunized during gestation. These lambs were referred to as "dummy lambs" because of their depressed sensorium and lack of response. They were also blind. Experimental studies of direct inoculation of this vaccine into fetal sheep have demonstrated that inoculation between 50 and 58 days' gestation consistently produced a severe necrotizing encephalitis that presented at term as hydranencephaly. Inoculation between 75 and 78 days' gestation produced multifocal encephalitis, which presented at term as porencephaly. This consists of congenital cystic cavities in the cerebrum that often communicate with the lateral ventricle. Inoculation after 100 days' gestation caused mild focal encephalitis with no resulting malformation. Thus the nature of the malformation depended on the gestational age at which infection of the fetus occurred.

The germinal cells of the telencephalon are especially susceptible to this infection, and are most abundant at the end of the first trimester in the lamb fetus. Necrosis of these cells in the first trimester prevents their contributing to the cerebral cortex and, along with the necrosis of the already differentiated cortical plate, leads to the cavitation typical of the malformation. By birth the inflammation has re-

solved, leaving the malformed tissue as the "scar" from the in utero infection.

Hydranencephaly also has been reported in calves; in these cases circumstantial evidence has incriminated the bluetongue virus as the cause.[45] Visual deficit, dullness ("dummy calves"), ataxia, and inability to suckle were the clinical signs. There was no history of clinical illness in the pregnant cattle, but the dams of the affected calves had high serum antibody titers to this virus, as did the affected calves that had not received colostrum. Elevated serum antibody levels in neonatal calves that did not receive colostrum are indicative of in utero infection which stimulated the production of specific antibodies.

In Australia, Japan, and Israel, hydranencephaly has been observed in ruminants, sometimes associated with arthrogryposis.[5, 10, 30, 35, 36, 52] The Akabane virus has been implicated in the pathogenesis of this disease by infection of the fetus during gestation.[17, 18, 20, 37, 43, 48] The malformation that results depends on the fetal age at infection and the degree of encephalomyelitis that occurs. Animals with hydranencephaly were usually infected early in gestation. Arthrogryposis was associated with loss of myelinated fibers in the white matter of the spinal cord, loss of ventral grey column neurons, and loss of fibers in ventral roots.

Hydranencephaly was observed in a 3-month old domestic short-haired kitten that had been blind and ataxic since birth.[14] The feline panleukopenia virus was implicated in the pathogenesis, based on direct immunofluorescence of the virus in the tissues. As a rule, the cerebellum is more severely affected by this virus, with few to no lesions in the cerebrum.

Unilateral hydranencephaly was found in an 8-month-old miniature poodle whose only clinical sign was a visual deficit. The lesion was limited to the neopallium nourished by the middle cerebral artery. No data were available to establish an in utero infection as the cause. In studying the pathogenesis of this malformation in human neurology, considerable emphasis has been placed on prenatal occlusion or agenesis of the carotid artery, and this has been produced experimentally in puppies.

Lissencephaly. Lissencephaly means a smooth brain without evidence of cerebrocortical folding to produce gyri and sulci. It is a congenital condition seen most commonly in the Lhasa Apso breed of dogs.[15, 55] The cerebral cortex is thick (pachygyria) owing to abnormal distribution of cell bodies. The lesion

presumably results from impaired neuronal migration. A genetic mechanism is presumed in this breed. In humans, intrauterine hypoxia or perfusion failure has been suggested as the pathogenetic mechanism.[49]

Clinical signs include difficulty in learning routine training programs, abnormal behavior, occasionally slow postural reactions and poor menace responses, and seizures. Seizures usually do not occur until the dogs are 10 to 12 months old.

I have seen this lesion associated with extensive symmetric cerebellar hypoplasia in a litter of wire-haired fox terriers and a litter of Irish setters. These dogs had a severe cerebellar ataxia.

CEREBELLAR DEGENERATION AND HYPOPLASIA

Abnormalities of the development of the cerebellum are discussed in the section on that organ system.

SPINAL CORD MALFORMATIONS

Meningomyelocele. Spina bifida (the failure of closure of one or more vertebral arches) associated with meningocele or meningomyelocele has been observed most commonly in Manx cats and brachiocephalic breeds of dogs, especially the English bulldog.[2, 7, 9, 22, 29, 31, 34, 37, 42, 54] This usually involves the sacral or last few lumbar vertebrae and the associated spinal cord. The owner's chief complaint usually is that the animal lacks control of its excretions. The tail, anus, and perineum are usually analgesic and may be atonic and areflexic. The pelvic limb gait may be normal or weak and ataxic. Cranial to the meningomyelocele various median plane—spinal cord abnormalities (myelodysplasia) are often found, with or without signs of abnormal pelvic limb function.

The caudal vertebral hypoplasia-aplasia and associated neural tube defect is inherited as an autosomal dominant factor in Manx cats. The homozygote is a prenatal lethal, whereas the clinically affected cats are heterozygotes with variable expression.

Myelodysplasia. Various forms of myelodysplasia have been observed in calves, sometimes associated with a malformed vertebral column.[6] The myelodysplasia has included bizarre overgrowth of spinal cord tissue, varying from a doubled or tripled dorsal grey column

in one segment of spinal cord, to two complete spinal cord segments side by side in one vertebral canal. The latter is referred to as diplomyelia. This usually has involved the caudal thoracic and lumbar spinal cord segments. Hydromyelia (dilated central canal), syringomyelia (cavitated white matter), or both, may accompany this. These conditions present with a nonprogressive difficulty in the use of the pelvic limbs from birth characterized by a marked, occasionally bizarre, incoordination of the pelvic limbs without obvious paresis. Pain perception and spinal reflexes usually are normal.

A newborn Holstein calf was observed with inability to stand on the pelvic limbs but had simultaneous protraction of the pelvic limbs if supported. The lumbosacral vertebrae were wider than normal and there were no caudal vertebrae. There was only a skin appendage for a tail. The lumbosacral vertebrae contained two vertebral canals separated by a bony partition, and each contained a separate spinal cord that joined at the first lumbar and caudal sacral segments. Each spinal cord had its own set of spinal nerves. The separation of two spinal cords by a bony partition is diastematomyelia.

SPINAL DYSRAPHISM. Spinal dysraphism has been reported as a hereditary disease in Weimaraner dogs.[32, 33] It is a form of myelodysplasia and is primarily an abnormality in development of the structures of the spinal cord along the median plane. There is no failure of the neural tube to close, as the term dysraphism connotes. The malformation includes aberrations in the dorsal median septum and the ventral median fissure, a dilated central canal (hydromyelia) or an absent central canal, cavitation in the white matter (syringomyelia), usually in the dorsal funiculi, and the abnormal presence of ventral grey column cells across the median plane between the central canal and the ventral median fissure. The signs are apparent by 4 to 6 weeks of age and do not progress. A characteristic symmetric simultaneous use of the pelvic limbs called "bunny hopping" is observed, along with some proprioceptive deficit. The spinal cord abnormality may be accompanied by scoliosis, abnormal dorsal cervical hair patterns, and a depression of the sternum on the median plane (koilosternia). The clinical signs are variable, depending on the degree of penetrance of the hypothesized codominant lethal gene. The homozygous condition is lethal, whereas the clinically affected dogs are heterozygotes.

The morphologic basis for the simultaneous-hopping-pelvic limb gait is unknown. The normal spinal cord generator of an alternating gait is thought to involve the ventral grey column general somatic efferent neurons and interneurons that cross between the ventral grey columns. This activity is influenced by afferent neurons and the associated dorsal grey columns. Experimentally a hopping gait followed irradiation of the nervous system of developing rats, which resulted in neuronal loss in the dorsal grey column.[19] In dysraphic Weimaraners, the abnormal location of neurons between the ventral grey columns may be involved in the failure to induce an alternating gait. In others there may be no visible morphologic disturbance.

A similar dysraphism was observed in 3 of a litter of 9 mixed husky dogs. Two others had an undefined malformation of the appendicular skeleton. These 3 puppies had shown simultaneous symmetric use of the pelvic limbs ("bunny hopping") since they had been able to walk. The signs had remained static. Myelodysplasia (spinal dysraphism) with or without spinal bifida occurs sporadically in other breeds of dogs.[12, 13, 54]

PATHOGENESIS

Whenever a malformation is diagnosed, owners immediately want to know if it is hereditary. This can only be determined by: (1) knowledge of the literature that documents the hereditary basis for that malformation in that species and breed; (2) careful documentation of that specific malformation in others in the breed that are all related in such a way as to establish an hereditary basis for the disease; and (3) careful planned repeated breeding of the parents of affected offspring, of affected offspring to their parents, or of affected offspring to each other. These latter two matings are dependent on the affected animals' surviving the malformation to a reproductive age and having the capability to reproduce.

Many malformations are sporadic, and there is no evidence of a similar malformation in the literature or in related offspring. However, it is important to document these because only then can other veterinarians appreciate the incidence of a malformation. What may be rare to an individual veterinarian may turn out to be more common when all of these individual experiences are documented and collated.

Such documentation of individual experiences has, in some instances, led to the establishment of an autosomal recessive inheritance as the cause of the condition. This is described in Chapter 13 for cerebellar cortical abiotrophy in two breeds of dog and in Holstein calves. Similarly, careful documentation of malformations may reveal a common environmental factor responsible for the condition.

The following is a case to show the value of the history, careful clinical and pathologic examinations, and knowledge of the literature in the understanding of disease. It is an example of an inherited malformation.

Case Report. Hereditary Hereford syndrome with brain, spinal cord, ocular, and muscle dysplasia.

Signalment. A 1-day-old Hereford calf.

Chief Complaint. Recumbent, blind with "white" eyes.

History. Following a normal parturition this calf was unable to get up. According to the owner the calf was representative of a herd problem of 3 years' duration. The herd consisted of 7 cows (6 of which traced back to 1 female) and 1 bull. Of the 7 calves born 2 years ago, 2 had been affected similarly. One year ago 5 out of 7 had been affected. This case was the second calf born this year. The other was normal.

Physical Examination. The calf was severely depressed (obtunded), recumbent, and unable to get up. Voluntary movements could be elicited from the limbs, along with normal spinal reflexes. The calf was blind. There were cataracts in both eyeballs ("white eyes") and the pupils were fixed and unresponsive to light. The eyeballs were deviated ventrally and an abnormal nystagmus could be elicited in some positions of the head.

Necropsy. Multiple lesions of malformation were observed. Both cerebral hemispheres were enlarged owing to the accumulation of an excessive amount of cerebrospinal fluid in widely dilated lateral ventricles (hydrocephalus). The third ventricle also was dilated. The cerebral gyri were smaller and more numerous than normal (polymicrogyria). The cerebellum was malformed and smaller than usual. Cerebellar cortical dysplasia and lack of myelin development were observed microscopically. The brain stem was bent in a sharp dorsal curve at the level of the midbrain. The colliculi were fused and projected caudally. The aqueduct was malformed and stenotic. The optic nerves and chiasm were small and cystic.

There were cataracts bilaterally, along with retinal dysplasia and a cone-shaped detachment of the retina bilaterally.

Muscular dystrophy and spinal cord-white matter dysplasia have been observed in similar Hereford calves reported in the literature. They were not studied in this calf.

Cause. Based on the herd history and previous published studies of a morphologically similar syndrome, it was assumed that the disease was inherited as an autosomal recessive.[3, 51]

FORAMEN MAGNUM—OCCIPITAL BONE

A dorsal notch or extension of the foramen magnum has been referred to as occipital dysplasia and has been related to clinical signs of congenital or acquired neurologic disease.[4, 26, 40, 41] This correlation has been made primarily in small and medium-sized brachycephalic breeds, but there is no conclusive evidence that the presumed bone malformation was the cause of the neurologic disease.

A study of a large number of normal dogs showed a considerable breed and individual variation in the shape and size of the foramen magnum.[53] A dorsal notch of the foramen magnum was frequently present in the skulls of small breeds of dogs. Usually a membrane covers the area of the notch not occupied by bone and dorsal to the foramen magnum. This dorsal notch develops as a result of incomplete ossification of the ventromedial part of the supraoccipital bone. It was concluded that this dorsal notch is a variation in the normal morphology of the occipital bone and is not related to disturbances of the nervous system.

REFERENCES

1. Amann, J.: The organization of spinal motoneurons and their relationship to corticospinal fibers in the racoon *(Procyon lotor)*. Ph.D. Thesis, Cornell University, 1971.
2. Bailey, C. S.: An embryological approach to the clinical significance of congenital vertebral and spinal cord abnormalities. J. Am. Anim. Hosp. Assoc., *11*:426, 1975.
3. Baker, M. L., Payne, L. C., and Baker, G. N.: The inheritance of hydrocephalus in cattle. J. Hered., *52*:135, 1961.
4. Bardens, J. W.: Congenital malformation of the foramen magnum in dogs. Southwest. Vet., *18*:295, 1965.
5. Bonner, R. B., Mylrea, P. J., and Doyle, B. J.: Arthrogryposis and hydranencephaly in calves. Aust. Vet. J., *37*:160, 1961.
6. Cho, D. Y., and Leipold, H. W.: Spina bifida and spinal dysraphism in calves. Zbl. Vet. Med. [A], *24*:680, 1977.
7. Clark, L., and Carlisle, C. H.: Spina bifida with syringomyelia and meningocele in a short-tailed cat. Aust. Vet. J., *51*:392, 1975.
8. Cordy, D. R., and Schultz, G.: Congenital subcortical encephalopathies in lambs. J. Neuropathol. Exp. Neurol., *20*:554, 1961.
9. DeForest, M. E., and Basrur, P. K.: Malformations and the Manx syndrome in cats. Can. Vet. J., *20*:304, 1979.
10. Della-Porta, A. J., Murray, M. D., and Cybinski, D. H.: Congenital bovine epizootic arthrogryposis and hydranencephaly in Australia. Aust. Vet. J., *52*:496, 1976.
11. Dennis, S. M., and Leipold, H. W.: Anencephaly in sheep. Cornell Vet., *62*:273, 1972.
12. Furneaux, R. W., Doige, C. E., and Kaye, M. M.: Syringomyelia and spina bifida occulta in a Samoyed dog. Can. Vet. J., *14*:317, 1973.
13. Geib, L. W., and Bistner, S. I.: Spinal cord dysraphism in a dog. J. Am. Vet. Med. Assoc., *150*:618, 1967.
14. Greene, C. E., Gorgacz, E. J., and Martin, C. L.: Hydranencephaly associated with feline panleukopenia. J. Am. Vet. Med. Assoc., *180*:767, 1982.
15. Greene, C. E., Vandevelde, M., and Braund, K.: Lissencephaly in two Lhasa Apso dogs. J. Am. Vet. Med. Assoc., *169*:405, 1976.
16. Halsey, J. H., Jr., Allen, N., and Chamberlain, H. R.: The morphogenesis of hydranencephaly. J. Neurol. Sci., *12*:187, 1971.
17. Hartley, W. J., De Sarem, W. G., Della-Porta, A. J., Snowdon, W. A., and Shepherd, N. C.: Pathology of congenital bovine epizootic arthrogryposis and hydranencephaly and its relationship to Akabane virus. Aust. Vet. J., *53*:319, 1977.
18. Hartley, W. J., Wanner, R. A., Della-Porta, A. J., and Snowdon, W. A.: Serological evidence for the association of Akabane virus with epizootic bovine congenital arthrogryposis and hydranencephaly syndromes in New South Wales. Aust. Vet. J., *51*:103, 1975.
19. Hicks, S. P., and D'Amato, C. J.: Development of the motor system: Hopping rats produced by prenatal irradiation. Exp. Neurol., *70*:24, 1980.
20. Inaba, Y., Kurogi, H., and Omori, T.: Akabane disease: Epizootic abortion, premature birth, stillbirth and congenital arthrogryposis-hydranencephaly in cattle, sheep, and goats caused by Akabane virus. Aust. Vet. J., *51*:584, 1975.
21. Jacobsen, M.: Developmental Neurobiology. New York, Holt, Rinehart, and Winston, 1970.
22. James, C. C. M., Lassman, L. P., and Tomlinson, B. E.: Congenital anomalies of the lower spine and spinal cord in Manx cats. J. Pathol., *97*:269, 1969.
23. Johnson, R. T.: Effects of viral infection on the developing nervous system. N. Engl. J. Med., *287*:599, 1972.
24. Johnson, R. T., and Mims, C. A.: Pathogenesis of viral infections of the nervous system. N. Engl. J. Med., *278*:23, 1968.
25. Kalter, H.: Teratology of the Central Nervous System. Chicago, University of Chicago Press, 1968.
26. Kelly, J. H.: Occipital dysplasia and hydrocephalus in a toy poodle. V. M. S. A. C., *70*:940, 1975.
27. Kitchen, H., Murray, R. E., and Cockrell, B. Y.: Spina bifida, sacral dysgenesis and myelocele. Am. J. Pathol., *68*:203, 1972.
28. Langman, J., Guerrant, R. L., and Freeman, B. G.: Behavior of neuroepithelial cells during closure of the neural tube. J. Comp. Neurol., *127*:399, 1966.
29. Leipold, H. W., Huston, K., Blauch, B., and Guffy, M. M.: Congenital defects of the caudal vertebral

column and spinal cord in Manx cats. J. Am. Vet. Med. Assoc., *164*:520, 1974.

30. Markusfeld, O., and Mayer, E.: An arthrogryposis and hydranencephaly syndrome in calves in Israel, 1969–1970. Epidemiological and clinical aspects. Refuah Vet., *28*:51, 1971.

31. Martin, A. H.: A congenital defect in the spinal cord of the Manx cat. Vet. Pathol., *8*:232, 1971.

32. McGrath, J. T.: Spinal dysraphism in the dog. Pathol. Vet., *2*[Suppl.]:1, 1965.

33. McGrath, J. T.: Spinal dysraphism. Comp. Pathol. Bull., *8*:2, 1976.

34. Michael James, C. C., Lassman, L. P., and Tomlinson, B. E.: Congenital anomalies of the lower spine and spinal cord in Manx cats. J. Pathol., *97*:269, 1969.

35. Moriguchi, R., Izawa, H., and Soekawa, M.: A pathological study on calves with arthrogryposis and hydranencephaly. Zbl. Vet. Med. [B], *23*:190, 1976.

36. Nobel, T. A., Klopfer, V., and Neumann, F.: Pathology of an arthrogryposis-hydranencephaly syndrome in domestic ruminants in Israel, 1969–1970. Refuah Vet., *28*:144, 1971.

37. Omori, T., Inaba, T., Kurogi, H., Miura, Y., Nobuto, K., Ohashi, Y., and Matsumoto, M.: Viral abortion, arthrogryposis-hydranencephaly syndrome in cattle in Japan, 1972–1974. Bull. Off. Int. Epix., *81*(5–6):447, 1974.

38. Osburn, B. I., Johnson, R. T., Silverstein, A. M., Prendergast, R. A., Jochim, M. M., and Levy, S. E.: Experimental viral-induced congenital encephalopathies. II. The pathogenesis of bluetongue vaccine virus infection in fetal lambs. Lab. Invest., *25*:206, 1971.

39. Osburn, B. I., Silverstein, A. M., Prendergast, R. A., Johnson, R. T., and Parshall, C. J., Jr.: Experimental viral-induced congenital encephalopathies. I. Pathology of hydranencephaly and porencephaly caused by bluetongue vaccine virus. Lab. Invest., *25*:197, 1971.

40. Parker, A. J., and Park, R. D.: Unusual deformity of the occipital bone in the dog. V. M. S. A. C., *69*:440, 1974.

41. Parker, A. J., and Park, R. D.: Occipital dysplasia in the dog. J. Am. Anim. Hosp. Assoc., *10*:520, 1974.

42. Parker, A. J., Park, R. D., Byerly, C. S., and Stowater, J. L.: Spina bifida with protrusion of

spinal cord tissue in a dog. J. Am. Vet. Med. Assoc., *163*:158, 1973.

43. Parsonson, I. M., Della-Porta, A. J., Snowdon, W. A., and Murray, M. D.: Congenital abnormalities in foetal lambs after inoculation of pregnant ewes with Akabane virus. Aust. Vet. J., *51*:585, 1975.

44. Püschner, H., and Fankhauser, R.: Drei seltene Gehirnmissbildungen beim Rind—"Duplicatas palli," einseitige Zystenzephalie und Mikroenzephalie mit Enzephalozele. Schweiz. Arch. Tierheilkd., *110*:198, 1968.

45. Richards, W. P. C., Crenshaw, G. L., and Bushnell, R. B.: Hydranencephaly of calves associated with natural bluetongue virus infection. Cornell Vet. *61*:336, 1971.

46. Schmidt, R. E., and Panciera, R. J.: Cerebral malformation in fetal lambs from a bluetongue enzootic flock. J. Am. Vet. Med. Assoc., *162*:567, 1973.

47. Scott, F. W., de Lahunta, A., Schultz, R. D., Bistner, S. I., and Riis, R. C.: Teratogenesis in cats associated with griseofulvin therapy. Teratology, *11*:79, 1975.

48. Shepherd, N. C., Gee, C. D., Jessep, T., Timmins, G., Carroll, S. N., and Bonner, R. B.: Congenital bovine arthrogryposis and hydranencephaly. Aust. Vet. J., *54*:470, 1978.

49. Stewart, R. M., Rickman, D. P., and Caviness, V. S., Jr.: Lissencephaly and pachygyria. Acta Neuropathol., *31*:1, 1975.

50. Trautwein, G., and Meyer, H.: Experimentelle Untersuchungen über erbliche Meningocele cerebralis beim Schwein. II. Pathomorphologie der Gehirnmissbildungen. Pathol. Vet., *3*:543, 1966.

51. Urman, H. K., and Grace, O. D.: Hereditary encephalopathy, a hydrocephalus syndrome in newborn calves. Cornell Vet., *54*:229, 1964.

52. Whittem, J. H.: Congenital abnormalities in calves: Arthrogryposis and hydranencephaly. J. Pathol. Bacteriol., *73*:375, 1957.

53. Watson, A. G.: The phylogeny and development of the occipito-atlas-axis complex in the dog. Ph.D. Thesis, Cornell University, 1981.

54. Wilson, J. H., Kurtz, H. J., Leipold, H. W., and Lees, G. E.: Spina bifida in the dog. Vet. Pathol., *16*:165, 1979.

55. Zaki, F.: Lissencephaly in Lhasa Apso dogs. J. Am. Vet. Med. Assoc., *169*:1165, 1976.

CEREBROSPINAL FLUID AND HYDROCEPHALUS

Cerebrospinal fluid (CSF) is a clear, colorless fluid that surrounds and permeates the entire central nervous system (CNS) and therefore protects, supports, and nourishes it. In general the CSF is produced by the choroid plexuses, circulates to the subarachnoid space, and is absorbed into the venous sinuses.[25, 58, 109]

PRODUCTION

More specifically, CSF originates from a number of sites. These include the choroid plexuses of the lateral, third, and fourth ventricles, directly from the brain by way of the ependymal lining of the ventricular system, directly from the brain by way of the pial-glial membrane covering its external surface, and from blood vessels in the pia-arachnoid (Fig. 3–1).[67, 68, 84] One study on total production of CSF in the dog revealed that 35 per cent derived from the third and lateral ventricles, 23 per cent from the fourth ventricle, and 42 per cent from the subarachnoid space. The result of these studies vary with the experimental model that is used.[13, 40, 61]

The method of production is both by ultrafiltration from the blood plasma and by active transport mechanisms that utilize energy. At the choroid plexus there are essentially two cell layers between blood plasma and ventricular CSF. The vascular endothelium is separated from the ependymal cells by a thin basement membrane and occasionally portions of meningeal cells. The ependymal cells of the choroid plexus are tall columnar cells with tight junctions near their apex. They have the characteristics of cells that function in the transcellular transport of materials: they have microvilli on their luminal surface and infoldings of the basal cytoplasm. This barrier is a semipermeable membrane that selectively and actively transports some materials and inhibits others.[21, 40] *(from kidneys)*

Compared with plasma ultrafiltrate, the CSF has less potassium and calcium, and more chloride, sodium, and especially magnesium. It has slightly less glucose, about 80 per cent of the blood level, and much less protein. In the dog, there is less than 25 mg per dl of protein, which is mostly albumin. Bile salts, penicillin, and products of the breakdown of hemoglobin are prevented from entering the CSF from the blood.

The rate of production varies with the species and method of determination. The following rates have been determined: dog—.047 cc per min, cat—.017 cc per min, man—0.5 cc per min.[14] In man this rate is equivalent to 3 to 5 times the total volume per day.

There is a continual turnover of CSF. There is evidence that it is produced at a constant flow rate despite the pressure of CSF in the ventricular system. In chronic obstructive hypertensive hydrocephalus, atrophy of the choroid plexus will decrease CSF production. The rate is independent of the hydrostatic pressure of the blood, but is influenced by the osmotic pressure of the blood. Hypertonic solutions in the blood will reduce the rate of formation. This has clinical application in head injuries with cerebral edema. An osmotic diuretic is

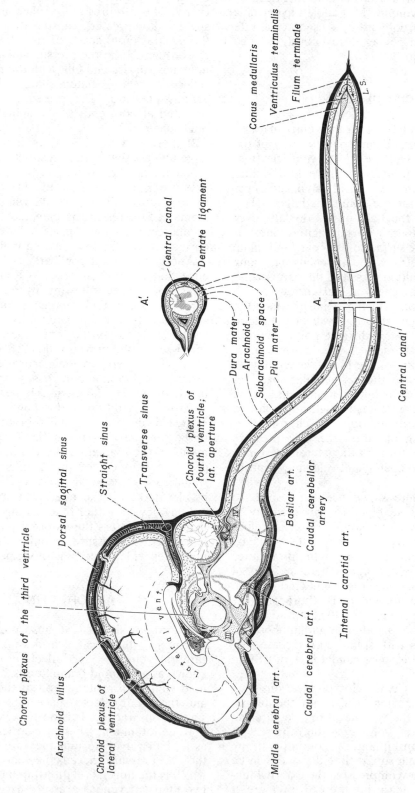

Figure 3–1. Relationship of meninges and subarachnoid space to ventricular system.

administered to decrease the rate of CSF formation and decrease intracranial pressure by reducing brain volume. Mannitol, a hypertonic solution of a carbohydrate, is used at the rate of 0.25 to 2 gm per kg intravenously as a 20 per cent solution.[34, 48]

CIRCULATION

The CSF circulates from the ventricular system to the subarachnoid space by way of the lateral apertures of the fourth ventricle (Fig. 3–2). In some individuals there is a similar passage between the central canal and subarachnoid space at the conus medullaris (Fig. 3–1). Much of the CSF passes dorsally over the cerebrum to the dorsal sagittal sinus. It covers the entire surface of the brain and spinal cord, and penetrates the parenchyma, along with the larger blood vessels in the perivascular spaces.[110] These spaces are extensions of the subarachnoid space to the point at which the pia mater reflects onto the wall of the blood vessel. This is not a distinct point, and for some distance the cells of the leptomeninges and the adventitia of the blood vessel may be closely related and the perivascular space reduced to small clefts between the cells.

The flow of the CSF is thought to be due to the pulsation of the blood in the choroid plexuses. With each pulsation the CSF pressure rises and surges towards the lateral apertures. The cilia on the ependymal cells may contribute to the flow.

In humans there is evidence that despite the erect posture, CSF tends to flow cranially as well as caudally. Radioiodinated serum albumin injected into the lumbar cistern can be followed by scanning radiographic procedures to the dorsum of the hemisphere in 12 to 24 hours. Radiopharmaceuticals injected into the lateral ventricle appear in the thoracolumbar subarachnoid space in 30 to 40 minutes.[28] Comparison of cerebellomedullary and lumbosacral CSF in animals with spinal cord disease suggests that there is some caudal flow of CSF in animals.

The cranial cavity is a closed space consisting of brain parenchyma, CSF, and the blood. Any change in the volume of one requires an adjustment in the volume of the others. This sensitive relationship and the continuity of the cranial and spinal subarachnoid spaces can be demonstrated by compressing the external jugular veins and measuring the CSF pressure at the cerebellomedullary cistern and the lumbar cistern. Venous compression causes an increase in venous blood volume in the cranial cavity. This requires more space and the CSF space is compressed, causing the pressure in the subarachnoid space to rise. For a similar reason the CSF in the pressure-measuring manometer will rise and fall, with the respirations reflecting the associated changes in thoracic venous pressure. The pressure elevation is reflected at both ends of the spinal subarachnoid space.

If there is a lesion such as a neoplasm or large abscess that obliterates the subarachnoid space along the spinal cord, and the CSF pressure is measured at the lumbar cistern, this pressure will not elevate when the intracranial CSF pressure is elevated by external jugular compression. This is called the Queckenstedt or jugular compression maneuver.

Another practical application of the knowledge that the cranial cavity is a closed space often can be seen following injury. One of the cardinal rules in the emergency room is to be sure the patient has a patent airway. This not only assures the proper oxygenation of blood for tissues, but prevents dilation of cerebral blood vessels. Hypercapnia causes cerebral arterial vasodilation and increases the volume of blood in the cranial cavity. If head injury is part of the syndrome, this augments the already existing problem of cerebral hemorrhage or edema that has taxed the space requirements in the cranial cavity. Similarly, when a dog is positioned for intracranial or cervical spinal cord surgery, the head and neck should be elevated and suspended from a specialized holding device, rather than resting on padding that will compress the external jugular veins. Normal CSF pressure is quite variable and fluctuates widely over a 24-hour period.

ABSORPTION

The major site of CSF absorption is at the arachnoid villus located in a venous sinus or cerebral vein.[2, 30, 76, 77] Collections of villi are known as arachnoid granulations.[41] The arachnoid villus is a prolongation of the arachnoid and the subarachnoid space into the venous sinus. The arachnoid tissue is covered by venous endothelium. These are structured to act as a "ball valve" so that they are open when the CSF pressure exceeds the venous pressure, which is the normal relationship between these two fluids. If venous pressure exceeds that of the CSF, these villi collapse. Flow is one way,

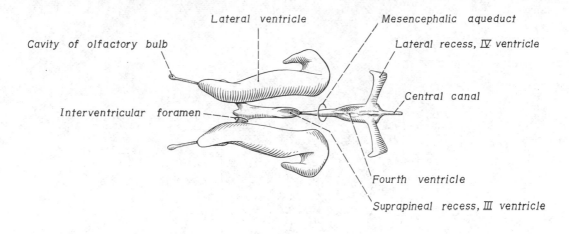

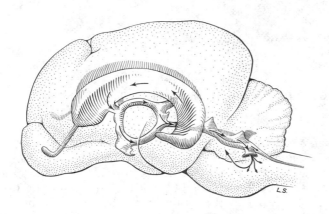

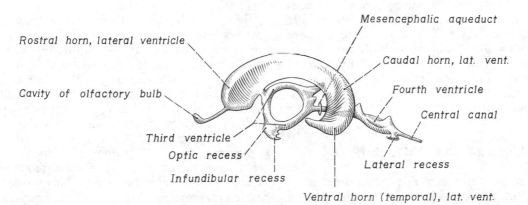

Figure 3–2. The canine ventricular system.

from CSF to blood. These villi are found in the venous sinuses and in some cerebral veins (Fig. 3–3).

Electron-microscopic studies of the endothelial cells lining the arachnoid villi have revealed transient transcellular channels that develop for the passage of materials from CSF to the venous system. These apparently develop only in response to a pressure gradient between the CSF and venous blood, and function as a "one-way valve" system.[94-96]

Other sites of absorption include the veins and lymphatics found around spinal nerve roots, and the spinal nerves and the first and

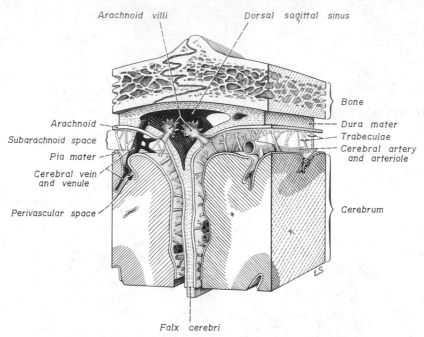

Figure 3–3.   Cerebral meninges and arachnoid villi.

second cranial nerves at the sites at which they leave the skull.[29] Some CSF may enter the brain parenchyma through the ependyma and be absorbed in blood vessels there. This probably occurs more often when intraventricular CSF pressure is elevated.[69]

Thus CSF is formed and absorbed throughout the ventricles and subarachnoid space, is in constant motion, and progresses generally toward the surface of the cerebral hemisphere and along the spinal cord. With the rate of production being independent of intracranial pressure, absorption is the primary homeostatic mechanism for maintenance of the intracranial pressure.

FLUID COMPARTMENTS

There are three extracellular fluid compartments in the cranial cavity associated with brain parenchyma: plasma, CSF, and the extracellular fluid (ECF). Exchanges between these are critical to the normal maintenance of brain function. There are unique features to the morphologic and physiologic barriers between these compartments.

The blood-brain barrier exists between plasma and ECF at the level of the capillaries.[73] It consists of a nonfenestrated, tightly joined layer of endothelial cells of the capillary wall, surrounded by a relatively complete layer of

foot processes from astrocytes and a thick basement membrane between them.[49] When this barrier is normal it prevents therapeutic levels of penicillin from entering the ECF of the brain parenchyma. Chloromycetin and some sulfonamides readily pass through this membrane to reach effective antibacterial levels in the ECF.

The blood-CSF barrier exists between plasma and ECF at the choroid plexus and consists of two cell layers separated by a thin basement membrane. The vascular endothelial layer has areas where only a thin cell membrane intervenes. These have been referred to as fenestrations or pores.[58] The choroidal epithelium consists of tall columnar cells with tight cell junctions at their apex, toward the ventricular lumen. Fragments of meningeal cells may be interspersed in the basement membrane between these cells. This serves as a semipermeable membrane between the plasma and CSF. In acid-base imbalances, CO_2 readily passes between plasma and CSF, whereas bicarbonate exchange is slow owing to the relative impermeability of this barrier to bicarbonate.[58]

The CSF-ECF barrier occurs over the outer surface of the brain and in the ventricles. In the ventricles there is a lining of ependymal cells that varies from columnar to squamous with incomplete intercellular junctions. There is no basement membrane, and subependymal glial cells lie under most of the ventricular ependymal cells. There is little barrier to exchange between CSF and ECF along this surface. The same relationship exists between CSF in the subarachnoid space over the outside of the brain and the adjacent ECF of the parenchyma. Here the barrier consists of a pial-glial membrane. A nearly complete layer of pia mater covers the outer surface of the brain. A basement membrane lies deep to this adjacent to a layer of astrocytic foot processes. There are no intercellular junctions in these cell layers. Thus, products in the CSF have ready access to the ECF of the parenchyma and are extremely important in maintaining normal brain function.

FUNCTION

CSF has a number of functions, including the protection and nourishment of the parenchyma and the maintenance of homeostasis. The brain is suspended in and buoyed by CSF, and thus is physically protected by it. CSF helps to modulate pressure changes that occur within the cranial cavity. In conjunction with cerebral blood flow, it helps regulate the intracranial pressure.

As a chemical buffer to the central nervous system, CSF helps maintain the proper ionic environment for the parenchyma. Being closely related to the "interstitial fluid" and in close proximity to the parenchyma, it provides a more stable and closely controlled ionic environment than the blood plasma. The pH of CSF has a direct influence on medullary function. A metabolic function may be served by CSF in acting as a medium for transport of metabolites and nutrients between the brain and the blood. It also may serve to transport neuroendocrine substances and neurotransmitters.

A clinical example of the importance of these functions is seen in the remarkable neurologic deficits that can accompany severe inflammation of the leptomeninges without direct involvement of the parenchyma. This is most commonly noted in cryptococcal meningitis of dogs and bacterial meningitis of calves.

CLINICAL APPLICATION OF CSF

CSF may be used in selected radiographic procedures, and may be analyzed for its cellular and chemical constituents.

Radiographic procedures utilizing a radiopaque dye or air are employed to demonstrate the shape of the CSF-containing system and reveal changes caused by disease.[71]

Myelography. A radiopaque material may be injected into the spinal subarachnoid space to determine if it has been altered by a space-occupying lesion in the vertebral canal, in the subarachnoid space, or in the spinal cord.[71, 92] Spinal cord diseases that cause parenchymal swelling will decrease the adjacent subarachnoid space and interfere with the flow and distribution of the radiopaque dye (Figs. 3–4, 3–5, 3–6).[18] Three contrast agents are used in veterinary medicine, although none is officially approved. These are metrizamide (Amipaque), sodium methiodal (Skiodan), and iophendylate (Pantopaque). Metrizamide and sodium methiodal are water-soluble and miscible with CSF. Iophendylate is fat-soluble and displaces CSF.

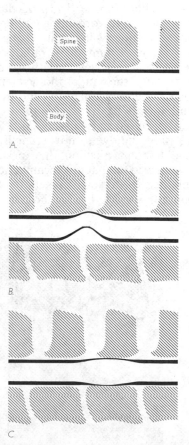

Figure 3–4. Myelographic interpretation, lateral view. *A:* normal; *B:* extradural compression; *C:* intradural enlargement (both views).

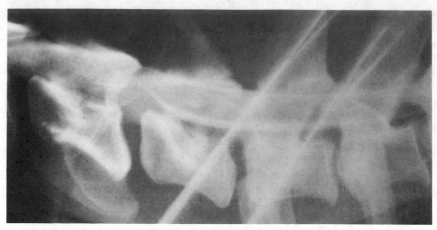

Figure 3–5. Skiodan myelogram of an extradural compression of the spinal cord at C6–C7 articulation in a 5-year-old Doberman pinscher. A protruded-proliferated intervertebral disk was presumed.

Metrizamide is the most commonly used material at the present.[9, 11, 36, 60, 72, 90] It is a relatively safe radiopaque dye that can be injected into the cerebellomedullary cistern and allowed to flow caudally the length of the spinal subarachnoid space. The procedure used is identical to that for obtaining CSF for analysis. One injection will usually persist long enough to allow a number of radiographs to be made of the area under concern. Sometimes the flow through the caudal thoracic and lumbar areas will be inadequate to confirm lesions here, and it will be necessary to inject the spinal subarachnoid space in the caudal lumbar area and allow the dye to flow cranially.

For the lumbar injection the anesthetized animal is placed in lateral recumbency with the trunk flexed. A spinal needle (3.5 inch, 20–22 gauge) is inserted along the cranial edge of the spine at L6 to penetrate the interarcuate ligament between L5 and L6. Rarely the subarachnoid space can be entered dorsal to the spinal cord to permit injection of dye. Usually the needle must be passed in a smooth motion through the spinal cord and into the subarachnoid space ventral to it. If you feel the needle strike the floor of the vertebral canal it can be backed off into this subarachnoid space. The ventral subarachnoid space at this site may provide enough CSF for analysis.

If you are unsuccessful at the L5–L6 site, the L4–L5 site may be used. In most dogs the subarachnoid space is too small at the lumbosacral site to permit it to be entered by a needle for CSF analysis or myelography.

Prior to the development of metrizamide, sodium methiodal (Skiodan) was routinely used.[18] However, this water-soluble dye is too

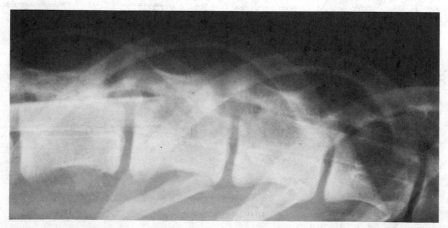

Figure 3–6. Skiodan myelogram (oblique view) of an intradural space-occupying lesion of T13 in a 3.5-year-old German shepherd. A neuroepithelioma was diagnosed.

toxic to the medullary centers to be injected at the cerebellomedullary cistern. Therefore, it is routinely injected by a lumbar puncture. This dye is rapidly absorbed and only persists in enough quantity to provide effective radiopacity for a few minutes. This limits the number of radiographs that can be made following one injection.

All of these procedures are done under general anesthesia. Following recovery from anesthesia for metrizamide myelography, seizures occasionally occur but can be readily controlled with diazepam (Valium).[24] This is more common in the larger breeds undergoing cisternal myelography for cervical lesions. This problem is much more common with sodium methiodal myelography. The patient will be depressed for at least one day following metrizamide myelography. A chemically induced meningitis occurs for a brief period but should not be a deterrent to the use of the procedure.

Iophendylate (Pantopaque) is an oil emulsion commonly used in humans via lumbar injections and most of it is removed following the procedure. It was used in veterinary medicine prior to the availability of the water-soluble dyes. It is relatively nontoxic and does not usually cause convulsions, but in animals it is difficult to remove. Because it is poorly absorbed from the subarachnoid space, it produces a severe persistent foreign body menin-

gitis.[105] This is not usually associated with clinical signs but it will make subsequent myelography difficult and CSF analysis useless.

Myelography is not an innocuous procedure, and it should be mostly reserved for those patients in which surgery is contemplated and specific lesion location is necessary.

Pneumoventriculography. This involves the injection of air directly into the lateral ventricle, allowing it to outline the ventricular system (see Fig. 3–2).[35, 47, 111] The site of injection is located by finding the half-way point between the external occipital protuberance and the lateral angle of the eyelids. Trace a line from there medially, perpendicular to the median plane of the skull. Enter the skull on that perpendicular line 3 to 5 mm from the median plane. A straight, pointed intramedullary bone pin about the size of the spinal needle may be used to bore a hole in the calvaria through which to pass the needle. On a lateral radiograph of the skull measure the depth of the cranial cavity. Do not insert the needle beyond half the distance from the calvaria to the floor of the cranial cavity. The normal ventricle may be difficult to enter. The widely dilated ventricle is entered immediately, but the pressure may be low enough to require aspiration to obtain the CSF. Withdraw a small amount of CSF (1 to 2 cc) and replace it with air. By rotating the patient, the

Figure 3–7. Pneumoventriculogram of a 3-month-old Manchester terrier with extensive dilation of the lateral ventricles.

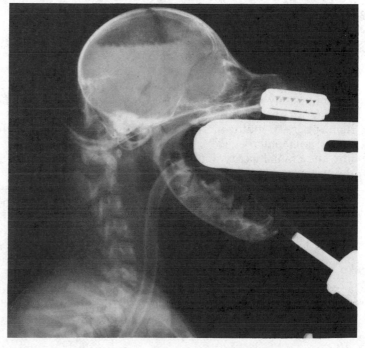

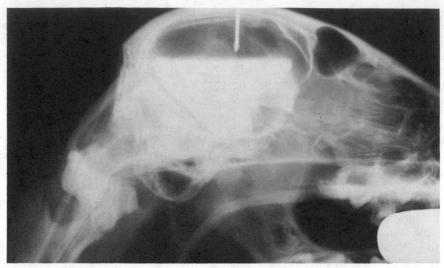

Figure 3–8. Air above contrast medium in the lateral ventricles of a 3-month-old miniature poodle with extensive hydrocephalus. The contrast medium can be visualized in the subarachnoid space in the vertebral canal, indicating the absence of any obstruction to flow through the ventricular system.

air can be moved in the ventricle so as to define all its borders. This is a safe procedure that can be done routinely on hospital patients with no aftereffects (Fig. 3–7).

Contrast Ventriculography. This may be performed by the same procedure using small amounts of meglumine iothalamate (Conray) or metrizamide, but it is less safe than air. It is especially useful to determine if there is a block in the ventricular system at the aqueduct or lateral aperture of the fourth ventricle. The latter cannot be determined at necropsy. The appearance of contrast medium in the cervical subarachnoid space from injection into the lateral ventricle confirms the patency of the system (Fig. 3–8).

Contrast Encephalography. Contrast encephalography will determine the presence or absence of the gyri and sulci of the cerebral hemisphere. If metrizamide is injected into the cerebellomedullary cistern and allowed to flow into the cranial cavity and over the surface of the brain, it will fill the sulci and permit their identification. Lissencephaly is a developmental failure of the neopallium to develop gyri and sulci and is most commonly observed in the Lhasa Apso. In some patients with severe hypertensive hydrocephalus, the neopallium is compressed to a smooth flat mantle eliminating the gyri. These lesions may be apparent in contrast encephalography.

Laboratory examination is performed on CSF because it often reflects disease processes that involve the parenchyma or meninges.

METHOD TO OBTAIN CSF

In the dog, the most reliable source of CSF for laboratory analysis is the cerebellomedullary cistern. The L5–L6 site used for myelography is good if an adequate amount of nontraumatized CSF can be obtained.[5] In the horse, cow, sheep, goat, and pig, both the atlanto-occipital and lumbosacral sites are useful sources of CSF. The following are detailed descriptions for the dog and horse that are applicable to the other species.

ATLANTO-OCCIPITAL (CEREBELLOMEDULLARY CISTERN) CEREBROSPINAL FLUID COLLECTION IN SMALL ANIMALS

With the patient under general anesthesia, surgically prepare the atlanto-occipital area between and caudal to the ears. For the right-handed individual, place the dog in left lateral recumbency with its skull and cervical vertebrae at the edge of the table. Have an assistant elevate the nose slightly so that it is parallel with the vertebral column, and flex the atlanto-occipital joint so that the median axis of the head is about at right angles to the median axis of the cervical vertebrae. Observe respirations continually, because vigorous flexion may bend the endotracheal tube and cause an obstructed airway.

If the tapping site is not palpated and the

needle is handled only at the hub, surgical gloves are not necessary. With the left hand, place the thumb on the external occipital protuberance and the first finger on the cranial edge of the right wing of the atlas. From these landmarks draw one imaginary line caudally along the dorsal median plane from the external occipital protuberance, and another transversely between the cranial edges of the wings of the atlas. The needle should be inserted where these two lines cross and be directed at the angle of the mandible.

A spinal needle with stilette that is 1.5 inches long and 20 gauge is adequate for most dogs and cats.[a] A 3-inch 20-gauge needle may be necessary in some dogs of the larger breeds. With the bevel directed to the side, insert the needle through the skin and into the underlying muscle and fascia. Direct it toward the angle of the mandible. Place the palm of the left hand on the skull for support and grasp the hub of the needle with thumb and first finger; do not release it until the procedure is completed. Remove the stilette with the right hand and observe for fluid. If none is seen, replace the stilette, and without releasing the left hand from the needle, continue to advance the needle 1 to 2 mm at a time. After each advancement remove the stilette and observe for fluid. In many instances a slight sudden loss of resistance may be felt as the atlantooccipital membrane and dura mater are penetrated simultaneously. Because it is not consistent, do *not* rely on this sign for the depth of your needle. Continual observation for fluid is the safest method. Slight rotation of the needle may produce fluid when the desired level has been reached but no fluid has emerged.

If the needle strikes bone at about the level you would expect fluid to appear, then the point of the needle must be walked gently caudally off the occipital bone or cranially off the atlas to reach the atlanto-occipital space. It is often preferable to withdraw the needle and start again, correcting for the slight error in direction of the first attempt. Do not advance the needle without the stilette. This will prevent occlusion of the needle with tissue, and there will be less damage if the nervous tissue is penetrated.

At all times maintain a firm grip on the needle with the left hand.

When fluid is observed, place the tip of the 3-way valve of the manometer[a] in the hub and measure the opening pressure when the CSF has reached its maximum height in the tube. Rotate the valve arm to close the connection to the tube and open the syringe. Withdraw 1 to 2 cc of CSF. Reopen the lumen to the manometer tube and measure the closing pressure. When this is determined close off the connection to the tapping needle, and remove the manometer and syringe unit. Replace the stilette and remove the needle in one motion.

In some small breeds of dogs and cats, if measurement of CSF pressure is not essential to the differential diagnosis it may be preferable not to attach the manometer unit to the needle, but to collect the fluid directly with a syringe. If the flow is slow, a direct sample may be collected most readily by letting the CSF drip from the hub into a test tube. Simultaneous jugular vein compression may hasten this flow.

The level at which the subarachnoid space is reached varies with the breed and the individual animal. In toy breeds and some cats it is often very close to the surface and is small. Caution is advised.

If whole blood appears in the spinal needle, withdraw the needle and obtain another sterile needle and repeat the procedure. Branches of the ventral internal vertebral venous plexus course close to the atlanto-occipital site and may be entered with the spinal needle. These are in the extradural space; therefore, the CSF in the subarachnoid space has not been contaminated with blood.

If there is blood in the CSF, this may be due to rupture of small blood vessels by the procedure or be part of the disease process. If it is due to the procedure, the blood should decrease as the CSF drips from the needle or as successive small quantities are removed by syringe. If the hemorrhage is part of the disease process, the amount will not change in the CSF as it is withdrawn. If you are uncertain, centrifugation will remove all of the blood from the sample, leaving a clear, colorless fluid if the hemorrhage was from the procedure. If it was part of the disease process, centrifugation will remove any erythrocytes that are present but the supernatant will have a yellow color (xanthochromia) from the hemoglobin breakdown products from the erythrocytes in the hemorrhage.

---

[a]Becton, Dickinson and Co., Rutherford, N.J. 07070.

[a]Manometer Tray, Pharmaseal Laboratories, Glendale, Calif. 91201.

Small amounts of iatrogenic hemorrhage will not interfere significantly with evaluation of the CSF.

ATLANTO-OCCIPITAL (CEREBELLOMEDULLARY CISTERN) CSF COLLECTION IN THE HORSE[63, 64]

The horse is given a general anesthetic of choice and placed in lateral recumbency. An area of the poll and neck (from between the ears to 6 to 8 inches caudally and approximately 3 to 4 inches on either side of the mane) is prepared surgically. The horse's head is flexed so that the median axis of the head is at right angles to the median axis of the cervical vertebrae. Such flexion of the atlanto-occipital joint can result in upper airway obstruction. A sterile fenestrated drape may be used to cover the site and sterile surgical gloves may be used to handle the 18- or 20-gauge 3.5-inch spinal needle.[a]

The site of skin penetration is located at the intersection of imaginary lines drawn between the cranial borders of the atlas and along the dorsal median plane (Fig. 3–9). Palpate the

---

[a]Becton, Dickinson and Co., Rutherford, N.J. 07070.

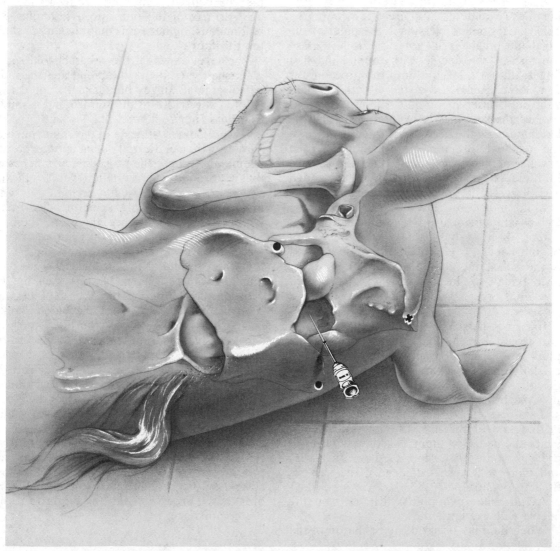

Figure 3–9.   Atlanto-occipital cerebrospinal fluid collection from the recumbent horse. Spinal needle in position with stilette removed. Palpable landmarks are the cranial borders of the atlas (● —— ●) and the external occipital protuberance (+) on the dorsal median plane.

wings of the atlas and define the site of skin penetration. It is important that the needle traverse the median plane during insertion, as it is possible to pass through the atlanto-occipital space and be too far lateral, thus missing the subarachnoid space. The needle usually is aimed at the lower jaw or lips (perpendicular to the cervical vertebrae), and the wrist of the hand holding the needle must rest on the sterile drape over the occipital area or dorsum of the neck so the needle can be moved slowly and with steady pressure. An initial thrust is often helpful to advance the needle the first inch through the thick skin and funicular part of the ligamentum nuchae. The needle is advanced until the dorsal atlanto-occipital membrane and cervical dura mater are penetrated. These tissues, being stretched with flexion of the head, often give rise to a clear "popping" sensation either of increased or sudden lack of resistance when penetrated. During insertion of the needle the stilette should be withdrawn whenever such a sensation is felt or whenever it is judged that a sufficient depth has been reached. Clear CSF appearing at the hub of the needle indicates a successful procedure. If no spinal fluid appears the needle is rotated 90 degrees, and if this is unsuccessful, the stilette is replaced and the needle advanced further.

The depth at which the subarachnoid space is entered and CSF obtained is normally between 2 and 3 inches. This depends on the size and weight of the horse, the angle of insertion of the spinal needle, and the degree of flexion of the atlanto-occipital joint. The needle must never be advanced without the stilette in place in order to prevent damage to neural tissue and plugging of the needle with tissue.

When CSF is obtained the opening pressure is measured immediately with a manometer, and the sample collected.[a] After the closing pressure is measured, the stilette is replaced and the needle withdrawn.

LUMBOSACRAL CSF COLLECTION IN THE HORSE (Method of I. Mayhew)[63]

The horse is lightly restrained in a standing position. Only in overtly excitable animals is use of a tranquilizer advised, as this tends to cause the horse to stand with most of the caudal weight supported on one pelvic limb with a resulting displacement of the utilized

landmarks. Lumbosacral CSF collection in the laterally recumbent horse (either tetraplegic or under general anesthesia) is generally more difficult than in the standing subject because of the resulting asymmetry of the palpable bony prominences.

The area is surgically prepared; a sterile drape and surgical gloves may be used in the procedure.

The site of skin penetration is found by attempting to correlate many different landmarks. This is because there are considerable individual and sex differences and often some of the landmarks cannot be palpated easily. The preferred site of skin penetration is within the depression bordered laterally by the medial rim of the tuber sacrale, cranially by the caudal edge of the sixth lumbar spine, and caudally by the cranial edge of the second sacral spine (Fig. 3–10). It is often one-quarter to one-half inch caudal to the cranial border of this depression and at the point of intersection of a line drawn between the cranial edge of each tuber sacrale and the dorsal median plane. The tuber sacrale of each side can be palpated a variable distance from the dorsal midline on a sagittal plane. The exact position and distance between each tuber sacrale vary. Generally these are more prominent and farther apart in mares. The first estimate of this site is the intersection at a line joining the caudal border of each tuber coxae with the dorsal midline. This often is between the highest points of the gluteal region. Palpate the lumbar spines and by moving caudally, the caudal edge of the spines of the fifth (L5) and sixth (L6) lumbar vertebrae can be palpated. Because the spine of L6 usually is shorter than that of L5, there is often palpable depression at the caudal edge of L5, and this is occasionally mistaken for the site. The first sacral spine is usually too short to palpate.

Following appropriate local analgesia, a small stab incision is made with a sterile surgical blade through the skin at this site. It is advisable to have a twitch available or lightly applied to the horse's upper lip. However, it is usually only during penetration of the dura mater that there is any response on the part of the horse, and generally this is restricted to a local response of tail movement, slight flexion of the pelvic limbs, and slight axial muscle contraction with evidence of conscious perception. An occasional horse will react with sudden violent movements, and if these cannot be predicted and prevented, an appropriate sedation or general anesthesia may be necessary.

[a]Manometer Tray, Pharmaseal Laboratories, Glendale, Calif. 91201.

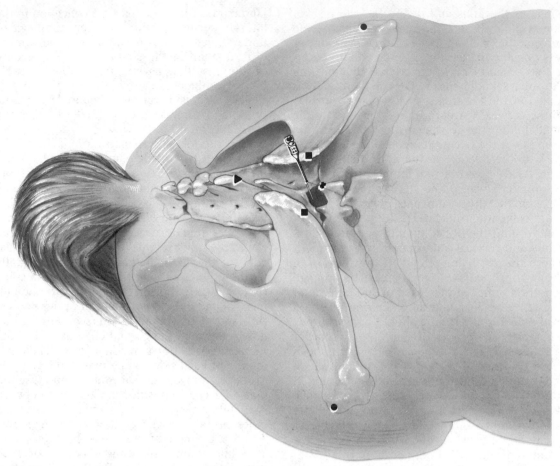

Figure 3–10. Lumbosacral cerebrospinal fluid collection from the standing horse. Spinal needle in position with stilette removed. Palpable landmarks are the caudal borders of each tuber coxae (● —— ●), the caudal edge of the spine of L6 (+), the cranial edge of the second sacral spine (▲), and the cranial edge of each tuber sacrale (■ —— ■).

A 3.5-inch 18- or 20-gauge spinal needle can be used in ponies and foals up to approximately 12 hands tall, and a 6.0-inch 18-gauge thin-wall needle with fitted stilette can be used on horses up to approximately 17 hands tall.[a] Occasionally, a special 8- or 9-inch spinal needle is required on very tall horses.

A right-handed person should stand on the horse's right side and rest the wrist of the right hand on the dorsal median plane of the horse cranial to the site of the previously made small skin incision. Holding the stilette firmly in place, advance the spinal needle along the median plane toward the lumbosacral space. The average depth of penetration of the needle to reach the subarachnoid space in a 450-kg horse is approximately 5 inches, and the di- ameter of the lumbosacral space is approximately 1.0 inch (Fig. 3–11).

The needle usually can be moved forward without much resistance. Penetration of the lumbosacral interarcuate ligament (ligamentum flavum) often is felt as a sudden loss of a slightly increased resistance, and the dura mater and arachnoid may be entered at the same time; otherwise, these membranes may be penetrated by advancing the needle a few millimeters, and this usually is accompanied by some local response on the part of the horse, as described. If CSF is not obtained, the needle can be advanced to the floor of the vertebral canal and then withdrawn, slowly rotating it a millimeter or less at a time. In this situation, the needle passes through the dorsal dura mater and subarachnoid space and conus medullaris, then through the ventral subarachnoid space and dura mater. It is imperative that the

[a]Becton, Dickinson and Co., Rutherford, N.J. 07070.

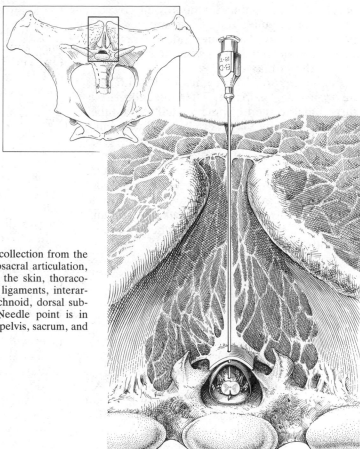

Figure 3–11. Lumbosacral spinal fluid collection from the horse. Transverse dissection through lumbosacral articulation, cranial view. Spinal needle passes through the skin, thoracolumbar fascia adjacent to the interspinous ligaments, interarcuate ligament, dorsal dura mater and arachnoid, dorsal subarachnoid space, and conus medullaris. Needle point is in ventral subarachnoid space. Cranial view of pelvis, sacrum, and area of dissection (insert).

hand holding the hub of the spinal needle rests very firmly on the horse whenever the needle is held or manipulated, and the stilette always must be in place during movement of the needle.

At each stage when the stilette is withdrawn to determine if the subarachnoid space is entered, several different efforts should be made to obtain CSF before the stilette is replaced and the needle advanced or withdrawn. First, an assistant should occlude both jugular veins to increase intracranial and thus intraspinal pressure. Then, the needle can be rotated up to 180° to stop any of the meninges or nerve roots from lying across and occluding the bevel of the needle point. Finally a small (5-ml) syringe can be applied to the needle hub and gentle suction pressure intermittently applied. (A heavy syringe tends to force the needle down farther, and continuous strong suction pressure also tends to promote hemorrhage and often occludes the needle with meninges

or cauda equina.) If the horse moves during collection, the jugular veins still can be readily occluded and CSF often can be aspirated from within the hub of the needle without connecting the syringe to it, thus reducing the chances of dislodging the needle from the subarachnoid space or initiating hemorrhage.

CSF COLLECTION IN CATTLE

Cisternal. The landmarks for a cisternal atlanto-occipital CSF collection are the same as for the other species. Calves may be restrained in lateral recumbency or may be mildly sedated. With the calf in lateral recumbency the clinician may kneel in front of the calf with its head flexed and held between the knees of the clinician. The clinician can lean over the calf to perform the procedure.

For the experienced clinician, adult cattle may be restrained sufficiently with a halter and noselead. The recumbent depressed cow can have its head pulled to the side and tied to the pelvic limb on that same side to permit a cisternal collection. Otherwise, heavy sedation or anesthesia may be necessary.

Lumbosacral. The spines of L5, L6, and S2 are usually palpable. The collection site is just caudal to the L6 spine medial to the tuber sacrale. This point is generally on a line joining the caudal edges of each tuber coxae. A 3.5 inch, 20 gauge spinal needle will be needed in adult cattle and a skin incision may facilitate passage of the needle. In some a slight decrease in resistance will be felt when the needle penetrates the interarcuate ligament. The animal or just its tail may move when the meninges are passed.

CEREBROSPINAL FLUID
EXAMINATION[3, 20, 26, 31, 32, 57, 66, 75, 87-89, 108]

Pressure

The pressure is only significant if it is elevated above normal. Occasionally in the normal animal there is insufficient pressure to cause the CSF to rise in the manometer. Although most dogs have a pressure of less than 170 mm H_2O under general anesthesia, some animals of the larger breeds have a higher normal pressure. This may be augmented by some gas anesthetics, especially if the anesthesia is prolonged prior to the pressure determination. (Normal CSF pressure in horses may reach 400 mm H_2O; Table 3–1.) Some of the conditions that cause an elevated CSF pressure are: (1) Space-occupying lesions—neoplasm, abscess, hemorrhages, noncommunicating hypertensive hydrocephalus. These compress the venous sinuses and prevent CSF absorption from the arachnoid villi. (2) Cerebral edema usually associated with brain injury. (3) Communicating hydrocephalus (occasionally). (4) Meningitis and (5) Vitamin A deficiency (see obstructive hydrocephalus, p. 48).

Physical

Normal CSF is clear and colorless. A red tinge appears if hemorrhage occurs during the tap. This should disappear as further aliquots of CSF are withdrawn. Centrifugation should leave a clear fluid. If the discoloration persists, then there has been previous hemorrhage into the CSF.

Although various ratios have been proposed to account for the extra leucocytes and protein in the CSF contributed by iatrogenic hemorrhage, one study has shown these to be unreliable.[106] No leucocytes and little to no protein will accompany the many thousands of red blood cells from this hemorrhage. Therefore, mild CSF contamination with hemorrhage will not alter the leucocyte and protein evaluations. When this hemorrhage contributes erythrocytes in excess of 10,000 per cmm these values may be altered and it is preferable to repeat the procedure. The tap can be repeated in 24 hours to obtain a fresh sample. The erythrocytes will be removed from the CSF within 24 hours. Whole blood may be obtained from epidural veins without entering the subarachnoid space. Repeat the procedure with a clean needle until CSF is obtained.

Xanthochromic (yellow) CSF usually is caused by free bilirubin of previous subarachnoid hemorrhage. This begins to appear about 12 hours after a hemorrhage occurs. Extremely high CSF total protein (more than 400 mg per 100 cc) or severe prolonged systemic icterus may cause xanthochromia. Centrifugation does not remove this color.

Turbidity is caused by an increase in the cell count (WBC or RBC or both) greater than 500 per cmm.

Foam that persists on the surface of the sample is indicative of an elevated protein content.

Fibrin clots occur with increased protein levels when fibrinogen is present, as in suppurative meningitis or profuse hemorrhage.

TABLE 3–1.　TABLE OF NORMAL VALUES

Species	Pressure (mm H_2O)	Protein (mg/dl)	Cells/cmm
Dog	<170	<25	<5
Cat	<100	<20	<5
Ox	<200	<40	<5
Sheep	<270	<40	<5
Pig	<145	<40	<5
Horse	<400	<70	<5

This may be prevented by using an anticoagulant in the sampling tube.

Cytologic-Biochemical[15, 65, 98]

Table 3–2 provides guidelines that relate the physical, cytologic, and chemical determinations in CSF with diseases of the nervous system. There are many exceptions. The CSF study must be evaluated in relation to the patient's history and the physical and neurologic examinations. Specific examples are shown in Table 3–3.

The CSF protein may increase without a concomitant increase in cells. This is sometimes called an albuminocytologic dissociation, and occurs under the following circumstances:

1. Extensive noninflammatory degeneration of brain parenchyma with tissue necrosis.

2. Vascular lesions with hemorrhage, or transudation from diseased blood vessels, or both.

3. Neoplasms that produce protein, interfere with blood vessel integrity, or produce necrosis of the adjacent parenchyma.

4. Some instances of viral nonsuppurative encephalitis such as canine distemper or leukoencephalomyelitis of goats. In canine distemper it has been shown that the globulin fraction of protein is increased.[23, 59]

The enzymes aspartate aminotransferase (AST) and creatine kinase (CK) may increase in CSF when extensive myelin degeneration has occurred.[50, 100, 104, 107] Lactic dehydrogenase (LDH) is increased in lymphosarcoma that directly involves the nervous system parenchyma.

CK is an enzyme limited to cardiac and skeletal muscle and nervous tissue. Elevations in serum CK reflect muscle disease, whereas elevations in CK in CSF reflect nervous system disease. The concentration of CK in CSF is usually independent of that in serum. Iatrogenic hemorrhage from attempts to obtain CSF will cause an elevation of CK in CSF from that present in the blood serum. A variety of neurologic diseases will cause an increase in CK in CSF. Although this evaluation is of little help in the differential diagnosis of neurologic diseases, significantly elevated CK in CSF usually indicates a guarded to poor prognosis.

Microbiologic

The fungus *Cryptococcus neoformans* and related fungi are the only agents that can be identified consistently in CSF. India ink staining of CSF may enhance their visibility. Bacteria may be observed in white blood cells in suppurative meningitis. Such cells should be Gram stained. All fluid that is turbid or any clots should be Gram stained and cultured. All

---

TABLE 3–2. CSF DETERMINATIONS AND DISEASES OF THE NERVOUS SYSTEM

Determination	Disease	
	Meningitis Bacterial Disease (suppurative inflammation)	Parenchymal Disease Tissue Necrosis: Neoplasia, Degenerations Viral Disease (nonsuppurative inflammation)
Physical	turbid, clot	clear, colorless
Cytologic (WBC)[51]		
Quantitative	large increase greater than 100/cmm	small increase less than 100/cmm
differential	mostly neutrophils	mostly mononuclear cells
Chemical		
Protein		
quantitative (total)	large increase greater than 100 mg/dl	small increase less than 100 mg/dl
qualitative (globulins)		
Pándy (phenol)	plus 2–4	0 to plus 1
Nonne Apelt (NH_3SO_4)	plus 2–4	0 to plus 1
Glucose—normally about 80% of blood level	normal or decreased to below 50% of the blood level	normal

TABLE 3-3. CLINICAL EXAMPLES OF ABNORMAL CEREBROSPINAL FLUID

Disease Process		Pressure mm H$_2$O	RBC/cmm	WBC/cmm	Protein mg/dl	Other
Inflammation:						
Viral Inflammation:						
Canine distemper encephalitis	1.	120	23	19–66% mononuclear	49	
	2.	65	–	4 mononuclear	88	
	3.	–	26	4 mononuclear	45	
Equine rhinopneumonitis		–	326	11 mononuclear	278	
Feline infectious peritonitis,						
meningoencephalitis	1.	–	–	500 mononuclear	185	
	2.	–	–	66–84% mono-nuclear, 26% neutrophils	404	
	3.	–	410	1144 mononuclear	498	
Fungal Inflammation:						
Canine cryptococcal meningo-encephalomyelitis						
1. Xanthochromic						
Organisms in CSF		too viscid	–	1353–mostly neutrophils	501	glucose–21 mg per dl blood glu-cose–67 mg per dl
2. Organisms in CSF		364	76	498–92% eosinophils	187	
3. Organisms in CSF		–	4670 (trauma)	280 mononuclear	154	
Protozoal Inflammation:						
Canine toxoplasma encephalitis						
1. Cerebral granuloma		256	2	17 mononuclear, 8 neutrophils	94	
2. Diffuse encephalitis		–	16	18 mononuclear	103	
Equine protozoal myelitis (lumbosacral)		–	–	29 mononuclear	51	
Bacterial Inflammation:						
Suppurative (bacterial) meningoencephalitis–calf		168	–	188–66% neutrophils	110	
Coliform meningoencephalitis–calf		–	650	2800–69% neutrophils	143	
Listeriosis-(meningo)encephalitis–bovine	1.	–	–	31 mononuclear mostly	79	
	2.	–	–	7 mononuclear mostly	27	
	3.	–	105	29–90% mononuclear	81	
Parasitic Inflammation:						
Cuterebra encephalitis (cat)		–	–	258–mostly neutrophils	89	
Cuterebra encephalitis (dog)		–	10	280–84% neutrophils, 16% mononuclears	98	
		–	24	20–50% neutrophils, 6% eosinophils, 44% mononuclear	38	
Parelaphostrongylus tenuis encephalomyelitis (goat)	1.	–	3340	50–70% mononuclear, 30% neutrophils	63	
	2.	–	2440	650–3% mononuclear, 97% eosinophils	71	
	3.	–	5040	70–61% mononuclear, 34% eosinophils, 5% neutrophils	92	
Neoplasia–Inflammation:						
Canine primary reticulosis	.1.	–	–	58 mononuclear	90	
	2.	–	–	324 mononuclear	360	
Neoplasia						
Ependymoma		237	–	13 mononuclear	110	
Choroid plexus carcinoma (lumbosacral roots)		–	5	2 mononuclear	42	
Choroid plexus papilloma (fourth ventricle)		170	30	4 mononuclear	54	
Reticulosarcoma		245	2	1 mononuclear	19	
Astrocytoma		410	–	10 mononuclear	20	
Ependymoblastoma		185	8	3 mononuclear	214	
Prostatic adenocarcinoma		–	–	9 mononuclear	67	
Degeneration						
Polioencephalomalacia–goat,		210	50	8 mononuclear	52	
cow		220	3800	30 mononuclear	135	
Focal myelomalacia (infarct)–dog		–	187	4 mononuclear	57	

fluid with neutrophils, or with moderate elevations of WBC, or both, should be cultured.

HYDROCEPHALUS[6, 7, 43, 82, 85]

In the broad use of the term, hydrocephalus is an increase in the volume of CSF. Terms often used in reference to hydrocephalus are:

Internal—Ventricular dilation.

External—Dilation of subarachnoid space.

Communicating—Extraventricular obstruction or compensatory hydrocephalus.

Noncommunicating — Intraventricular obstruction preventing communication of the entire ventricular system with the cerebellomedullary cistern of the subarachnoid space.

Normotensive—Normal CSF pressure.

Hypertensive—Increased CSF pressure.

Two major categories of hydrocephalus are compensatory and obstructive.

Compensatory. CSF accumulates in space in the cranial cavity not occupied by brain parenchyma. Examples include malformation with hypoplasia of tissue, and destruction of tissue from degeneration associated with ischemia, inflammation, or injury. The bluetongue and Akabane viruses destroy developing cerebrocortical tissue, producing hydranencephaly and a massive accumulation of CSF. The bovine virus diarrhea virus destroys fetal cerebellar tissue, leaving cystic CSF-filled spaces. Thrombosis of the middle cerebral artery causes infarction of a large portion of the cerebrum. CSF accumulates and fills in the area of destroyed tissue. This is seen in ischemic encephalopathy in cats. The same occurs in severe polioencephalomalacia (cerebrocortical necrosis) in ruminants.

These are examples of normotensive communicating compensatory hydrocephalus.

Obstructive. Obstruction to flow or absorption of CSF causes ventricular dilation, especially of the lateral ventricles, with more loss of the white matter than grey matter. The cerebral cortex is relatively spared. The obstruction can be caused by a number of conditions. CSF pressure varies with the disease process.

1. Neoplasia may interfere directly with flow through the interventricular foramen, third ventricle, mesencephalic aqueduct, or lateral apertures. This produces a noncommunicating hypertensive hydrocephalus in the lateral ventricles. CSF pressure may be normal at the cerebellomedullary site. The degree of hydrocephalus is variable but often minimal.

2. Neoplasia may interfere indirectly with absorption through the arachnoid villi because of its compressive effect on the venous sinuses. CSF pressure is usually hypertensive at the cerebellomedullary cistern. The degree of hydrocephalus is usually minimal.

3. Inflammation of the ependyma of the mesencephalic aqueduct causes obstruction to flow and a noncommunicating hypertensive hydrocephalus of the third and lateral ventricles.[51-54]

Example: Experimental inoculation of neonatal hamsters or ferrets with human myxoviruses including mumps virus or the type 1 reovirus results in an acute ependymitis, which in the healing stage causes obstruction to CSF flow through the mesencephalic aqueduct, and subsequent noncommunicating hydrocephalus. The signs are observed 2 to 4 weeks after the inoculation. At necropsy there is a loss of ependyma or abnormalities of the ependyma, with partial or complete obstruction. The lesions of active inflammation have disappeared.

Experimental intracerebral inoculation of canine parainfluenza virus into gnotobiotic puppies produces encephalitis.[10] In puppies studied 1 to 6 months after inoculation, hydrocephalus was observed with dilated lateral and third ventricles. Subependymal and aqueductal lesions were observed in some of these puppies. The exact relationship between the viral encephalitis and the hydrocephalus remains to be determined.

Feline infectious peritonitis virus may cause a severe meningitis and ependymitis. The latter may occlude the aqueduct, producing hydrocephalus.[22, 86]

4. Inflammation of the meninges may interfere with flow through the lateral apertures, or with absorption through the arachnoid villi.[19, 42, 86]

An acquired hydrocephalus and associated periventricular encephalitis has been described in 6- to 8-week-old dogs with rapidly progressing clinical signs.[46] The presence of a periventricular, choroidal, and meningeal inflammation with fibrinous exudate and neutrophilic and mononuclear cell infiltrate strongly suggested a primary bacterial infection.

5. Malformation of the mesencephalic aqueduct produces a noncommunicating obstructive hydrocephalus.[8, 52-55, 62, 93] A failure of a continuous aqueduct to develop causes permanent obstruction to flow and a noncommunicating, obstructive hypertensive hydrocephalus with severe dilation of the third and lateral ventricles. This may be accompanied by a massive expansion of the cranial cavity and large nonossified portions of the calvaria. In

puppies it is common to have hydrocephalus with widely dilated lateral ventricles that is normotensive at the lateral ventricle and cerebellomedullary cistern. The cranial cavity may be normal or expanded. Clinical signs are often static. At necropsy no obstruction to flow can be found. It is hypothesized that this condition may result if during a critical period in fetal development the aqueduct is inadequate to accommodate the total flow of CSF produced in the third and lateral ventricles. A partial but critical obstruction occurs, and the lateral ventricles expand at the expense of the extremely delicate fetal cerebral tissue. With growth the aqueduct expands to accommodate the CSF produced rostral to it, and pressures are normalized. However, the damage has been done, and the expanded lateral ventricles covered by attenuated cerebral cortex persist. This hypothesis remains to be proved.

6. Malformation of the arachnoid villi in number or structure or both produces a communicating hydrocephalus. This also may be the critical defect in some dogs that are seen with hydrocephalus early in life. There is a critical point above which CSF pressure will not induce an increase in absorption owing to the lack of function of the absorptive mechanism. There are no more valves to open. This critical point may be within the normal range of physiologic CSF pressures. A functional obstruction exists and the ventricles dilate. The ventricular and cisternal pressures generally are normal. This hypothesis also has not been substantiated.

These two hypothesized mechanisms—inadequate aqueductal flow during a critical period of development, and arachnoid villi malformation—may account for the so-called congenital or constitutional hydrocephalus common among small breeds of dogs with large skulls (Chihuahua, Yorkshire terrier, Manchester terrier, toy poodle) and among the brachiocephalic breeds (Boston terrier, Pekingese, English bulldog).

A syndrome of late-onset hydrocephalus that is referred to as occult or normal pressure hydrocephalus occurs in humans.[19, 39, 61] It is a progressive disorder despite the lack of CSF hypertension, and is related to inadequate CSF circulation to the cerebral arachnoid villi for absorption. It is readily treated by surgical shunting procedures. Most hydrocephalic puppies with or without progressive signs have normal CSF cisternal and ventricular pressures. The pathogenesis of these two diseases may be related.

Under all of the preceding circumstances CSF production usually continues at a constant rate regardless of the intraventricular CSF pressure. CSF flow volume may be constant regardless of the CSF pressure. Production decreases only when the choroid plexus becomes altered by the hypertension. Intraventricular pressure is not constant but varies continuously.

Numerous studies have been done on the pathophysiology of hydrocephalus.[61, 74, 80-82, 91] Light and electron-microscopic studies of the cerebrum adjacent to the lateral ventricle indicate that during the hypertensive phase CSF may pass into the parenchyma.[101] There is also evidence that CSF absorption may occur through the choroid plexus.[69]

7. Vitamin A deficiency interferes with the absorption of CSF at the arachnoid villi. CSF pressure elevates but ventricular dilation is not common. Experimentally the level of vitamin A deficiency can be correlated with the increase in CSF pressure caused by this absorptive obstruction. This is mostly a clinical problem in young beef cattle (6 to 8 months) kept for a number of months on dry, vitamin A-deficient pastures.[14, 70] This results in seizures. Their CSF pressure is elevated and their plasma vitamin A levels are abnormally low. This condition can be corrected with vitamin A therapy.[14]

CLINICAL SIGNS

Clinical signs are variable.[4, 27, 82] They are mostly referable to disturbance of the cerebral hemispheres. No signs may be seen in the presence of considerable ventricular dilatation. The following signs should be looked for.

1. Disturbed consciousness, with lethargy to severe depression (obtundation), tendency to sleep, hypoactivity, propulsive circling, head pressing, convulsions, changes in behavior, dementia.

2. Motor signs include a spastic paresis, especially if the brain stem is involved. With severe cerebral disturbance the gait may be normal if the brain stem is normal. Hypermetric ataxia occurs if the cerebellum is involved. An abnormal position of the eyeballs—strabismus—with a ventral and lateral deviation may occur from pressure on the oculomotor nerve or from a malformation of the orbit owing to changes in the shape of the skull bones.

The strabismus in most of these patients is thought to be due to the orbital malformation because both eyeballs will abduct and adduct on moving the head from side to side and there is no pupillary dilation, which also would be expected with oculomotor nerve compression.

3. Sensory signs include ataxia and blindness. A bilateral visual deficit with normal pupillary response is the most common and consistent clinical sign observed in these patients. This reflects the attenuation of the cerebral white matter (optic radiation) and visual cortex. A mild, general proprioceptive ataxia occasionally occurs if the brain stem is involved. Postural reactions are consistently slow when there is disturbance of the sensorimotor portion of the cerebrum.

4. Abnormal shape of the skull, with an enlarged calvaria with open sutures (fontanelles).

The attenuated cerebral tissue is apparently quite susceptible to injury. Occasionally exacerbation of clinical signs has been associated with hemorrhage into the ventricular CSF and tearing of sheets of white matter from the wall of the lateral ventricle.

Hydromyelia and/or syringomyelia commonly accompany the dilated ventricles in congenital obstructive hydrocephalus but rarely produce clinical signs.

A 3-month-old Great Pyrenees was examined for a progressive gait abnormality that mostly reflected a cervical spinal cord lesion. In addition there were signs of bilateral cerebral and cerebellar abnormality. Contrast ventriculography revealed widely dilated lateral and fourth ventricles. The failure of dye to enter the subarachnoid space from the fourth ventricle indicated a failure of the lateral apertures to form. At autopsy this ventricular dilation was confirmed. In addition there was extensive cavitation of the dorsal funiculi from C2 to C8. The syrinx did not obviously communicate with the central canal in the sections studied. The spinal cord was enlarged and the parenchyma was compressed adjacent to the syrinx. A cervical vertebral scoliosis developed as the neurologic signs progressed. Similar spinal cord lesions have been observed in experimental noncommunicating hypertensive hydrocephalus with inflammatory obstruction of the lateral apertures and arachnoid villi. It is hypothesized that the spinal lesions are a reflection of the increased pressure from the ventricles to the central canal.[44, 45, 102, 103]

ANCILLARY EXAMINATION

Radiography. Plain radiographs may show a diffuse homogeneous "ground glass" opacity of the cranial cavity from the fluid contents. The gyral pattern of the calvaria may be absent and open sutures may be apparent.

Pneumoventriculography. This is performed best by direct injection of air into the lateral ventricle, as described under the uses of CSF. Air injected into the cerebellomedullary cistern may pass through the lateral apertures into the ventricular system, but this procedure is not dependable. Contrast ventriculography by direct injection of meglumine iothalamate (Conray) or metrizamide determines the degree of ventricular dilation and the integrity of the aqueduct and lateral apertures.

Electroencephalography. The EEG pattern in hydrocephalus is usually consistent and characteristic. In all leads there is a diffuse slowing of the normal pattern with a remarkable increase in amplitude.[18, 27, 56, 78]

TREATMENT

The treatment for hydrocephalus depends on the cause.[4] In cases of obstructive hydrocephalus a direct lateral ventricular tap may confirm the diagnosis and provide temporary relief from some of the signs.[83]

Medical therapy with corticosteroids (1 to 2 mg per lb of dexamethasone or Azium) may provide temporary relief in patients with exacerbated or progressive clinical signs. Lower doses of steroids may be effective (0.25 to 1 mg per day for several or on alternate days). Corticosteroids will decrease the production of CSF.

Surgical therapy for more permanent relief involves a procedure for draining the fluid from the lateral ventricle.[33, 37, 38] Most shunt this fluid into the vascular system such as the jugular vein or right atrium (the ventriculoatrial shunt). Others shunt the CSF into the peritoneal cavity. A one-way valve is installed so that only CSF can flow out of the ventricle.

REFERENCES

1. Adams, R. D., Fisher, C. M., Hakim, S., Ojemann, R. G., and Sweet, W. H.: Symptomatic occult hydrocephalus with "normal" cerebrospinal fluid pressure: A treatable disease. N. Engl. J. Med., *273*:117, 1965.
2. Andres, K. H.: Zur Feinstruktur der Arachnoidalzotten bei Mammalia. Z. Zellforsch. Mikrosk. Anat., *82*:92, 1967.
3. Averill, D. A., Jr.: Examination of the cerebrospinal fluid. *In* Kirk, R. W. (ed.): Current Veterinary Therapy V: Small Animal Practice. Philadelphia, W. B. Saunders Co., 1974.

4. Averill, D. R., Jr.: Diagnosis and treatment of hydrocephalus in the dog. *In* Proceedings of the Kal Kan Symposium 1978.

5. Bailey, C. S.: Lumbar puncture for collection of CSF. *In* Proceedings of the 40th Annual Meeting of the American Animal Hospital Association, 1973.

6. Baker, M. L., Payne, C. A., and Baker, G. N.: The inheritance of hydrocephalus in cattle. J. Hered., *52*:135, 1961.

7. Banks, W. C., and Monlux, W. S.: Canine hydrocephalus. J. Am. Vet. Med. Assoc., *121*:453, 1952.

8. Barlow, R. M., and Donald, L. G.: Hydrocephalus in calves associated with unusual lesions in the mesencephalon. J. Comp. Pathol., *73*:410, 1963.

9. Bartels, J. E., Braund, K., and Redding, R. W.: An experimental evaluation of a non-ionic agent Amipaque (metrizamide) as a neuroradiologic medium in the dog. J. Am. Vet. Radiol. Soc., *4*:117, 1977.

10. Baumgärtner, W. K., Krakowka, S., Koestner, A., and Evermann, J.: Acute encephalitis and hydrocephalus in dogs caused by canine parainfluenza virus. Vet. Pathol., *19*:1979, 1982.

11. Beech, J.: Metrizamide myelography in .horses. J. Am. Vet. Radiol. Soc., *20*:22, 1979.

12. Benson, D. F., LeMay, M., Patten, D. H., and Rubens, A. B.: Diagnosis of normal-pressure hydrocephalus. N. Engl. J. Med., *283*:609, 1970.

13. Bering, E. A., Jr., and Sato, O.: Hydrocephalus: Changes in formation and absorption of cerebrospinal fluid within the cerebral ventricles. J. Neurosurg., *20*:1050, 1963.

14. Blood, D. C., Henderson, J. A., and Radostits, O. M.: Veterinary Medicine. 5th ed. Philadelphia, Lea and Febiger, 1979.

15. Bosch, I., and Oehmichen, M.: Eosinophilic granulocytes in cerebrospinal fluid: Analysis of 94 cerebrospinal fluid specimens and review of the literature. J. Neurol., *219*:93, 1978.

16. Bowster, D.: Cerebrospinal Fluid Dynamics in Health and Disease. Springfield, Ill., Charles C Thomas, 1960.

17. Brass, W., and Horzinek, I.: Klinik und Elektronenencephalogramm des Hydrocephalus internus beim Hund. Deutsch Tiererztl. Wochenschr., *78*:42, 1971.

18. Bullock, L. P., and Zook, B. C.: Myelography in dogs using water-soluble contrast mediums. J. Am. Vet. Med. Assoc., *151*:321, 1967.

19. Cammermeyer, J.: The frequency of meningoencephalitis and hydrocephalus in dogs. J. Neuropathol. Exp. Neurol., *20*:386, 1961.

20. Coles, E. H.: Cerebrospinal fluid. *In* Kaneko, J. J., and Cornelius, C. E. (eds.): Clinical Biochemistry of Domestic Animals. 2nd ed., vol. II. New York, Academic Press, 1970.

21. Cserr, H. F.: Physiology of the choroid plexus. Physiol. Rev., *51*:273, 1971.

22. Csiza, C. K., Scott, F. W., de Lahunta, A., and Gillespie, J. H.: Feline viruses. XIV. Transplacental infections in spontaneous panleukopenia of cats. Cornell Vet., *61*:423, 1971.

23. Cutler, R. W. P., and Averill, D. R., Jr.: Cerebrospinal fluid gamma globulins in canine distemper encephalitis. Neurology, *19*:1111, 1969.

24. Davis, E. M., Glickman, L., Rendano, V. T., Quick, C. B., and Short, C. E.: Seizures in dogs following metrizamide myelography. J. Am. Anim. Hosp. Assoc., *17*:642, 1981.

25. Davson, H.: Physiology of the Cerebrospinal Fluid. London, J. & A. Churchill, 1967.

26. deLahunta, A.: Examination of the cerebrospinal fluid. *In* Kirk, R. W., (ed.): Current Veterinary Therapy III. Philadelphia, W. B. Saunders Co., 1970.

27. de Lahunta, A., and Cummings, J. F.: The clinical and electroencephalographic features of hydrocephalus in three dogs. J. Am. Vet. Med. Assoc., *146*:954, 1965.

28. Di Chiro, G., Hammock, M. K., and Bleyer, W. A.: Spinal descent of cerebrospinal fluid in man. Neurology, *26*:1, 1976.

29. DiChiro, G., Stein, S. C., and Harrington, T.: Spontaneous cerebrospinal fluid rhinorrhea in normal dogs. Radioisotope studies of an alternate pathway of CSF drainage. J. Neuropathol. Exp. Neurol., *31*:447, 1972.

30. Donner, F. R.: Basic physiology of cerebrospinal fluid outflow. Exp. Eye Res. [Suppl.]:323, 1977.

31. Fankhauser, R.: The cerebrospinal fluid. *In* Innes, J. R. M., and Saunders, L. S. (eds.): Comparative Neuropathology. New York, Academic Press, 1962.

32. Fedotov, A. I.: Cerebrospinal fluid of domestic animals. Russian Scientific Translation Program, Division of General Medical Services. National Institute of Health, Washington, D.C., U.S. Department of Health, Education, and Welfare, 1960.

33. Few, A. B.: The diagnosis and surgical treatment of canine hydrocephalus. J. Am. Vet. Med. Assoc., *149*:286, 1966.

34. Fishman, R. A.: Brain edema. N. Engl. J. Med., *293*:706, 1975.

35. Fitzgerald, T. C.: Anatomy of cerebral ventricles of domestic animals. Vet. Med., *56*:38, 1961.

36. Funkquist, B.: Myelographic localization of spinal cord compression in dogs: A comparison between cisternal and lumbar injections of metrizamide "Amipaque" in diagnosing and locating spinal cord compression. Acta Vet. Scand., *10*:269, 1975.

37. Gage, E. D.: Surgical treatment of canine hydrocephalus. J. Am. Vet. Med. Assoc., *157*:1729, 1970.

38. Gage, E. D., and Hoerlein, B. F.: Surgical treatment of canine hydrocephalus by ventriculo-atrial shunting. J. Am. Vet. Med. Assoc., *153*:1418, 1968.

39. Geschwind, N.: The mechanism of normal pressure hydrocephalus. J. Neurol. Sci., *7*:481, 1968.

40. Gomez, D. G., and Potts, D. G.: The choroid plexus of the dog. Anat. Rec., *181*:363, 1975.

41. Gomez, D. G., Potts, D. G., and Deonarine, V.: Arachnoid granulations of the sheep. Arch. Neurol., *30*:169, 1974.

42. Greene, H. J., Leipold, H. W., and Vestwebor, J. E.: Experimentally induced hydrocephalus in calves. Am. J. Vet. Res., *35*:945, 1974.

43. Greene, H. J., Leipold, H. W., and Hobbs, C. M.: Bovine congenital defects: Variations of internal hydrocephalus. Cornell Vet., *64*:596, 1974.

44. Hall, P. V., Kalsbeck, J. E., Wellman, H. N., Campbell, R. L., and Lewis, S.: Radioisotope evaluation of experimental hydrosyringomyelia. J. Neurosurg., *45*:181, 1976.

45. Hall, P., Turner, M., Aichinger, S., Bendick, P., and Campbell, R.: Experimental syringomyelia: The relationship between intraventricular and intrasyrinx pressures. J. Neurosurg., *52*:812, 1980.

46. Higgins, R. J., Vandevelde, M., and Braund, K. G.: Internal hydrocephalus and associated periventricular encephalitis in young dogs. Vet. Pathol., *14*:236, 1977.

47. Hoerlein, B. F., and Petty, M. F.: Contrast encephalography and ventriculography in the dog—preliminary studies. Am. J. Vet. Res., *22*:1041, 1961.

48. Hooshmand, H., Dove, J., Houff, S., and Suter, C.: Effects of diuretics and steroids on CSF pressure. Arch. Neurol., *21*:499, 1969.

49. Iida, T.: Elektronenmikroskopiche Untersuchungen am Oberflächlichen Anteil des Gehirns bei Hund und Katze. Arch. Histol. Jpn., *27*:267, 1966.

50. Indrieri, R. J., Holliday, T. A., and Keen, C. L.: Critical evaluation of creatine phosphokinase in cerebrospinal fluid of dogs with neurologic disease. Am. J. Vet. Res., *41*:1299, 1980.

51. Johnson, R. T.: Hydrocephalus and viral infections. Review article. Dev. Med. Child Neurol., *17*:807, 1975.

52. Johnson, R. T., and Johnson, K. P.: Hydrocephalus as a sequela of experimental myxovirus infections. Exp. Mol. Pathol., *10*:68, 1969.

53. Johnson, R. T., and Johnson, K. P.: Hydrocephalus following viral infection: The pathology of aqueductal stenosis developing after experimental mumps virus infection. J. Neuropathol. Exp. Neurol., *27*:591, 1968.

54. Johnson, R. T., Johnson, K. P., and Edmonds, C. J.: Virus-induced hydrocephalus: Development of aqueductal stenosis in hamsters after mumps infection. Science, *157*:1066, 1967.

55. Kilham, L., and Margolis, G.: Hydrocephalus in hamsters, ferrets, rats and mice following inoculations with reovirus type I. I. Virologic studies. Lab. Invest., *21*:183, 1969.

56. Klemm, W. R., and Hall, C. L.: Electroencephalograms on anesthetized dogs with hydrocephalus. Am. J. Vet. Res., *32*:1859, 1971.

57. Kornegay, J. N.: Cerebrospinal fluid collection, examination, and interpretation in dogs and cats. Compend. Contin. Ed., *3*:85, 1981.

58. Lewis, A. J.: Mechanisms of Neurologic Disease. Boston, Little, Brown Co., 1976.

59. Long, J. F., Jacoby, R. O., Olson, M., and Koestner, A.: Beta-glucuronidase activity and levels of protein and protein fractions in serum and cerebrospinal fluid of dogs with distemper-associated demyelinating encephalopathy. Acta Neuropathol. (Berlin), *25*:179, 1973.

60. Lord, P. F., and Olsson, S-E.: Myelography with metrizamide in the dog: A clinical study on its use for the demonstration of spinal cord lesions other than those caused by intervertebral disk protrusions. J. Am. Vet. Radiol. Soc., *17*:42, 1976.

61. Lorenzo, A. V., Page, L. K., and Watters, G. V.: Relationship between cerebrospinal fluid formation, absorption, and pressure in human hydrocephalus. Brain, *93*:679, 1970.

62. Margolis, G., and Kilham, L.: Hydrocephalus in hamsters, ferrets, rats, and mice following inoculations with reovirus type I. II. Pathologic studies. Lab. Invest., *21*:189, 1969.

63. Mayhew, I. G.: Collection of cerebrospinal fluid from the horse. Cornell Vet., *65*:500, 1975.

64. Mayhew, I. G.: Cerebrospinal fluid collection from the horse. Equine Pract., *1*:45, 1979.

65. Mayhew, I. G., and Beal, C. R.: Technique of analyses of cerebrospinal fluid. Vet. Clin. North Am., *10*:155, 1980.

66. Mayhew, I. G., Whitlock, R. H., and Tasker, J. B.: Equine cerebrospinal fluid: Reference values of normal horses. Am. J. Vet. Res., *38*:1271, 1977.

67. Milhorat, T. H.: The choroid plexus and cerebrospinal fluid production. Science, *166*:1514, 1969.

68. Milhorat, T. H., Hammock, M. K., Fenstermacher, J. D., Rall, D. F., and Levin, V. A.: Cerebrospinal fluid production by the choroid plexus and brain. Science, *173*:330, 1971.

69. Milhorat, T. H., Mosher, M. B., Hammock, M. K., and Murphy, C. F.: Evidence for choroid plexus absorption in hydrocephalus. N. Engl. J. Med., *283*:286, 1970.

70. Mills, J. H. L., Nielsen, S. W., Rousseau, J. E., Woelfel, C. G., and Eaton, H. D.: Experimental pathology of dairy calves ingesting one-third the daily requirement of carotene. Acta Vet. Scand., *8*:324, 1967.

71. Morgan, J. P., Suter, P. F., and Holliday, T. A.: Myelography with water-soluble contrast medium radiographic interpretation of disc herniation in dogs. Acta Radiol. [Suppl.] *319*:217, 1971.

72. Nyland, T. G., Blythe, L. L., Pool, R. R., Helphrey, M. G., and O'Brien, T. R.: Metrizamide myelography in the horse: Clinical, radiographic, and pathologic changes. Am. J. Vet. Res., *41*:204, 1980.

73. Oldendorf, W. H.: The blood-brain barrier. Exp. Eye Res. [Suppl.]: 177, 1977.

74. Oppelt, W., Patlack, C., and Rall, D.: Effect of certain drugs on cerebrospinal fluid production in the dog. Am. J. Physiol., *206*:247, 1964.

75. Parker, A. J.: The diagnostic uses of cerebrospinal fluid. J. Small Anim. Pract., *13*:607, 1972.

76. Pollay, M., and Welch, K.: The function and structure of the canine arachnoid villi. J. Surg. Res., *2*:307, 1962.

77. Potts, D. G., and Deonarine, V.: Effect of positional changes and jugular vein compression on the pressure gradient across the arachnoid villi and granulations of the dog. J. Neurosurg., *38*:722, 1973.

78. Prynn, R. B., and Redding, R. W.: Electroencephalogram in occult canine hydrocephalus. J. Am. Vet. Med. Assoc., *152*:1651, 1968.

79. Roszel, J. F.: Membrane filtration of canine and feline cerebrospinal fluid for cytologic evaluation. J. Am. Vet. Med. Assoc., *160*:720, 1972.

80. Russell, D. S.: Observations on the pathology of hydrocephalus. London, England, Medical Research Council Report No. 265, 1949.

81. Sahar, A., Hochwald, G. M., and Ransohoff, J.: Experimental hydrocephalus: Cerebrospinal fluid formation and ventricular size as a function of intraventricular pressure. J. Neurol. Sci., *11*:81, 1970.

82. Sahar, A., Hochwald, G. M., Kay, W. J., and Ransohoff, J.: Spontaneous canine hydrocephalus: Cerebrospinal fluid dynamics. J. Neurol. Neurosurg. Psychiatry, *34*:308, 1971.

83. Savell, C. M.: Cerebral ventricular tap: An aid to diagnosis and treatment of hydrocephalus in the dog. Am. Anim. Assoc. Proc., 532, 1974.

84. Segal, M. B., and Pollay, M.: The secretion of cerebrospinal fluid. Exp. Eye Res. [Suppl.]:127, 1977.

85. Selby, L. A., Hayes, H. M., and Becker, S. V.:

Epizootologic features of canine hydrocephalus. Am. J. Vet. Res., *40*:411, 1979.

86. Slauson, D. O., and Finn, J. P.: Meningoencephalitis and panophthalmitis in feline infectious peritonitis. J. Am. Vet. Med. Assoc., *160*:729, 1972.

87. Slesingr, L., and Hrazdira, C. L.: Untersuchungen der Zerebrospinalflüsigkeit von Hunden und Pferden. Zentralbl. Veterinaer Med., *17*:338, 1970.

88. Smith, M. C.: The diagnostic value of caprine cerebrospinal fluid analysis. *In* International Goat and Sheep Research, (in press).

89. Steinberg, S.: Cerebrospinal fluid. *In* Medway, W., Prier, J. E., and Wilkinson, J. S. (eds.): Textbook of Veterinary Clinical Pathology. Baltimore, Williams & Wilkins, 1969.

90. Stowater, J. L., and Kneller, S. K.: Clinical evaluation of metrizamide as a myelographic agent in the dog. J. Am. Vet. Med. Assoc., *175*:191, 1979.

91. Strecker, E. P., Bush, M., and James, A. E., Jr.: Cerebrospinal fluid imaging as a method to evaluate communicating hydrocephalus in dogs. Am. J. Vet. Res., *34*:101, 1973.

92. Suter, P. F., Morgan, J. P., Holliday, T. A., and O'Brien, T. R.: Myelography in the dog: Diagnosis of tumors of the spinal cord and vertebrae. J. Am. Radiol. Soc., *12*:29, 1971.

93. Timmonds, G. D., and Johnson, K. D.: Aqueductal stenosis and hydrocephalus after mumps encephalitis. N. Engl. J. Med., *283*:1505, 1970.

94. Tripathi, R. C.: The functional morphology of the outflow systems of ocular and cerebrospinal fluids. Exp. Eye Res. [Suppl.]:65, 1977.

95. Tripathi, B. J., and Tripathi, R. C.: Vascular transcellular channels as the drainage pathway of cerebrospinal fluid. J. Physiol. (London), *239*:195, 1973.

96. Tripathi, R.: Tracing the bulk outflow of cerebrospinal fluid by transmission and scanning electron microscopy. Brain Res., *80*:503, 1974.

97. Urman, H. K., and Grace, O. D.: Hereditary encephalomyopathy. A hydrocephalus syndrome in newborn calves. Cornell Vet., *54*:229, 1964.

98. Vandevelde, M and Spano, J. S.: Cerebrospinal fluid cytology in canine neurologic disease. Am. J. Vet. Res., *38*:1827, 1977.

99. Vermeulen, H. A.: Über den Conus Medullaris der Haustiere sein besonders verhalten beim Pferd und desen Bedeutung, Berl. Munch. Tierarztl. Wochenschr., *2*:13, 1916.

100. Wakim, K. G., and Fleisher, G. A.: The effect of experimental cerebral infarction on transaminase activity in serum, cerebrospinal fluid and infarcted tissue. Mayo Clin. Proc., *31*:391, 1956.

101. Weller, R. O., Wisniewski, H., Shulman, K., and Terry, R. D.: Experimental hydrocephalus in young dogs. Histological and ultrastructural study of the brain tissue damage. J. Neuropathol. Exp. Neurol., *30*:613, 1971.

102. Williams, B.: Experimental communicating syringomyelia in dogs after cisternal kaolin injection. Part 2: Pressure studies. J. Neurol. Sci., *48*:109, 1980.

103. Williams, B., and Bentley, J.; Experimental communicating syringomyelia in dogs after cisternal kaolin injection. Part 1: Morphology. J. Neurol. Sci., *48*:93, 1980.

104. Wilson, J. W.: Clinical application of cerebrospinal fluid creatine phosphokinase determination. J. Am. Vet. Med. Assoc., *171*:200, 1977.

105. Wilson, J. W., Bahr, R. J., Leipold, H. W., and Guffy, M. M.: Acute leptomeningeal reaction to subarachnoid injection of ethyl iodophenylundecylate in dogs. J. Am. Vet. Med. Assoc., *169*:415, 1975.

106. Wilson, J. W., and Stevens, J. B.: Effects of blood contamination on cerebrospinal fluid analysis. J. Am. Vet. Med. Assoc., *171*:256, 1977.

107. Wilson, J. W., and Wilterout, S. K.: Cerebrospinal fluid creatine phosphokinase in the normal dog. Am. J. Vet. Res., *37*:1099, 1976.

108. Wright, J. A.: Evaluation of cerebrospinal fluid in the dog. Vet. Rec., *103*:48, 1978.

109. Wolstenholme, G. E. W., and O'Connor, C. M. (eds.): The Cerebrospinal Fluid. Boston, CIBA Symposium, Little Brown Co., 1958.

110. Woolam, D. H. M., and Miller, J. W.: The perivascular spaces of the mammalian central nervous system and their relation to the perineuronal and subarachnoid spaces. J. Anat., *89*:193, 1955.

111. Yaghmai, J., Deonarine, V., Deck, M. D. F., and Potts, D. G.: Air ventriculography in the dog brain, utilizing tomography. Am. J. Vet. Res., *32*:319, 1971.

LOWER MOTOR NEURON— GENERAL SOMATIC EFFERENT SYSTEM

LOWER MOTOR NEURON

This is the efferent neuron of the peripheral nervous system that connects the central nervous system with the muscle to be innervated. The entire function of the central nervous system is manifested through the lower motor neuron. The lower motor neuron system (LMN) includes three components: the general somatic efferent system (GSE), the general visceral efferent system (GVE), and the special visceral efferent system (SVE).

GENERAL SOMATIC EFFERENT SYSTEM (GSE)

This system of the lower motor neuron includes neurons that innervate striated voluntary skeletal muscle derived from somites, somatic mesoderm of body wall (limb buds), and head myotomes. These neurons are located in all the spinal nerves and cranial nerves III, IV, VI, and XII.

SPINAL NERVE DIVISION

The cell bodies are located in the ventral grey column throughout the entire spinal cord. The shape and size of the ventral grey column reflect the number of neurons present. The ventral grey column is topographically organized.[3] The GSE neurons innervating the axial musculature populate the medial portion of the column. The GSE neurons that innervate the appendicular musculature are located laterally and cause the lateral bulge of the ventral grey column that is evident at the cervical and lumbosacral intumescences (Fig. 4–1). These lateral portions of the ventral grey column can be subdivided further into motonuclear columns representative of muscle groups, or the peripheral nerves present in the limbs. Neurons that innervate proximal limb muscles are located in the ventral portion of the lateral part of the ventral grey column. Those to the distal limb muscles are in the dorsal portion. These motonuclear columns have been identified by sectioning peripheral nerves or ablating specific muscles, and then observing in the spinal cord ventral grey column the retrograde chromatolysis of the cell bodies whose axons were destroyed by the experimental procedure. (horseradish peroxidase)

The dendritic zone of the multipolar general somatic efferent neuron is confined to the grey matter of the spinal cord. The axon courses through the white matter between lateral and ventral funiculi to leave the spinal cord as part of a ventral rootlet. It continues in a ventral root, through the spinal nerve, and into the limbs as part of a specific peripheral nerve, which is distributed to a specific group of muscles (Fig. 4–2).

At the level of the muscle cells each axon

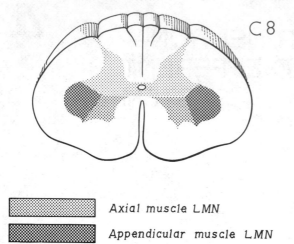

Axial muscle LMN

Appendicular muscle LMN

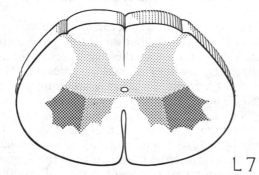

Figure 4–1. Spinal cord topography depicted at the cervical (C8) and lumbar (L7) intumescences.

of a general somatic efferent neuron divides into several branches. Each of these axonal branches ends on a muscle cell at a motor endplate. Each muscle cell is usually only innervated by the axon of one neuron. In the fetus and newborn, more than one neuron may innervate the motor end-plate of a muscle cell, but during early postnatal development this polyneuronal innervation is reduced to a single neuron.[115, 154] The number of muscle cells innervated by one motoneuron is called the motor unit. It varies from 100 to 150 cells in the proximal appendicular muscles to 3 to 4 cells in extraocular muscles. Muscles involved in functions that require a large degree of coordination are innervated by motoneurons with small motor units (only a few muscle cells per neuron). The strength of a muscle contraction depends on the number of motor units activated in a muscle.

At the motor end-plate the myelin is lost and the axon terminates in several small branches that form a cluster in a localized area

near the longitudinal center of the muscle cell. Each of these branches terminates on a specialized modification of the sarcolemma. This terminal is called the neuromuscular ending, junction, or synapse (Fig. 4–3).

The neuromuscular junction consists of a distended axonal terminal covered by a Schwann cell (lemmocyte) that has not formed myelin up to the point at which the axon extends into a sarcoplasmic trough on the surface of the muscle cell. The endoneurium of the neuron and the endomysium of the muscle cell are continuous outside the trough. Inside the trough the axolemma and sarcolemma are juxtaposed. The axon terminal contains numerous mitochondria and synaptic vesicles that are presumed to be the source of the neurotransmitter substance, acetylcholine.

The sarcoplasmic trough is located on an area of the muscle cell at which the sarcoplasm has accumulated. This is called the sole plate, and abounds with muscle-cell nuclei and mitochondria. The sarcoplasmic trough is extended further by invaginations of the sarcoplasm to form postsynaptic membrane folds (subneural clefts). The synaptic cleft between the presynaptic membrane (axolemma) and postsynaptic membrane (sarcolemma) is about 200Å.

Portions of the muscle cell membrane at the tops of these folds in the sarcoplasmic trough comprise the muscle receptor sites which will bind the acetylcholine released from the axon terminal. This muscle receptor is a glycoprotein consisting of polypeptide subunits. Acetylcholine is released from the axon terminal in packets (quanta) upon the stimulus of depolarization of the neuron. Calcium is important in this release process. This binding of acetylcholine and its receptor results in depolarization of the entire muscle cell membrane. Acetylcholinesterase is located in the depths of the folds and acts to degrade the acetylcholine molecule.

SPINAL CORD SEGMENTS—
VERTEBRAL COLUMN

For clinical purposes it is important to know in which segments of the spinal cord the cell bodies of general somatic efferent motor neurons are found whose axons are in specific peripheral nerves.

In the dog the spinal cord is composed of about 36 segments: 8 cervical, 13 thoracic, 7 lumbar, 3 sacral, and usually 5 caudal. Each

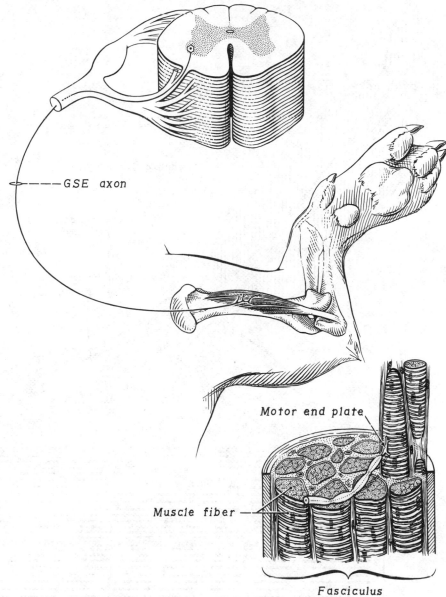

GSE axon

Motor end plate

Muscle fiber

Fasciculus

Figure 4–2.   Lower motor neuron–GSE innervation of the medial head of the triceps brachii.

segment has a number of dorsal and ventral rootlets that arise from the dorsolateral and ventrolateral aspects of each of its sides. They join to form a dorsal and ventral root on each side. The segmental spinal ganglion is found in the dorsal root at the level of the intervertebral foramen. Just beyond this, the dorsal and ventral roots join and intermix to form the spinal nerve. Thus, each spinal cord segment is connected to the tissues of the body by a spinal nerve on each side.

The development of the spinal cord segments and the vertebral column in the embryo are closely related events, which accounts for the manner in which the roots of each spinal cord segment are distributed between the vertebrae. The roots of the first cervical spinal cord segment leave the canal through the lateral vertebral foramina in the arch of the atlas. The roots of the second to the seventh cervical segments leave the canal through the intervertebral foramina cranial to the vertebrae of the same number. The roots of the eighth cervical segment exit cranial to the first thoracic vertebra. All the remaining roots leave the canal through the intervertebral foramina

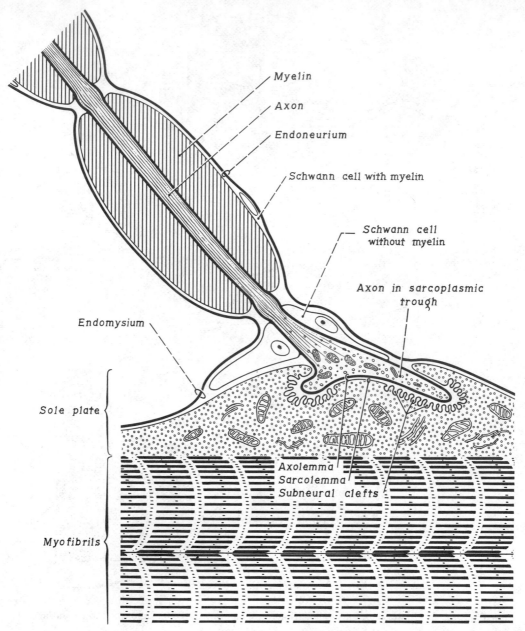

Myelin

Axon

Endoneurium

Schwann cell with myelin

Schwann cell without myelin

Axon in sarcoplasmic trough

Endomysium

Sole plate

Axolemma
Sarcolemma
Subneural clefts

Myofibrils

Figure 4–3. Neuromuscular junction of a motor end-plate.

caudal to the vertebrae of the same number. Because of the greater growth in length of the vertebral column the relationship of the spinal cord segments and vertebrae is somewhat altered. In the dog only the first and occasionally second cervical spinal cord segments, and the last two thoracic and first two or three lumbar segments lie in the vertebral column within the vertebrae of the same number, but all the remaining segments reside in the canal cranial to the vertebrae of the same number (Figs. 4–4, 4–5).

The more cranial the location of a spinal cord segment is from its corresponding vertebra, the longer the roots are to reach the appropriate intervertebral foramina. This is particularly evident in the lumbosacral region of the spinal cord of the dog, in which the last three lumbar segments reside approximately over the fourth lumbar vertebral body and the three sacral segments are within the fifth lumbar vertebra. The spinal cord usually ends within the cranial half of the seventh lumbar vertebra. In small breeds of dogs these rela-

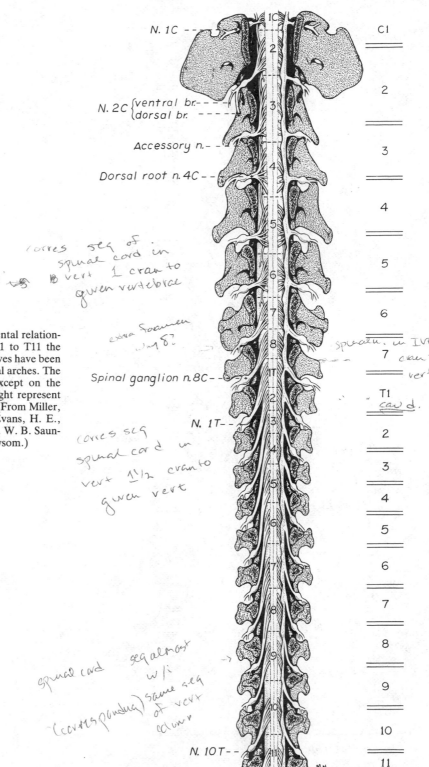

Figure 4–4. Spinal cord segmental relationship to vertebral bodies. From C1 to T11 the spinal cord, roots, ganglia, and nerves have been exposed by removal of the vertebral arches. The dura mater has been removed except on the right side. The numbers on the right represent the levels of the vertebral bodies. (From Miller, M. E., Christensen, G. C., and Evans, H. E., Anatomy of the Dog. Philadelphia. W. B. Saunders Co., 1964. Drawn by M. Newsom.)

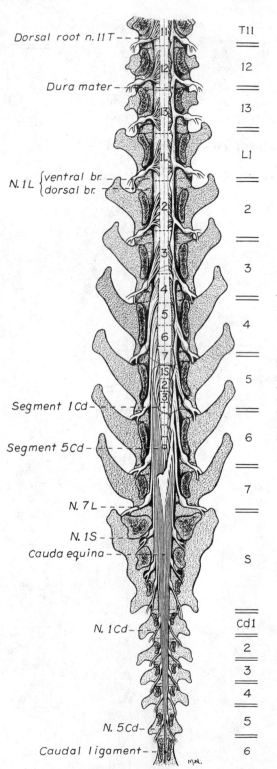

Dorsal root n.11T
Dura mater
N.1L {ventral br. / dorsal br.
Segment 1Cd
Segment 5Cd
N. 7L
N. 1S
Cauda equina
N. 1Cd
N. 5Cd
Caudal ligament

T11
12
13
L1
2
3
4
5
6
7
S
Cd1
2
3
4
5
6

Figure 4–5. Spinal cord segmental relationship to vertebral bodies. From T11 through the caudal segments the spinal cord, roots, ganglia, and nerves have been exposed by removal of the vertebral arches. The dura mater has been removed except on the right side. The numbers on the right represent the levels of the vertebral bodies. (From Miller, M. E., Christensen, G. C., and Evans, H. E., Anatomy of the Dog. Philadelphia, W. B. Saunders Co., 1964. Drawn by M. Newsom.)

tionships may shift caudally by one half of a vertebra. Each species varies in this relationship.[94] In my experience, in the mature cat the three sacral segments may be found in the vertebral canal over the body of L6 and the spinal cord usually ends over the body of L7. Some literature states the spinal cord may extend as far caudally as S3 in the adult cat.

As a rule in adult horses the first 3 sacral segments are over the body of L6 and the last 2 sacral and first few caudal segments are over the body of S1. The spinal cord ends over S2. In adult cattle the 5 sacral segments are usually over the body of L6 and the caudal segments are over S1. In the calf the spinal cord will extend caudally over S3.[94]

Knowledge of the location of the lumbosacral segments is helpful in performing lumbar myelography or obtaining CSF from the lumbosacral area.

FUNCTION

The general somatic efferent portion of the lower motor neuron comprises the motor component of the spinal reflexes that are tested in the neurologic examination. Knowledge of the anatomy of this system is helpful in localizing lesions to portions of the peripheral nervous system or spinal cord. The general somatic afferent (GSA) or general proprioceptive (GP) system contains the sensory component of these reflexes. It consists of a dendritic zone (receptor) in the skin or neuromuscular spindle, and an axon that courses through a specific peripheral nerve, spinal nerve, and dorsal root, entering the dorsal grey column of the corresponding spinal cord segment, and terminating in a telodendron on a second neuron, usually in the dorsal grey column. The cell body of the general somatic afferent neuron is located in the respective spinal ganglion at the distal end of the dorsal root.

In the patellar tendon reflex the sensory neuron terminates directly on the GSE neuron in the ventral grey column. For most other spinal reflexes the sensory neuron telodendron ends on an interneuron in the grey matter that in turn terminates on the GSE neuron (Fig. 4–6).

Spinal reflexes need only the peripheral components and involved segments of the spinal cord to function. They will function even if the spinal cord segments have been cut off and isolated from the rest of the central nervous system.

In order to interpret the spinal reflexes properly, their anatomic components must be understood (Table 4–1).

Thoracic Limb Reflexes

The thoracic limbs are innervated primarily from the sixth cervical (C6) to the first thoracic (T1) segment. Small contributions come from the C5 and T2 segments. The spinal nerves from these segments intertwine to form the brachial plexus, out of which course the specific peripheral nerves of the thoracic limbs. The flexor reflex is performed by pinching a toe. This may be done with the fingers, but a pair of forceps applied to the base of the nail is more reliable. The subsequent prompt flexion or withdrawal of the limb requires the integrity of the roots and grey matter of the spinal cord from C6 to T1. The axillary, musculocutaneous, median, ulnar, and part of the radial peripheral nerves function in this reflex (Fig. 4–7).

Two tendon reflexes can be tested in the thoracic limbs. They are not always present in normal animals. The biceps reflex is elicited by ballottement of the first finger placed on the distal end of the biceps brachii and brachialis on the medial side of the elbow. Contraction of these muscles may be palpated and flexion of the elbow observed. This reflex is mediated entirely by the musculocutaneous nerve (C6, 7, 8). The triceps reflex tests the radial nerve (C7, 8, T1, 2), and is elicited by tapping the triceps tendon just proximal to its insertion on the olecranon. Extension of the elbow is observed. The absence of these reflexes is not significant. Their presence indicates that the involved anatomic components can function. If they are increased, it indicates a possible upper motor neuron (UMN) disease.

The cutaneous trunci reflex may involve a much larger portion of the spinal cord. Light irritation or pricking the skin of the trunk with a pin causes contraction of the cutaneous trunci and a quick movement of the skin. This reflex is mediated through the segmental sensory neurons, in which the stimulus is elicited. The impulse enters the corresponding segment of the spinal cord and through interneurons is passed cranially through the spinal cord white matter to the T1 and C8 spinal cord segments, where the general somatic efferent neurons of the lateral thoracic nerve are located. Stimulation of these causes contraction of the cutaneous trunci muscle. This reflex requires vigorous repetitive sensory stimulation in some

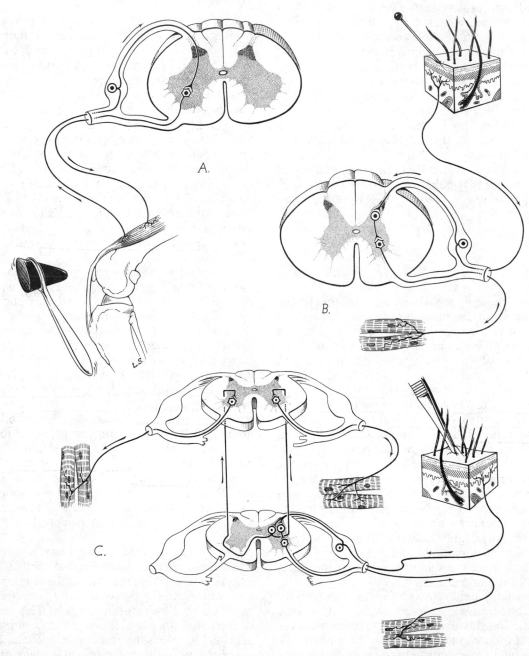

Figure 4–6. Spinal segmental reflexes: *A*: monosynaptic myotatic-patellar reflex; *B*: polysynaptic flexor reflex to a noxious stimulus; *C*: polysynaptic flexor reflex with intersegmental transmission of impulses.

**TABLE 4–1. TOPOGRAPHIC ANATOMY OF SPINAL REFLEX
TESTING IN DOGS**

	Reflex	Peripheral Nerve	Spinal Cord Segments	Level in Vertebral Canal
Thoracic Limb	Flexor	All peripheral nerves of thoracic limb	C6–T2	C5–T1
	Biceps*	Musculocutaneous	C6–8	C5–7
	Triceps*	Radial	C7–T2	C6–T1
	Extensor carpi radialis*	Radial	C7–T2	C6–T1
Pelvic Limb	Flexor	Sciatic	L6–S1	L4–5
	Patellar	Femoral	L4–6	L3–4
	Cranial tibial*	Peroneal	L6–7	L4
	Gastrocnemius*	Tibial	L7–S1	L4–5

*Not always present in normal dogs

dogs and occasionally cannot be elicited.[11] The most caudal extent over the back where this reflex can be elicted varies. In most dogs this is at least midlumbar; in many it reaches the lumbosacral articulation.

Pelvic Limb Reflexes

The pelvic limbs are innervated from the L4 to S1 segments of the spinal cord.[72] Muscles that flex the hip joint receive innervation from as far cranial as the L1 segment. The spinal nerves from the L4 to S3 segments join to form the lumbosacral plexus. The peripheral nerves to the perineum and pelvic limbs are derived from this plexus. The flexor reflex of the pelvic limbs depends on the integrity of the sciatic nerve, whose roots and cell bodies are associated with the L6 to S1 segments of the spinal cord. The patellar reflex is the only reliable tendon reflex. When the patient is relaxed, a light tap of the patellar tendon elicits a brisk extension of the stifle. If present, the reflex can be observed for its briskness, degree of activity, or the presence of clonus. The peripheral nerve controlling this reflex is the femoral nerve, whose roots and cell bodies are located in the L4 to L6 spinal cord segments. The L5 ventral root is the most significant motor component of this reflex.[191] The patellar reflex is graded plus 2 for normal, plus 1 for depressed, 0 for absent, plus 3 for hyperactive, and plus 4 for clonus (Fig. 4–8).

The perineal reflex is elicited by light stimulation of the perineum with a pin or forceps. The normal response is a sharp contraction of the anal sphincter and flexion of the tail. This reflex depends on the integrity of the sacral and caudal segments of the spinal cord.

LOWER MOTOR NEURON DISEASE SIGNS

Abnormalities of any part of the general somatic efferent lower motor neuron cause signs of muscle weakness—paresis or paralysis, along with hyporeflexia or areflexia, hypotonia or atonia, and neurogenic atrophy.

Spinal reflexes are depressed or absent when there is a loss of the motor component of the reflex arc. Muscle tone is dependent on a continual contraction of a small, regulated number of muscle cells. When their motor innervation is lost, there can be no contraction to maintain muscle tone. This condition is ascertained best by passive manipulation of the limb of the recumbent animal. Palpation of the anus and manipulation of the tail also help to detect hypotonia or atonia.

Denervation implies interruption of the lower motor neuron. Muscle cells that are denervated degenerate. Muscle protein is lost rapidly, and over a long period of time the cell eventually dies and is replaced by connective tissue. As the cell degenerates and loses protein, it atrophies. This occurs rapidly, being observed within 1 week of denervation, and is referred to as neurogenic atrophy. The rate and degree of atrophy vary with the species and the muscle that is denervated. Denervated muscles may be atrophic for weeks and return

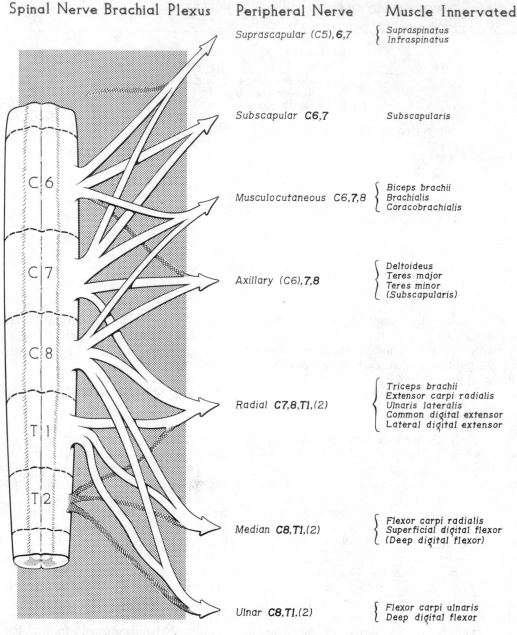

Spinal Nerve Brachial Plexus	Peripheral Nerve	Muscle Innervated
	Suprascapular (C5),**6**,**7**	Supraspinatus Infraspinatus
	Subscapular **C6,7**	Subscapularis
	Musculocutaneous C6,7,8	Biceps brachii Brachialis Coracobrachialis
	Axillary (C6),**7,8**	Deltoideus Teres major Teres minor (Subscapularis)
	Radial **C7,8,**T1,(2)	Triceps brachii Extensor carpi radialis Ulnaris lateralis Common digital extensor Lateral digital extensor
	Median **C8,T1,**(2)	Flexor carpi radialis Superficial digital flexor (Deep digital flexor)
	Ulnar **C8,T1,**(2)	Flexor carpi ulnaris Deep digital flexor

Flexor reflex: Sensory: varies with area stimulated
                 Motor: musculocutaneous, axillary, median, ulnar, radial
Biceps reflex: Sensory and Motor: musculocutaneous
Triceps reflex: Sensory and Motor: radial

Figure 4–7.   Segmental innervation from cervical intumescence of thoracic limb muscles in the dog.

to normal size when reinnervated. A good example of this phenomenon is coonhound paralysis (acute polyradiculoneuritis).

The clinical presentation depends on how much of the general somatic efferent lower motor neuron is affected. The abnormality may occur at any point along the lower motor neuron: at the cell body in the ventral grey column, in the ventral root, spinal nerve, or peripheral nerve, or at the neuromuscular junction. Ischemic necrosis of the ventral grey column, segmental demyelinization of the ven-

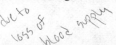

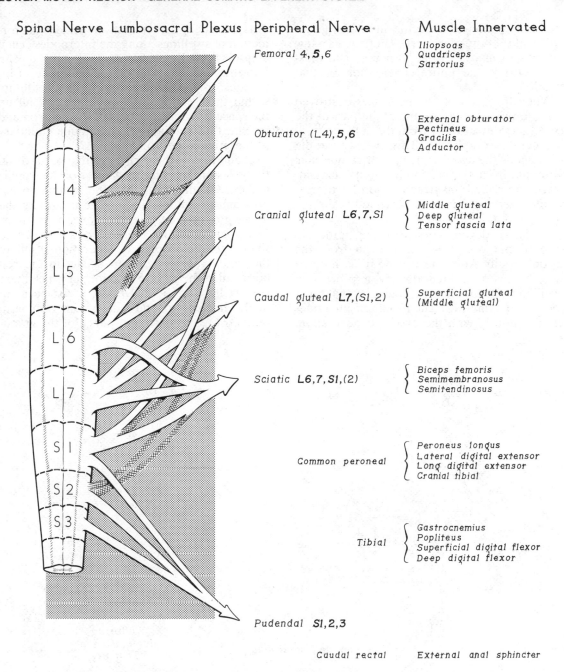

Spinal Nerve Lumbosacral Plexus Peripheral Nerve   Muscle Innervated

Femoral 4,**5**,6
{ Iliopsoas
  Quadriceps
  Sartorius

Obturator (L4),**5**,**6**
{ External obturator
  Pectineus
  Gracilis
  Adductor

Cranial gluteal **L6**,7,S1
{ Middle gluteal
  Deep gluteal
  Tensor fascia lata

Caudal gluteal **L7**,(S1,2)
{ Superficial gluteal
  (Middle gluteal)

Sciatic **L6**,7,S1,(2)
{ Biceps femoris
  Semimembranosus
  Semitendinosus

Common peroneal
{ Peroneus longus
  Lateral digital extensor
  Long digital extensor
  Cranial tibial

Tibial
{ Gastrocnemius
  Popliteus
  Superficial digital flexor
  Deep digital flexor

Pudendal **S1**,2,3

Caudal rectal   External anal sphincter

Flexor reflex: Sensory and Motor: Sciatic nerve
Patellar reflex: Sensory and Motor: Femoral nerve
Perineal reflex: Sensory and Motor: Pudendal nerve

Figure 4–8. Segmental innervation from lumbosacral intumescence of pelvic limb muscles in the dog.

tral roots, traumatic avulsion of selected dorsal and ventral roots, neoplasia of a spinal nerve, contusion to a peripheral nerve, inflammation of the peripheral nerves, and ineffective transmission at the neuromuscular junction are all examples of diseases of the GSE lower motor neuron that produce the characteristic signs, but with differing degrees of severity. The dysfunction caused by destruction of an entire peripheral nerve exceeds that caused by destruction of an entire root or spinal nerve. This is because the peripheral nerve supplies the total innervation of a specific muscle, whereas a ventral root or spinal nerve contributes a few neurons to many peripheral nerves and muscles but not the entire innervation of that muscle.

When the axon of any neuron is destroyed at some point along its course, the part of the axon that courses away from the cell body will degenerate completely. This is because the axon needs the axoplasmic flow of cytoplasmic materials from the cell body for its survival. Waller described this degeneration for the peripheral nerves; therefore it is called Wallerian degeneration (Fig. 4–9).

Wallerian degeneration is a trophic degeneration that occurs in the neuron from the lesion distally from the cell body as follows: (1) The axon disintegrates by a process of swelling and subsequent granulation that takes about 3 to 4 days. (2) The myelin disintegrates simultaneously with the axonal degeneration.

This secondary demyelination includes the formation of swellings along the internodes called ellipsoids, and the fragmentation of myelin into droplets. (3) The motor end-plate disintegrates. (4) The Schwann cells proliferate within their endoneurial covering and fill up the space previously occupied by the axon and myelin, thus retaining the anatomic boundary of the original neuron.

In addition to these changes that occur distal to the lesion, because of the loss of the trophic influence of the cell body other changes occur proximal to the lesion. (1) The trauma of the injury produces degeneration over a few internodes proximal to the lesion in a manner similar to the trophic degeneration distal to the lesion. (2) A reaction occurs in the cell body called the axonal reaction, in which there is a swelling of the cell body, a displacement of the nucleus to one side of the cytoplasm (eccentric), and partial dispersal of the granu-

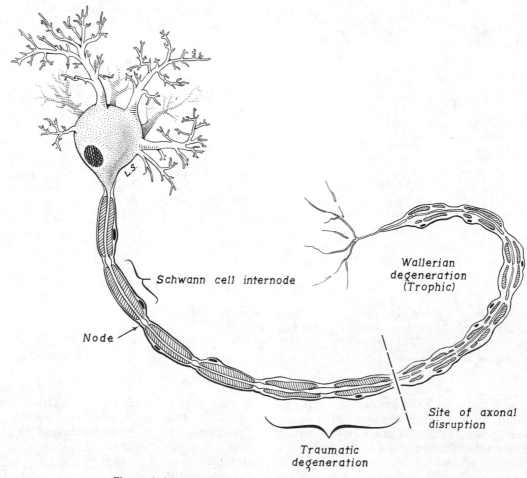

Figure 4–9. Wallerian degeneration of a lower motor neuron.

lar endoplasmic reticulum (Nissl substance) in the region around the nucleus and center of the cell body, or central chromatolysis. These changes represent regenerative efforts by the cell body.

Regeneration begins in about 7 days, starting at the site of the axonal degeneration where normal axonal materal exists. Each axon grows out a number of processes called axonal buds, which grow into the existing cords of proliferated Schwann cells and the endoneurium that provides a pathway for them. The rate of growth is approximately 1 to 4 mm per day. This process is dependent on the proximity of the severed stumps of the neurons and the absence of any impediment to the growth of these axonal buds, such as the proliferation of fibrous connective tissue secondary to the tissue destruction that destroyed the neurons.

When the axonal buds cannot find a pathway to the distally located bands of Schwann cells, they grow in a haphazard manner and form an observable swelling known as a neuroma. These are often a sequel to the neurectomies that are performed in the distal extremities of horses and may be a source of irritation to the patient.[62]

ELECTRODIAGNOSTIC TECHNIQUES IN NEUROMUSCULAR DISEASE

Electromyography (EMG) is the study of the electrical activity of muscle by insertion of a recording electrode into the muscle and recording the electrical activity by means of an amplifier on an oscilloscope.[18, 25, 32, 33, 89, 140, 168] An audible signal accompanies this recording. It is used clinically to determine if the lower motor neuron, its myelin, or the muscle fibers themselves are the site of the lesion. Like any other ancillary procedure, it is used to confirm a clinical observation of peripheral nerve or muscle disease and may contribute to the prognosis.

Normal resting muscle does not show observable electrical activity on the electromyograph once the electrode placement is stabilized. There also is no audible signal given. This is the resting potential. In lower motor neuron disease muscle cells may become denervated. About 5 days following such denervation in the dog continuous spontaneous potentials called fibrillations develop, with amplitudes usually less than 200 μv. They are biphasic, of 1 to 2 msec (less than 7 msec) in

duration and produce a sound like eggs frying. They may occur as often as 2 to 30 per sec. Fibrillations are said to represent the spontaneous action potential or contraction of a single denervated muscle cell. Denervation disturbs the muscle cell metabolism that is thought to account for its spontaneous activity. The prevalence of fibrillations in denervated muscle may decrease after a 3-week period. Positive sharp waves (potentials) also accompany the denervation of lower motor neuron disease and are characterized by an initial low voltage sharp positive deflection with a slow return to the baseline. Voltage is variable, ranging from 50 to 1000 μv. The duration is usually several times longer than a fibrillation, and these have a dull sound. Spontaneous contraction of single motor units is often visible on the muscle surface and is called a fasciculation. It varies from 300 to 2000 μv in amplitude and lasts from 4 to 10 msec. This also may accompany the denervation of lower motor neuron disease. It occasionally occurs in normal muscle. Because fibrillations and positive sharp waves occur with denervation, their presence implies axonal degeneration in the neuromuscular disease. Severe myelin abnormality will impair the rate of impulse transmission and motor nerve conduction will be slow.

Motor nerve conduction can be determined by the same electromyographic instruments, and the evoked potential of the muscle can be observed.[25, 89, 123, 162, 163, 168, 174] For practical purposes this usually is performed in the thoracic limb by stimulating the ulnar nerve at the elbow and in the carpal canal, and recording from the interosseous muscles. In the pelvic limbs the tibial nerve is stimulated at the stifle and proximal to the tarsus and the responses are recorded from the interosseous muscles. Other motor nerves and the muscles they innervate may be used. Normal conduction time varies between 50 and 60 m per sec. Nerves that have been injured and avulsed and have undergone Wallerian degeneration (from 4 to 5 days) will not conduct an impulse.[2, 88] Decreased conduction times usually occur in nerves with severe loss of their myelin. The evoked potential resulting from motor nerve stimulation is the summated motor unit potential recorded on the oscilloscope. Normally it is a smooth bi- or triphasic wave, 5 to 10 msec in duration, varying in amplitude but often greater than 3000 μv. In lower motor neuron disease the evoked potential may be polyphasic and prolonged if some nerve fibers are conducting slowly. Loss of some motor units prevents smooth summation of response. Polyphasic potentials of decreased amplitude also may occur in myositis. If the inflammation involves the neuromuscular ending, denervation potentials may accompany this. Sensory nerve conduction velocities may also be determined.[99]

Sensory nerve conduction velocity may be determined by stimulating a sensory nerve distally and recording the response at some point proximally in the same nerve. Superficial branches of the radial nerve are used in the thoracic limb and the superficial peroneal nerve in the pelvic limb.

Myotonia is defined as the continued active contraction of a muscle that persists after the stimulation or voluntary effort has stopped. On the electromyograph, it is stimulated by the needle insertion and appears as a repetitive, high frequency discharge that initially increases in amplitude and frequency and then decreases over 4 to 5 seconds. On the loudspeaker this produces a distinct sound that waxes and wanes and is described as the "dive-bomber sound" because of the resemblance. This is a nonspecific change that occurs with many forms of muscle disease. It presumably results from a hyperexcitable muscle-cell membrane.[84, 187] Bizarre high frequency potentials, or pseudomyotonia, have a sudden onset upon needle insertion, persist for a variable period, and stop suddenly without a waxing and waning effect. These also result from disturbances of the muscle cell membrane.

NEUROMUSCULAR DISEASE

DISEASES OF THE GSE LOWER MOTOR NEURON (Table 4–2)

Neuromuscular diseases may be defined as disorders of the motor unit of skeletal muscles, i.e., the entire GSE lower motor neuron and the muscle cells it innervates. These diseases often include the SVE lower motor neurons to striated visceral muscle of the larynx, pharynx, and esophagus. Therefore, this includes diseases of the cell bodies in the central nervous system; the axons in spinal and cranial nerve roots, in spinal and cranial nerves, and in peripheral nerves and their Schwann cells and associated myelin; the neuromuscular junction and the muscle cells it innervates.

Neuromuscular diseases may be classified anatomically as neuropathies, junctionopa-

TABLE 4–2. NEUROMUSCULAR DISEASES

Diseases of the GSE Lower Motor Neuron

Neuromuscular Junction
   Botulism
   Tick paralysis
   Myasthenia gravis

Peripheral Nerve
   Trauma
   Neoplasia
   Ischemia—caudal aortic thrombosis-embolism

Spinal Roots and Nerves
   Trauma—root avulsion
   Lumbosacral stenosis—cauda equina syndrome
   Neoplasia-neurofibroma
   Inflammation

Spinal Roots and/or Nerves and Peripheral Nerves
   Inflammation

   Acute Polyneuritis-Polyneuropathy
   Dog: Idiopathic polyradiculoneuritis–Coonhound
      paralysis
      Acute idiopathic polyneuropathy
      Post-rabies vaccination
      Distal denervating disease
      Brachial plexus neuritis
   Other Species: Cat, goat, cattle

   Chronic Polyneuritis-Polyneuropathy
   Dog: Chronic polyneuritis
      Inherited hypertrophic neuropathy
      Giant axonal neuropathy
      Distal symmetric polyneuropathy
      Metabolic neuropathy
   Horse: Chronic equine polyneuritis (neuritis of
      cauda equina)

Spinal Cord
   Focal myelopathy from compression
   Acute ischemic myelopathy—fibrocartilaginous emboli
   Diffuse myelomalacia
   Poliomyelomalacia in pigs
   Inflammations: viral, protozoal
   Hereditary neuronal abiotrophy in Swedish Lapland
      dogs
   Hereditary spinal muscular atrophy in Brittany spaniels
   Stockard's paralysis

Muscle Disease

Myositis
   Infectious
   Idiopathic-Immune mediated
      Masticatory
      Polymyositis

Myotonia
   Hereditary myopathic myotonia of young animals
   Acquired myopathic myotonia of old dogs

Myopathy

thies, myopathies, and neuromyopathies. Neuropathies include central motoneuron diseases of the cell bodies and peripheral motoneuron disease that affects the axon, its myelin (primary demyelination), or both axons and Schwann cells.

The following examples of general somatic efferent lower motor neuron disease are organized topographically starting with the neuromuscular junction and progressing proximally toward the spinal cord. Some include other systems of the lower motor neuron and others include lesions of the peripheral sensory neurons as well. They are discussed here because of the recognizable deficit of GSE function.

Neuromuscular Junction

Botulism, tick paralysis, and myasthenia gravis all are diseases that affect the function of the neuromuscular junction. Myasthenia gravis is characterized by episodic occurrences of lower motor neuron weakness associated with exercise, and is responsive to anticholinesterase therapy. Botulism and tick paralysis are rapidly progressive, sometimes fatal, lower motor neuron paralytic diseases that are not significantly responsive to such therapy.

Botulism. Botulism is a LMN paralysis caused by the toxin produced by the bacterium *Clostridium botulinum.* The toxin may be ingested in feed or carrion in which this organism is growing and producing toxin, or the agent may infect a wound and produce toxin that presumably gains entrance to the blood stream and ultimately reaches neuromuscular junctions, in which it is thought to interfere with acetylcholine release and function.[136] There are significant species differences in susceptibility to botulism. Some are dependent on the type of toxin to which the animal is exposed. Dogs and pigs are the most resistant to this disease. Dogs are most susceptible to the type C toxin.[10, 14, 16, 48] Ruminants are most susceptible to types C and D toxins,[161] and types B and C toxins most commonly affect horses.

At the New York State College of Veterinary Medicine, botulism has been diagnosed presumptively as a herd problem in cattle and in individual horses and dogs. In these situations it has not been possible to prove the diagnosis. Usually, once the signs are recognized in large animals the disease is fatal. Dogs may recover.

Cattle assumed to have this disease show a weak, unsteady gait without ataxia and often become recumbent in 24 to 48 hours.[9, 71, 165] Some cattle die without obvious signs.[78] It is important to recognize the lack of ataxia in order to differentiate this condition from a spinal cord lesion. All muscles are hypotonic and weak. This includes the tail, anus, limbs, ears, eyelids, lips, tongue, and pharynx. Palpation of facial muscles and testing tongue strength by pulling it from the mouth are helpful in determining the signs of diffuse lower motor neuron disease. Dysphagia, or difficulty in swallowing, is a prominent sign and may be confused with anorexia. Death is caused by respiratory paralysis. The source is often difficult to prove. Contaminated high moisture corn silage has been implicated in one herd.[144]

Some forms of organophosphate poisoning may mimic botulism, except that pelvic limb weakness may be more apparent than thoracic limb weakness before the animal becomes recumbent.[139] The tail may be carried slightly elevated, and the animal constantly urinates small quantities. Diffuse neuromuscular paresis prevails, and late in the disease, includes cranial nerves with lower motor neuron function. Cattle become recumbent and die from respiratory paralysis. Careful study of spinal cord and peripheral nerves may reveal degeneration of axons, myelin, and cell bodies. The neuropathy is described as a dying back of the axon. Triorthocresyl phosphate and triorthotolyl phosphate can produce these lesions.[31, 153]

HORSE

Foals. A diffuse rapidly progessive neuromuscular paresis occurs in foals 2 to 8 weeks old.[131, 157, 175, 176] These are usually fast-growing foals that suddenly develop a stiff, short-strided gait and muscle tremors. Because of the severe tremors that develop as they try to support weight on weakening limbs, these foals have been called "shaker foals." They have difficulty rising and can stand only for a few minutes before collapsing. Dysphagia is common and milk runs out the nostrils following attempts to nurse. Mydriasis with slowly responsive pupils, constipation, and frequent urination of small quantities of urine may occur. Terminally these foals become dyspneic, extend their head and neck, and develop a tachycardia. Death can occur in a few hours to 72 hours or more. Mortality is high. A few recover spontaneously in a 3- to 4- week period.

Clostridium botulinum type B can be isolated from organs with necrotic lesions. These include gastric ulcers, small areas of liver necrosis, umbilical abscesses, skin wounds, and lung abscesses. The horse is extremely susceptible to minute amounts of toxin produced by *Clostridium botulinum.* This small amount diluted by serum has no effect when injected into laboratory mice. Type C toxicoinfectious botulism has also been implicated in a foal.[102]

Adults. A similar disease is observed in adult horses as sporadic cases or herd outbreaks.[175, 176] Acute onset of dysphagia, severe limb paresis with trembling, and rapid progression to recumbency are usually observed. These horses may be quite depressed. Recumbent horses that can support on their sternum often rest their chin on the floor to support their head. Death can occur in a few hours. If the onset is slow, chances for recovery after a few days to a week are good. Horses that can walk have a stilted short-strided gait without ataxia.

No lesions are observed in the nervous system. Occasionally gastric ulcers or other necrotic lesions that harbor *Clostridium botulinum* are found, similar to foals with the same syndrome. In others, no lesions are found as a source of the toxin. Although the feed is suspect in these patients, no specific source of toxin has been implicated. Involvement of the multiple horses on one property would suggest a point source of toxin in the environment and not an infection in these horses.

Experimentally the disease can be reproduced by infecting necrotic lesions with *Clostridium botulinum* spores. Steroids enhance the development of the disease; therefore, stress is thought to be important in the pathogenesis. Affected foals are usually fast-growing and are nursing mares that are fed an excessively nutritious diet.

Some clinicians believe that frequent administration of an anticholinesterase—neostigmine, 2 mg in foals or 5–10 mg per 1000 lb, every 1 to 2 hours—may help these patients improve. Antibiotics should be administered for possible clostridial infection of a lesion in the horse.

There is evidence that the botulinum toxin interferes with the release of acetylcholine by altering the function of calcium in this mechanism. A number of drugs have been studied that will increase the availability of calcium at the neuromuscular junction. Oral quinidine has been used in humans, cattle, and horses without clear evidence of its efficacy in the domestic animals. 4-Aminopyridine showed the best response in experimental animals with botulism.[130] We have administered 4-aminopyridine intravenously to horses that were recumbent with the clinical diagnosis of botulism. It produced excessive muscular twitching, salivation, anxiety, and rapid respirations, but did not significantly alter the course of the disease. This drug needs further study.

DOGS. The usual source of toxin for the dog is carrion that harbors the growing organism.[10, 14, 16, 48] The onset of signs may be from a few hours to a few days after ingestion of the toxin. Signs consist of a rapidly developing paresis that progresses from pelvic limbs to thoracic limbs and usually cranial nerve muscles innervated by cranial nerves. Early in the disease the gait will be stiff and short-strided. Dogs may use their hindlimbs simultaneously and hop like a rabbit. The limbs may tremble as they attempt to support weight on the weakening limbs. Weakness is usually evident in muscles of the face, jaw, pharynx, and occasionally the esophagus. These dogs drool and cough, and have difficulty prehending and swallowing. Regurgitation is associated with a megaesophagus.

There is no ataxia–general proprioceptive deficit. Postural reactions are poorly performed in the very weak animal. If the weight is held by the examiner and the paw lightly placed on the ground, the patient will hop rapidly and accurately unless the weakness is too severe. This dog is aware of its limb position. The recumbent, severely weak dog will be very hypotonic, with no patellar reflexes and weak flexor reflexes. Pain sensation is normal but the voice is weak. Hyperesthesia is not evident (Table 4–3).

On EMG there are usually no denervation potentials. The evoked motor potential to a single supramaximal stimulus is markedly reduced.

Most dogs recover in 1 to 3 weeks with only nursing care. Inhalation pneumonia is a serious potential complication in dysphagic dogs with megaesophagus.

Type C toxin may be identified in the serum or feces of affected dogs.

Tick Paralysis. Tick paralysis, most commonly observed in dogs and children, can affect all species in those areas in which the appropriate tick is located.[14] The common wood tick, *Dermacentor variabilis,* and *Dermacentor andersoni* are incriminated most often. Signs can result from the feeding of one female tick. The tick is presumed to elaborate a salivary neurotoxin that circulates and interferes with acetylcholine liberation at the neuromuscular junction. The toxin may act by interfering with the function of calcium in the release of acetylcholine. Signs occur 5 to 9 days after tick infestation, with a rapid onset of lower motor neuron paresis. Dogs often first appear weak in the pelvic limbs, and then become recumbent in 24 to 72 hours. Spinal reflexes are depressed or absent. Pain is perceived normally and there is no evidence of hyperesthesia. The lower motor neurons of the cranial nerves are not affected significantly. Occasionally mild facial and jaw muscle weakness occurs. Death may occur in 1 to 5 days from respiratory paralysis. Direct removal of the tick or ticks or dipping the animal in an insecticide solution to kill them is followed by recovery in 24 to 72 hours (Table 4–3).

In eastern Australia *Ixodes holocyclus* produces a severe lower motor neuron paralysis that rapidly progresses from pelvic to thoracic limbs in all species of domestic animals and in humans.[104] Signs often include sialosis, emesis, and mydriasis. A slow respiratory rate and dyspnea are common. Death from respiratory paralysis may occur despite insecticide dips and tick removal. Hyperimmune serum is administered intravenously.[35]

Myasthenia Gravis. Myasthenia gravis (grave muscle weakness) is a common disease in humans. A similar syndrome has been reported in the dog[66, 73, 112, 129, 147-149, 192] and cat.[50, 135] The disease has been described in two forms: a congenital non-autoimmune form and an acquired autoimmune form. The congenital form occurs in puppies with onset from 3 to 8 weeks of age. This has been observed in litters of springer spaniels,[107] smooth-haired fox terriers,[106, 137] and Jack Russell terriers.[150, 151] I have observed it in a litter of Samoyeds. In the Jack Russell terriers and fox terriers there is presumptive evidence that the disease is inherited. The acquired form has been reported more commonly in young adults of the larger breeds of dogs, but any age and breed are susceptible. There is no sex predilection.

The clinical signs are episodic, associated with exercise, and recover with rest. The owner often complains that the animal tires easily. The severity varies but usually increases progressively if the disease is not treated. The episodic nature of this disease is in distinct contrast to the other diseases affecting the neuromuscular junction and to acute polyneuritis.

In the acquired disease, both spinal and cranial nerve neuromuscular junctions are affected and reflected in the clinical signs. Upon exercise, the gait, which initially is normal, develops shorter and shorter strides, which may appear stiff or stilted. There is decreased ability to support, possibly culminating in complete collapse. This may occur primarily in the pelvic limbs or the thoracic limbs or equally in all four limbs. When the signs are severe, postural reactions cannot be performed. How-

ever, if most of the weight is held by the examiner the patient will usually attempt to hop, place, or replace the turned-over paw very rapidly, indicating no deficiency in proprioception. Normal spinal reflexes are usually retained. Axial muscle weakness will be evident by the ventral flexion posture of the neck and inability to extend it.

Cranial nerve signs will consist of difficulty prehending food and water, dysphagia, and postprandial regurgitation. Facial muscle weakness may be profound, with constant drooling and inability to close the eyelids. Weak jaw tone, weak tongue retraction, and a weak gag reflex may be palpated. Wheezing and gagging may be heard during respirations and attempts to swallow. Laryngeal paresis may be severe enough to cause inspiratory dyspnea and a hypoxic cyanosis. A megaesophagus is usually present on thoracic radiographs. Aspiration pneumonia is a serious sequelae of this disease.

In the congenital form signs are first observed around 3 to 8 weeks of age when the puppies are beginning to walk. Affected puppies are less active than their normal littermates. Usually the pelvic limbs show the first weakness, followed by the forelimbs, neck, and sometimes pharyngeal muscles and muscles of mastication. The dog may become unable to stand or hold up its head and may choke on food. Megaesophagus has not been observed.

Because the anatomic abnormality is limited to the neuromuscular junction, there is no sensory abnormality in this disease. The acquired disease is considered an immune-mediated disease consisting of antigen-antibody complexes that block some of the muscle cell receptors from availability to the normal amounts of acetylcholine released at the axon terminal. This complex involves immunoglobulin-G antibodies specific for muscle-cell receptor and the C3 complement. Antimuscle-cell receptor and antistriational antibodies have been detected in sera of affected dogs with the acquired disease, but not in the congenital form.[46, 66, 77, 124] Thymomas have been observed in some myasthenic persons and rarely in dogs.[95]

In the congenital form, assays have determined a deficiency of acetylcholine muscle receptor in the muscle cell membranes. The reason for this is still unknown. It may reflect a developmental failure to synthesize sufficient receptor or the formation of an abnormal receptor that does not bind normally with acetylcholine or form a normal neuromuscular junction, or it may reflect accelerated degradation of the receptor.

There is one report of myasthenia gravis in a 7-week-old Yorkshire terrier–Jack Russell terrier crossbreed in which reduced levels of acetylcholine muscle receptors were associated with autoantibodies to these receptors. Complete recovery followed 8 months of therapy. Neonatal myasthenia occurs in children born to myasthenic mothers, presumably from passage of antibodies across the placenta. The same could potentially occur in puppies after ingestion of colostral antibodies. This has not yet been reported in animals.

Diagnosis and therapy primarily involve the administration of anticholinesterases to permit the acetylcholine released from the axon terminals to be available longer and have more opportunity to bind with a muscle receptor and initiate an action potential.

For diagnosis, the preferred anticholinesterase is edrophonium (Tensilon) at 0.5 to 5 mg intravenously, depending upon the size of the dog. In puppies with the congenital form, 0.1 to 0.5 mg is sufficient. The effect occurs within seconds and lasts only about 5 minutes. This effect can be dramatic and in seconds can restore a collapsed recumbent dog to complete normality that lasts a few minutes before the weakness recurs. Because of the short duration of the effect, toxicity is less of a problem and pretreatment with atropine to prevent muscarinic side effects is unnecessary. Intramuscular neostigmine methylsulfate at 0.04 to 0.06 mg per kg body weight will require 10 to 15 minutes to produce an effect, and repeated injections may be necessary.

Toxicity may occur in the normal dog or in the overdosed patient and result in paralysis from the depolarizing action of excessive acetylcholine in the muscle. Atropine and oxygen should be available to treat this toxicity. Pretreatment with atropine at 0.05 mg per kg may alleviate some of the muscarinic side effects which include sialosis, vomiting, and diarrhea.

If electrodiagnostic equipment is available, the diagnosis may be confirmed by the demonstration of a decremental muscle response to repetitive motor nerve stimulation and a reduction or elimination of the decrement following administration of an anticholinesterase.

The long-acting anticholinesterase pyridostigmine (Mestinon) is recommended for oral treatment at a dose of 30 to 60 mg, 2 to 3 times per day. Puppies with congenital myasthenia may only need 7.5 mg, but response to treatment may be erratic. Sudden death occasionally occurs. Neostigmine bromide (Prostigmine) may also be effective at 0.5 mg per kg, 2 to 3 times per day. Adrenocorticosterids are indicated in the acquired disease and may be used alone or in combination with anticholinesterase therapy. This therapy is usually reserved for those dogs that do not respond well to anticholinesterase therapy or become refractory to it.

Spontaneous recovery has occurred in some dogs with the acquired disease after a few weeks to months of therapy and therapy has been discontinued. Relapse may occur subsequently. Permanent spontaneous recovery may occur in some dogs with the congenital form. This has been observed in springer spaniels and Samoyeds.

The megaesophagus rarely responds to therapy, and postprandial regurgitation may be a persistent problem with the continual threat of aspiration pneumonia. It is important to feed these dogs when their strength is the best after therapy. These dogs may be better if fed a moist food or slurry frequently in small quantities and from an elevated position.

Keep these dogs warm, as a cold environment will induce shivering, which will create increased demands for acetylcholine in the muscle.

If the acetylcholine neurotransmitter is rapidly depleted the animal can suddenly become paralyzed. This is referred to as a myasthenic crisis and can be difficult to differentiate from a cholinergic crisis, which occurs if the animal is overdosed with anticholinesterase. The nicotinic effect of the overdosage results in depolarization of muscle, fasciculations, and paralysis. The muscarinic effect produces sialosis, vomiting, diarrhea, miosis, and bradycardia. Intravenous edrophonium will restore the animal in a myasthenic crisis to normal and briefly exacerbate the cholinergic crisis. The cholinergic crisis should be treated with atropine.

Peripheral Nerves

Trauma. Individual nerves or groups of peripheral nerves are susceptible to injury.[15, 116, 118, 184, 196] The following is an enumeration of these nerves and the signs to be expected. These signs include the general somatic afferent deficit as well as loss of function of the general somatic efferent lower motor neuron.

THORACIC LIMB

Radial Paralysis—Distal Brachium. The limb can support weight, but often only on the dorsum of the paw. The carpus and digits do not extend properly, occasionally causing the paw to be placed on the ground on its dorsal surface (knuckled). The dog may compensate by flipping the paw forward when the elbow is quickly flexed. There is analgesia of a portion of the cranial and lateral antebrachium and dorsal paw (see Fig. 9–4). This injury often follows fractures of the distal humerus.[74, 103, 173]

Radial Paralysis—Proximal Brachium.[156] The limb cannot support weight, and collapses on the dorsal surface of the paw. Initially the elbow is "dropped," a position more ventral than normal owing to the loss of shoulder flexion function of the long head of the triceps. The limb often is carried off the ground with the elbow flexed (musculocutaneous). There is analgesia of a portion of the cranial and lateral antebrachium and dorsal paw. In the calf there also may be difficulty in advancing the limb.

Radial, Axillary, and Thoracodorsal Paralysis. In addition to the signs of a proximal radial paralysis, the elbow is permanently in a posture more ventral than normal (dropped) because of the paralysis of almost all the flexors of the shoulder.[116, 118] There is analgesia of a portion of the dorsal paw, cranial and lateral antebrachium (radial), and a small area of the lateral brachium and caudal scapular region.

Median and Ulnar Paralysis. The gait is normal, but the carpus is more extended than usual and therefore slightly closer to the ground surface as a result of the lack of contraction in the flexors of the carpus and digits.

There is analgesia of the caudal antebrachium, lateral paw, and possibly the palmar paw. The latter area may have innervation from the branch of the musculocutaneous nerve that joins the median nerve near the elbow.

In the calf, the gait appears slightly stiff owing to the extension of the carpus, fetlock, and pastern joints.

Musculocutaneous Paralysis. The gait is normal in the dog. The elbow may be slightly straight (overextended), and the paralysis of elbow flexion may make it difficult to raise the paw to a table surface. There is analgesia of the medial antebrachium.

Supracapsular Paralysis. No clinical signs are evident in the dog. In the calf only slight abduction of the limb occurs, causing a slight circumduction of the limb.

In the horse signs of acute suprascapular nerve injury are variable. Clinical patients often show abduction of the shoulder on bearing weight. The subsequent atrophy confined to the supraspinatus and infraspinatus muscles implicates this nerve in the injury. Pectoral nerve involvement cannot be excluded but no subsequent pectoral muscle atrophy is evident. Experimental neurectomy in small horses causes no signs of a gait deficit. Draft horses with chronic suprascapular nerve injury ("sweeney") related to the collar portion of the harness only show neurogenic atrophy. The gait is normal.

Pectoral Paralysis. In the horse the elbow abducts when weight is borne by the affected limb.

PELVIC LIMB

Femoral Paralysis. There is inability to support weight, and the limb collapses. The dog learns to walk bearing most of its weight on the normal limb and only making a short stride on the affected limb. In the horse when the stifle collapses (flexes), the tarsus and digit automatically suddenly flex.

There is analgesia of the medial side of the thigh, leg, and paw (saphenous). The horse rests with all the joints of the affected limb flexed, and the affected hip region appears more ventral than normal. Femoral nerve paralysis has been observed in calves born following dystocia caused by a hip or stifle lock position that resulted in a stretching of the femoral nerve.[180]

Peroneal Paralysis. The paw often is placed with its dorsal surface on the ground (knuckled) and the tarsus is overextended straighter than normal. There is analgesia of the cranial leg and dorsal paw areas.[13]

This occurs in cattle that are recumbent and lie with pressure on the lateral side of the tibia, where this nerve courses subcutaneously. Peroneal nerve compression has been documented. (See obturator paralysis.)

Tibial Paralysis. On bearing weight the paw sinks and is closer to the ground owing to the lack of tarsal extension. There is analgesia of the caudal leg and plantar paw area. In the calf the fetlock also is "knuckled forward."

Sciatic Paralysis. The limb can support weight and be advanced, but the tarsus is overflexed and sinks close to the ground surface, and the paw is dragged on its dorsal surface and placed with the dorsal surface on the ground. Hip flexion and stifle extension are normal. There is analgesia of the limb distal to the stifle, except for the medial surface.[12]

The sciatic nerve is subject to fractures of the ilium at the greater sciatic notch and fractures of the femur with caudal displacement of a fractured portion. It is susceptible to injury by closed intramedullary bone pinning through the trochanteric fossa. Sciatic nerve entrapment may occur subsequent to injury in the region and the development of scar tissue.[84, 183]

Intramuscular injections of drugs into this nerve at the hip or caudal to the femur cause varying degrees of sciatic paralysis that usually is transient but may be permanent. These are especially common in calves given prophylactic injections of antibiotics and/or vitamin E-selenium preparations in the gluteal or caudal thigh muscles. The protective muscle mass is small in these animals, and the sciatic nerve or its branches are easily injured. Intramuscular injections in calves should be placed in the epaxial muscles of the neck.

Obturator Paralysis. The paralyzed limb slides out or abducts on a smooth surface. The gait is normal on the surface that provides a grip for the dog. Similar signs occasionally are seen in cattle following dystocia.

Massive rectal impaction may compress the obturator nerves in the cat.

In the calf, unilateral or bilateral obturator nerve section causes no alteration in the standing posture, but on walking or running the affected limb or limbs are noticeably abducted. In the adult cow, unilateral obturator nerve section causes slight abduction when the animal is standing or walking. The limb often slides laterally when the cow stands up. This will depend on the nature of the ground surface on which the animal is located. Bilateral neurectomy causes total abduction and collapse of the cow; it is unable to stand unassisted.

There is clinical and experimental evidence to support that most nerve injuries associated with calving involve the sixth lumbar spinal nerve contribution to the sciatic nerve.[37] After leaving the intervertebral foramen this nerve courses ventral to the prominent ridge on the sacrum before passing laterally to join the first two sacral spinal nerves. The sixth lumbar spinal nerve is readily compressed against this bony ridge and injured. This spinal nerve contributes a significant number of neurons to the peroneal nerve branch of the sciatic nerve. Therefore, these cattle stand on the dorsal surface of the foot. This clinical sign cannot be explained by an obturator nerve paralysis.

The sixth lumbar spinal nerve also contributes to the adductor muscles in the thigh, which accounts for some difficulty in standing without abducting the limb. This lesion is probably the major cause of the neurologic difficulty observed in cattle in using their pelvic limbs normally after calving. Recumbent cattle often suffer extensive muscle necrosis, which contributes to this deficit.

Cranial Gluteal Paralysis. In the supporting-propulsive phase of the stride, as all the weight is borne on the affected limb and this phase is completed, the stifle is observed to abduct or rotate so that its cranial surface is directed laterally. This has been observed in dogs following automobile injuries, and in horses with focal lesions of protozoal myelitis in the lumbosacral intumescence.

Neoplasia. Nonneural neoplasms may compress one or more peripheral nerves, causing lower motor neuron paresis. In parakeets renal adenocarcinoma may compress the sciatic and/or femoral nerves that course dorsal to the kidney. Sciatic paralysis in the bird prevents the normal perching mechanism from functioning, and causes hyporeflexia, atrophy, and hypalgesia.

An osteogenic sarcoma of the ventral aspect of the sacrum may compress the sacral nerves and caudal lumbar nerves that form the sciatic nerve. Paralysis of the anus, bladder and rectum, and caudal thigh and leg muscles results. The tail is spared if the vertebral canal is not invaded by the mass. Such a lesion can be diagnosed by rectal examination.

Ischemic Neuromyopathy. Caudal aortic thrombosis or embolism is common in cats[91, 142] and occasionally is observed in dogs and horses.[29] There is complete pelvic limb paralysis (paraplegia), except for hip flexion in some patients. The pelvic limbs are cold; the affected muscles may be firm on palpation and no femoral pulse is present. The portion of the limbs distal to the stifle are most profoundly affected. The caudal leg muscles are often swollen, firm, and painful. In addition to the lack of muscle function owing to the interference with their circulation, the peripheral nerves also become ischemic. This can be determined by the sensory deficit that is also present. The spinal cord is not ischemic in these cases unless the thrombosis is proximal to the renal arteries. Innervation to the tail, anus, perineum, bladder, and rectum is not affected.

The prognosis is generally poor. In cats it most usually is associated with a bacterial endocarditis or cardiomyopathy.[179] Surgical removal has had variable success. Conservatively treated cats may improve. It is usual for some function to return within three weeks. Further ischemic episodes are a possibility.

In dogs, heartworms in the femoral artery have produced an ischemic neuromyopathy in the limb supplied by that vessel.[28, 164]

Spinal Roots and Nerves

Trauma. The spinal roots are susceptible to injury by fractured vertebrae. Usually the signs observed reflect the damage done in the spinal cord. The exceptions to this are caudal lumbar, sacral, and caudal fractures that injure the roots of the cauda equina caudal to the end of the spinal cord. For example, a fracture and luxation of L7 may spare the spinal cord parenchyma or only affect the caudal segments, and yet may severely injure the roots of L6 and L7 and all the sacral and caudal roots that pass through the displaced vertebral foramen of L7. This could produce a denervated tail, anus, perineum, bladder, and rectum, and sciatic nerve paralysis bilaterally. The dog can stand and walk by hip flexion and stifle extension, but bears weight on the dorsal surface of the paws. The tail and anus are atonic, unresponsive to the perineal reflex, and analgesic. The pelvic limb paws are analgesic except for the medial side, which is innervated by the saphenous nerve (L4, L5, L6). Noxious pressure applied to digits 2 (lateral side), 3, 4 and 5 elicits no pain response or flexor reflex. Similar stimulation of the first digit produces pain and hip flexion, but no flexion of the stifle, tarsus, or digits.

In cattle, injury to the caudal lumbar, sacral, and caudal nerves may occur from sacrocaudal fractures and compression from the mounting and riding activity of bulls or other cows. In severe cases the tail head will appear depressed and pushed into the perineum. Anal and tail tone will be depressed. Rarely they show evidence of bilateral peroneal paresis with walking on the dorsal surface of the hind digits.

ROOT AVULSION. Avulsion of the roots of the brachial plexus is the most common cause of the ipsilateral thoracic limb paralysis that occurs following an animal's being struck by a car.[82, 83] When the proximal thoracic limb is forced caudally along the trunk strain is put on the spinal roots, especially at C8 and T1. Excessive strain causes them to rip off the spinal cord or pull apart intrinsically. Occasionally the entire spinal nerve will be torn off of the dura. The rootlets are more vulnerable to injury because of their minimal amount of supporting connective tissue as compared with the rest of the peripheral nervous system outside of the dura.

The signs vary depending on the severity of the lesion and the number and type of roots involved. Occasionally either the dorsal or ventral roots of a spinal nerve will be spared. Usually for signs to occur the roots of two or more spinal cord segments must be involved. In total dysfunction, the roots of segments C6 through T1 are involved. In the latter case all muscles are paralyzed and the limb is dragged constantly along the ground on the dorsal surface of the paw, completely unable to be moved or support weight. Analgesia is variable but may be present over all aspects of the paw, antebrachium, and the distal half of the brachium. With incomplete involvement of these roots the area of analgesia does not correspond to specific peripheral nerves, but is probably dermatomal in distribution.

If the roots of the more caudal segments (C8 and T1) are avulsed, sparing C6 and C7, shoulder and elbow function may be spared and the motor signs are similar to those of proximal radial paralysis.

The ipsilateral cutaneous trunci reflex is absent in all cases with the C8 and T1 roots avulsed. A contralateral response is observed. Normally, sensory stimulation of the skin over the thorax or abdomen induces a bilateral contraction of the cutaneous trunci. The impulses enter the spinal cord at the level of the stimulus. They are passed cranially through the white matter to the grey matter at T1 and C8, where the neurons of the lateral thoracic nerve are activated to cause the cutaneous trunci to contract.

Avulsion of the T1 roots also causes ipsilateral miosis (partial Horner's syndrome).

Surgery is not justified when there is evidence of a brachial plexus root avulsion. Although rare, recovery has been reported, especially when the clinical signs do not indicate a complete functional deficit of all of the components of the brachial plexus. If the injury consists of a contusion, recovery may occur by 1 to 2 weeks. Severe lesions that have some rootlets still attached to the spinal cord and some rootlets with intact axons may improve by regeneration of axons from the injury site, or intact axons may sprout collaterals to reinnervate adjacent denervated muscle cells. This may account for the few patients that have shown some recovery after many weeks to months. Serial studies of the EMG on the triceps brachii and motor nerve conduction velocity in the radial nerve may help to determine the potential for recovery.[167]

With signs of a severe lesion and no improvement after 4 to 6 weeks, amputation of the affected limb should be considered.

If the physical and neurologic examination suggests contusion of the brachial plexus itself or if radiographs show skeletal injury at this site, the brachial plexus can be explored surgically. This approach has been described for the dog[117] and horse.[97]

Avulsion of the lumbosacral roots is rare. One case was observed in a cat in which the roots of L5, L6, L7, and S1 were avulsed traumatically from the spinal cord on one side or severely contused. There were associated femoral and sciatic paralyses of the ipsilateral limb.

LUMBOSACRAL STENOSIS—CAUDA EQUINA SYNDROME. Lumbosacral stenosis occurs in adult dogs and is more common in older dogs of the larger breeds. A lumbosacral malformation, malarticulation of longstanding, is hypothesized as the pathogenesis. Similar signs can occur at this site from injuries with subluxation, compressing neoplasms, intervertebral disk extrusions, or diskospondylitis.

Narrowing of the vertebral canal between L7 and S1 can affect all or part of the caudal and sacral nerves passing through that part of the canal and may affect the seventh lumbar spinal nerves passing laterally through the intervertebral foramina between L7 and S1. Clinical signs are variable, with the most common being pain. Evidence of this varies from resentment to handling or palpation to hypersensitivity over the lumbosacral area and to mild to vicious chewing of the skin innervated by the affected sensory nerves. Incontinence of urine and feces is frequently observed. The tail and anus may be weak, hypotonic, and hyporeflexic. The gait may be normal, cautious from pain, lame from pain or paresis, or obviously paretic. The paresis reflects a partial sciatic nerve problem from compression of the seventh lumbar and/or first sacral spinal nerves. Lameness may be intermittent. Muscle atrophy may reflect a chronic partial denervation of muscles.

This is a chronic, slowly progressive disorder. Plain radiography may be diagnostic if the lesions involving the intervertebral disk and mineralized tissue are advanced enough. Intervertebral disk extrusion, ventrolateral spondylosis, and/or subluxation of the sacrum ventral to L7 may be observed. Tomography may

help in diagnosing the stenosis. Soft tissue proliferation involving the intervertebral disk and/or interarcuate ligament may require myelography or interosseous vertebral venography. Surgical decompression is the treatment of choice.

Neoplasia. Neurofibroma may affect one spinal nerve without producing significant neurologic deficit. Clinical signs usually occur when the spinal cord becomes compressed by the mass lesion or when multiple spinal nerves are involved.

Inflammation. Rarely, a neuritis occurs in the spinal roots in dogs, caused by the protozoa *Toxoplasma gondii.*[6] This organism can affect any portion of the central nervous system, as well as the roots of the spinal nerves. The clinical signs reflect the areas in which the most damage has taken place.

Spinal Roots and/or Nerves and Peripheral Nerves

Acute Polyneuritis-Polyneuropathy
DOG

Idiopathic Polyradiculoneuritis. Acute idiopathic polyradiculoneuritis, the lesion of coonhound paralysis, is the most common inflammation of multiple portions of the peripheral nervous system in dogs.[40, 42, 45, 183] It usually predominates in the ventral roots but can affect any portion of the nervous system covered by peripheral myelin, occasionally even the cranial nerves.

This disease affects dogs of any breed, both sexes, and usually of adult age. Puppies are less commonly affected. The disease is most common in dogs used to hunt raccoons or where dogs have exposure to raccoons. However, a clinically similar paralysis can occur in dogs with no possible exposure to raccoons.

The initial chief complaint from the owner is a progressive weakness and occasionally a change or loss of voice in hunting dogs. Weakness usually begins in the pelvic limbs and thoracic limb weakness rapidly follows. Occasionally thoracic limb weakness precedes that in the pelvic limbs. Weakness is symmetric, but occasionally in the early stages one limb is weaker than the other. Weakness in a dog that can still walk will look like lameness and consist of a rapid, short, sometimes stilted stride. When all four limbs are affected the dog appears as if it were walking on a hot surface. Ataxia does not usually occur.

The limb paresis usually progresses rapidly and makes an animal unable to get up by a few hours to a few days. Dogs have been found recumbent and completely paralyzed with this disease in a 12- to 24-hour period from the first observation of weakness. More often it takes a few days to reach this stage. A few dogs remain ambulatory when the disease runs a shorter course.

When history of exposure to raccoons is available, it usually occurred 7 to 12 days prior to the onset of the neurologic signs.

The signs observed on neurologic examination depend on the stage of the illness and the degree of paresis that is present. All dogs are alert and responsive. Cranial nerves are normal except for a small percentage of severely affected dogs that have a bilateral facial paresis. Prehension and swallowing are normal. Recumbent dogs will have to be supported to eat and drink.

The dog that is weak but still can walk will have short quick strides with the limbs kept under the trunk. The back may be arched (flexed) to help do this. No abduction, hypermetria, prolonged protraction or standing on the dorsum of the paw will be observed. The pelvic limbs may be slightly crouched. Postural reactions will be absent if the animal cannot support all of its weight on the limb being tested and it will collapse. If the dog's weight is borne by the examiner, the limb responses are often very rapid, demonstrating that the dog has normal sensory function and knows where the limb is located. Severely affected dogs have no response to postural reaction testing.

As a rule muscle tone and spinal reflexes will all be decreased or absent, but this depends on the stage and severity of the disease. The patient that can still walk will look stiff, or hypertonic, because it is using all the muscle function it has to remain standing and walking. This patient will not be hypertonic on limb manipulation when it is placed in lateral recumbency and is relaxed. Its spinal reflexes may be normal or depressed. Usually the patellar reflex disappears before the flexor reflex but this is variable.

The severely paralyzed patient is atonic. When picked up and held with the trunk supported, the neck and limbs hang limp and useless with no tone generated and no movement observed. This contrasts with the observations in a dog paralyzed by a severe cranial cervical spinal cord lesion. That lesion causes upper motor neuron paralysis and spasticity and that dog's limbs are hypertonic and rigidly extended but with severely reduced or no motion.

All spinal reflexes are usually absent in the recumbent paralyzed patient with polyneuritis. The tail may also be paralyzed but usually retains some tone. The severely paralyzed patient cannot move its neck or tail. The perineal reflex is always normal.

Pain sensation is always normal and many patients seem hyperesthetic to sensory stimuli that normally would not bother them. They move their head and jaws and try to bark when only modest pressure is exerted on the digits with forceps or upon moderate muscle palpation. Weakness of the voice is obvious. This hyperesthesia is a feature of polyradiculoneuritis that does not occur with botulism or tick paralysis. It is not evident in all patients (Table 4–3).

A possible explanation for this apparent paradox of mild dorsal root lesions associated with hyperesthesia is as follows. There are cell bodies in the dorsal grey column whose axons comprise the spinothalamic tracts of the pain projection pathway. Their activity is modulated by inhibitory neurons in the substantia gelatinosa in the dorsal aspect of the dorsal grey column. These inhibitory interneurons are inhibited by small neurons primarily concerned with noxious stimuli and generation of the pain pathway. These inhibitory interneurons are activated by the larger neurons primarily concerned with proprioceptive function. Pain projection is therefore a summation of activity of the large and small neurons in the dorsal roots that terminate in the substantial gelatinosa and central projection nuclei of the dorsal grey column. Loss of the larger neurons lowers the threshold to response of the dorsal grey column cell bodies for the spinothalamic pathway and may be the basis for the hyperesthesia that is observed in polyradiculoneuritis. Other possible explanations include a decreased stimulus threshold of unmyelinated afferent fibers which have been described in ventral roots where the lesion is most severe.[34]

Bladder and rectal paralysis are not observed. In the first few days of acute paralysis, retention may be observed owing to the overall recumbent state of the animal. Within a short while the dog will excrete normally.

Electromyography 6 to 7 days after the onset will show excessive fibrillation and positive sharp waves in those dogs with significant axonal involvement and denervation. Widespread primary demyelination will cause a delayed motor nerve conduction velocity. When there is significant evidence of axonal degeneration there may be a significantly slower rate of recovery; thus the density of denervation potentials may have prognostic value. Lumbosacral CSF may have an elevated protein level without a significant pleocytosis.

Usually after a week of clinical signs, muscle atrophy is present. This will have to be palpated in long-haired dogs. Muscle atrophy will rapidly progress and become very severe in most all the appendicular and axial muscles. It is especially prominent in the proximal limb muscles. No atrophy occurs in the head muscles.

The duration of paresis or paralysis is variable. A few dogs show rapid recovery in a few days to a week. Most tetraplegic dogs require 3 to 8 weeks to become ambulatory. A few may require 3 to 4 months to become ambulatory and still completely recover, including return of muscle mass. A few have residual muscle wasting and may have lack of endurance. Recovery in most dogs follows the reverse order of the onset of signs. If pelvic limb weakness occurred first followed by thoracic limb weakness, recovery will first occur in the thoracic limbs. When these dogs first start to walk they show the characteristic short-strided "lame" gait of a dog with partial paresis.

An occasional patient dies of this disease from respiratory paralysis. These are more often the dogs with an acute onset of recumbency and total paralysis. Careful monitoring of oxygen levels in the blood will determine the patient that should be placed on a respirator. A rare patient remains recumbent without recovery.

There is no specific treatment for this disease in dogs because the cause of the disease is still not specifically known. Some clinicians use large doses of steroids, but there is no clear indication that such treatment is associated with a faster recovery rate. The same observation has been made in humans for the Landry-Guillain-Barré syndrome, which is an acute polyradiculoneuritis similar to this one in dogs.[45, 93] Good nursing care is essential. The recumbent patient is maintained best on a water bed. Skin sores over bony prominences are rare in dogs that are kept on water beds and are frequently turned. A 3- to 4-ft deep bedding of straw or hay is nearly as effective if the animal is turned frequently. It is important to be sure these dogs evacuate their bowels and bladder and are kept clean of any excrement.

Protection from future attacks of this disease is apparently short-lived or nonexistent, for quite a few patients have full recovery only to have the disease occur again on subsequent exposure to another raccoon. As many as five separate episodes of this disease have been recorded in several dogs, and dogs with two or three episodes are common. The severity of the subsequent episodes is variable and they do not necessarily become progressively worse each time.

The lesion of polyradiculoneuritis is primarily in the ventral roots and peripheral nerves, which accounts for the lower motor neuron–general somatic efferent signs that predominate in the clinical disease. It consists of primary segmental demyelination and axonal degeneration.[42] The larger, more heavily myelinated axons are the most affected in this disease. Mononuclear interstitial cellular infiltrates occur in affected nerves. The extent and composition of these infiltrates vary. Lymphocytes and plasma cells are the most common.

Pathogenic studies suggest that this is an immune-mediated disease. Electromicroscopic studies suggest that the primary demyelination does not require macrophage involvement and that it may be mediated by humoral mechanisms. A similar mechanism is proposed for the axonal degeneration. Increased levels of immunoglobulin G have been determined in the serum and CSF of dogs with acute polyradiculoneuritis.

Experimental reproduction of the disease has been difficult. On one occasion the same clinical disease was produced following injection of raccoon saliva intradermally into a coonhound that previously had the natural disease and had recovered.[101] It is assumed that the limiting factor is some unique immunologic factor present in the susceptible animal. The specific source or health of the raccoon is less important.

In one study, a very severe experimental allergic neuritis was produced in the littermate offspring of patients that had recovered from the natural disease.[98, 100] Intradermal inoculation of aliquots of the same emulsion of canine sciatic nerve and Freund's complete adjuvant into random source dogs produced only minimal disease in a few dogs. This suggested a genetic predisposition of dogs susceptible to this immune-mediated disease.

Coonhound paralysis may be a useful model for the study of the human disease, the Landry-Guillain-Barré syndrome, which is identical in its clinical features and similar in its pathologic features. The cause of the human disorder remains unknown, but it is thought to be an immune-mediated disease that may be indirectly related to a primary viral disease in another system. The human disease usually follows another infection, such as upper respiratory infections, infectious mononucleosis, and other systemic diseases, by 7 to 10 days.

Acute Idiopathic Polyneuropathy. A progressive lower motor neuron tetraparesis has been recognized in otherwise healthy dogs with no history of prior illness or exposure to raccoons.[24, 141] The lower motor neuron paresis progressed from pelvic to thoracic limbs and reached its peak in from 1 to 21 days. Spinal reflexes were depressed or absent. Pain perception was retained and hyperesthesia was not evident. No signs of cranial nerve deficit were observed.

Denervation potentials and slow motor nerve conduction velocity were observed in varying degrees. CSF was normal in those dogs from which it was obtained.

Dogs without secondary complications usually recovered in about 3 to 6 weeks.

Fascicular biopsies of peripheral nerves revealed minimal degenerative changes. One autopsy showed demyelination with extensive mononuclear inflammatory cell infiltrate in roots and proximal nerves. The lesion appears to be a polyneuritis of unknown cause. More study is necessary to determine its clinical and pathologic comparison to coonhound paralysis.

Post-Rabies Vaccination. Rarely a dog will develop the clinical signs of an acute polyneuritis or polyneuropathy 7 to 10 days following rabies vaccination. Some of these are known to be inactivated vaccines of mouse brain origin. This disease seems to be clinically similar to coonhound paralysis and acute polyneuropathy. Recovery usually occurs similar to these diseases. The relationship to the rabies vaccination remains to be proven. It is not thought to be a direct effect of the virus and is a different syndrome from the rare case of acute polioencephalomyelitis due to rabies vaccine virus.

Distal Denervating Disease. Distal denervating disease is a degenerative neuropathy that affects the distal terminal motor axons of dogs.[90] There is no obvious sex, age, or breed predilection. It is a common neuropathy in the United Kingdom. A lower motor neuron tetraparesis or tetraplegia develops acutely over a few days or more slowly over 3 to 4 weeks. The signs of paresis are limited to limb and trunk muscles plus a loss of bark in some dogs. The progressive weakness is accompanied by loss of tone and spinal reflexes. Muscle atrophy becomes severe especially in proximal extensor muscles. Proprioception and pain sensation are normal. Hyperesthesia is not reported and signs of cranial nerve deficit are not usually evident.

Denervation potentials are present in almost all appendicular muscles and in some axial muscles. Motor nerve conduction velocity may be reduced, as is the evoked muscle action potential.

Most dogs recover completely in 4 to 6 weeks following development of maximum weakness. Some may take longer.

The lesion consists of a diffuse degeneration of distal intramuscular axons and myelin with collateral sprouting. A toxic cause is proposed but remains unknown.

This disease is remarkably similar to acute polyradiculoneuritis (coonhound paralysis) and acute idiopathic polyneuropathy. Thorough electrodiagnostic and biopsy studies will be necessary to differentiate these diseases.

Brachial Plexus Neuritis-Neuropathy. A syndrome has been recognized in the dog similar to brachial plexus neuropathy in humans, which in some instances follows prophylactic inoculations such as tetanus antiserum.[1, 41, 181] Such cases have been referred to as serum neuritis. The disease is characterized by a sudden onset of pain and paresis in the thoracic limbs. Signs of paresis progress rapidly and are limited to muscles innervated by the brachial plexus. It is proposed that the allergic condi-

TABLE 4–3. DIFFERENTIAL FEATURES OF ACUTE DIFFUSE LOWER MOTOR NEURON PARALYSIS[14]

Polyradiculoneuritis
Exposure to raccoons
Minimal cranial nerve signs
  Occasional facial paresis
Hyperesthesia
Protein in lumbosacral CSF
Muscle atrophy after 5 to 7 days

Tick Paralysis
Tick infestation
Response to tick removal
Minimum cranial nerve signs
  Occasional facial paresis
No hyperesthesia
No atrophy

Botulism
Exposure to spoiled food
Significant cranial nerve signs
  Weak facial and jaw muscles
  Dysphagia, regurgitation (megaesophagus)
No hyperesthesia
Mydriasis, if severe
No atrophy

tion causes a swelling of the spinal nerves that compress the nerves where they pass through the intervertebral foramina. Destruction of axons at that point causes Wallerian degeneration in the rest of the peripheral nerves distal to the foramina. The prognosis for functional recovery in man is considered good, but it may take up to 3 years or longer for the destroyed axons to regenerate and reinnervate the paralyzed muscles. In some patients with brachial plexus neuropathy, other illnesses or strenuous exercise preceded the onset of neurologic signs. In others, there has been no history to associate with this disease.

A 9-month-old female Great Dane suddenly developed severe paresis of the thoracic limbs, preceded by 2 allergic episodes with facial edema and generalized urticaria over a 48-hour period. A diet of horse meat had been instituted 2 weeks prior to the first allergic attack. Severe lower motor neuron deficit was found in both thoracic limbs. Flexor reflexes were depressed and neurogenic atrophy developed rapidly in all thoracic limb muscles. The signs were bilateral but not symmetric. Pelvic limb function was essentially normal, but patellar reflexes were depressed. Facial paresis was present on one side. Electromyography showed evidence of denervation. Biopsy of the sensory branches of the radial nerve in the forearm revealed extensive Wallerian degeneration. Skin testing showed hypersensitivity to horse serum. Over a period of 9 weeks no change was noted, and a necropsy was performed. Severe axonal and myelin degeneration had occurred in many of the peripheral nerves, leaving only cords of collagen, fibroblasts, and Schwann cells. The degenerative lesions were limited to the peripheral nerves of the thoracic limbs and could be followed proximally to the level of the spinal nerve component.

CAT. I have observed a lower motor neuron paralysis in an adult cat similar to acute canine polyradiculoneuritis. Tetraplegia developed with atonia, areflexia, and atrophy. There were no cranial nerve signs. The cat completely recovered in a few weeks after developing complete tetraplegia.

GOAT. A 6-week-old Alpine goat was studied for a progressive pelvic limb paresis and ataxia. At necropsy segmental demyelination was observed in the spinal roots accompanied by a mononuclear cell inflammation. A polyradiculoneuritis was diagnosed.[132]

CATTLE. There has been speculation that beef calves may develop a syndrome resembling polyneuritis following strain-19 Brucella vaccination. The signs referred to were limited to the pelvic limbs, and the calves did not recover.[155]

I have observed a clinical syndrome of rapidly progressive diffuse neuromuscular weakness in a 4-month-old female Hereford with onset of signs 1 day after strain-19 Brucella vaccination. The heifer went down on the second day with profound weakness and no evidence of ataxia. Voluntary movement, tone, and spinal reflexes were retained. She became able to stand 10 days later and made a nearly normal recovery. Muscle enzymes were normal throughout the illness. The nature of this disease and its relationship to Brucella vaccination remains to be determined.

Chronic Polyneuritis-Polyneuropathy
DOG

Chronic Polyneuritis.[40, 41, 44] A number of mature dogs have been observed with a slowly progressive weakness of one or more limbs, and occasionally with facial paresis and a loss of voice volume. Asymmetry of signs is common but not constant. If advanced lesions are present, the animal may be unable to support its weight and its limbs may slide out from under it. In the early stages of chronic canine polyneuritis the resemblance of the lower motor neuron paresis to the lame gait caused by musculoskeletal disease often has confused the diagnosis. Normal joint palpation, the lack of joint or bone pain, the presence of neurogenic atrophy and sometimes hyporeflexia, and the demonstration of paresis on postural reaction testing help to establish the signs as neurogenic. Ataxia generally is not observed in peripheral nerve disorders.

Electromyography, conduction times and biopsy of nerve tissue help confirm the diagnosis. If there is nerve root involvement, an albuminocytologic dissociation may be present in the CSF.

Pathologic changes are variable and suggest a diverse pathogenesis.[60, 61]

Inherited Hypertrophic Neuropathy in Tibetan Mastiffs. An autosomal recessive inherited hypertrophic neuropathy has been recognized in Tibetan Mastiff dogs.[39, 166] The rapidly progressive weakness begins between 7 and 12 weeks of age. Weakness first occurs in the pelvic limbs and in most dogs involves the thoracic limbs in a few days. In some only the pelvic limbs are primarily affected. Pelvic limb weakness is evident by the decreased ability to support weight with a prominent lack of tarsal extension causing a crouched, plantigrade appearance of the limbs. Hypotonia is evident. Patellar reflexes are absent and flexor reflexes are mildly depressed. Pain sensation is normal. Mild muscle wasting occurs, but severe neurogenic atrophy is not evident.

Severely affected dogs become recumbent within 3 weeks of the onset of signs. Some voluntary movement is retained in the limbs but it is insufficient for standing and walking. Limb contractures frequently occur in the recumbent dogs. A few improve after 6 to 7 weeks and retain the ability to stand and walk but retain the shuffling plantigrade gait in the pelvic limbs.

Electromyography shows rare denervation potentials, but motor nerve conduction velocities are markedly slow. This suggests a significant myelin abnormality. Cerebrospinal fluid has normal cell values but elevated protein.

Light and electron microscopic study of peripheral nerves and roots reveals widespread primary demyelination and Schwann cell hyperplasia, producing "onion bulbs" with relatively little early degeneration of axons. Mild axonal degeneration also occurs in chronic lesions.

Pedigree analysis of affected puppies from one kennel substantiated an autosomal recessive inheritance for this disease.[166] The initial study showed that all 15 affected puppies were produced by breeding of 3 sires and 5 dams, all of which were clinically normal. Ten litters from these breedings contained a total of 62 puppies, of which 15 were affected. In the United States, the Tibetan Mastiff breed has developed through intensive breeding and now includes only about 280 animals.

These initial studies suggest an inherited inborn defect in the ability of Schwann cells to form or maintain a stable myelin sheath.

Giant Axonal Neuropathy (GAN). Giant axonal neuropathy is a presumed autosomal recessive inherited disease of young German Shepherds.[52, 55, 56] Clinical signs begin around 15 months of age and slowly progress. Gait abnormalities are limited to the pelvic limbs, with a symmetric paresis and ataxia. Over a few months there is decreased ability to remain standing, accompanied by loss of patellar reflexes, distal muscle atrophy, and hypalgesia in the pelvic limbs. The flexor reflex is retained. By 21 months fecal incontinence may occur but bladder control is normal. Loss of the bark and regurgitation may occur between 16 and 20 months. Progressive loss of esophageal motility is responsible for the regurgitation.

Electrophysiologic abnormalities precede the onset of clinical signs and consist of decreased amplitude of evoked muscle action potentials and sensory nerve action potentials. Denervation potentials occur later.

Lesions are widespread in the central and peripheral nervous system. Focal axonal swelling containing neurofilaments are observed in the distal portions of peripheral nerves and in central neurons, which is the basis for the name of the disease. Secondary demyelination is associated with this axonal lesion. Morphologic and chemical studies show that the accumulated neurofilaments are normal.

The clinical signs are thought to be primarily the result of the peripheral nervous system lesions. Spontaneous improvement or recovery does not occur.

Distal Symmetric Polyneuropathy. A 1.3-year-old Great Dane dog is described at Auburn, Alabama, with a distal symmetric polyneuropathy.[23] A similar patient was studied in Australia.[68] After 4 weeks of progressive gait abnormality, neurologic examination revealed a hypermetric, ataxic pelvic limb gait with atrophy of the muscles distal to both stifles. Postural reactions were depressed in all four limbs. Tone and spinal reflexes were normal. After 4 more weeks of progression, muscle atrophy was evident in both forearms and in the muscles of mastication.

Denervation potentials occurred in atrophic appendicular muscles. Sciatic and ulnar nerve stimulation did not evoke any action potentials of distal muscles.

Axonal and myelin degeneration were severe in the distal parts of peripheral nerves in all limbs. The lesions suggested a dying-back process of unknown etiology.

Metabolic Neuropathy. Peripheral neuropathy accompanies chronic diabetes mellitus and chronic renal failure in humans. Diabetes mellitus, chronic nephritis, hyperadrenocorticism, and hypothyroidism are common in dogs and cats. Neuromyopathy associated with these metabolic disorders has been suggested in domestic animals, but a specific relationship between lesions, clinical signs, and the metabolic defect remains to be described.

We have observed a presumed diabetic neuropathy in cats. These cats with diabetes mellitus developed weakness of tarsal extension and walked with a plantigrade gait. Electrophysiologic studies supported a neurogenic basis for the paresis. Improvement followed therapy for the diabetes mellitus.

A myopathy has been observed in dogs with

hyperadrenocorticism and hypothyroidism and has been suggested for diabetes mellitus. No peripheral nerve lesions were seen in 7 dogs with chronic diabetes mellitus.[21]

Adult hypothyroid dogs have been observed with slowly progressive neuromuscular weakness associated with scapular and masticatory muscle atrophy. A myopathy is apparent on biopsy. Improvement in strength follows thyroid therapy.

Mild facial paresis and/or peripheral vestibular abnormalities have been observed in hypothyroid dogs secondary to pituitary neoplasia with little response to thyroid therapy. Severe inspiratory dyspnea from laryngeal paresis and mild regurgitation associated with megaesophagus have been observed in hypothyroid dogs that may show some response to thyroid therapy. Others require laryngeal surgery. Polymyositis has been observed in dogs with lymphocytic thyroiditis. Myopathy with myotonia occurs in dogs with hyperadrenocorticism and rarely in hypothyroid dogs.

Malignant neoplasms, especially carcinomas, are associated with neuromyopathy in humans and should be investigated in domestic animals.

HORSE

Equine Polyneuritis—Neuritis of the Cauda Equina. This is a disease of horses that affects adult horses of either sex and of any breed.[43, 47, 63, 81, 133, 134, 145, 146, 172] The signs are usually progressive with an acute or chronic course and reflect the anatomic components most profoundly affected, the cauda equina.

Most patients have a profound loss of all function of the caudal nerves to the tail and sacral nerves to the anus, perineum, rectum, and bladder. The tail will be weak to totally paralyzed, atonic, and areflexic. The anus will be hypotonic or atonic and widely dilated and areflexic. The rectum will be full and require manual evacuation. The bladder will be full and urine will dribble from the vulva or penis. Patients with signs of lower motor neuron paralysis to these regions will have complete sensory deficit and will be analgesic in the tail, anus, perineum, and laterally in the area of skin innervated by the most cranially affected sacral nerve.

The external prepuce or sheath will have normal sensation. This is supplied by the second to fourth lumbar spinal nerves that comprise the genitofemoral nerve. The skin on the surface of the protruded relaxed penis will be analgesic if the perineum is analgesic, as it receives sensory supply from a branch of the pudendal nerve from the sacral plexus.

The earliest signs include a limp tail and a failure to excrete normally and sometimes an apparent paresthesia with the horse rubbing its tail or buttocks on objects.

As the disease progresses a mild paresis and ataxia may occur in the pelvic limbs, reflecting more cranial involvement of sacral and lumbar rootlets and spinal nerves. The signs are usually symmetric. Atrophy and/or increased sensitivity to palpation may be evident in the gluteal muscles. Rarely there is evidence of thoracic limb deficit due to involvement of spinal nerves to the brachial plexus.

In a few horses cranial nerve deficits are observed. Most commonly these reflect involvement of the facial and vestibulocochlear nerves and rarely the trigeminal nerve. These signs are usually asymmetric and consist of a unilateral facial paresis and ipsilateral peripheral vestibular deficit.

This disease may be progressive only in its early development and may remain static with no change in the signs due to the sacral and caudal nerve lesion. Rarely the cranial nerve signs may recover on one side and appear on the other side.

The lesions consist of a remarkable proliferation of inflammatory cells and connective tissue elements in the extradural components of the affected sacral and caudal nerves. This is a granulomatous inflammation with extensive fibrosis that abounds with lymphocytes and plasma cells and often has eosinophils, giant cells, and microabscesses present. This is associated with extensive degeneration of axons and myelin. This inflammatory proliferation is so extensive that it causes these nerves to adhere together and may nearly fill the remaining space in the vertebral canal. Sometimes the granulomatous lesion extends through the intervertebral foramina into the adjacent axial muscles. This gross and microscopic granulomatous lesion is only apparent outside the dura. The intradural components of these affected spinal nerves have no gross lesions but have a microscopic lesion consisting of areas of inflammation with infiltration by lymphocytes, plasma cells, and macrophages. Demyelination is most extensive in the area of cell infiltrates but also occurs in the absence of penetrating macrophages. Axonal degeneration is not as profound as in the extradural nerves. The inflammatory segmental demyelination may precede the irreversible axonal degeneration.

The intradural lesion most resembles the lesions seen in canine polyradiculoneuritis and may result from an immune-mediated disease.

Immunologic studies have determined the presence of anti-P_2 bovine myelin basic protein antibodies in the sera of horses with neuritis of the cauda equina, which suggests an autoimmune basis for this disease.[109] Extensive culturing of the intradural and extradural granulomatous lesions has not revealed a pathogenic agent. There is speculation that this lesion may be indirectly related to a persistent infection with the equine herpes virus I agent or, less likely, equine viral arteritis. This remains to be proven.

Spinal Cord

Lesions that affect the cell bodies of the general somatic efferent lower motor neuron in the spinal cord produce similar signs of lower motor neuron disease that are specific to the area unnervated.

Focal Myelopathy from Compression. A neoplasm, extruded intervertebral disk, or vertebral fracture that compresses spinal cord segments L4, L5, and L6 produces a paresis or paralysis of the pelvic limbs due to the spinal cord dysfunction. This is accompanied by a bilateral femoral nerve paralysis and loss of the patellar reflex as a result of the direct injury to the cell bodies of these femoral nerve neurons.

A similar lesion between T3 and L3 causes paresis and ataxia or paralysis of the pelvic limbs with normal or hyperactive pelvic limb reflexes and no clinical signs of lower motor neuron disease in the neurologic examination. This is because spinal cord segments L4 through S1 are not involved directly with the lesion. There may be destruction of general somatic efferent lower motor neuron cell bodies in one or more segments, but unless they supply limb muscles their region of denervation is difficult to detect except by means of electromyography. EMG of the axial muscles may find the level of the lesion by showing denervation potentials in the muscles innervated by the affected segment.

Embolic Myelopathy. Embolic myelopathy has been associated with fibrocartilaginous emboli in both arteries and veins in the parenchyma and leptomeninges at all levels of the spinal cord.[51, 70, 79, 85, 86, 96, 113, 199] The signs are sudden in onset and usually stabilize within 24 hours. Rarely, signs progress from 48 to 72 hours. From then on, they remain unchanged or improve, depending on the degree of ischemic compromise of the tissue.

Although this disease is more common in adult dogs of the larger breeds, it has been observed in small breeds and in dogs as young as 3 months old.[138] It has only been seen in nonchondrodystrophic breeds. Any portion of the spinal cord can be affected, unilaterally or bilaterally. Usually the lesion is confined to a few adjacent segments. No lesions are seen in the brain or in other organs.

The infarcts that occur may be ischemic or hemorrhagic and usually affect both grey and white matter at the level of the lesion. Clinical signs reflect the location of the lesion. If the infarction occurs on the right side of the spinal cord from the sixth through the eighth cervical spinal cord segments, the loss of the cell bodies in the lateral portion of the ventral grey columns causes a lower motor neuron paralysis of the ipsilateral thoracic limb. The adjacent white matter lesion causes ataxia and spastic paresis, or paralysis of the ipsilateral pelvic limb. Ordinarily dogs do not show evidence of a painful experience associated with the development of this lesion. Usually no pain is elicited on vertebral manipulation.

In some dogs the emboli may cause almost total infarction of the caudal, sacral, and caudal lumbar and middle lumbar spinal cord segments. This results in complete lower motor neuron paralysis of the tail, perineum, bladder, rectum, and pelvic limbs. Tone and spinal reflexes are all absent. In addition, there is analgesia of the affected area due to loss of the spinal cord portion of the general somatic afferent neurons entering from the dorsal roots, as well as of the cell bodies of the neurons in the dorsal grey column. Despite the destruction of the spinal cord white matter, the clinical signs reflect the grey matter destruction. Cases such as these with signs of extensive grey matter destruction have a very poor prognosis.

The major diseases to differentiate from this one when there is such a peracute focal spinal cord disorder are external injury and internal injury from intervertebral disk extrusion. The history should permit external injury to be ruled out. If the dog acts as if it is in pain or is painful to vertebral palpation, an extruded intervertebral disk should be suspected. This clinical sign alone will not permit differentiation of these two diseases. Immediate radiography and myelography are essential because the disk extrusion should be considered for surgical removal, whereas the fibrocartilaginous embolic disease is not a surgical disease.

Plain radiographs are normal. At the onset slight swelling of the parenchyma may be observed on a myelogram. Within the first few hours cerebrospinal fluid may show an elevated neutrophil count along with mild elevation of protein levels. After 24 to 48 hours cell counts are normal, or there is a slight elevation of mononuclear cells and the protein typically remains elevated.

Therapy consists of corticosteroids as they would be used to treat any spinal cord injury. Prognosis depends on the severity of the lesion. Animals with total dysfunction and significant grey matter involvement have a poor prognosis. As a rule, if any recovery is to occur there will be some indication of improvement in the 7 to 10 days following the onset of the clinical signs. It may take a few weeks to regain a functional gait. Approximately half of the patients we have diagnosed with this disease have improved to be functional pets.

In order to produce the ischemic myelopathy that is observed it is necessary to simultaneously compromise many closely associated small blood vessels to the same region of the spinal cord. This would require multiple emboli, and many emboli are usually observed at autopsy. Because the embolic material found in arteries and/or veins of the affected parenchyma or leptomeninges stains like fibrocartilage, it is assumed that the source of the fibrocartilage must be from degenerating nucleus pulposus.[197] In some patients intervertebral disk material has been found projecting into the ventral internal vertebral venous plexus that is adjacent to the dorsolateral aspect of the disks.[96] In other patients branches of the spinal arteries have been found growing into a chronic intervertebral disk protrusion, and fibrocartilage has been observed in the lumen of these vessels.[96] In many patients there is no good evidence of intervertebral disk degeneration, protrusion, or extrusion. This may reflect how careful or complete the examination is. Although common in humans, intervertebral disk extrusion into the adjacent marrow of the vertebral body is rare or nonexistent in the domestic animal.

Fibrocartilaginous emboli have not been found in vessels associated with spinal cord infarcts in the chondrodystrophic breeds with intervertebral disk extrusions. All reports and my experience have been in nonchondrodystrophic breeds. The clinical disease is more common in young adults but it has been observed at almost any age, including dogs as young as 3 months. A few dogs have a history of related trauma but this can be clearly denied in many patients. It is difficult to rationalize

the intervertebral disk as the source of the fibrocartilage in dogs of nonchondrodystrophic breeds that are less than 1 year of age without a history of trauma. More careful study of the intervertebral disks plus related vasculature is necessary in these patients.

Fibrocartilaginous embolic myelopathy has also been reported in the cat[198] and the horse[178] with evidence of intervertebral disk protrusion and in a sow with fracture at a vertebral epiphyseal growth plate.[152]

Diffuse Myelomalacia. A diffuse progressive myelomalacia occasionally can be found following an acute intervertebral disk extrusion at any level of the thoracolumbar vertebral column.[84] It also was observed in one patient in which a neurofibroma was compressing the lumbar spinal cord; it occasionally follows the focal myelomalacia caused by external injury. In a few patients no associated vertebral column lesion could be identified. The lesion is a combination of ischemic and hemorrhagic infarction of the entire parenchyma of the spinal cord, but the roots in the leptomeninges are spared. Hemorrhage often occurs in the subarachnoid space. The spinal cord lesion has been termed hematomyelia, but this is not accurate. The parenchymal bleeding that occurs is secondary to the infarction. Despite the severe ischemic lesion, no significant lesions of the vessels have been observed. Necrosis of the vessels takes place in the infarct, but this is assumed to be secondary to the ischemic lesion. The lesion appears to be the result of a sudden and progressive occlusion of all the microvasculature to the spinal cord parenchyma. This may be due to a progressive release of catecholamines or similar vasoconstrictor substance.

Careful study of a patient from the start shows that the myelomalacia first occurs at the site of the disk extrusion, and then typically descends and ascends from that site. Occasionally it only descends or only ascends through the adjacent spinal cord segments. In a few instances a portion of a spinal cord segment is normal between areas of myelomalacia, indicating that this is not just a pressure-induced phenomenon.

Usually, at the cranial extent of the lesion in the cervical spinal cord there is a core of necrosis in the central canal and ventral aspect of the dorsal funiculi.

The typical patient with ascending and descending myelomalacia secondary to protrusion of an intervertebral disk at any site along the thoracolumbar vertebral column begins with a sudden onset of complete paraplegia. At the initial examination of the pelvic limbs the reflexes may be intact and hyperactive (spastic). Later examination (48 to 72 hours) reveals a flaccid paraplegia with atonia and total areflexia of the muscles of the pelvic limbs. The tail is flaccid and the anus is dilated and unresponsive to stimuli. There is no pain perception from any of these areas. The abdomen is flaccid. At that time or within the next few days the animal begins to act paretic and ataxic in the thoracic limbs. It prefers to lie in lateral recumbency with the thoracic limbs extended, and demonstrates exquisite pain when handled in the thoracic or cervical region. Reflexes persist in the thoracic limbs at this time. A line of analgesia usually can be located in the cranial thoracic region. Bilateral Horner's syndrome may occur. Respirations progressively become more diaphragmatic. Death often occurs in 7 to 10 days from the onset of signs and is caused by respiratory paralysis. There is no treatment for this condition.

Occasionally the myelomalacia only descends and therefore death does not occur, but no therapy is known that will bring about recovery once these lesions occur.

This extensive lower motor neuron disease with analgesia is not difficult to recognize, and patients should not be subject to surgical therapy. The lesion has developed following immediate decompressive laminectomy of the acute extrusion and prior to recognizable signs of progressive myelomalacia; thus it would seem that such surgery is not preventive.

Poliomyelomalacia in Pigs. A poliomyelomalacia has been observed in young pigs, 6 weeks to 5 months old.[102, 143] The disease usually occurs over a short period of time as an outbreak in several pigs that are kept in the same environment. The signs occur suddenly and include ataxia and paresis of all four limbs. Pigs rapidly become too weak to stand and have loss of patellar and flexor reflexes.

The lesion is bilaterally symmetric in the spinal cord grey matter and predominates in the cervical and lumbar spinal cord segments. Similar lesions and signs occur when an acute nicotinamide deficiency is induced by injecting 6 aminonicotinamide intraperitoneally into pigs.[144] A natural acute nicotinamide deficiency is proposed caused by ingestion of an antimetabolite of nicotinamide. Selenium toxicosis produces similar lesions experimentally in pigs and has been documented in the feed of nat-

urally affected pigs.[200] How this relates to nicotinamide deficiency remains to be proven.

Inflammations. These may affect focal or diffuse areas of the spinal cord grey matter and produce associated signs of lower motor neuron disease.

Polioencephalomyelitis caused by an enterovirus in young pigs (Teschen's, Talfan's, or Ontario disease) has a predilection for spinal cord grey matter.

Rabies encephalomyelitis also may produce an ascending type of lower motor neuron paralysis, since it destroys more of the spinal cord grey matter. The signs of this disease are extremely variable but one should be on the lookout for it when lower motor neuron signs accompany the ataxia, paresis, and indications of cerebral disturbance. A hypotonic tail often is found in rabid cattle. Horses with rabies often present with spinal cord signs.

Vaccine-induced rabies in cats initially produces an LMN paresis in the limb that is injected. These LMN signs rapidly progress to both pelvic limbs, tail, anus, and bladder. The poliomyelitis of the lumbosacral intumescence results from the rabies virus entering the spinal cord from the axons at the site of the injection.

A polioencephalomyelitis of unknown cause has been reported in cats with severe spinal cord lesions affecting grey and white matter.[98, 182] These cats ranged in age from 3 months to 6 years old. Clinical signs of chronic progressive spinal cord disease predominated but seizures occasionally occurred.

Occasionally, the canine distemper virus or *Toxoplasma gondii* in dogs destroys enough spinal cord grey matter to produce lower motor neuron signs along with the signs of destruction of white matter. Although toxoplasmosis can affect any portion of the central nervous system with focal or diffuse lesions, these lesions may predominate in the grey matter of the lumbosacral intumescence in puppies. These are usually chronic, slowly progressive lesions that cause LMN signs with paresis, hypotonia, hyporeflexia to areflexia, and muscle atrophy. As the pelvic limb muscles become denervated, a remarkable contracture of the denervated muscles may produce rigidly extended limbs that cannot be flexed manually. This is especially apparent if the quadriceps femoris muscle is affected by an L4 to L6 ventral grey column lesion and may be unilateral or bilateral. These puppies also often have a myositis due to the toxoplasma infection. It is assumed that the muscle contracture is a sequela to the denervation in young, rapidly growing puppies. However, the primary muscle lesion may also be involved. These puppies may not have other signs of systemic toxoplasmosis and may be alert, eat well, and act healthy except for the neuromuscular signs. Toxoplasmosis should always be suspected when signs of progressive neurologic and muscle disease are present. Abnormal CSF and elevated serum creatine kinase will help to confirm these observations. Serum toxoplasma antibody titers may be absent, which supports immunosuppression as the reason for the susceptibility to this disease.

Motor Neuron Disease—Abiotrophy

HEREDITARY NEURONAL ABIOTROPHY IN THE SWEDISH LAPLAND DOG. An autosomal recessive hereditary disease of young Swedish Lapland dogs characterized by neuronal abiotrophy causes tetraplegia, muscle atrophy, and severe limb contractures.[158] The onset is around 5 weeks of age. The paralysis involves the general somatic efferent lower motor neuron system, especially to appendicular muscles, and is rapidly progressive. The neurogenic atrophy is accompanied by severe limb deformity and arthrogryposis related to the young age and rapid growth of the animal.

Neuronal cell body degeneration occurs in the ventral grey column of the spinal cord. This predominates in the lateral portion at the intumescences, which accounts for the clinical signs. The neuronal degeneration is diffuse, involving spinal ganglion cell bodies, cerebellar Purkinje neurons, myelin and axons in spinocerebellar tracts, dorsal funiculi, and the central portions of vestibulocochlear, optic, and trigeminal nerves. Only the loss of general somatic efferent neurons is reflected in the clinical signs.

HEREDITARY SPINAL MUSCULAR ATROPHY IN BRITTANY SPANIELS. A progressive weakness and muscle atrophy occurs in Brittany Spaniels that have an inherited degeneration of ventral grey column and brain stem motor neurons.[36, 128] Most dogs are affected by 4 to 5 months of age. A few have onset before 2 months or not until 8 months. Weakness first occurs in proximal appendicular and axial muscles. Pelvic limb signs are more pronounced with a wide-based, crouched posture, and waddling gait. Fatigue rapidly follows mild exercise. Weakness progresses to the thoracic limbs. The head may droop or bob and swing side to side during walking. After months of progression they may become unable to stand. The period to tetraplegia varies from 4 to 26 months.

Reflexes become depressed in more severely affected muscles. Atrophy is most pronounced in the proximal appendicular muscles and epaxial muscles adjacent to the vertebral spines. Weakness develops in the facial and tongue muscles and the gag reflex may be depressed. Atrophy of facial muscles may cause elevation of the ears and wrinkling of the face. Masticatory muscle atrophy may occur.

On EMG denervation potentials are most pronounced in the axial muscles. Nerve conduction velocities are normal.

The lesion consists of a loss of motoneurons from the spinal cord ventral grey column and brain stem nuclei. Degenerative changes are evident in some of the remaining motoneurons.

Pedigree analysis suggests that this motoneuron abiotrophy is inherited as an autosomal recessive abnormality.

STOCKARD'S PARALYSIS. Stockard's paralysis is a progressive paraparesis in young dogs from selected matings of Great Danes and Bloodhounds or Great Danes and Saint Bernards.[171] At 11 to 14 weeks these puppies develop rapidly progressive pelvic limb paresis that evolves over a few days. Some become paraplegic. The distal pelvic limb muscles are most severely affected.

This disease was described as a complex hereditary lethal (abiotrophy) for localized lumbar somatic motoneurons and preganglionic motoneurons resulting in paralysis. These matings were all carried out in a laboratory. To my knowledge this disease has not been observed outside this experimental setting.

Muscle Disease[30]

Myositis.

This disease is described here because muscle is the effector organ in the neuromuscular system and, when the muscle is diseased, the clinical signs may resemble those of lower motor neuron disease.[30]

INFECTIOUS MYOSITIS. Bacterial myositis is uncommon in small animals. *Toxoplasma gondii* produces a myositis that is often associated with encephalomyelitis. It is most common in puppies. Progressive weakness may be followed by a severe muscle atrophy with shortening of the muscles resulting in rigidly extended limbs. *Leptospira icterohaemorrhagica* can cause a generalized hemorrhagic necrotizing myopathy as part of a systemic infection.

IDIOPATHIC OR IMMUNE-MEDIATED MYOSITIS. Although the idiopathic or immune-mediated myositis is divided into separate diseases for discussion, they probably represent clinical and pathologic variations of a single primary muscle inflammatory disease. This polymyositis may present as a masticatory, pharyngeal-esophageal, focal appendicular, or a diffuse muscular clinical problem, depending on where the lesion is most profound.[7, 57, 58, 64, 114, 190]

Masticatory Myositis. This is the most commonly recognized myositis and occurs in acute and chronic forms.

Acute: The acute form is most common in adult German Shepherds, although any breed is susceptible. These dogs present with acutely swollen and painful muscles of mastication. This severe swelling may cause the eyes to bulge. The dog will not open or close its mouth and will vigorously resent your attempts to manipulate it. The dog may have a fever and swollen tonsils and mandibular lymph nodes. There often is a leukocytosis, usually with a neutrophilia and occasionally eosinophilia. Serum CK is significantly elevated during the active acute phase.

The lesion consists of severe necrosis of muscle cells and massive amounts of hemorrhage, edema, macrophages, lymphocytes, plasma cells, occasionally neutrophils, and sometimes eosinophils. This disease has been called eosinophilic myositis because of a peripheral blood eosinophilia and the presence of eosinophils in the lesion. However, eosinophils may not be present in either location.

An autoimmune disease is suspected because of the nature of the lesion and elevated serum gamma globulins. After one or more acute episodes of this myositis, the muscles atrophy. This atrophy may be so severe that the dog may be unable to open its mouth. At no time does paralysis occur. The disease is usually bilateral, but rarely it is limited to one side.

Chronic: The chronic form has been referred to as atrophic myositis and is characterized by a progressive severe atrophy of the muscles of mastication. This may follow one or more episodes of the acute disease. More often it occurs unrelated to the acute form. The atrophy is accompanied by increasing difficulty in opening the mouth (trismus) and may be severe enough to prevent eating. The disease is normally bilateral but occasionally it is unilateral.

Small foci of inflammatory cells are present in these atrophied muscles. These are predominantly lymphocytes and plasma cells. Connective tissue elements are more abundant.

In some dogs with the acute or chronic form of masticatory myositis, similar lesions will be seen in other muscles with or without clinical signs related to them. This supports this disease as a polymyositis that in the masticatory form may have a predilection for muscles of branchial arch origin.

For treatment, immunosuppresive doses of corticosteroids should be administered in the acute disease until CK levels are normal and clinical improvement is evident. The acute disease is usually quite responsive to 0.5 to 1.0 mg per kg of prednisone or prednisolone 2 times a day. After remission occurs the dose can be decreased by 50 percent and administered on alternate days. The therapy should not be terminated abruptly.

Recurrence of the disease is common; therefore, it is recommended to maintain these dogs on long-term, low-dose, alternate-day therapy (2.5 to 5.0 mg total dose every other day).

Corticosteroids may also help the atrophied dog unable to open its jaw. The response to steroids will not be dramatic. The initial high dose should be maintained for about 2 weeks and then halved by changing to alternate-day therapy. With improvement the dose can be slowly decreased. Usually this will avoid the necessity to use surgical methods or forceful traction on the jaws to open them. Complete return of normal muscle mass should not be expected.

Polymyositis. When the same lesion described in the muscles of mastication is more widespread, the chief complaint and signs will reflect the main areas of muscle affected. This may include the masticatory muscles. The chief complaint may be a lame or stiff gait or an obviously weak gait with poor endurance, swallowing difficulties with regurgitation and occasionally inhalation pneumonia, or generalized atrophy of muscles. Dogs may have one or more of these problems.

Weakness can be present in all four limbs or just the pelvic limbs. The gait will consist of short, stiff, shuffling strides. The mildly affected dog will walk with a lame or stiff gait. There is no proprioceptive deficit and spinal reflexes are usually normal. Pain may be evident on muscle palpation. Acutely inflamed muscles may be swollen. Exercise may exacerbate the weakness. Esophageal involvement will produce a megaesophagus and regurgitation, and occasionally dysphagia occurs. Fever may occur in the acute disease. In prolonged disease atrophy is common. Slow, subtle wasting may result from a chronic polymyositis.

CK and aldolase are often elevated in the

serum of dogs in the acute stage of the disease. Electromyography may reveal denervation potentials if motor end-plates are involved in the lesion. There will often be a decreased duration and amplitude of the motor unit action potential. Bizarre high frequency discharges (pseudomyotonia) occasionally may be present.

The most common lesion is a plasma and lymphoid cell interstitial inflammation with a necrosis of muscle cells and occasionally arterioles. Some patients have hypergammaglobulinemia, positive antinuclear antibodies, and circulating antimuscle antibodies. Polymyositis has been described in a dog with systemic lupus erythematosus.[122, 126] For these reasons polymyositis is presumed to be an autoimmune disease. Occasionally polymyositis occurs in dogs with severe hypothyroidism from a primary lymphocytic thyroiditis, which in itself is an immune-mediated disease. This suggests a common factor responsible for these autoimmune conditions. Thyroid function should be evaluated in those patients suspected of having polymyositis.

Treatment should consist of corticosteroids similar to that recommended for the masticatory myositis.

FELINE POLYMYOSITIS-POLYMYOPATHY. A polymyopathy has been recognized in mature cats 10 months to 13 years old, of different breeds, and both sexes.[8] These cats have a unique posture that is characteristic for this disease. This consists of a persistent flexion of the head, apparently due to weak cervical epaxial muscles. Limb weakness was worse in the forelimbs than the hindlimbs. These cats often became fatigued after a few steps and lay down. CK and aldolase are consistently elevated in the serum. Some of the cats recovered while on corticosteroid therapy and one recovered spontaneously. Recovery occurred in 1 to 6 weeks, but recurrent episodes occurred in a few of these cats. On EMG there were fibrillations and positive sharp waves, bizarre high frequency potentials, and myotonic discharges in one cat. Study of muscle revealed patchy areas of necrosis of individual muscle cells with macrophages, wide variation in fiber size, basophilia, interstitial lymphocytic infiltration, and mild fibrosis. The cause remains unknown.

Myotonia. Myotonia is the clinical sign of a skeletal muscle cell abnormality that results in a delay in relaxation following a normal stimulus for contraction. It consists of a series of repetitive action potentials in the muscle cells in response to depolarization that produces continual contraction following a voluntary effort or electrical stimulaton. The basic defect is thought to be in the muscle cell membrane.

Clinically it is manifested predominantly in the extensor muscles of the limbs, resulting in a stiff gait and firm muscles. Proximal limb muscles feel firm and slightly enlarged. This clinical sign may be most evident at the start of activity after a period of rest and in some instances slowly decreases following a period of moderate activity such as walking. On electromyography, needle insertion stimulates a myotonic reaction, which is a continuous series of repetitive motor unit action potentials that increase and then decrease in amplitude and frequency. This is accompanied by a characteristic loud, high-pitched sound that increases and decreases like a "dive bomber." A similar needle stimulation of a continuous series of high frequency discharge that is persistent and does not wax and wane is called a bizarre high frequency potential, or pseudomyotonia. Both EMG forms of myotonia reflect an abnormal muscle cell membrane. Pseudomyotonia is more common in myopathy or myositis. In some disorders this myotonic reaction can be elicited by lightly tapping the muscle with a finger or blunt instrument. The sudden local contraction of muscle may cause a depression referred to as the myotonic dimple.

Myotonia is classically described as a congenital disease, or in young patients associated with degenerative muscle disease that may be hereditary, or in older patients associated with high levels of circulating corticosteroids that may be acquired or iatrogenic. Rarely it may occur in hypothyroidism. It is a common sign of degenerative muscle disease and is occasionally observed on electromyographic evaluation of animals with myositis.

At the present most all domestic animal diseases that show myotonia are associated with varying degrees of myopathy.[53, 54] In young animals most of these myopathies are familial. In older animals they are associated with an endocrine abnormality. Attempts to classify myotonia of domestic animals similar to that of humans has confused the terminology. The following domestic animal diseases have been grouped according to age of onset and cause.

HEREDITARY MYOPATHIC MYOTONIA OF YOUNG ANIMALS

Goat. Classic myotonia occurring in the goat has been referred to as a fainting disease;

however, there is no disturbance of the animal's sensorium.[23, 27, 110] This myotonia is observed shortly after birth and usually involves almost all the voluntary striated skeletal muscles of the body. The myotonia may be so severe at the onset that the animal falls on its side with rigidly extended limbs. The myotonia slowly decreases with rest or mild exercise. During this period the gait is extremely stiff. There is considerable day-to-day variation in the severity of signs. Percussion dimples can be elicited. This is thought to be inherited as either an autosomal dominant or an autosomal recessive disease.[26] Abnormal muscle histochemistry and ultrastructure are described. Decreased chloride conductance and increased calcium uptake have also been associated with this disease. The clinical signs and chloride abnormality are similar to those of Thomsen's disease in humans.

Horse. A much less dramatic myotonia has been reported in young horses, which may cause a mild stiffness in the gait, especially in the pelvic limbs. The most obvious sign, however, is focal irregular swellings-bulges of the proximal caudal thigh muscles due to severe myotonia of these cells.[170] This is usually bilateral. Light percussion exacerbates these dimples. Onset of signs varies from a few weeks to 5 to 6 months of age. Progressive signs beyond 6 or 7 months of age have been minimal. No abnormal chloride ion conductance has been associated with this. Muscle studies have been incomplete and inconclusive. Data are insufficient to implicate inheritance in this disease.

Chow Chow. A severe myotonic syndrome affecting almost all skeletal muscles has been observed around 2 to 3 months of age in related Chow Chows in the United Kingdom,[53] New Zealand,[108] Australia,[6, 69] and Holland.[187] The myotonic signs resemble those observed in the goat. The dogs have a sawhorse posture, and the limbs are extremely stiff and splay out to the side. Adduction and forelimb protraction are difficult. Laryngeal spasm and dyspnea may occur at onset of movement. Proximal limb and neck muscles are hypertrophied. Signs slowly decrease with persistent mild activity and are worse in cold weather. Occasionally prehension is difficult, and some dysphagia may occur. Myotonic dimples are reported in limb or tongue muscles. Serum CK may be mildly elevated. The associated myopathy is mild, consisting of some variations from normal in the diameter of muscle fibers, fiber necrosis, and an increase in sarcolemmal nu-

clei. Oral administration of procainamide may reduce the signs. An autosomal recessive inheritance is suspected.

Golden Retriever, Irish Terrier. Young male golden retrievers and Irish terriers have been observed to develop an abnormal gait and dysphagia at 6 to 8 weeks of age, which progress in a few weeks to a severe gait abnormality with remarkable stiffness due to myotonia. These dogs tire easily on minimal exercise. They occasionally have respiratory distress and rarely become cyanotic. They have a stiff short stride and a unique rolling motion of the forequarters as they swing their trunk side to side to help protract the thoracic limbs. There is limitation to the degree of jaw opening. Except for the signs of muscle disease, there are no other abnormalities on neurologic examination. Spinal reflexes are normal. Muscle atrophy occurs as the disease progresses. After a few weeks the clinical signs may stabilize with no further change.

Significant elevations of muscle cell enzymes occur in the serum of these dogs (LDH, AST, CK). Lesions consist of patchy areas of extensive muscle cell necrosis, with phagocytosis and calcification. The clinical signs and pathologic lesions are identical in the two breeds. Breeding studies with the Irish terriers support an autosomal recessive, sex-linked hereditary basis for the disease. Similar studies are lacking in the golden retrievers. I have studied 2 affected male golden retriever littermates in New York, and it has been observed in golden retrievers in California and Massachusetts. All cases have been observed in male dogs.

Labrador Retrievers. A familial myopathy has been reported in Labrador retrievers with the onset of weakness at 3 to 6 months of age.[120] An early sign is inability to hold the head up. The weakness progresses to the limb muscles accompanied by stiffness and resulting in very short strides and hopping movements. Signs decrease with rest and increase with exercise, excitement, or cold. As the dog matures the progression of signs abates but muscle atrophy is severe. The myopathy consists of a specific absence of type II fibers in the affected skeletal muscles. An autosomal recessive inheritance has been proposed from breeding studies.[121]

ACQUIRED MYOPATHIC MYOTONIA OF ADULT DOGS. A mild myopathy with myotonia has been observed in dogs with hyperadrenocorticoidism (canine Cushing's disease).[4, 17, 59, 80, 87] The hyperadrenocorticoidism has been associated with bilateral adrenocortical hyperplasia with or without a pituitary neoplasm, adrenocortical adenoma, and prolonged exposure to treatment with corticosteroids.[19, 160]

These are usually older dogs of either sex and several breeds; they begin to develop a slowly progressive weak but stiff gait that is often more marked in the pelvic limbs. The myotonia is usually symmetric but occasionally one limb is more affected. Muscle atrophy is apparent but proximal limb muscles feel enlarged and firm. Myotonic dimples occur in hypertrophied muscles. Mild elevations in serum CK may accompany the myopathy, which consists of myofiber atrophy, especially the type II fibers, occasional fiber necrosis, and increased sarcolemmal nuclei. Mild evidence of neuropathy has also been observed.

Treatment of adrenocortical hyperplasia with o, p′DDD (Mitotane, Lysodren) has been effective in some patients as has removal of steroid therapy in the iatrogenic cases.

In some dogs with hyperadrenocorticoidism, clinical signs of myotonic myopathy are not present but electromyographic studies have revealed myotonia.[20]

I have observed a similar myotonia in one dog with clinical signs of hypothyroidism including subnormal T3, T4, and TSH response evaluations. Adrenal function was normal.[185]

Myopathy

EXERTIONAL MYOPATHY. Exertional myopathy occurs in racing greyhounds and horses. Clinical signs are usually only apparent during intensive training or during a race. In dogs, abrupt stiffness and limb hyperextension occur accompanied by swollen and/or firm, painful muscles.[75, 76] The epaxial muscles are most often involved. Cyanosis may occur if the problem is generalized. In patients with severe acute signs, the rhabdomyolysis is severe enough to cause myoglobinuria.

It is proposed that this is a metabolic disorder with a sequence of events that involves uncontrolled acidosis at the muscle cell, swelling of muscles, local ischemia, muscle cell necrosis, and myoglobinuria.

Therapy should include intravenous fluids with bicarbonate, corticosteroids, antibiotics, cooling, and rest.

A similar problem occurs in working horses that are rested a few days but kept on a full working feed ration. Shortly after starting to work after this rest, they develop severe myopathy, especially of lumbar, epaxial, and hindlimb muscles accompanied by profound weakness, often with rigidly extended limbs and myoglobinuria. Recumbency and death are common.

NUTRITIONAL MYOPATHY. This disease is most common in young ruminants, occasionally foals, and rarely dogs.[110] It is known as white muscle disease owing to the gross lesions that result from the muscle necrosis. It is related to a nutritional deficiency of vitamin E and/or selenium.

Young puppies were described as slow to rise and having a stiff, stilted gait with generalized muscular weakness. Exercise will exacerbate the signs. This is especially true in foals with a predisposition for this disease. After confinement, if they are turned outside with the mare for exercise, the signs will suddenly appear or become much worse. The same exacerbation by exercise and excitement is observed in ruminants. In dogs, the EMG may demonstrate myotonia. Serum muscle enzymes are greatly increased because of the widespread muscle necrosis.

Episodic Weakness

Episodic weakness waxes and wanes and usually is exacerbated by exercise.[67, 111, 127, 160, 195] When the animal is at rest it may be mild or not apparent. It is a clinical sign of several pathophysiologic conditions. The differential diagnosis primarily involves four major categories of disease: brain, neuromuscular, metabolic, and cardiovascular. Some of the following have been described previously in this chapter.

Brain Disease. Structural lesions of the nervous system usually do not produce episodic weakness. The signs will be persistent, slowly improve, or slowly progress. Generalized seizure disorders will produce rapid collapse associated with tonic-clonic limb activity, mastication, salivation, loss of consciousness, and other signs of uncontrolled impulse activity in the brain. This is readily distinguished from the alert responsive animal whose only clinical problem is episodes of weakness.

CATAPLEXY. Cataplexy is an idiopathic disorder of the sleep-wake mechanism in the brain which may produce few to many episodes per day of sudden collapse. During these episodes of a few second's duration, the animal will be completely paralyzed with atonic limbs. Partial attacks cause the animal to lose some muscle tone, making it unable to support weight and stumble. These are brief episodes that suddenly occur in a normal animal, and the animal suddenly returns to complete normality after the brief episode. (See Chapter 17.)

Diagnosis. In many patients these episodes can be stopped with intravenous imipramine (Tofranil) at 0.5 mg per kg.

Neuromuscular Diseases

MYASTHENIA GRAVIS. Myasthenia gravis probably is the most classic disease whose signs are characterized by weakness following exertion. In addition to the appendicular weakness that may cause collapse, there may be facial, laryngeal, pharyngeal, and esophageal muscle weakness resulting in sialosis, dysphagia, occasional regurgitation and inspiratory dyspnea. There may be incontinence and a weak voice. Ataxia does not occur in this disease. This disease occurs in puppies and adults.

Diagnosis. Response to intravenous edrophonium (Tensilon)-0.5 to 5 mg.

POLYMYOSITIS. Some dogs with polymyositis may show exacerbation of their weakness during exercise. The clinical signs may be manifested in the pelvic limbs alone or in all four limbs. The gait may be stiff, short-strided, symmetric or asymmetric, but not ataxic. Other signs of muscle involvement include dysphagia, postprandial regurgitation, difficulty in chewing, and a hoarse bark. Proximal limb muscles may be painful on palpation.

Diagnosis. Elevated serum muscle enzymes, EMG, muscle biopsy.

Metabolic Disease

HYPOGLYCEMIA. Weakness, or ataxia and lethargy, or both, may occur with hypoglycemia and be increased by exertion. Hypoglycemia may result from increased utilization of glucose when there are neoplasms of pancreatic beta cells. These usually occur in the older dog.

Decreased synthesis may cause hypoglycemia. This occurs in the glycogen storage diseases of toy breed puppies, in functional hypoglycemia of hunting dogs, in adrenocortical insufficiency, and in hepatic insufficiency.

Diagnosis. Blood glucose (resting, fasting, after exercise), serum insulin.

HYPERKALEMIA. Hyperkalemia may occur in primary or secondary adrenocortical insufficiency, diabetes mellitus, acute renal failure, or severe acidosis. Weakness that may be episodic results, accompanied by the more characteristic signs of these diseases.

Diagnosis. Serum sodium and potassium, ECG, plasma cortisol, ACTH response, blood glucose, urinalysis, BUN, creatinine, blood pH.

HYPOKALEMIA. Hypokalemia resulting from severe vomiting, diarrhea, urinary loss, excessive fluid therapy, or insulin therapy is uncommon. However, it may produce an episodic weakness.

Diagnosis. Serum potassium.

Cardiovascular Disease. Cardiovascular diseases may produce episodic weakness, ataxia, lethargy, and syncope. The diseases most commonly implicated are cardiac arrhythmias (atrial fibrillation, ventricular tachycardia, sinus arrest, atrial standstill), conduction blocks, congestive heart failure, and heartworm. All of these conditions may cause a decreased cardiac output and peripheral anoxia, which is the basis for the episodic weakness.

Diagnosis. ECG, heartworm tests, thoracic radiographs.

Hemangiosarcomas that periodically bleed into the abdomen will cause recurrent weakness and/or collapse.

Diagnosis. Palpation, abdominal radiographs, abdominocentesis, hemogram.

DATA BASE. A minimum data base should be obtained from laboratory work that includes a hemogram, urinalysis, fasting blood glucose, serum electrolytes, and serum enzymes (CK, AST, LDH). An electrocardiogram should be done on all of these patients. Additional data may include heartworm examination, thoracic radiographs, response to imipramine, response to edrophonium, and muscle biopsy.

REFERENCES

1. Alexander, J. W., de Lahunta, A., and Scott, D. W.: A case of brachial plexus neuropathy in a dog. J. Am. Anim. Hosp. Assoc., *10*:515, 1974.
2. Allam, M. W., Nulsen, F. E., and Lewey, F. H.: Electrical intraneural bipolar stimulation of peripheral nerves in the dog. J. Am. Vet. Med. Assoc., *114*:87, 1949.
3. Amann, J. F.: The organization of spinal motoneurons and their relationship to corticospinal fibers in the raccoon (*Procyon lotor*). Ph.D. thesis, Cornell University, 1971.
4. Arnold, S.: An endocrine abnormality in a dog. Senior seminar, Flower Library, New York State College of Veterinary Medicine, 1974.
5. Averill, D. A., Jr.: Polymyositis in the dog. *In* Kirk, R. W. (ed.): Current Veterinary Therapy V: Small Animal Practice. Philadelphia, W. B. Saunders Co., 1974.
6. Averill, D. A., Jr., and de Lahunta, A.: Toxoplasmosis of the canine nervous system: Clinicopathologic findings in four cases. J. Am. Vet. Med. Assoc., *159*:1134, 1971.
7. Averill, D. A., Jr.: Diseases of the muscle. Vet. Clin. North Am., *10*:223, 1980.

8. Averill, D. A., Jr.: The nervous system. *In* Holzworth, J. (ed.): Diseases of the Cat. Philadelphia, W. B. Saunders Co., (in press).

9. Bargai, V., Cohen, A., and Benado, A.: An outbreak of botulism in a dairy herd. Refuah Vet., *30*:135, 1973.

10. Barsanti, J. A., Walser, M., Hatheway, C. L., Bowen, J. M., and Crowell, W.: Type C botulism in American Foxhounds. J. Am. Vet. Med. Assoc., *172*:809, 1978.

11. Bässler, H. P.: Die Reflex Untersuchung beim Hund. Arch. Exp. Vet. Med., *15*:100, 1961.

12. Bennett, D.: An anatomical and histological study of the sciatic nerve relating to peripheral nerve injuries in the dog and cat. J. Small Anim. Pract., *17*:379, 1976.

13. Bennett, D., and Vaughan, L. C.: Peroneal paralysis in the cat and dog: An experimental study. J. Small Anim. Pract., *17*:499, 1976.

14. Barsanti, J. A.: Botulism, tick paralysis, and acute polyradiculoneuritis (coonhound paralysis). *In* Kirk, R. W. (ed.): Current Veterinary Therapy VII: Small Animal Practice. Philadelphia, W. B. Saunders Co., 1980.

15. Bennett, D., and Vaughan, L. C.: The use of muscle relocation techniques in the treatment of peripheral nerve injuries in dogs and cats. J. Small Anim. Pract., *17*:99, 1976.

16. Blakemore, W. F., Rees-Evans, E. T., and Wheeler, P. E. G.: Botulism in foxhounds. Vet. Rec., *100*:57, 1977.

17. Bluvas, P.: Myotonia in a case of canine Cushing's disease. Senior seminar. Flower Library, New York State College of Veterinary Medicine, 1974.

18. Bowen, J. M.: Electrodiagnostic testing and electromyography. *In* Hoerlein, B. F. (ed.): Canine Neurology. 2nd ed. Philadelphia, W. B. Saunders Co., 1971.

19. Braund, K. G., Dillon, A. R., and Mikeal, R. L.: Experimental investigation of glucocorticoid-induced myopathy in the dog. Exp. Neurol., *68*:50, 1980.

20. Braund, K. G., Dillon, A. R., Mikeal, R. L., and August, J. R.: Subclinical myopathy associated with hyperadrenocorticisim in the dog. Vet. Pathol., *17*:134, 1980.

21. Braund, K. G., Dillon, A. R., and Pidgeon, G. L.: Neuromuscular changes in dogs with spontaneous diabetes mellitus. *In* Proceedings of the American College of Veterinary Internal Medicine Scientific Seminar, 1981.

22. Braund, K. G., Luttgen, P. J., Redding, R. W., and Rumph, P. F.: Distal symmetrical polyneuropathy in a dog. Vet. Pathol., *17*:422, 1980.

23. Brown, G. L., and Harvey, A. M.: Congenital myotonia in the goat. Brain, *62*:24, 1939.

24. Brown, M. J., and Northington, J. N.: Acute canine idiopathic polyneuropathy (ACIP): A new model of the Guillain-Barré syndrome. Peripheral Nerve Study Group, Lexington, Ky., 1981.

25. Brown, N. O., and Zaki, F. A.: Electrodiagnostic testing for evaluation of neuromuscular disorders in dogs and cats. J. Am. Vet. Med. Assoc. *174*:86, 1979.

26. Bryant, S. H.: Myotonia in the goat. Ann. N.Y. Acad. Sci., *317*:314, 1979.

27. Bryant, S. H., Lipicky, R. J., and Herzog, W. H.: Variability of myotonic signs in myotonic goats. Am. J. Vet. Res., *29*:2371, 1968.

28. Burt, J. K., Lipowitz, A. J., and Harris, J. A.:

Femoral artery occlusion by *Dirofilaria immitis* in a dog. J. Am. Vet. Radiol. Soc., *18*:166, 1977.

29. Butler, H. C.: An investigation into the relationship of an aortic embolus to posterior paralysis in the cat. J. Small Anim. Pract., *12*:141, 1971.

30. Cardinet, G. H., and Holliday, T. A.: Neuromuscular diseases of domestic animals: A summary of muscle biopsies from 159 cases. Ann. N.Y. Acad. Sci., *317*:290, 1979.

31. Cavanagh, J. B.: Peripheral nerve changes in orthocresyl phosphate poisoning in the cat. J. Pathol. Bacteriol., *87*:365, 1964.

32. Chrisman, C. L.: Electromyography in the localization of spinal cord and nerve root neoplasia in dogs and cats. J. Am. Vet. Med. Assoc., *166*:1074, 1975.

33. Chrisman, C. L., Bunt, J. R., Wood, P. K., and Johnson, E. W.: Electromyography in small animal neurology. J. Am. Vet. Med. Assoc., *160*:311, 1972.

34. Coggeshall, R. E., and Langford, L. A.: Branching of axons in dorsal root and peripheral nerve. Peripheral Nerve Study Group, Lexington, Ky., 1981.

35. Cooper, B. J.: Studies on the pathogenesis of tick paralysis. Ph.D. thesis, University of Sydney, Sydney, Australia, 1976.

36. Cork, L. C., Griffin, J. W., Munnell, J. F., Lorenz, M. D., Adams, R. J., and Price, D. L.: Hereditary canine spinal muscular atrophy. J. Neuropathol. Exp. Neurol., *38*:209, 1979.

37. Cox, V. S., Breazile, J. E., and Hoover, T. R.: Surgical and anatomic study of calving paralysis. Am. J. Vet. Res., *36*:427, 1975.

38. Cox, V. S., and Martin, C. E.: Peroneal nerve paralysis in a heifer. J. Am. Vet. Med. Assoc., *167*:142, 1975.

39. Cummings, J. F., Cooper, B. J., de Lahunta, A., and Van Winkle, T. J.: Canine inherited hypertrophic neuropathy. Acta Neuropathol., *53*:137, 1981.

40. Cummings, J. F., and de Lahunta, A.: Canine polyneuritis. *In* Kirk, R. W. (ed.): Current Veterinary Therapy V: Small Animal Practice. Philadelphia, W. B. Saunders Co., 1974.

41. Cummings, J. F., and de Lahunta, A.: Chronic relapsing polyradiculoneuritis in a dog. A clinical, light, and electron-microscopic study. Acta Neuropathol., *28*:191, 1974.

42. Cummings, J. F., de Lahunta, A., Holmes, D. F., et al.: Coonhound paralysis: Further clinical studies and electron microscopic observations. Acta Neuropathol., *56*:167, 1982.

43. Cummings, J. F., de Lahunta, A., and Timoney, J. F.: Neuritis of the cauda equina, a chronic idiopathic polyradiculoneuritis in the horse. Acta Neuropathol., *46*:17, 1979.

44. Cummings, J. F., and de Lahunta, A.: Hypertrophic neuropathy in a dog. Acta Neuropathol., *29*:325, 1974.

45. Cummings, J. F., and Haas, D. C.: Coonhound paralysis. An acute idiopathic polyradiculoneuritis in dogs resembling the Landry-Gullain-Barré syndrome. J. Neurol. Sci., *4*:51, 1967.

46. Cummings, J. F., de Lahunta, A., Lorenz, M. D., and Washington, L. D.: Canine brachial plexus neuritis: A syndrome resembling serum neuritis in man. Cornell Vet., *63*:590, 1973.

47. Dahme, E., and Deutschländer, N.: Die Neuritis der Cauda Equina beim Pferd in Elektronenmikros-

kopischen Bild. Zentrallblat. Vet. Med. [A], 23:502, 1976.

48. Darke, P. G. G., Roberts, T. A., Smart, J. L., and Bradshaw, P. R.: Suspected botulism in foxhounds. Vet. Rec., 99:98, 1976.

49. Daw, P. C., Yano, C. S., and Ettinger, S. J.: Antibody to acetylcholine receptor in canine and human myasthenia gravis: Differential cross reactivity with human and rabbit receptor. Neurology, 29:1065, 1979.

50. Dawson, J. R. B.: Myasthenia gravis in a cat. Vet. Rec., 86:562, 1970.

51. de Lahunta, A., and Alexander, J. W.: Ischemic myelopathy secondary to presumed fibrocartilaginous embolism in nine dogs. J. Am. Anim. Hosp. Assoc., 12:37, 1976.

52. Duncan, I. D.: Peripheral nerve disease in the dog and cat. Vet. Clin. North Am., 10:177, 1980.

53. Duncan, I. D.: Myotonia in the dog. In Kirk, R. W. (ed.): Current Veterinary Therapy VII. Philadelphia, W. B. Saunders Co., 1980.

54. Duncan, I. D.: Myotonia in the dog. In Kirk, R. W. (ed.): Current Veterinary Therapy VIII: Small Animal Practice. Philadelphia, W. B. Saunders Co., 1983.

55. Duncan, I. D., and Griffiths, I. R.: Canine giant axonal neuropathy. Vet. Rec., 101:438, 1977.

56. Duncan, I. D., and Griffiths, I. R.: Peripheral nervous system in a case of canine giant axonal neuropathy. Neuropathol. Appl. Neurobiol., 5:25, 1979.

57. Duncan, I. D., and Griffiths, I. R.: Inflammatory muscle disease in the dog. In Kirk, R. W. (ed.): Current Veterinary Therapy VII: Small Animal Practice. Philadelphia, W. B. Saunders Co., 1980.

58. Duncan, I. D., and Griffiths, I. R.: Inflammatory muscle disease in the dog. In Kirk, R. W. (ed.): Current Veterinary Therapy VII: Small Animal Practice. Philadelphia, W. B. Saunders Co., 1980.

59. Duncan, I. D., Griffiths, I. R., and McQueen, A.: A myopathy associated with myotonia in the dog. Acta Neuropathol., 31:297, 1975.

60. Dyck, P. J., and Lambert, E. H.: Polyneuropathy associated with hypothyroidism. J. Neuropathol. Exp. Neurol., 29:631, 1970.

61. Dyck, P. J., Johnson, W. J., Lambert, E. H., and O'Brien, P. C.: Segmental demyelination secondary to axonal degeneration in uremic neuropathy. Mayo Clin. Proc., 46:400, 1971.

62. Evans, L. H., Campbell, J. H., Pinner-Poole, B., and Jenny, J.: Prevention of painful neuromas in horses. J. Am. Vet. Med. Assoc., 153:313, 1968.

63. Fankhauser, R., Gerber, H., Cravero, G. C., and Straub, R.: Klinik und Pathologie der Neuritis Caudae equina (NCE) des Pferdes. Schweiz. Arch. Tierheilk., 117:675, 1975.

64. Farnbach, G. C.: Myositis in the dog. Compend. Contin. Ed., 1:183, 1979.

65. Farnbach, G. C.: Clinical electrophysiology in veterinary neurology. Parts I and II. Compend. Contin. Ed., 2:791 and 843, 1980.

66. Farrow, B. R. H.: Myasthenia, myotonia, and storage disease. In Proceedings of the Kal-Kan Symposium, 1978.

67. Farrow, B. R. H.: Episodic weakness. In Kirk, R. W. (ed.): Current Veterinary Therapy VII: Small Animal Practice. Philadelphia, W. B. Saunders Co., 1980.

68. Farrow, B., Personal communication, 1982.

69. Farrow, B. R. H., and Malik, R.: Hereditary my-otonia in the Chow Chow. J. Small Anim. Pract., 22:451, 1981.

70. Feigin, I., Popoff, N., and Adachi, M.: Fibrocartilaginous venous emboli to the spinal cord with necrotic myelopathy. J. Neuropathol. Exp. Neurol., 24:63, 1965.

71. Fjolstad, M., and Klund, T.: An outbreak of botulism among ruminants in connection with ensilage feeding. Nord. Vet.-Med., 21:609, 1969.

72. Fletcher, T. F.: Lumbosacral plexus and pelvic limb myotomes of the dog. Am. J. Vet. Res., 31:35, 1970.

73. Fraser, D. C., Palmer, A. C., and Senior, J. E. B.: Myasthenia gravis in the dog. J. Neurol. Neurosurg. Psychiatry, 33:431, 1970.

74. Frost, W. W., and Lumb, W. V.: Radiocarpal arthrodesis: A surgical approach to brachial paralysis. J. Am. Vet. Med. Assoc., 149:1073, 1966.

75. Gannon, J. R.: External rhabdomyolysis (myoglobinuria) in the racing Greyhound. In Kirk, R. W. (ed.): Current Veterinary Therapy VII: Small Animal Practice. Philadelphia, W. B. Saunders Co., 1980.

76. Gannon, J. R.: Exertional rhabdomyolysis (myoglobinuria) in the racing Greyhound. In Kirk, R. W. (ed.): Current Veterinary Therapy VIII: Small Animal Practice. Philadelphia, W. B. Saunders Co., 1983.

77. Garlepp, M., Farrow, B., Kay, P., and Dawkins, R. L.: Antibodies to acetylcholine receptor in myasthenic dogs. Immunology, 37:807, 1979.

78. Gray, T. C., and Bulgin, M. S.: Botulism in an Oregon dairy cow herd. J. Am. Vet. Med. Assoc., 180:160, 1982.

79. Greene, C. E., and Higgins, R. J.: Fibrocartilaginous emboli as the cause of ischemic myelopathy in a dog. Cornell Vet., 66:131, 1976.

80. Greene, C. E., Lorenz, M. D., Munnell, J. F., Prasse, K. W., White, N. A., and Bowen, J. M.: Myopathy associated with hyperadrenocorticism in the dog. J. Am. Vet. Med. Assoc., 174:1310, 1979.

81. Greenwood, A. G., Barker, J., and McLeish, I.: Neuritis of the cauda equina in a horse. Equine Vet. J., 5:111, 1973.

82. Griffiths, I. R.: Avulsion of the brachial plexus. 1. Neuropathology of the spinal cord and peripheral nerves. J. Small Anim. Pract., 15:165, 1974.

83. Griffiths, I. R.: Avulsion of the brachial plexus. 2. Clinical aspects. J. Small Anim. Pract., 15:177, 1974.

84. Griffiths, I. R.: The extensive myelopathy of intervertebral disc protrusions in dogs (the ascending syndrome). J. Small Anim. Pract., 13:425, 1972.

85. Griffiths, I. R.: Spinal cord infarction due to emboli arising from the intervertebral discs in the dog. J. Comp. Pathol., 83:225, 1973.

86. Griffiths, I. R., Barker, J., and Palmer, A. C.: Cholesterol masses in association with spinal cord infarction due to intervertebral disk emboli. Acta Neuropathol., 33:85, 1975.

87. Griffiths, I. R., and Duncan, I. D.: Myotonia in the dog: A report of four cases. Vet. Rec., 93:184, 1973.

88. Griffiths, I. R., and Duncan, I. D.: Some studies of the clinical neurophysiology of denervation in the dog. Res. Vet. Sci., 17:377, 1974.

89. Griffiths, I. R., and Duncan, I. D.: The use of electromyography and nerve conduction studies in the evaluation of lower motor neurone disease or injury. J. Small Anim. Pract., 19:329, 1978.

90. Griffiths, I. R., and Duncan, I. D.: Distal denervating disease. A degenerative neuropathy of the distal motor axon in dogs. J. Small Anim. Pract., 20:579, 1979.
91. Griffiths, I. R., and Duncan, I. D.: Ischemic neuromyopathy in cats. Vet. Rec., 104:518, 1979.
92. Griffiths, I. R., Duncan, I. D., McQueen, A., Quirk, C., and Miller, R.: Neuromuscular disease in dogs: Some aspects of its investigation and diagnosis. J. Small Anim. Pract., 14:533, 1973.
93. Grose, C., Henle, W., Henle, G., and Feorino, P. M.: Primary Epstein-Barr virus infections in acute neurologic diseases. N. Engl. J. Med., 292:392, 1975.
94. Habel, R. E.: Applied Veterinary Anatomy. Ithaca, N.Y., R. E. Habel, 1975.
95. Hall, G. A., Howell, J. McC., and Lewis, D. G.: Thymoma with myasthenia gravis in a dog. J. Pathol., 108:177, 1972.
96. Hayes, M. A., Creighton, S. R., Boysen, B. G., and Holfeld, N.: Acute necrotizing myelopathy from nucleus pulposus embolism of arteries and veins in large dogs with early disk degeneration. J. Am. Vet. Med. Assoc., 173:289, 1978.
97. Henry, R. W., Diesem, C. D., Hunter, M. A., and Rankin, J. S.: Surgical approach to the equine brachial plexus. J. Am. Vet. Med. Assoc., 171:190, 1977.
98. Hoff, E. J., and Vandevelde, M.: Non-suppurative encephalomyelitis in cats suggestive of a viral origin. Vet. Pathol., 18:170, 1981.
99. Holliday, T. A., Ealand, B. G., and Weldon, N. E.: Sensory nerve conduction velocity: Technical requirements and normal values for branches of the radial and ulnar nerves of the dog. Am. J. Vet. Res., 38:1543, 1977.
100. Holmes, D. F., and de Lahunta, A.: Experimental allergic neuritis in the dog and its comparison with the naturally occurring disease: Coonhound paralysis. Acta Neuropathol., 30:329, 1974.
101. Holmes, D. F., Schultz, R. D., Cummings, J. F., and de Lahunta, A.: Experimental coonhound paralysis, an animal model for Guillain-Barré syndrome. Neurology, 29:1186, 1979.
102. Hopkinson, W. I.: Syringomyelia in pigs. Aust. Vet. J., 56:506, 1980.
103. Hussain, S., and Pettit, G. D.: Tendon transplantation to compensate for radial nerve paralysis. Am. J. Vet. Res., 28:336, 1967.
104. Ilkiw, J. E.: Tick paralysis in Australia. In Kirk, R. W. (ed.): Current Veterinary Therapy VII: Small Animal Practice. Philadelphia, W. B. Saunders Co., 1980.
105. Innes, J. R. M., and Saunders, L. Z.: Comparative Neuropathology. New York, Academic Press, 1962.
106. Jenkins, W. L., Van Dyke, E., and McDonald, C. B.: Myasthenia gravis in a Fox Terrier litter. J. S. Afr. Vet. Assoc., 47:59, 1976.
107. Johnson, R. P., Watson, A. D. J., Smith, J., and Cooper, B.: Myasthenia in Springer Spaniel littermates. J. Small Anim. Pract., 16:641, 1975.
108. Jones, B. R., Anderson, L. J., Barnes, G. R. G., Johnstone, A. C., and Juby, W. D.: Myotonia in related Chow Chow dogs. N.Z. Vet. J., 25:217, 1977.
109. Kadlubowski, M., Hughes, R. A. C., and Dalleywater, C.: Antibodies to P₂ in experimental allergic neuritis (EAN) and equine cauda equina neuritis but not Marek's disease or Guillain-Barré syndrome (GBS). Peripheral Nerve Study Group, Lexington, Ky., 1981.
110. Kaspar, L. U., and Lombard, L. S.: Nutritional myodegeneration in a litter of beagle dogs. J. Am. Vet. Med. Assoc., 143:284, 1963.
111. Kelly, M. J.: Periodic weakness. In Proceedings of the 45th Annual Meeting of the American Animal Hospital Association, 1978.
112. Kelly, M. J.: Myasthenia gravis—a receptor disease. Compend. Contin. Ed., 3:544, 1981.
113. Kornegay, J. N.: Ischemic myelopathy due to fibrocartilaginous embolism. Compend. Contin. Ed., 11:402, 1980.
114. Kornegay, J. N., Gorgacz, E. J., Dawe, D. L., Bowen, J. M., White, N. A., and DeBuysscher, E. V.: Polymyositis in dogs. J. Am. Vet. Med. Assoc., 176:431, 1980.
115. Korneliussen, H., and Jansen, J. K. S.: Morphological aspects of the elimination of polyneuronal innervation of skeletal muscle fibres in newborn rats. J. Neurocytol., 5:591, 1976.
116. Knecht, C. D.: Radial-brachial paralysis. In Kirk, R. W. (ed): Current Veterinary Therapy V: Small Animal Practice. Philadelphia, W. B. Saunders Co., 1974.
117. Knecht, C. D., and Greene, J. A.: Surgical approaches to the brachial plexus in small animals. J. Am. Anim. Hosp. Assoc., 13:592, 1977.
118. Knecht, C. D., and St. Claire, L. E.: The radial-brachial paralysis syndrome in the dog. J. Am. Vet. Med. Assoc., 154:653, 1969.
119. Kolb, L. C.: Congenital myotonia in goats. Bull. Johns Hopkins Hosp., 63:221, 1938.
120. Kramer, J. W., Hegreberg, G. A., Bryan, G. M., Meyers, K., and Ott, R. L.: A muscle disorder of Labrador retrievers characterized by deficiency of Type II muscle fibers. J. Am. Vet. Med. Assoc., 169:817, 1976.
121. Kramer, J. W., Hegreberg, G. A., and Hamilton, M. J.: Inheritance of a neuromuscular disorder of Labrador Retriever dogs. J. Am. Vet. Med. Assoc., 179:380, 1981.
122. Krum, S. H., Cardinet, G. H., Andersen, B. C., Holliday, T. A.: Polymyositis and polyarthritis associated with systemic lupus erythematosus in a dog. J. Am. Vet. Med. Assoc., 170:61, 1977.
123. Lee, A. F., and Bowen, J. M.: Evaluation of motor nerve conduction velocity in the dog. Am. J. Vet. Res., 31:1361, 1970.
124. Lennon, V. A., Palmer, A. C., Pflugfelder, C., and Indrieri, R. C.: Myasthenia gravis in dogs: Acetylcholine receptor deficiency with and without anti-receptor autoantibiodies. In Rose, N. R., Bigazzi, P. E., and Werner, N. L. (eds.): Genetic Control of Autoimmune Disease. New York, Elsevier North Holland Inc., 1978.
125. Levin, M.: Paroxysmal hypertonia induced by affect: A symptom in man and animals. Arch. Neurol. Psychiatry, 32:1286, 1934.
126. Lewis, R. M.: Systemic lupus erythematosus. In Kirk, R. W. (ed.): Current Veterinary Therapy V: Small Animal Practice. Philadelphia, W. B. Saunders Co., 1974.
127. Lorenz, M. D.: Episodic weakness in the dog. In Kirk, R. W. (ed.): Current Veterinary Therapy V: Small Animal Practice. Philadelphia, W. B. Saunders Co., 1974.
128. Lorenz, M. D., Cork, L. C., Griffin, J. W., Adams,

R. J., and Price, D. L.: Hereditary spinal muscular atrophy in Brittany Spaniels: Clinical manifestations. J. Am. Vet. Med. Assoc., *175*:833, 1979.

129. Lorenz, M. D., de Lahunta, A., and Almstrom, D. H.: Neostigmine-responsive weakness in the dog similar to myasthenia gravis. J. Am. Vet. Med. Assoc., *161*:705, 1972.

130. Lundh, H., Leander, S., and Thesleff, S.: Antagonism of the paralysis produced by botulinum toxin in the rat. J. Neurol. Sci., *32*:29, 1977.

131. MacKay, R. D., and Berkhoff, G. A.: Type C toxicoinfectious botulism in a foal. J. Am. Vet. Med. Assoc., *180*:163, 1982.

132. MacLachlan, N. J., Gribble, D. H., and East, N. E.: Polyradiculoneuritis in a goat. J. Am. Vet. Med. Assoc., *180*:166, 1982.

133. Manning, J. P., and Gosser, H. S.: Neuritis of the cauda equina in horses. VM/SAC, *68*:1162, 1973.

134. Martens, R., Stewart, J., and Eicholtz, D.: Clinicopathologic Conference-University of Pennsylvania. J. Am. Vet. Med. Assoc., *156*:478, 1970.

135. Mason, K. V.: A case of myasthenia gravis in a cat. J. Small Anim. Pract., *17*:467, 1976.

136. Merson, M. H., and Dowell, V. R., Jr.: Epidemiologic, clinical and laboratory aspects of wound botulism. N. Engl. J. Med., *289*:1005, 1973.

137. Miller, L. M.: Personal communication, 1982.

138. Nafe, L.: Personal communication, 1982.

139. Nicholson, S. S.: Bovine posterior paralysis due to organophosphate poisoning. J. Am. Vet. Med. Assoc., *165*:280, 1974.

140. Norris, F. H.: The EMG. New York, Grune & Stratton, 1963

141. Northington, J. W., Brown, M. J., Farnbach, G. C., and Steinberg, S. A.: Acute idiopathic polyneuropathy in the dog. J. Am. Vet. Med. Assoc., *179*:375, 1981.

142. Olmstead, M. L., and Butler, H. C.: Five hydroxytryptamine antagonists and feline aortic embolism. J. Small Anim. Pract., *18*:247, 1977.

143. O'Sullivan, B. M., and Blakemore, W. F.: Acute nicotinamide deficiency in pigs. Vet. Rec., *103*:543, 1978.

144. O'Sullivan, B. M., and Blakemore, W. F.: Acute nicotinamide deficiency in the pig induced by 6-aminonicotinamide. Vet. Pathol., *17*:748, 1980.

145. Pallaske, G.: Zur Pathologie der chronischen Neuritis der Cauda Equina. Dtsch. Tierarztl. Wochenschr., *73*:415, 1966.

146. Pallaske, G.: Zur pathologie der chronischen Neuritis der Cauda Equina. Dtsch. Tierarztl. Wochenschr., *73*:415, 1966.

147. Palmer, A. C.: Myasthenia gravis. Vet. Clin. North Am., *10*:213, 1980.

148. Palmer, A. C., and Barker, J.: Myasthenia in the dog. Vet. Rec., *95*:452, 1974.

149. Palmer, A. C., and Barker, J.: Myasthenia in the dog. Vet. Rec., *95*:452, 1974.

150. Palmer, A. C., and Goodyear, J. V.: Congenital myasthenia in the Jack Russell Terrier. Vet. Rec., *103*:433, 1978.

151. Palmer, A. C., Lennon, V. A., Beadle, C., and Goodyear, J. N.: Autoimmune form of myasthenia gravis in a juvenile Yorkshire Terrier X Jack Russell Terrier hybrid contrasted with congenital (non-autoimmune) myasthenia gravis of the Jack Russell Terrier. J. Small Anim. Pract., *21*:359, 1980.

152. Pass, D. A.: Posterior paralysis in a sow due to cartilaginous emboli in the spinal cord. Aust. Vet. J., *54*:100, 1978.

153. Prineas, J.: The pathogenesis of dying-back polyneuropathies. Part I. An ultrastructural study of experimental triorthocresylphosphate intoxication in the cat. J. Neuropathol. Exp. Neurol., *28*:571, 1969.

154. Riley, D. A: Multiple axon branches innervating single endplates of kitten soleus myofibers. Brain Res., *110*:158, 1976.

155. Roberts, S. J., Squire, R. A., and Gilman, H. L.: Deaths in two calves following vaccination with Brucella abortus strain 19 vaccine. Cornell Vet., *52*:592, 1962.

156. Rooney, J. R.: Radial paralysis in the horse. Cornell Vet., *53*:328, 1963.

157. Rooney, J. R., and Prickett, M. E.: The shaker foal syndrome. Mod. Vet. Pract., *48*:44, 1967.

158. Sandefelt, E., Cummings, J. C., de Lahunta, A., Bjork, G., and Krook, L.: Hereditary neuronal abiotrophy in the Swedish Lapland dog. Cornell Vet. *63*(Suppl. 3):1, 1973.

159. Scott, D. W., and de Lahunta, A.: Eosinophilic polymyositis in a dog. Cornell Vet., *64*:47, 1974.

160. Scott, D. W., and Greene, C. E.: Iatrogenic secondary adrenocortical insufficiency in dogs. J. Am. Anim. Hosp. Assoc., *10*:555, 1974.

161. Simmons, G. C., and Tammemage, L.: Clostridium botulism type D as a cause of bovine botulism in Queensland. Aust. Vet. J., *40*:123, 1964.

162. Sims, M. H., and Redding, R. W.: Failure of neuromuscular transmission after complete nerve section in the dog. Am. J. Vet. Res., *40*:931, 1979.

163. Sims, M. H., and Redding, R. W.: Maturation of nerve conduction velocity and the evoked muscle potential in the dog. Am. J. Vet. Res., *41*:1247, 1980.

164. Slonka, G. F., Castleman, W., and Krum, S.: Adult heartworms in arteries and veins of a dog. J. Am. Vet. Med. Assoc., *170*:717, 1977.

165. Smart, J. L., and Roberts, T. A.: Bovine botulism. Vet. Rec., *101*:201, 1977.

166. Sponenberg, D. P., and de Lahunta, A.: Hereditary hypertrophic neuropathy in Tibetan Mastiff dogs. J. Heredity, *72*:287, 1981.

167. Steinberg, S. S.: The use of electrodiagnostic techniques in evaluating traumatic brachial plexus root injuries. J. Am. Anim. Hosp. Assoc., *15*:621, 1979.

168. Steinberg, H. S.: A review of electromyographic and motor nerve conduction velocity techniques. J. Am. Anim. Hosp. Assoc., *15*:613, 1979.

169. Steinberg, S., and Botelho, S.: Myotonia in a horse. Science, *137*:979, 1962.

170. Steinberg, S., and Botelho, S.: Myotonia in a horse. Science, *137*:979, 1962.

171. Stockard, C. R.: An hereditary lethal for localized motor and preganglionic neurones with a resulting paralysis in the dog. Am. J. Anat., *59*:1, 1936.

172. Stünzi, H., and Pohlenz, J.: Zur Pathologie der Neuritis Caudae Equinae beim Pferd. Schweiz. Arch. Tierheilkd., *116*:533, 1974.

173. Swaim, S. F.: Peripheral nerve surgery in the dog. J. Am. Vet. Med. Assoc., *161*:905, 1972.

174. Swallow, J. S., and Griffiths, I. R.: Age related changes in the motor nerve conduction velocity in dogs. Res. Vet. Sci., *23*:29, 1977.

175. Swerczek, T. W.: Experimentally induced toxicoinfectious botulism in horses and foals. Am. J. Vet. Res., 41:348, 1980.

176. Swerczek, T. W.: Toxicoinfectious botulism in foals and adult horses. J. Am. Vet. Med. Assoc., 176:217, 1980.

178. Taylor, H. W., Vandevelde, M., and Firth, E. C.: Ischemic myelopathy caused by fibrocartilaginous emboli in a horse. Vet. Pathol., 14:479, 1977.

179. Tilley, L. P., and Liu, S-k.: Cardiomyopathy and thromboembolism in the cat. Fel. Pract., 5:32, 1975.

180. Tryphonas, L., Hamilton, G. F., and Rhodes, C. S.: Perinatal femoral nerve degeneration and neurogenic atrophy of quadriceps femoris muscle in calves. J. Am. Vet. Med. Assoc., 164:801, 1974.

181. Tsairis, P., Dyck, P. J., and Mulder, D. W.: Natural history of brachial plexus neuropathy. Arch. Neurol., 27:109, 1972.

182. Vandevelde, M., Braund, K. G.: Polioencephalomyelitis in cats. Vet. Pathol., 16:420, 1979.

183. Vandevelde, M., Oettli, P., Fatzer, R., and Rohr, M.: Polyradikuloneuritis beim Hund. Klinische, histologische und ultrastrukturelle Beobachtungen. Schw. Arch. Tier., 123:207, 1981.

184. Vaughan, L. C.: Peripheral nerve injuries: An experimental study in cattle. Vet. Rec., 76:1293, 1964.

185. Venables, G. S., Bates, D., and Shaw, D. A.: Hypothyroidism with true myotonia. J. Neurol. Neurosurg. Psychiatry, 41:1013, 1978.

186. Walker, T. L.: Ischiatic nerve entrapment. J. Am. Vet. Med. Assoc., 178:1284, 1981.

187. Wentink, G. H., Hartman, W., and Koeman, J. P.: Three cases of myotonia in a family of chows. Tijdschr. Diergeneeskd., 14:729, 1974.

188. Wentink, G. H., Van der Linde-Sipman, J. S., Meijer, A. E. F. H., Kamphiusen, H. A. C., Van Vorsteinbosch. C. J. A. H. V., Hartman, W., and Hendricks, H. J.: Myopathy with a possible recessive X-linked inheritance in a litter of Irish terriers. Vet. Pathol., 9:328, 1972.

189. White, G. R., and Plaskett, J.: Nervous, stiff-legged or fainting goats. Am. Vet. Rev., 28:556, 1904.

190. Whitney, J. C.: Eosinophilic myositis in dogs. Vet. Rec., 67:1140, 1955.

191. Wilson, J. W.: Relationship of the patellar tendon reflex to the ventral branch of the fifth lumbar spinal nerve in the dog. Am. J. Vet. Res., 39:1174, 1978.

192. Withrow, S. J., and Amis, T. C.: Sciatic nerve injury associated with intramedullary fixation of femoral fractures. J. Am. Anim. Hosp. Assoc., 13:562, 1977.

193. Witt, W. M., and Ludwig, R. D.: Anticholinesterase-responsive weakness in the canine similar to myasthenia gravis of man. J. Am. Anim. Hosp. Assoc., 14:137, 1978.

194. Woods, C. B., and Lorenz, M. D.: Episodic weakness: A problem-oriented case study. J. Am. Anim. Hosp. Assoc., 11:473, 1975.

195. Woods, C. B., and Lorenz, M. D.: Episodic weakness: A problem-oriented case study. J. Am. Anim. Hosp. Assoc., 11:473, 1975.

196. Worthman, R. P.: Demonstration of specific nerve paralyses in the dog. J. Am. Vet. Med. Assoc., 131:174, 1957.

197. Zaki, F., and Prata, R. G.: Necrotizing myelopathy secondary to embolization of herniated intervertebral disk material in the dog. J. Am. Vet. Med. Assoc., 169:222, 1976.

198. Zaki, F. A., and Prata, R. G.: Necrotizing myelopathy in a cat. J. Am. Vet. Med. Assoc., 169:228, 1976.

199. Zaki, F., Prata, R. G., and Kay, W. J.: Necrotizing myelopathy in five Great Danes, J. Am. Vet. Med. Assoc., 165:1080, 1974.

200. Wilson, T. M., and Drake, T. R.: Porcine focal symmetrical poliomyelomalacia. Can. J. Comp. Med., 46:218, 1982.

CRANIAL NERVE—LOWER MOTOR NEURON: GENERAL SOMATIC EFFERENT SYSTEM, SPECIAL VISCERAL EFFERENT SYSTEM

GENERAL SOMATIC EFFERENT— GSE

The cranial nerve general somatic efferent neurons innervate the striated voluntary musculature derived from occipital somites (tongue muscles) and head myotomes (extraocular muscles). They are found in cranial nerves III, IV, VI, and XII. As is the case with spinal nerves, this is not the only function of these cranial nerves. Cranial nerve III also contains general visceral efferent neurons, and all of these nerves contain sensory neurons, mostly of a proprioceptive nature.

The nuclei that contain the general somatic efferent neurons in the brain stem are located in an incomplete longitudinal column from caudal medulla to rostral midbrain. This column is adjacent to the midline ventral to the floor of the ventricular system (Fig. 5–1). Except for cranial nerve IV, the nerves emerge from the brain stem in a longitudinal row near the ventral median plane.

CRANIAL NERVE XII—HYPOGLOSSAL NEURONS

Anatomy. The general somatic efferent neuronal cell bodies are located in the hypoglossal nucleus in the medulla (Plates 3, 4). The nucleus is adjacent to the midline and floor of the fourth ventricle. It is a long nucleus (3 to 5 mm), extending from the obex caudally nearly to the level of the acoustic stria rostrally (Fig. 5–2).

The axons pass directly ventrally and slightly laterally through the reticular formation across the lateral portion of the olivary nucleus. They emerge lateral to the pyramid as a longitudinal series of small roots. The row of hypoglossal roots merges at the small hypoglossal canal to form the hypoglossal nerve. The neurons course to the extrinsic tongue muscles (styloglossus, hyoglossus, and genioglossus), the intrinsic tongue muscles, and the geniohyoideus. A recent study of the dog showed that the cell bodies of a few neurons to intrinsic lingual muscles are located in the caudal pole of the facial nucleus, and each genioglossus muscle is innervated by neurons from both hypoglossal nuclei.[68] The hypoglossal nerve is much smaller inside the cranial cavity than outside the skull. This is due to the increase in myelination and connective tissue that occurs after the nerve emerges from the hypoglossal canal.

Clinical Signs. Lesions of any part of the neurons result in impairment of the function of the tongue in deglutition, prehension, mastication, and speech. With unilateral lesions

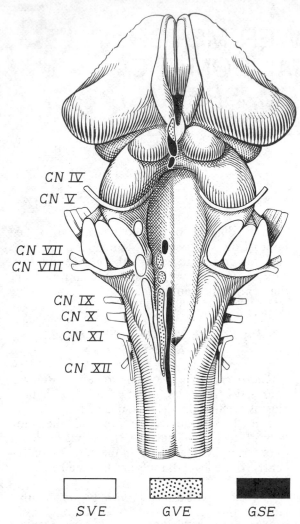

CN IV

CN V

CN VII
CN VIII

CN IX
CN X
CN XI

CN XII

| SVE | GVE | GSE |

Figure 5–1. Functional organization of cranial nerve nuclei in brain stem: special visceral efferent (SVE), general visceral efferent (GVE), general somatic efferent (GSE).

the tongue, when protruded, deviates toward the side of the lesion. The normally functioning genioglossus and intrinsic muscles protrude the tongue toward the affected side. The weight of the atonic paralyzed half also contributes to this deviation. The animal may be observed to lick its lips only on the paralyzed side. The most reliable feature of unilateral tongue paralysis is atrophy of the ipsilateral half of the tongue.

CRANIAL NERVE VI—ABDUCENT NEURONS

Anatomy. The general somatic efferent neuronal cell bodies are located in the abdu-

cent nucleus (Plate 6). This is a small nucleus located in the rostral medulla in the GSE neuron column at the level where the caudal cerebellar peduncles merge with the cerebellum. It is adjacent to the midline ventral to the floor of the fourth ventricle. The axons of the genu of the facial special visceral efferent neurons pass over this nucleus (see Figs. 5–2, 5–6).

The axons of the cell bodies in the abducent nucleus pass directly ventrally through the reticular formation medial to the distinct dorsal nucleus of the trapezoid body, and emerge through the trapezoid body lateral to the pyramid. The abducent nerve leaves the cranial cavity through the orbital fissure, and within the periorbita innervates the lateral rectus and retractor bulbi muscles.

The clinical signs caused by lesions of these neurons will be discussed after the anatomy of all three cranial nerves to the extraocular muscles is considered.

CRANIAL NERVE IV—TROCHLEAR NEURONS

Anatomy. The general somatic efferent neuronal cell bodies are located in a small nucleus in the caudal mesencephalon at the level of the caudal colliculi (Plate 10). This trochlear nucleus is adjacent to the midline in the ventral part of the central grey substance that surrounds the mesencephalic aqueduct. It is caudal to the oculomotor nucleus, which is in the same functional column. The medial longitudinal fasciculus is medial and ventral to the trochlear nucleus (Fig. 5–3).

The axons course dorsally around the central grey substance and caudally to reach the rostral medullary velum between the two caudal colliculi (Plate 9). Here the axons cross to the opposite side and emerge from the velum caudal to the caudal colliculus, where they pass rostroventrally over the side of the mesencephalon to reach the floor of the cranial cavity. These axons leave the cranial cavity through the orbital fissure, and within the caudal periorbita innervate the dorsal oblique muscle.

CRANIAL NERVE III—OCULOMOTOR NEURONS

Anatomy. These general somatic efferent neuronal cell bodies are located in the oculo-

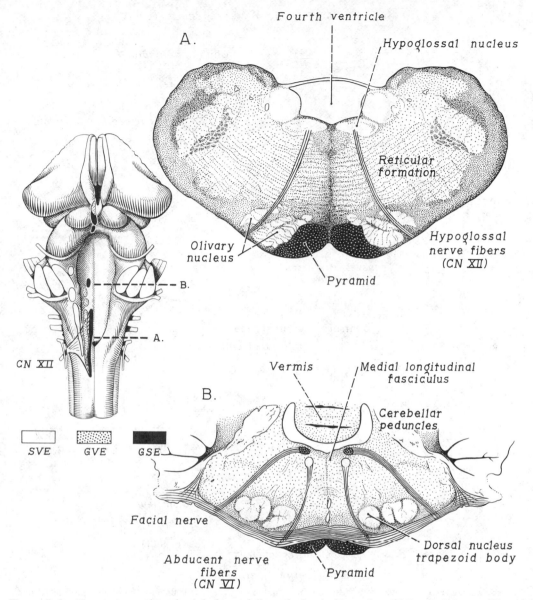

Figure 5–2. Transverse sections through the medulla at the level of hypoglossal *(A)* and abducent *(B)* nuclei.

motor nucleus in the rostral mesencephalon at the level of the rostral colliculus (Plates 11, 12). The nucleus is adjacent to the midline within the ventral part of the central grey substance that surrounds the mesencephalic aqueduct. In primates this nucleus has been subdivided into the groups of neurons that innervate specific muscles. It extends caudally to the trochlear nucleus and rostrally to the level of the pretectal area. It is dorsal to the red nucleus. The medial longitudinal fasciculus is located ventral and medial to this nucleus.

This longitudinal fasciculus serves to interconnect the general somatic efferent nuclei of the neurons innervating the extraocular muscles, and functions in their coordinated conjugated movements (see Fig. 5–3).

The axons of the oculomotor neurons pass ventrally through the reticular formation of the tegmentum medial to the red nucleus, substantia nigra, and crus cerebri. They emerge on the lateral side of the intercrural fossa and course rostrally lateral to the hypophysis and through the orbital fissure.

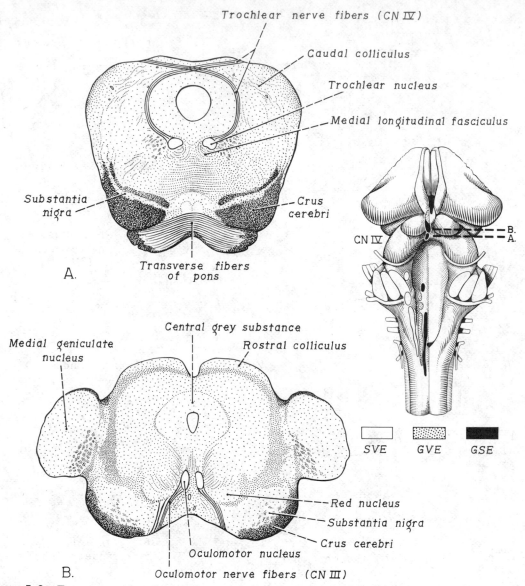

Figure 5–3. Transverse sections through the mesencephalon at level of trochlear *(A)* and oculomotor *(B)* nuclei.

Within the periorbita they innervate the dorsal and ventral recti, medial rectus, ventral oblique, and levator palpebrae muscles.

Function. In order to understand the signs that result from lesions of one or more of the three cranial nerves that innervate the extra-ocular muscles, the normal action of the muscles on the eyeball must be understood. If the eyeball is assumed to have three axes for rotation, the muscles can be grouped into three opposing pairs. Around a horizontal axis through the center of the eyeball the dorsal rectus elevates the eyeball and the ventral rectus depresses it. Around a vertical axis through the center of the eyeball the medial rectus adducts and the lateral rectus abducts the eyeball. Around the anterior-posterior axis through the center of the eyeball the dorsal oblique intorts the eyeball or rotates the dorsal portion medioventrally toward the nose, and the ventral oblique extorts the eyeball or moves the same point lateroventrally away from the nose. These muscles do not function alone, but continually act together in a synergistic or antagonistic manner to provide for conjugate movement of both eyeballs in the same direction at the same time. This is exemplified most easily by the action of the medial and lateral recti in horizontal conjugate movement (Fig. 5–4).

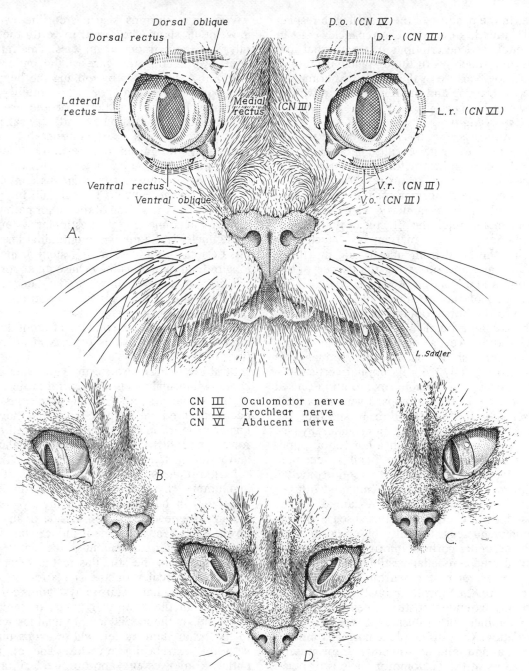

Figure 5–4. Functional anatomy of the extraocular muscles *(A)*. Directions of strabismus following paralysis of the oculomotor *(B)*, abducent *(C)*, and trochlear *(D)* neurons.

When the eyeballs move conjugately to the right, this requires facilitation of abducent neurons to the lateral rectus of the right eyeball and inhibition to those of the left eyeball, simultaneous with facilitation of the oculomotor neurons to the medial rectus of the left eyeball and inhibition to those of the right eyeball. The medial longitudinal fasciculus functions in this coordinated activity.

The function of any one muscle at a specific time depends on the position of the eyeball. The functions of the extraocular muscles in domestic animals do not compare exactly with those in humans because of anatomic differences in the position of the eyeball with respect to the muscle insertion. Discrepancies exist in the published descriptions of the normal and abnormal functions of the extraocular muscles in the dog because of the lack of experimental data for the dog and the reliance upon what is known in humans.

Clinical Signs

STRABISMUS (Fig. 5–4). Lesions of the abducent nucleus or nerve cause paralysis of the lateral rectus and retractor bulbi muscles. Paralysis of the lateral rectus results in a medial strabismus, an abnormal position of that eyeball resulting in asymmetry. Compared with the normal eyeball, the affected eyeball cannot be abducted fully. This can be detected by moving the head from side to side in a horizontal plane and observing the degree of abduction and adduction of each eyeball.

Lesions of the trochlear nucleus or nerve paralyze the dorsal oblique muscle. In species with a round pupil, no strabismus may be observed; however, ophthalmoscopic examination may show the superior retinal vein deviated laterally from its normal vertical position because of the abnormal rotation caused by the tone in the unopposed ventral oblique muscle. In the cat the dorsal aspect of the vertical pupil would be positioned laterally (see Fig. 5–4). In the calf with a horizontal pupil, the medial aspect of the pupil is deviated dorsally. This is referred to as dorsomedial strabismus, and is seen in ruminants with polioencephalomalacia. It is assumed to be caused by the effects of this disease on the trochlear nucleus. It is also observed in cattle with cerebellar cortical abiotrophy presumably from altered cerebellar-vestibular tonic control over the lower motor neuron. It is important to be sure the bovine animal's head is in a normally extended posture when the eyeballs are examined for strabismus. Extension of the head above the normal plane normally induces a ventral and mild dorsomedial strabismus.

Lesions of the oculomotor nucleus or nerve produce a lateral and ventral strabismus due to the paralysis of the extraocular muscles, and ptosis due to the paralysis of the levator palpebrae muscle. In addition, the loss of function of the general visceral efferent neurons which are also a component of this nerve results in a dilated pupil that is unresponsive to light stimulus. There is experimental evidence to support the direction of this strabismus, although it is difficult to explain the ventral deviation on the basis of the anatomy of the oblique muscles.

When a strabismus is suspected, the eyeball movements should be tested to verify the paralysis of the extraocular muscles. This can be done by directing the gaze of the patient in different positions, or by moving the head of the patient vertically or horizontally and watching for the symmetry of the eyeball movements. The vestibular and cervical proprioceptive systems exert considerable influence over the nuclei of the cranial nerves innervating extraocular muscles. Movements of the head require a simultaneous conjugate response by the eyeballs to maintain the normal plane of vision. One of the major pathways involved in connecting the vestibular system to these nuclei is the medial longitudinal fasciculus. Lesions of the vestibular system or medial longitudinal fasciculus may cause an abnormal position of an eyeball when the head is in certain positions. This appears as a strabismus, but usually can be corrected by repositioning the head. A general somatic efferent lower motor neuron strabismus persists in all positions of the head.

Strabismus may also occur with some congenital abnormalities in the central projections of the visual system. Medial strabismus has been observed in Siamese cats that have a higher proportion of retinal ganglion cell neurons that project to the contralateral thalamus and visual cortex.[69]

NORMAL NYSTAGMUS. Nystagmus is an involuntary rhythmic movement of the eyeballs. It can be induced normally by slowly moving the head from side to side or up and down. Such head movement induces impulses in the vestibular component of the eighth cranial nerve from the stimulus to the receptors in the semicircular ducts. The afferent neuronal pathway that results in nystagmus continues through the vestibular nuclei in the medulla and via the medial longitudinal fasciculus to the brain stem nuclei, whose axons innervate the extraocular muscles. The efferent pathway involves the appropriate facilitation and inhibition of general somatic efferent neurons of cranial nerves III, IV, and VI to move the eyeballs.

This is tested best in domestic animals by slowly moving the head from side to side and observing the limbus to note the nystagmus. This form of nystagmus has a rapid phase in the direction of movement and a slow phase in the opposite direction. The direction of the nystagmus is defined by the direction of the rapid phase.

This form of normal nystagmus is called

vestibular, or physiologic, nystagmus because it is induced by head movements that initiate activity in the vestibular system. Some refer to this normal response as a "doll's eye" response or movement. The rapid phase or direction of the nystagmus is in the same direction as the movement of the head. Moving the head to the left causes a left nystagmus. Moving the head ventrally causes a ventral nystagmus. This occurs only as the head is being moved. Both eyeballs are affected similarly and move simultaneously, in conjugate fashion. It is abnormal if a nystagmus persists after the head movement is stopped. If the entire animal is rotated rapidly and then stopped, a brief normal postrotatory nystagmus occurs usually for less than 10 seconds. This nystagmus is opposite to the direction of the rotation. It is assumed that the slow movement is induced by the stimulation of the receptors in the vestibular system. The fast movement is a nonvestibular reflex resetting of the eyeball induced by a pontine reticular formation mechanism.

Lesions that destroy the vestibular system, the medial longitudinal fasciculus, or the neurons of cranial nerves III, IV, and VI cause a loss of normal vestibular nystagmus. In the neurologic evaluation of a patient following intracranial injury, it is important to distinguish between the signs of diffuse cerebral edema and those of brain stem contusion. A loss of the normal vestibular nystagmus indicates a severe lesion in the brain stem affecting the vestibular nuclei, or the medial longitudinal fasciculus, or both.

Observation of the eyeball response in normal vestibular nystagmus also allows evaluation of the function of specific extraocular muscles. In an animal with a right abducent nerve paralysis, there would be a medial strabismus of the right eyeball. In testing for normal vestibular nystagmus, the right eyeball would fail to abduct fully on moving the head to the right.

SPECIAL VISCERAL EFFERENT— SVE

The neurons of the special visceral efferent portion of the lower motor neuron generally innervate striated voluntary muscle derived from branchial arch mesoderm that is associated with visceral structures of the respiratory and digestive systems. These neurons are found in cranial nerves V, VII, IX, X, and XI. The muscles innervated include the muscles of mastication (V), facial muscles (VII), the muscles of the palate, pharynx, larynx, and esophagus (IX, X, XI), and cervical muscles (XI). The nuclei that contain the SVE neurons in the brain stem are located in an incomplete longitudinal column in a ventrolateral position from the pons to the caudal medulla. In the embryo these are located ventral to the floor of the fourth ventricle between the general somatic efferent and general visceral efferent immature neurons. This SVE column migrates ventrolaterally to a position closer to its main source of afferent stimuli from the trigeminal system. This phenomenon is called neurobiotaxis. An additional special visceral efferent nucleus is located in the ventral grey column of the cervical spinal cord.

CRANIAL NERVE V—TRIGEMINAL NEURONS

The SVE neuronal cell bodies are located in the motor nucleus of the trigeminal nerve in the pons (Plate 7). The nucleus is found at the level of the rostral cerebellar peduncle in the lateral reticular formation, medial to the pontine sensory nucleus of the trigeminal nerve and dorsal to the dorsal nucleus of the trapezoid body. This nucleus lacks a distinct boundary (Fig. 5–5).

The axons pass laterally and slightly ventrally through the middle cerebellar peduncle to join the sensory neurons of the trigeminal nerve. Between the pons and the trigeminal canal these motor neurons often can be seen as a separate nerve (the motor root) on the medial aspect of the sensory part of the trigeminal nerve. These motor neurons pass through the trigeminal ganglion in the trigeminal canal of the petrosal bone, join the mandibular nerve, and pass through the oval foramen to be distributed to the muscles of mastication: masseter, temporal, pterygoids, rostral digastricus, and mylohyoid.

Clinical Signs. Bilateral disease of these motor neurons causes a dropped jaw that cannot be closed. There is difficulty prehending food or retaining it in the oral cavity. Manipulation of the jaw reveals the muscle atonia. Neurogenic atrophy follows if the paralysis persists. Unilateral disease may be difficult to discover until the muscle atrophy appears. The lower jaw may be directed toward the side of

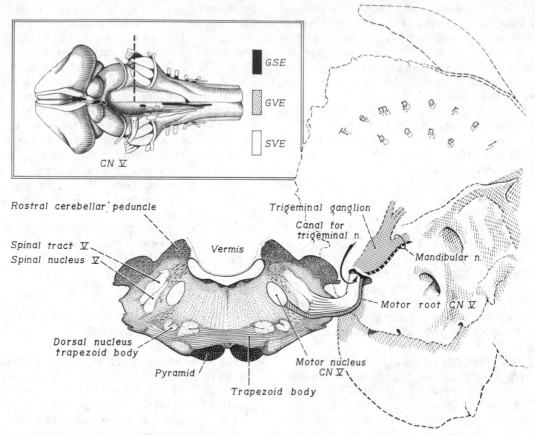

Figure 5–5. Transverse section of pons at level of motor nucleus of trigeminal nerve.

the lesion by the unopposed tone in the normal pterygoids and chewing may be asymmetric, but this is difficult to detect.

CRANIAL NERVE VII—FACIAL NEURONS

These special visceral efferent neuronal cell bodies are located in the facial nucleus in the medulla caudal to the trapezoid body and the level of attachment of the caudal cerebellar peduncle to the cerebellum (Plate 5). The nucleus is ventrolateral in the medulla midway between the pyramid and the spinal tract of the trigeminal nerve. It is caudal to the dorsal nucleus of the trapezoid body and rostral to the olivary nucleus (Fig. 5–6).

The axons pass dorsomedially to the midline of the floor of the fourth ventricle. Here they pass rostrally over the abducent nucleus in the genu of the facial nerve, then course ventrolaterally through the medulla medial to the spinal nucleus and tract of the trigeminal nerve

and lateral to the dorsal nucleus of the trapezoid body (Plate 6). The axons emerge through the trapezoid body on the ventral side of the vestibulocochlear nerve. The facial nerve passes into the internal acoustic meatus of the petrosal bone on the dorsal side of the vestibulocochlear nerve. The facial nerve passes through the facial canal in the petrosal bone and emerges through the stylomastoid foramen. Branches of the facial nerve are distributed to the muscles of facial expression, that is, the muscles of the ear, eyelids, nose, cheeks, lips, and the caudal portion of the digastricus muscle.

Clinical Signs. Lesions of the nucleus or the nerve up to the level of its termination into the branches that supply the different muscle groups result in a complete facial paresis or paralysis, with inability to move these muscles normally. The paralysis can be seen in the asymmetric position of the ears, eyelids, lips, and nose. The ear may droop in those animals with a normally erect aural posture. If the ear cartilage is stiff, as in most cats and

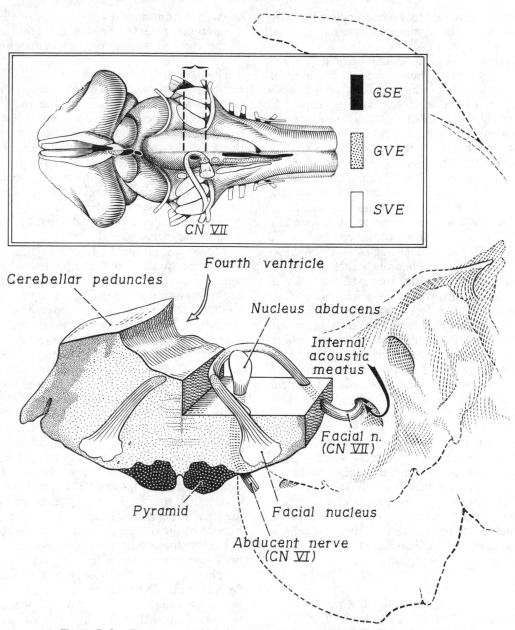

Figure 5–6. Transverse section of medulla at level of facial and abducent nuclei.

dogs, it may keep the ear erect despite the muscular paralysis. The lip may droop on the affected side, allowing saliva to drip from the corner of the mouth. It is helpful to extend the head with a finger between the mandible and examine the corner of the lips for asymmetry. On the paralyzed side more mucosa is exposed, and drooling may be apparent. The nose may be pulled toward the normal side owing to the unopposed nasal muscles. This deviation is remarkable in the horse and obvious in sheep and goats. In the dog and cat there is only a slight deviation of the philtrum from its normally vertical position. During inspiration the nostril may not be opened as wide as usual on the affected side. The palpebral fissure in small animals is often slightly wider than average and fails to close on stimulation of the cornea or eyelids (corneal and palpebral reflexes). In facial paresis this closure is weak. In large animals the loss of tone in the frontalis muscle which contributes fibers that elevate the dorsal eyelid causes slight ptosis. The eyelids of both sides should be palpated simultaneously for strength of closure in examining for asymmetry in cases of facial paresis.

Lesions of the individual branches of the facial nerve along their course to the muscles they innervate produce paresis or paralysis restricted to those muscle groups. Injury to the buccal branches of the facial nerve on the side of the masseter muscle causes the lips to droop and the nose to be pulled toward the normal side. This occurs in horses that are tabled for surgery for a prolonged period of time without proper padding of the head. Eyelid and ear function are normal. Injury to the auriculopalpebral nerve at the zygomatic arch only causes paresis of the ear and eyelid muscles. Cattle that struggle in a stanchion may injure the palpebral branch where it crosses the zygomatic arch. This results in unilateral or bilateral eyelid paralysis.

Because of the close association of the facial and vestibulocochlear nerves, they often are affected simultaneously by the same lesion. This can happen in or on the medulla or in the petrosal bone.[2] It is important to distinguish between the two locations because of the difference in the therapy and prognosis. Both a medullary neoplasm and otitis media-interna can affect the function of these two cranial nerves. The former usually affects the function of other brain stem structures, which aids in the location of the lesion. These structures include the upper motor neuron, causing tetra- or hemiparesis; general proprioception, producing ataxia; ascending reticular activating system, resulting in signs ranging from depression to coma; and the abducent nucleus, bringing about medial strabismus.

CRANIAL NERVES IX, X, AND XI— GLOSSOPHARYNGEAL, VAGUS, AND ACCESSORY NEURONS

These three will be considered together because their special visceral efferent neuronal cell bodies are all located in one nucleus, nucleus ambiguus.[8] They are topographically organized, with the SVE neuronal cell bodies of the glossopharyngeal nerve the most rostral and those of the accessory nerve the most caudal. Nucleus ambiguus is an ill-defined column of neurons located ventrolateral in the medulla medial to the spinal tract and nucleus of the trigeminal nerve (Plates 3, 4). It extends from the facial nucleus rostrally through the caudal medulla to a level slightly caudal to the obex. It is continued by the motor nucleus of the accessory nerve through the grey matter of the cervical spinal cord segments (Fig. 5–7).

The axons of the neuronal cell bodies in the rostral part of nucleus ambiguus arch slightly dorsally and ventrolaterally, to emerge with the general visceral efferent axons of the glossopharyngeal nerve along the lateral aspect of the medulla caudal to the vestibulocochlear nerve. The glossopharyngeal nerve traverses the jugular foramen and the tympanooccipital fissure. Its special visceral efferent axons innervate the stylopharyngeus and may be distributed to other pharyngeal muscles by way of the pharyngeal plexus.

The axons of the SVE cell bodies in the middle portion of nucleus ambiguus take a similar course and emerge with the GVE axons of the vagus nerve on the lateral aspect of the medulla caudal to the glossopharyngeal roots.[11, 20] The SVE axons pass in the vagus nerve through the jugular foramen and tympanooccipital fissure. Some join the pharyngeal plexus with the glossopharyngeal neurons to innervate muscles of the palate and pharynx and cervical esophagus. Others leave the vagus in the cranial laryngeal nerve to innervate the cricothyroid muscle. The recurrent laryngeal nerve and its caudal laryngeal branch innervate all the other muscles of the larynx and cervical and cranial thoracic esophagus. In the cat and in humans, these latter SVE axons have been determined to arise from the caudal portion of nucleus ambiguus, and they pass to the vagus by way of the internal branch of the accessory nerve. As the vagus nerve courses through the neck and thorax, branches supply the striated esophageal muscle. These branches contain SVE neurons from nucleus ambiguus. Studies with horseradish peroxidase on esophageal innervation show that cell bodies in the nucleus ambiguus innervate the entire length of the esophagus.[39]

The axons of the SVE neuronal cell bodies in the caudal portion of nucleus ambiguus arch slightly dorsally and course ventrolaterally to emerge from the lateral aspect of the medulla with the GVE axons of the cranial roots of the accessory nerve. These are caudal to the vagal SVE and GVE axons. The cranial roots join to form the internal branch of the accessory nerve. The internal branch passes laterally and joins the external branch of the accessory nerve, which courses rostrally along the cervical spinal cord and medulla. For a short distance these SVE neurons form part of the

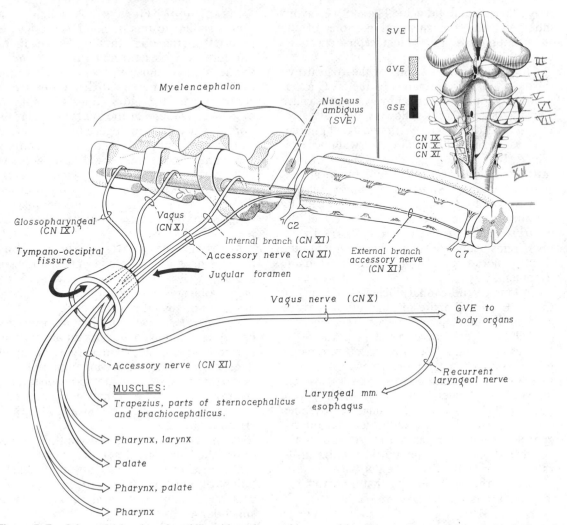

Figure 5–7. Schematic drawing of medulla with nucleus ambiguus and its efferent neurons and cervical spinal cord with external branch of accessory nerve.

accessory nerve as it enters the jugular foramen. As the accessory nerve traverses the jugular foramen and tympanooccipital fissure, the internal branch leaves the accessory nerve and joins the vagus nerve. The SVE axons of this internal branch are thought to innervate the muscles of the larynx and cervical and cranial thoracic esophagus by way of the recurrent laryngeal nerve branch of the vagus nerve.[66] Electromyographic studies in the anesthetized horse show that the cricoarytenoideus dorsalis and cricothyroid muscles are most active during inspiration. The other intrinsic laryngeal muscles are more active during expiration.[29]

The SVE neuronal cell bodies of the external branch of the accessory nerve are located in the motor nucleus of the accessory nerve in the lateral portion of the ventral grey column, from the first to sixth or seventh cervical spinal cord segments.

The axons pass laterally to emerge from the lateral side of the spinal cord as the spinal roots of the accessory nerve. These join to form a common bundle—the external branch of the accessory nerve—which courses cranially dorsal to the denticulate ligament between the segmental dorsal and ventral rootlets of the cervical spinal nerves (see Fig. 5–7). More SVE axons are added to it from each successive cervical segment. The external branch passes rostrally through the foramen magnum into the cranial cavity. The internal branch joins with it temporarily as it passes through the jugular foramen. The accessory nerve emerging from the tympanooccipital fissure contains only its external branch. These SVE axons innervate the trapezius and portions of the sternocephalicus and brachiocephalicus muscles.

Clinical Signs. Lesions of the rostral two thirds of nucleus ambiguus or the SVE axons in the glossopharyngeal and vagal nerves cause varying degrees of swallowing difficulty, referred to as dysphagia. With unilateral pharyngeal paralysis partial ability to swallow is retained, but choking, gagging, and loss of food through the nostrils occurs. With bilateral pharyngeal paralysis swallowing cannot be performed, and attempts are accompanied by choking and the appearance of food at the nostrils. The gag reflex is absent. Normal swallowing has been thoroughly documented in the dog by cineradiography[65] as a basis for studying dysphagia.[60]

Lesions of the caudal nucleus ambiguus or the SVE axons in the internal branch of the accessory nerve, vagus nerve, recurrent or caudal laryngeal nerve result in paralysis of the laryngeal muscles.[33] Laryngeal hemiplegia is proposed to occur more frequently in mature, long-necked horses from constant stretching of the longer left recurrent laryngeal nerve.[43, 44] This causes an inspiratory dyspnea (roaring), owing to the failure of the left cricoarytenoideus dorsalis muscle to abduct the vocal fold and dilate the glottis. Similar inspiratory dyspnea is seen in the dog with bilateral disease of the SVE neurons that innervate the laryngeal muscle.

DISEASES

The following are examples of diseases that affect one or more of the cranial nerve general somatic efferent neurons and special visceral efferent lower motor neurons.

Neuromuscular Junction

BOTULISM. The toxin produced by *Clostridium botulinum* affects all the neuromuscular junctions of striated muscle, interfering with the release of acetylcholine. Multiple cranial nerve deficits accompany the generalized GSE spinal nerve deficit. Facial, hypoglossal, pharyngeal, and esophageal paresis all occur. Dysphagia is a common sign. Regurgitation from megaesophagus may occur in dogs. Extraocular muscle paresis often is not obvious to the examiner. Cattle probably are the most susceptible among domestic animals, and the dog the least susceptible. A more complete description of this disease can be found in Chapter 4.

MYASTHENIA GRAVIS. A clinical syndrome similar to this human disease has been reported in the dog. In this disease there is interference with neuromuscular transmission at the striated muscle receptor. This affects both the spinal nerve GSE neurons and the cranial nerve GSE and SVE neurons that elaborate acetylcholine at the neuromuscular junction. Dysphagia and regurgitation associated with megaesophagus have been seen most commonly. Facial and hypoglossal paresis with abnormal prehension and laryngeal paralysis with inspiratory dyspnea resulting in cyanosis also have been found. A more complete description of this disease can be found in Chapter 4.

MYOSITIS—MYOPATHY. Primary muscle diseases may affect the pharyngeal and esophageal muscles and result in dysphagia and megaesophagus with regurgitation. These diseases are discussed in Chapter 4.

Peripheral Nerves. Peripheral nerves can be injured, involved in inflammatory or neoplastic lesions of adjacent tissues, or undergo degeneration from direct inflammation of the nerve (neuritis) or from metabolic disturbances (neuropathy). These cranial nerve lesions are presented in a caudal to rostral order (XII to III).

1. Injury: A fractured hyoid bone could injure the hypoglossal nerve and cause ipsilateral paresis of the tongue. Strenuous manipulation of the tongue has been reported to produce a temporary paralysis in horses and small dogs.

2. Laryngeal Hemiplegia-Paralysis: Horse — Laryngeal hemiplegia is the cause of the so-called "roarer horse." It is usually more profound on the left side and involves paralysis of all the muscles innervated by the left recurrent laryngeal nerve. Paralysis of the cricoarytenoideus dorsalis causes inability to abduct the vocal fold; on inspiration this interferes with the flow of air, creating an audible sound— roaring. Expiration takes place without an audible sound, since the vocal fold is moved aside passively by the air. The position of the laryngeal ventricle, with its opening cranial to the vocal fold, augments the inspiratory dyspnea.

Pathologic studies on the laryngeal muscles and recurrent laryngeal nerves have confirmed that the muscle lesions consist of neurogenic atrophy caused by denervation.[20-23] The most profound peripheral nerve lesions occur at the level of the larynx, with both myelin and axon degenerations.[12] More proximally, in the recurrent laryngeal nerve there is segmental demyelination and remyelination of normal-appearing axons. This lesion has been described as a dying-back of the axon. Many subclinical patients have been described.[19]

A number of explanations have been offered for this unique asymmetric lesion based on the longer intrathoracic course of the left recurrent laryngeal nerve and its relationship to the arch of the aorta. Early explanations emphasized the greater exposure of the left recurrent laryngeal nerve to inflammatory diseases in the thorax affecting lymph nodes and pleura adjacent to the nerve.[31]

The disease is reported to occur predominantly in the larger breeds or the larger individuals of the light horse breeds (15 to 17 hands).[41, 43, 44] Based on this observation, the following hypothesis was suggested:[55, 56]

The left recurrent laryngeal nerve passes caudal to the aortic arch and is longer and farther ventral from the vertebral column than the right recurrent laryngeal nerve, which passes around the costocervical artery of the right subclavian artery. If the center of rotation of the head and neck is considered to be the cervicothoracic junction, and both recurrent nerves are fixed cranially at the larynx and caudally at the respective arteries that they pass around, the right recurrent laryngeal nerve is closer to the center of rotation and is more congruent with the axis of the cervical vertebrae. Therefore, when the neck is extended or flexed to the right, greater tension is exerted on the left recurrent laryngeal nerve. Continual tension on this left nerve directly or on its blood supply may cause the nerve to degenerate by interfering with axon flow at this point. This would produce the most severe neuropathy distally at the larynx and explain the dying-back of the axons. This happens more commonly in large, mature horses with long necks and deep chests, because the left nerve is displaced further from the cervicothoracic junction and the vertebral axis and is more susceptible to tension in this position.

Study of the left recurrent laryngeal nerve where it courses around the aorta in clinically affected patients has not revealed any compressive or ischemic lesion at this site. Although the exceedingly long length of the left recurrent laryngeal nerve may be important in the pathogenesis of the distal axon degeneration, the specific mechanism remains unknown. The higher incidence of clinical disease in longer-necked horses may relate only to the longer length of the nerve and not to its specific relationship to the aorta.

Laryngeal paralysis has been reported in Arabian foals, associated with the administration of oral haloxon starting at 2 days old.[67]

Dog—Laryngeal paresis has been noted in dogs with chronic polyneuritis-polyneuropathy.[47] Excessive manipulation of the vagal nerves or their fibrosis subsequent to surgery for fenestration of cervical intervertebral disks may cause laryngeal paresis or paralysis and regurgitation due to esophageal malfunction.[33] In thyroidectomy the recurrent laryngeal nerve is often interrupted or fibrosed. The nerve passes cranially on the dorsal edge of the thyroid gland. Bilateral involvement causes laryngeal paralysis with episodes of gagging, cyanosis, and collapse. Laryngeal hemiplegia and dysphagia occurred in a cat with extensive involvement of one vagus nerve and its distal ganglion with lymphosarcoma.[46]

Laryngeal paresis alone or with megaesophagus has been observed in hypothyroid dogs.

3. Guttural Pouch Mycosis: In horses, mycotic inflammation of the dorsal wall of the guttural pouch is the most common cause of dysphagia and epistaxis (nosebleed).[13-15, 27, 42] This pouch is a sac-like ventral diverticulum of the auditory tube that is situated dorsal to the pharynx on each side, ventral to the cranium and atlas (Fig. 5–8). As they course to the pharyngeal muscles, the glossopharyngeal nerve and pharyngeal branch of the vagus nerve are associated closely with the caudodorsal and lateral walls of the medial compartment of the guttural pouch. Involvement of these nerves in the mycotic inflammation causes ipsilateral dysphagia. If the inflammation erodes the internal carotid artery, which also courses along the caudodorsal and mediodorsal walls of the medial compartment, bleeding occurs into the pouch and out the pharyngeal opening into the nasopharynx. This is the source of the epistaxis. The same lesion that affects the internal carotid artery may involve the associated internal carotid nerve, which consists of postganglionic sympathetic axons passing to structures in the head, including the contents of the orbit. Paralysis of the smooth muscle of the orbit results in Horner's syndrome. Extensive inflammation also can involve the adjacent facial nerve, producing facial paralysis, or the vagus nerve, producing laryngeal hemiplegia. Proliferative lesions are commonly observed in the proximal end of the stylohyoid bone and its articulation through the tympanohyoid with the petrosal bone in these horses with guttural pouch mycosis. Although these lesions frequently involve the

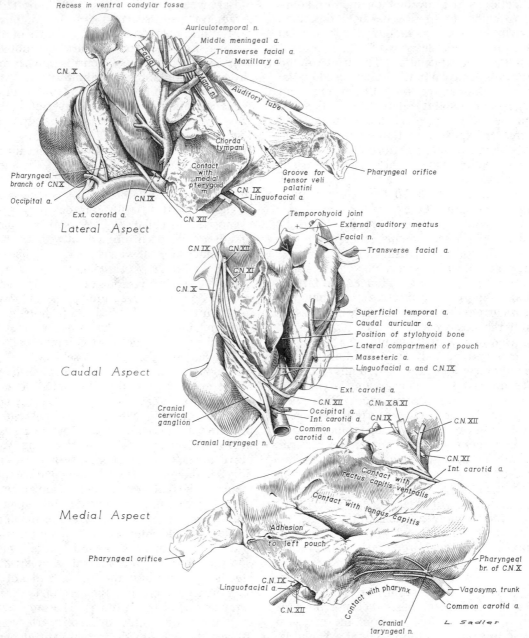

Figure 5–8. Dissection of the right guttural pouch of a horse with its associated cranial nerves and vessels. (From Habel, R. E.: Applied Veterinary Anatomy. Ithaca, N.Y., R. E. Habel, 1975.)

wall of the tympanic bulla, only rarely do peripheral vestibular signs occur with this disease.

It is hypothesized that a fungus, a species of *Aspergillus* that is normally a harmless contaminant of the guttural pouch, invades the tissues of the wall of the pouch when they are injured by trauma associated with the hyoid bone. Therapy for this disease is difficult. Systemic and local applications of various fungicidal agents have been used. Local lavage of the guttural pouch with iodine solutions has been the most effective. A surgical procedure has been described to prevent hemorrhage from the involved portion of the internal carotid artery.[28] This involves placement of a catheter with an inflatable balloon in the internal carotid artery. The balloon is placed beyond the site of the lesion to occlude the retrograde flow of blood from the cerebral arterial circle when the internal carotid artery is occluded at its origin from the common carotid artery.

4. Neoplasia: Neoplastic involvement of the nerves along their course can affect their function. These neoplasms can be external to the skull, involving only the peripheral nerves, or inside the cranial cavity, involving bone or meninges and the peripheral nerves passing through them. Signs of involvement of the adjacent brain stem aid in locating the mass within the cranial cavity.

Beware of dogs that present with the chief complaint of chronic gagging and coughing in the absence of a pharyngeal, laryngeal, or palatal lesion as an explanation. If the problem persists, be sure to consider a paresis or paralysis of the nerves to these muscles on one side. An inflammatory or neoplastic involvement of these nerves in their extracranial course could explain a chronic syndrome of gagging and coughing. A neoplastic lesion may be palpated through the mouth just ventral to the area of the tympanic bulla.

Meningioma of the meninges ventral to the medulla, and mostly on the right side, resulted in progressive partial hypoglossal paresis (XII), right-sided vestibular signs (VIII), paresis more on the right side of the body (right hemiparesis) with deficient postural reactions (upper motor neuron and general proprioception), and depression (ascending reticular activating system—ARAS) in a 9-year-old spaniel dog.

Osteogenic sarcoma of the right petrous temporal and basioccipital bone caused dysphagia in a 1-year-old German shepherd from involvement of the glossopharyngeal nerve and vagus nerve.

A carotid body neoplasm in a 9-year-old wire-haired fox terrier involved the hypoglossal nerve and produced an ipsilateral paresis of the tongue.[4]

A 4-year-old female Norwegian elkhound developed bilateral paralysis and atrophy of the muscles of mastication, complete inability to move the eyeballs, and blindness with dilated unresponsive pupils. This was caused by a diffuse meningioma in the middle and rostral cranial fossae that destroyed cranial nerves II, III, IV, V, and VI as they coursed to their appropriate foramina.

Two aged cats, 10 and 13 years old, had unilateral facial paralysis, sympathetic paralysis of the head, and peripheral vestibular disturbance all on one side.[50] Each had radiographic evidence of neoplastic involvement of the tympanic portion of the temporal bone. One neoplasm was a fibrosarcoma; the other was a squamous cell carcinoma.

5. Otitis Media-Interna: Otitis media in all species occasionally involves the facial nerve as it traverses the facial canal in the petrosal bone.[2] In its course through this canal, a portion of the nerve is separated from the cavity of the tympanic bulla (middle ear) only by a small amount of loose connective tissue. Paresis or paralysis is observed in the entire area of distribution of the facial nerve. These usually are associated with signs of vestibular ataxia caused by the disturbance of the vestibulocochlear nerve in the inner ear. In small animals, Horner's syndrome may accompany inflammatory lesions of the middle ear from involvement of the postganglionic sympathetic axons that pass through the middle ear.

In adult horses a syndrome of facial and vestibular nerve paresis to paralysis has been observed associated with radiographic evidence of bony enlargement of the proximal end of the stylohyoid bone. This increased area of radiopacity usually surrounds the area of the tympanic bulla. There is no evidence of mycosis in the adjacent guttural pouch of these horses. The relationship of the chronic otitis media to the periosteal bone proliferation along the stylohyoid bone remains to be determined. There is no osteomyelitis. Despite the guarded prognosis due to the degree of bone involvement, complete recovery from the clinical neurologic signs has been observed following prolonged antibiotic therapy. Facial paralysis and peripheral vestibular disturbance were reported in four horses with radiographic evidence of tympanosclerosis; two of these also had a prior history of cranial injury.[24]

6. Hemifacial Spasm: A constant contraction of all the facial muscles on one side of the head, called hemifacial spasm, has been observed in dogs. On the affected side of the face the nose will be pulled caudally and the lips will feel hypertonic. The palpebral fissure will be smaller owing to partial closure of the eyelids, and the ear will be slightly elevated. In most dogs, some slight movement can be stimulated in the eyelids and sometimes the ear and nose. The facial muscles on the opposite side function normally.

This syndrome has been observed and described in patients with otitis media with or without signs of vestibular system disturbance and Horner's syndrome. A hyperirritability of the facial nerve has been offered as the explanation for the signs observed.[26, 52]

I have observed patients with spontaneous hemifacial spasm with no prior history of neurologic signs and no other signs suggestive of an otitis, and I have observed one dog in which this syndrome followed a complete facial paralysis of unknown cause.

General anesthesia or local anesthesia of branches of the involved facial nerve will decrease these clinical signs. This means that the signs are not the result of a complete facial paralysis followed by neurogenic atrophy and contraction of the facial muscles from the shortened atrophied muscle cells. A hyperirritability from a facial neuritis is presumed to be involved in these dogs. Once these signs develop they usually persist unaltered, despite antibiotic and/or corticosteroid therapy. Hemifacial spasm that precedes signs of progressive central nervous system disease has not yet been observed.

One mature dog had episodes of hemifacial spasm and Horner's syndrome every 3 to 4 weeks following head trauma from an automobile that caused rupture of the ipsilateral tympanum.

In humans hemifacial spasm is reported with peripheral nerve disorders and with intramedullary neoplasms of the mesencephalon, pons, and medulla.[48] It is proposed that the latter lesion isolates the facial nuclear motoneurons from the upper motor neuron and inhibitory interneuronal activity. Mild hemifacial spasm was noted in a mature horse with a proliferative nonsuppurative focal encephalitis of the medulla thought to be caused by a protozoal agent. Spasms of muscles innervated by cranial nerves III, V, VII and XII all on one side were reported in one dog with a focal gliotic lesion in the medulla.[49]

7. Injury to the petrosal bone may cause hemorrhage in the middle and inner ears and bleeding from the external ear canal through a ruptured tympanum. This usually is associated with a fracture of the basioccipital or petrosal bone. Facial nerve function may be sacrificed, along with that of the vestibulocochlear nerve.

8. Facial paresis can accompany the signs of polyneuritis of coonhound paralysis, of brachial plexus neuritis, or of neuritis of the cauda equina in horses. The signs are usually those of paresis, not paralysis.

9. Idiopathic facial paralysis occurs in the dog. The onset is generally sudden and the course variable. Improvement may take place in a few weeks. Complete recovery may never occur. There are no other signs of neurologic disease. Pathologic studies of fascicular biopsies of the facial nerve in the dog have revealed axonal degeneration and secondary demyelination of the larger neurons. This occurred proximally as far as the stylomastoid foramen. The inability to close the eyelids may lead to secondary corneal lesions from improper lubrication with lacrimal secretions. In humans this is referred to as Bell's palsy and is postulated to be a facial neuritis. It is treated with corticosteroids.[1]

Unilateral or bilateral facial paresis or paralysis in dogs may be caused by a neuropathy associated with chronic hypothyroidism, or pituitary neoplasia, or both. Signs of peripheral vestibular disturbance often are associated with this. In experimental studies of hypothyroidism the signs of facial and vestibular nerve disturbance have resolved following thyroid hormone therapy. Results have been less remarkable in clinical cases. The reason for the predominant involvement of cranial nerves VII and VIII in this endocrinopathy is unknown.

In a few instances bilateral facial paralysis with unilateral or bilateral vestibular signs unrelated to hypothyroidism has resolved spontaneously. Steroid therapy has been used, but its efficacy is unknown. It is suspected that the lesion is a polyneuritis of cranial nerves VII and VIII.

10. Trigeminal Neuritis: Bilateral paralysis of the muscles of mastication (motor V palsy) is found in dogs and cats. There is a fairly sudden onset of inability to close the jaw, and it hangs loose with the mouth open. Food cannot be prehended. Swallowing is usually normal, although occasionally some dysphagia has been suspected. No obvious deficit of sensory perception from the head has been observed, although it would be expected with complete involvement of the trigeminal nerve. In a few dogs unilateral Horner's syndrome has occurred, presumably from involvement of the postganglionic sympathetic axons coursing in the ophthalmic nerve. Recovery usually occurs in 2 to 3 weeks. The dog or cat may have to be tube-fed during part of this time. Necropsy has revealed an extensive bilateral nonsuppurative neuritis of all portions of the trigeminal nerve and ganglion, but no involvement of the brain stem. Demyelination was more prominent than axonal degeneration. The cause is unknown. Recovery is assumed to follow remyelination. In a few dogs atrophy has occurred in the masticatory muscles during the recovery stage; the muscles have later returned to normal. At no time has trismus been observed.

An identical clinical syndrome in the dog has been described as mandibular neurapraxia and ascribed to traumatic stretching, pinching, or ischemia of the nerve.[53] There is no confirmation of these lesions. There is no history or evidence of trauma in the patients I have studied, and this would be most unlikely without skeletal damage.

11. Compression of the oculomotor nerve on the ventral surface of the cranial cavity in cases of extensive hydrocephalus involving the lateral ventricles may be the cause of a ventrolateral strabismus. However, in most instances the apparent strabismus is due to the malformation of the orbits that accompanies the skull deformity.

Brain Stem Neurons. Disease in the brain stem can destroy the cell bodies or the intramedullary axons of these neurons.

1. Abiotrophy–Hereditary Laryngeal Paralysis in Bouviers: Spontaneous laryngeal paralysis occurs in young Bouviers, with onset around 4 to 6 months of age.[61, 63, 64] Clinical signs consist of increasing loss of endurance, increasing laryngeal stridor, and dyspnea on exertion. During stress, hyperthermia, cyanosis, vomiting, and collapse may occur. Dysfunction of the laryngeal abductor muscles can be observed on laryngoscopy. EMG of intrinsic laryngeal muscles demonstrates denervation potentials. On necropsy neurogenic atrophy is present in laryngeal muscles and Wallerian degeneration in the recurrent laryngeal nerves. Studies of the nucleus ambiguus show a decreased number of neuronal cell bodies and degeneration of cell bodies bilaterally. Pedigree and breeding studies support an autosomal dominant inheritance.[62]

2. Esophageal hypomotility will result from loss of neurons in the nucleus ambiguus that innervate the esophageal striated muscle. Canine esophageal achalasia, megaesophagus, and esophageal neuromuscular disease are synonyms for a disease that is common in dogs and occasionally occurs in cats.[9, 17, 32, 37, 54, 58] It has been reported in almost all breeds of dogs including mixed breeds, but occurs predominantly in the German shepherd. It is reported as an inherited disease in wire-haired fox terriers and miniature schnauzers.[11, 16] The congenital form usually becomes apparent in the young animal when it is weaned. It also occurs as an acquired disease in older dogs.[36] There is one report of a foal with congenital megaesophagus.[3]

The salient clinical features are postprandial regurgitation of undigested food, with radiographic evidence of megaesophagus to the level of the diaphragm. Contrast radiography demonstrates abnormal esophageal motility, with failure of the gastroesophageal junction to dilate when swallowing is initiated. Often if the dog is stood on its pelvic limbs, the added weight of the esophageal contents aids movement through this junction, which is not hypertonic. In most cases there is no true achalasia or primary failure of the gastroesophageal junction to relax.

The pathogenesis is unknown, but experimental studies suggest that the disturbance is neural, not muscular.[8, 30, 50, 59] Myenteric ganglion cells appear to be present in normal numbers.[5, 7] One study in one dog demonstrated a lack of the normal number of neuronal cell bodies in the nucleus ambiguus.[10] A similar study in 3 cats did not show any abnormality in the nucleus ambiguus or the parasympathetic nucleus of the vagus.[6] Further investigations of a similar nature are needed. It has been shown in dogs that the striated muscle of the esophagus is innervated by special visceral efferent neurons that course from the nucleus ambiguus to the esophagus in the vagus nerves.[39]

Unilateral vagus nerve lesions or vagotomy usually is not associated with clinical signs in dogs. Bilateral cervical vagal disease or vagotomy causes paralysis of the larynx with inspiratory dyspnea and cyanosis, and abnormal esophageal swallowing with regurgitation and megaesophagus. In response to swallowing there is absence of normal esophageal peristalsis and failure of the gastroesophageal junction (sphincter) to relax. Food accumulates in the distal esophagus, which dilates. Bilateral cranial thoracic vagal disease or vagotomy that spares the recurrent laryngeal nerves produces abnormal function of the thoracic esophagus with regurgitation of undigested food and megaesophagus. These signs closely resemble the natural disease in dogs and cats most often referred to as achalasia. Electrolytic lesions of the nucleus ambiguus in dogs and of the parasympathetic nucleus of the vagus in cats produce esophageal dysfunction similar to the clinical syndrome.[34]

3. Listeriosis is a bacterial disease of the brain caused by *Listeria monocytogenes*. It is seen primarily in ruminants and has a predilection for the brain stem, in which it produces foci of necrosis and inflammation. These usually consist of a mixture of mononuclear cells and foci of neutrophils in the parenchyma. Occasionally, it is entirely a mononuclear inflammation.

Multiple neurologic signs are produced that may include unilateral facial paresis or paralysis, abducent paralysis, trigeminal paralysis, especially the motor component, and pharyngeal paralysis. Signs of disturbance to consciousness (ARAS), circling (SP), and paresis to paralysis of the limbs (UMN) indicate that the lesion is confined to the central nervous system. Vestibular signs (SP) often accompany the lesion because of the involvement of the vestibular nuclei in the medulla. CSF is often abnormal, with changes characteristic of non-suppurative disease despite the fact that this is a bacterial disease, often with many neutrophils in the lesion. (Example: a 2-year-old cow with 31 mononuclear cells per cu mm and 79 mg of protein per dl.) The most common signs are facial paresis, head tilt and ataxia, dysphagia, weak jaw, paresis of limbs, and depression.

4. Leukoencephalomyelitis occurs most commonly in young goats and is caused by a type C retrovirus (CAE virus), which also produces arthritis in older goats. Lesions can occur anywhere in the spinal cord or brain. Occasionally lesions are limited to or predominate in the pons and medulla and produce signs similar to those described for listeriosis.

5. Rabies is caused by a virus that primarily destroys neuronal cell bodies. Although there are textbook descriptions of the furious and dumb forms of this disease, there is nothing typical about the way it presents. Involvement of the cell bodies of these lower motor neurons in the brain stem can cause deficits in their function. Pharyngeal paralysis (nucleus ambiguus) and paralysis of the muscles of mastication with a dropped jaw (motor nucleus of cranial nerve V) are the lower motor neuron signs most commonly seen.

6. Focal protozoal encephalitis of the medulla of horses may produce signs similar to those of listeriosis in ruminants.

7. Neoplasms of the brain stem may involve the intramedullary portion of these neurons. Other signs of brain stem involvement accompany the lower motor neuron.

8. In polioencephalomalacia in ruminants the only suggestion of cranial neuronal involvement is strabismus, with the medial aspect of the eyeball deviated dorsally.[38] This is thought to be the result of a peculiar sensitivity of trochlear neurons to this degenerative metabolic disease.

9. Leukoencephalomalacia occurs in horses that feed on moldy corn for an extended period of time. The lesion is primarily in the cerebral white matter, but all parts of the neuraxis can be affected by the necrosis and the edema. Pharyngeal paralysis often accompanies the signs of cerebral disturbance (lethargy, dementia, visual deficit, circling). This dysphagia actually may be caused by the acute disturbance of upper motor neuron control of the brain stem centers for swallowing.[35]

DIFFERENTIAL DIAGNOSIS OF PHARYNGEAL PARALYSIS IN THE HORSE

Pharyngeal paresis or paralysis is a common clinical sign in the horse. The following is a differential diagnosis for this clinical deficit, in order of site of lesion.

Pharyngeal Muscles. There are no accompanying signs to suggest involvement of the brain. Myositis of pharyngeal muscles may be accompanied by myositis of the muscles of the tongue, mastication, or heart. Inflammation of heart muscles causes the patient's sudden demise. Muscle cell enzyme levels may be elevated in the serum.

Pharyngeal Nerves (Glossopharyngeal and Vagus Nerves). There are no accompanying signs to suggest involvement of the brain. Pathogenesis is as follows:

1. Botulism is a common cause of dysphagia. The dysphagia is associated with other signs of the lower motor neuron–neuromuscular ending dysfunction of cranial and spinal nerves. It is helpful for diagnosis if more than one animal is affected.

2. Guttural pouch mycosis may lead to pharyngeal hemiplegia, laryngeal hemiplegia, or both, accompanied by an epistaxis. Visual examination of the interior of the pouch may be diagnostic.

3. Polyneuritis with pharyngeal, laryngeal, facial, and hypoglossal nerve involvement may accompany a neuritis of the cauda equina. The latter causes lower motor neuron paresis or paralysis of the tail, anus, bladder, and rectum, with hypalgesia or analgesia of the same areas. Pelvic limb function may be abnormal.

4. Polyneuropathy with pharyngeal and laryngeal nerve involvement occurs in chronic lead poisoning.

5. Injury: Dysphagia and laryngeal hemiplegia following injury to cranial nerves IX, X, and XI were caused by rupture of the longus capitis and the rectus capitis ventralis muscles from hyperextension.[40] This occurred when a horse fell over backwards while exercising on a mechanical horse-walker.

Nucleus Ambiguus or the Swallowing Center in the Medulla. Pharyngeal paralysis is accompanied by other signs of a focal (medullary) or diffuse (brain stem–cerebral) lesion. Pathogenesis is as follows:

1. Suppurative meningitis around the brain stem or a focal abscess in this area.

2. Encephalitis: rabies, equine viral encephalitides (VEE, EEE, WEE), or protozoal encephalitis.

3. Encephalomalacia: moldy corn poisoning.

4. Acute liver necrosis or chronic liver necrosis in the advanced stages, with encephalopathy.

Pharyngeal paralysis frequently accompanies severe cerebral disease without a specific lesion of the nucleus ambiguus or swallowing center, suggesting that higher centers are involved in this function.[35] This is referred to as a pseudobulbar palsy, for there is no specific lesion in the nuclei in the medulla (bulb). The lesion has destroyed the upper motor neurons in the cerebrum that influence the activity of the medullary nuclei, and dysphagia results.

REFERENCES

1. Adoor, K. K., Wingerd, J., Bell, D. N., Manning, J. J., and Hurley, J. P.: Prednisone treatment for idiopathic facial paralysis (Bell's palsy). N. Engl. J. Med., 287:1268, 1972.

2. Blauch, B., and Strafuss, A. C.: Histologic relationships of the facial (7th) and vestibulocochlear (8th) cranial nerves within the petrous temporal bone in the dog. Am. J. Vet. Res., 35:481, 1974.

3. Bowman, K. F., Vaughan, J. T., Quick, C. B., Hankes, C. H., Redding, R. W., Purohit, R. C., Rumph, P. F., Powers, R. D., and Harper, N. K.: Megaesophagus in a colt. J. Am. Vet. Med. Assoc., 172:334, 1978.

4. Chrisman, C. L.: Electromyography in the localization of spinal cord and nerve root neoplasia in dogs and cats. J. Am. Vet. Med. Assoc., 166:1074, 1975.

5. Clifford, D. H.: Myenteric ganglion cells of the esophagus in cats with achalasia of the esophagus. Am. J. Vet. Res., 34:1333, 1973.

6. Clifford, D. H., Barboza, P. F. T., and Pirsch, J. G.: The motor nuclei of the vagus nerve in cats with and without congenital achalasia of the esophagus. Br. Vet. J., 136:74, 1980.

7. Clifford, D. H., and Gyorkey, F.: Myenteric ganglion cells in dogs with and without hereditary achalasia of the esophagus. Am. J. Vet. Res., 32:615, 1971.

8. Clifford, D. H., Lee, M. O., Byun, K. W., and Lee, D. C.: Effects of autonomic drugs on the cardiovascular system: Dogs with achalasia (under halothane anesthesia). Am. J. Vet. Res., 38:323, 1977.

9. Clifford, D. H., Lee, M. O., Lee, D. C., and Ross, J. N. Jr.: Classification of congenital neuromuscular dysfunction of the canine esophagus. J. Am. Vet. Radiol. Soc., 17:98, 1976.

10. Clifford, D. H., Pirsch, J. G., and Mauldin, M. L.: Comparison of motor nuclei of the vagus nerve in dogs with and without esophageal achalasia. Proc. Soc. Exp. Biol. Med., 142:878, 1973.

11. Clifford, D. H., Waddell, E. D., Patterson, D. R., Wilson, C. F., and Thompson, H. L.: Management of esophageal achalasia in miniature schnauzers. J. Am. Vet. Med. Assoc., 161:1012, 1972.

12. Cole, C. R.: Changes in the equine larynx associated with laryngeal hemiplegia. Am. J. Vet. Res., 7:69, 1946.

13. Cook, W. R.: The clinical features of guttural pouch mycosis in the horse. Vet. Rec., 83:336, 1968.

14. Cook, W. R.: Observations on the etiology of epistaxis and cranial nerve paralysis in the horse. Vet. Rec., 78:396, 1966.

15. Cook, W. R., Campbell, R. S. F., and Dawson, C.: The pathology and etiology of guttural pouch mycosis in the horse. Vet. Rec., 83:422, 1968.

16. Cox, V. S., Wallace, L. J., Anderson, V. E., and Rushnea, R. A.: Hereditary esophageal dysfunction in the Miniature Schnauzer dog. Am. J. Vet. Res., 41:326, 1980.

17. Diamant, N., Szizepanski, M., and Meci, H.: Manometric characteristics of idiopathic megaesophagus in the dog: An unsuitable animal model for achalasia in man. Gastroenterology, 65:216, 1973.

18. Dubois, F. S., and Foley, J. O.: Experimental studies on vagus and spinal accessory nerves in the cat. Anat. Rec., 64:285, 1936.

19. Duncan, I. D., Baker, G. J., Heffron, C. J., and Griffiths, I. R.: A correlation of the endoscopic and pathological changes in subclinical pathology of the horse's larynx. Equine Vet. J., 9:220, 1977.

20. Duncan, I. D., Griffiths, I. R., and Madrid, R. E.: A light and electron microscopic study of the neuropathy of equine idiopathic laryngeal hemiplegia. Neuropathol. Appl. Neurobiol., 4:483, 1978.

21. Duncan, I. D., and Griffiths, I. R.: Pathological changes in equine laryngeal muscles and nerves. Proc. Am. Assoc. Equine Pract., 19:97, 1973.

22. Duncan, I. D., Griffiths, I. R., McQueen, A., and Baker, G. O.: The pathology of equine laryngeal hemiplegia. Acta Neuropathol., 27:337, 1974.

23. Duncan, I. D., Griffiths, I. R., McQueen, A., and Baker, G. O.: The pathology of equine laryngeal hemiplegia. Acta Neuropathol., 27:337, 1974.

24. Firth, E. C.: Vestibular disease and its relationship to facial paralysis in the horse: A clinical study of 7 cases. Aust. Vet. J., 53:560, 1977.

25. Flieger, S.: The nerve centers of the nervus laryngicus cranialis and caudalis and their participation in the innervation of the larynx. Polskie Archiwum Weterynaryjne, 14:467, 1971.

26. Fox, M. W.: A canine neuropathy resembling facial hemiatrophy and spasms in man. Mod. Vet. Pract., 44:64, 1963.

27. Freeman, D. E.: Diagnosis and treatment of diseases of the guttural pouch (Part 1). Compend. Contin. Ed., 2:53, 1980.

28. Freeman, D. E., and Donawick, W. J.: Occlusion of internal carotid artery in the horse by means of a balloon-tipped catheter: Evaluation of a method designed to prevent epistaxis caused by guttural pouch mycosis. J. Am. Vet. Med. Assoc., 176:232, 1980.

29. Goulden, B. E., Barnes, G. R. G., and Quinlan, T. J.: The electromyographic activity of intrinsic laryngeal muscles during quiet breathing in the anesthetized horse. N.Z. Vet. J., 24:157, 1976.

30. Gray, G. W.: Acute experiments on neuroeffector function in canine esophageal achalasia. Am. J. Vet. Res., 35:1075, 1974.

31. Habel, R. E.: Applied Veterinary Anatomy. Ithaca, N.Y., R. E. Habel, 1975.

32. Harvey, C. E., O'Brien, J. A., Durie, V. R., Miller, D. J., and Veenena, R.: Megaesophagus in the dog: A clinical survey of 79 cases. J. Am. Vet. Med. Assoc., 165:443, 1974.

33. Higgs, B., and Ellis, F. H., Jr.: The effect of bilateral supranodosal vagotomy on canine esophageal function. Surgery, 58:828, 1965.

34. Higgs, B., Kerr, F. W. L., and Ellis, F. H., Jr.: The

experimental production of esophageal achalasia by electrolytic lesions in the medulla. J. Thorac. Cardiovasc. Surg., 50:613, 1965.

35. Hockman, C. H., Bieger, D., and Weerasuriya, A.: Supranuclear pathways of swallowing. Prog. Neurobiol., 12:15, 1979.

36. Hoffer, R. E., MacCoy, D. M., Quick, C. B., Barclay, S. M., and Rendano, V. T.: Management of acquired achalasia in dogs. J. Am. Vet. Med. Assoc., 175:814, 1979.

37. Hoffer, R. E., Valdes-Dapena, A., and Bane, A. E.: A comparative study of naturally occurring canine achalasia. Arch. Surg., 95:83, 1967.

38. Howard, J. R.: Neurological examination of cattle. Scope, 13:2, 1968.

39. Hudson, L. C.: The origins of innervation of the esophagus and the caudal pharyngeal muscles with histochemical and ultrastructural observations on the esophagus of the dog. Ph.D. Thesis, Cornell University, Ithaca, N.Y., 1982.

40. Knight, A. P.: Dysphagia resulting from unilateral rupture of the rectus capitis ventralis muscles in a horse. J. Am. Vet. Med. Assoc., 170:735, 1977.

41. Koch, C.: Diseases of the larynx and pharynx of the horse. Compend. Contin. Ed., 2:73, 1980.

42. Leemann, W., and Seiferle, E.: Mykosen des Luftsackes beim Pferd. Schweiz. Arch. Tierheilk., 112:627, 1970.

43. Marks, D., Mackey-Smith, M. P., Cushing, L. S., and Leslie, J. A.: Etiology and diagnosis of laryngeal hemiplegia in horses. J. Am. Vet. Med. Assoc., 157:429, 1970.

44. Marks, D., Mackey-Smith, M. P., Cushing, L. S., and Leslie, J. A.: Observations on laryngeal hemiplegia in the horse and treatment by abductor muscle prosthesis. Equine Vet. J., 2:159, 1970.

45. McGrath, J. T.: Neurologic Examination of the Dog. 2nd Ed. Philadelphia, Lea and Febiger, 1960.

47. O'Brien, J. A., Harvey, C. E., Kelly, A. M., and Tucker, J. T.: Neurogenic atrophy of the laryngeal muscles of the dog. J. Small. Anim. Pract., 14:521, 1973.

48. O'Connor, P. J., Parry, C. B., and Davies, R.: Continuous muscle spasm in intramedullary tumors of the neuraxis. J. Neurol. Neurosurg. Psychiatry, 29:310, 1966.

49. Parker, A. J., Cusick, B. K., Park, R. D., and Small, E.: Hemifacial spasms in a dog. Vet. Rec., 93:514, 1973.

50. Rendano, V. T., de Lahunta, A., and King, J. M.: Extracranial neoplasia with facial nerve paralysis in two cats. J. Am. Anim. Hosp. Assoc., 16:921, 1980.

51. Rethi, A.: Histological analysis of the experimental degenerated vagus nerve. Acta Morphol. (Budapest), 1:221, 1951.

52. Roberts, S. A., and Vainisi, S. J.: Hemifacial spasm in dogs. J. Am. Vet. Med. Assoc., 150:381, 1967.

53. Robins, G.: Dropped jaw—mandibular neurapraxia in the dog. J. Small Anim. Pract., 17:753, 1976.

54. Rogers, W. A., Fenner, W. R., and Sherding, R. G.: Electromyographic and esophagomanometric findings in clinically normal dogs and dogs with idiopathic megaesophagus. J. Am. Vet. Med. Assoc., 174:181, 1979.

55. Rooney, J. R.: Autopsy of the Horse. Baltimore, Williams & Wilkins, 1970.

56. Rooney, J. R., and Delaney, F. M.: Laryngeal hemiplegia in horses, a theoretical analysis. Proc. AAEP, 15:13, 1969.

57. Schaer, M., Zaki, F. A., and Harvey, H. J.: Laryngeal hemiplegia due to neoplasia of the vagus nerve in a cat. J. Am. Vet. Med. Assoc., 174:513, 1979.

58. Sokolovsky, V.: Achalasia and paralysis of the canine esophagus. J. Am. Vet. Med. Assoc., 160:943, 1972.

59. Strombeck, D. R., and Troya, L.: Evaluation of lower motor neuron function in two dogs with megaesophagus. J. Am. Vet. Med. Assoc., 169:411, 1976.

60. Suter, P. F., and Watrous, B. J.: Oropharyngeal dysphagias in the dog: A cinefluorographic analysis of experimentally induced and spontaneously occurring swallowing disorders. Vet. Radiol., 21:24, 1980.

61. Venker-van Haagen, A. J.: Investigations on the pathogenesis of hereditary laryngeal paralysis in the Bouvier. Thesis, University of Utrecht, 1980.

62. Venker-van Haagen, A. J., Bouw, J., and Hartman, W.: Hereditary transmission of laryngeal paralysis in Bouviers. J. Am. Anim. Hosp. Assoc., 17:75, 1981.

63. Venker-van Haagen, A. J., Hartman, W., and Goedegebuure, S. A.: Spontaneous laryngeal paralysis in young Bouviers. J. Am. Anim. Hosp. Assoc., 14:714, 1978.

64. Venker-van Haagen, A. J., Hartman, W., Goedegebuure, A., and Wentink, G. J.: The source of normal motor unit potentials in supposedly denervated laryngeal muscles of dogs. Zbl. Vet. Med. [A], 25:751, 1978.

65. Watrous, B. J., and Suter, P. F.: Normal swallowing in the dog: A cineradiographic study. J. Am. Vet. Radiol. Soc., 20:99, 1979.

66. Watson, A. G.: Some aspects of the vagal innervation of the canine esophagus. An anatomical study. M. S. thesis, Massey University, New Zealand, 1974.

67. Rose, R. J., Hartley, W. J., and Baker, W.: Laryngeal paralysis in Arabian foals associated with oral haloxon administration. Equine Vet. J., 13:171, 1981.

68. Chibuzo, G. A., and Cummings, J. F.: An enzyme tracer study of the organization of the somatic motor center for the innervation of different muscles of the tongue: Evidence for two sources. J. Comp. Neurol., 205:273, 1982.

69. Stone, J., Campion, J. E., and Leicester, J.: The nasotemporal division of retina in the Siamese cat. J. Comp. Neurol., 180:783, 1978.

LOWER MOTOR NEURON— GENERAL VISCERAL EFFERENT SYSTEM

This group of lower motor neurons innervates the smooth muscle associated with blood vessels and visceral structures, glands, and cardiac muscle. It is an involuntary system and represents the lower motor neuron for the autonomic nervous system. The autonomic nervous system is a physiologic and anatomic system with central and peripheral components. It includes higher centers situated in the hypothalamus, midbrain, pons, and medulla. The hypothalamus is the primary integrating center for the autonomic nervous system. Nuclei in its rostral portion subserve the parasympathetic division of the general visceral efferent lower motor neuron, whereas the nuclei in its caudal portion subserve the sympathetic division of the general visceral efferent lower motor neuron. These hypothalamic nuclei receive afferents from the cerebrum by way of numerous pathways, from thalamic nuclei, and from ascending general visceral afferent (GVA) pathways. The hypothalamus influences the activity of the metabolic centers in

the reticular formation of the midbrain, pons, and medulla. These centers influence visceral smooth muscle, cardiac muscle, and glandular activity by means of the general visceral efferent lower motor neuron located in specific cranial and spinal nerves. This autonomic nervous system is concerned with emergency mechanisms and the repair and preservation of a constant internal environment. The concept of maintaining a steady state in the internal environment for continuous efficient function of the body is referred to as homeostasis. The peripheral part of the autonomic nervous system includes the sensory neurons mostly from the body viscera, the GVA system, and a lower motor neuron, the GVE system.

The GVE lower motor neuron is composed of two neurons interposed between the central nervous system and the organ innervated. The first neuron has its cell body located in the grey matter of the CNS, and its axon courses through a cranial or spinal nerve to a peripheral ganglion, where it synapses with the cell body of the second neuron. The first neuron with its telodendron in a peripheral ganglion is called the preganglionic neuron. The second neuron has its cell body and dendritic zone in a peripheral ganglion and its axon, the postganglionic axon, terminates in the structure to be innervated.

The GVE system is grouped into two divisions physiologically and anatomically. The sympathetic system, the thoracolumbar system, has the cell bodies of the preganglionic neuron located in the intermediate grey column of the spinal cord from approximately the first thoracic to fifth lumbar spinal cord segment. With a few exceptions, the neurotransmitter elaborated at the telodendron of the postganglionic axon is norepinephrine. The parasympathetic system, the craniosacral system, has the cell bodies of the preganglionic neuron located in the sacral segments of the spinal cord and in nuclei of the brain stem associated with cranial nerves III, VII, IX, X, and XI. Acetylcholine is the neurotransmitter released at the telodendron of the postganglionic axon.

CONTROL OF PUPILS

In clinical neurology knowledge of this GVE system is important in the understanding of pupillary size and responsiveness to light and excitement. The parasympathetic GVE innervation of the eyeball responds to the afferent modality of light, whereas the sympathetic GVE innervation is stimulated by the factors that elicit excitement, fear, or anger.

SYMPATHETIC GVE LOWER MOTOR NEURON INNERVATION OF THE EYEBALL

The preganglionic cell bodies are located in the intermediate grey column of the first three or four segments of the thoracic spinal cord. The axons pass through the ventral grey column and adjacent white matter to join the ventral roots of these segments and the proximal portion of the segmental spinal nerve. Before the spinal nerve branches, these preganglionic axons leave the spinal nerve in the segmental ramus communicans, which joins the thoracic sympathetic trunk inside the thorax ventrolateral to the vertebral column. The axons usually pass cranially without synapse in a trunk ganglion. They pass through the cervicothoracic and middle cervical ganglia and course cranially in the cervical sympathetic trunk, where the latter is part of the vagosympathetic trunk. Medial to the origin of the digastricus muscle and ventromedial to the tympanic bulla, the cervical sympathetic trunk separates from the vagus and terminates in the cranial cervical ganglion. Here the preganglionic axons synapse on the cell bodies of the second neuron in this two-neuron LMN system. The cell body of the postganglionic axon is in the cranial cervical ganglion. The axons for ocular innervation in the cat and dog course

rostrally through the tympanooccipital fissure with the internal carotid artery, and pass between the tympanic bulla and the petrosal bone into the middle ear cavity, closely associated with the ventral surface of the petrosal bone.[2] The axons continue rostrally between the petrosal bone and the basisphenoid to join the ventral surface of the trigeminal ganglion and the ophthalmic nerve. The ophthalmic nerve enters the periorbita through the orbital fissure. The postganglionic sympathetic axons are distributed by way of ophthalmic nerve branches to the smooth muscle of the periorbita, the eyelids, including the third eyelid, and the iris muscles, particularly the dilator of the pupil[1, 7, 39, 46] (Fig. 6–1). In large animals most of these axons follow the internal carotid artery in the internal carotid nerve and reach the orbital smooth muscle by way of its blood vessels. Normal tone in these orbital smooth muscles keeps the eyeball protruded, the palpebral fissure widened, the third eyelid retracted, and the pupil partially dilated. Other axons leave the cranial cervical ganglion and course with blood vessels and cranial and spinal nerves to the blood vessels and sweat glands of the skin of the head and cranial cervical area.

Clinical Signs. Loss of this innervation causes a lack of tone in the periorbital smooth muscle so that the eyeball retracts slightly, producing enophthalmos. Loss of tone in the eyelid muscle results in slight narrowing of the palpebral fissure. This is most evident in the upper eyelid, which droops, a condition called ptosis. Lack of retraction of the third eyelid allows it to protrude, and lack of pupillary dilation in response to painful stimuli, excitement, or stress causes the pupil at rest to be smaller than the opposite, normal pupil. A small pupil is referred to as miosis. Changes in the amount of light stimulating the retina alter the size of the pupil by the activation of the pupillary constrictor muscle. In the absence of light a small amount of dilation occurs in the pupil that is miotic from lack of sympathetic innervation. These signs are referred to as Horner's syndrome and are associated with

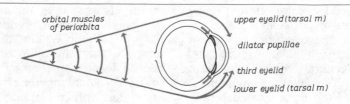

orbital muscles of periorbita

upper eyelid (tarsal m)

dilator pupillae

third eyelid

lower eyelid (tarsal m)

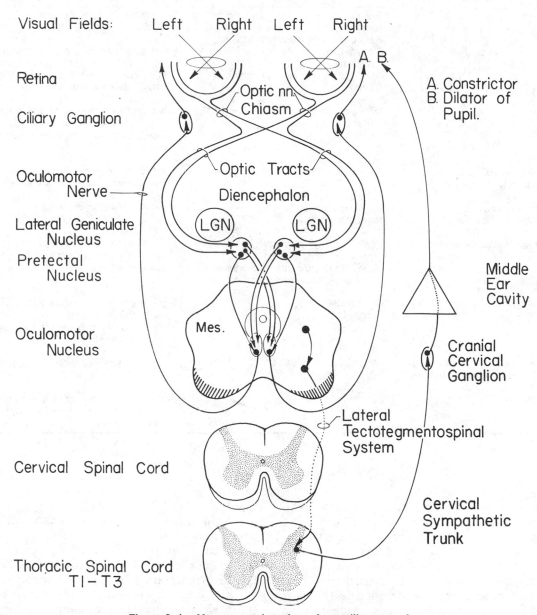

Pathway for Pupillary Control

Visual Fields: Left Right Left Right

Retina

Ciliary Ganglion

A. B.
A. Constrictor
B. Dilator of Pupil.

Optic nn. Chiasm

Optic Tracts

Oculomotor Nerve

Diencephalon

Lateral Geniculate Nucleus

LGN   LGN

Pretectal Nucleus

Middle Ear Cavity

Oculomotor Nucleus

Mes.

Cranial Cervical Ganglion

Lateral Tectotegmentospinal System

Cervical Spinal Cord

Cervical Sympathetic Trunk

Thoracic Spinal Cord
TI—T3

Figure 6–1. Neuroanatomic pathway for pupillary control.

lesions in any portion of this lower motor neuron pathway from the cranial thoracic spinal cord segments to the orbit (Table 6–1).

In addition to these signs of denervation of orbital smooth muscle, peripheral vasodilation takes place and may cause increased warmth, a pink color to the skin that may be observed best in the ear, and congestion of the nasal muscosa on the side of the lesion. In all animals except the horse, loss of sympathetic innerva-

tion causes decreased sweating, or anhidrosis. This sign is usually difficult to observe.

Pre- or postganglionic destruction of the sympathetic innervation of the head of horses is followed immediately by profuse sweating of the ipsilateral half of the face and cranial neck.[10, 33, 43] Although there is sympathetic cholinergic innervation of sweat glands in the horse, the sweat glands are also extremely responsive to blood flow.[3] The increased blood

TABLE 6–1. HORNER'S SYNDROME—SUMMARY OF LESIONS

Location	Lesion	Associated Neurologic Deficit
Cervical spinal cord	External injury Focal leukomyelomalacia (embolic infarct, disk compression)	Tetraplegia—spastic, dyspnea Hemiplegia–ipsilateral, spastic
T1–T3 spinal cord	External injury Neoplasm Focal poliomyelomalacia (embolic infarct)	Pelvic and thoracic limb paresis or paralysis with lower motor neuron deficit in thoracic limbs and upper motor neuron deficit in pelvic limbs
	Diffuse myelomalacia (ascending and descending)	Lower motor neuron deficit and analgesia of tail, anus, pelvic limbs, abdomen, and thorax with paretic thoracic limbs
T1–T3 ventral roots Proximal spinal nerves	Avulsion of roots of brachial plexus	Brachial plexus paresis or paralysis of the thoracic limb on the same side
Cranial thoracic sympathetic trunk	Lymphosarcomna Neurofibroma	None if confined to the trunk
Cervical sympathetic trunk	Injury from surgical intervention in the area, or from dog bites Neoplasm (thyroid adenocarcinoma, neurofibroma, lymphosarcoma)	None if unilateral. Bilateral lesions interfere with laryngeal and esophageal function because of vagal involvement
Middle ear cavity (small animals)	Otitis media Neoplasia	Signs of peripheral vestibular disturbance: ipsilateral ataxia, head tilt, nystagmus, and sometimes facial palsy, or hemifacial spasm
Cranial cervical ganglion—internal carotid nerve (horses)	Guttural pouch mycosis	Dysphagia, laryngeal hemiplegia, facial paresis
Retrobulbar	Contusion Neoplasia	Varies with degree of contusion to the optic and oculomotor nerves, which also influence pupillary size

flow that results from loss of peripheral vasoconstriction in sympathetic paralysis causes profuse sweating in the area of denervation. The same area of vasodilation is hyperthermic,[36] and the nasal and conjunctival mucosae are congested. The hyperthermia can best be determined by palpation of the ears, and the sweating may be most evident at the base of the ears. If the paralysis persists, the sweating may disappear. There is a prominent ptosis of the upper eyelid, but only a slight third eyelid protrusion and slight miosis.

The clinical sign of sweating in horses with sympathetic denervation may be helpful in localizing thoracolumbar spinal cord lesions. For example, if a caudal thoracic fracture causes an extensive lesion in one or two adjacent segments, the severe paraparesis and pelvic limb ataxia may be accompanied by a focal band of sweating coursing transversely on both sides of the trunk. This is caused by the focal damage to cell bodies of the preganglionic sympathetic neurons in the spinal cord or their axons in the associated spinal nerves.

In cattle, sheep, and goats,[43] the most constant signs of sympathetic paralysis of the head are the hyperthermia detected on ear palpation and the upper eyelid ptosis. The miosis and third eyelid protrusion are subtle. In cattle, the anhidrosis characteristic of all species except the horse is evidenced by less sweating visible on the surface of the nose on the denervated side.

Some examples of lesions that disturb this GVE lower neuron system follow (Table 6–1).

Diseases

1. Injury, infarction, or neoplastic involvement of the cranial thoracic spinal cord causes signs of paresis or paralysis of the pelvic limbs and mild deficits in the thoracic limbs, in addition to ipsilateral Horner's syndrome.

2. Avulsion of the roots or spinal nerves of

the brachial plexus in dogs and cats commonly results from automobile accidents. The finding of Horner's syndrome on the same side as the paralyzed thoracic limb indicates that the injury to the nerves innervating the thoracic limb is at the level of the vertebral column.

3. Thoracic inlet or cranial mediastinal lesions such as lymphosarcoma that involve the cranial thoracic sympathetic trunk, or caudal cervical sympathetic trunk, or both may lead to Horner's syndrome, with no other signs of neurologic deficit.[12]

4. Injury to the cervical sympathetic trunk from a dog bite or from the surgical exposure of the cervical intervertebral disks may result in an ipsilateral Horner's syndrome that usually is transient. Neoplastic involvement of the cervical sympathetic trunk along its course is another cause. Lymphosarcoma or neurofibroma may directly involve the vagosympathetic trunk. Thyroid adenocarcinoma may incorporate the adjacent vagosympathetic trunk.

5. Mycosis of the guttural pouch in horses may involve the cranial cervical ganglion or internal carotid nerve and produce Horner's syndrome.

6. In small animals otitis media may produce Horner's syndrome, often accompanied by signs of peripheral vestibular disturbance, with or without facial paresis, or hemifacial spasm.

7. Retrobulbar injury, neoplasia, or abscess may cause this syndrome.

The sympathetic GVE lower motor neuron is influenced by pathways descending from the higher centers of the autonomic nervous system in the brain stem. In humans such a pathway is described that affects the sympathetic GVE innervation of these orbital smooth muscles. This pathway begins in the rostral colliculus and tegmentum of the midbrain, where it is influenced by the hypothalamus. It descends through the lateral pons, medulla, and lateral funiculus of the cervical spinal cord to the thoracolumbar spinal cord segments, where it synapses in the grey matter, influencing the activity of all of the sympathetic preganglionic cell bodies in the intermediate grey column. This is called the lateral tectotegmentospinal system or the upper motor neuron for the sympathetic system. Pain stimuli or emotional responses that cause pupillary dilation do so by activating the sympathetic GVE of the cranial thoracic spinal cord by way of this lateral tectotegmentospinal system. This system is activated by ascending spinotectal and spinothalamic (pain) pathways, or direct cor-

ticotectal pathways, or both, or indirectly by corticohypothalamic pathways and the dorsal longitudinal fasciculus from the hypothalamus to the tectum.

In humans, lesions in any part of the lateral tectotegmentospinal system cause a miotic pupil on the affected side that does not respond to stress stimuli, but passively dilates a small amount in response to the reduction of light. In domestic animals upper motor neuron lesions that result in Horner's syndrome are less common. Horner's syndrome has been observed with cervical spinal cord lesions that cause extensive destruction in the lateral funiculus. If these lesions are bilateral, Horner's syndrome is bilateral and there usually is respiratory distress from the severity of the involvement of the upper motor neuron for respiration. I have observed bilateral Horner's syndrome for about 48 hours following severe injury to the spinal cord bilaterally that produced tetraplegia and respiratory embarrassment. In dogs unilateral infarction from fibrocartilaginous emboli[8, 13] and unilateral compression from an acute disk extrusion on that side have produced ipsilateral hemiplegia and Horner's syndrome. If skin temperature is measured it will be increased over the entire half of the body on the paralyzed side. This is evidence of the loss of influence of the upper motor neuron for the sympathetic system on the entire thoracolumbar intermediate grey column where the preganglionic cell bodies are located. A similar relationship is more obvious in the horse, where an upper motor neuron sympathetic paralysis results in sweating over the entire ipsilateral half of the body from the nose to the tail.[21] This has been observed in horses with extensive lesions of protozoal myelitis in the lateral funiculus of cervical spinal cord segments. The signs observed are hemiparesis and ataxia of the limbs on the same side and ipsilateral sweating.

Horner's syndrome has also been observed with space-occupying lesions that compress the hypothalamus.[22] These are usually pituitary neoplasms or meningiomas. It is not a common clinical sign of pituitary-hypothalamic neoplasia.

Pharmacologic testing may be used to help locate the lesion responsible for Horner's syndrome.[4, 42] Indirect-acting sympathomimetic drugs such as dextroamphetamine cause release of endogenous norepinephrine from intact second neurons in the LMN. If Horner's syndrome is due to a lesion in the UMN for the sympathetic system or the first (preganglionic) neuron of the LMN, normal mydriasis will occur following the instillation of 1 to 2 drops of 1 per cent hydroxyamphetamine. If the lesion is in the second neuron of the LMN, dilation will not occur or will be incomplete. With second neuron lesions there are no stores of norepinephrine to be released.

When the smooth muscle is denervated by lesions of the second neurons of the LMN, this muscle becomes supersensitive to neurotransmitter available to it. This phenomenon is called denervation hypersensitivity. This denervated muscle will respond to low concentrations of direct-acting sympathomimetic drugs that normally would be ineffective. Ten per cent phenylephrine will produce mydriasis when the dilator of the pupil has been denervated by a lesion of the second neuron of the LMN. Similarly, intraocular application of 0.1 cc of 0.001 per cent epinephrine will produce pupillary dilation in about 20 minutes with lesions in the second neuron of the LMN but will take 38 to 40 minutes with lesions in the first (preganglionic) neuron or sympathetic UMN.

PARASYMPATHETIC GVE LOWER MOTOR NEURON INNERVATION OF THE EYEBALL (CRANIAL NERVE III— OCULOMOTOR NEURONS)

The cell bodies are located in the parasympathetic oculomotor nucleus rostral to the general somatic efferent component of this nucleus at the level of the rostral part of the rostral colliculus and pretectal area (Plates 12 and 13). This portion of the oculomotor nucleus is called the Edinger-Westphal nucleus in humans and is located in the ventral part of the central grey substance next to the midline ventral to the rostral part of the mesencephalic aqueduct. The axons course ventrally with the general somatic efferent axons, and leave the mesencephalon medial to the crus cerebri in the lateral part of the intercrural fossa. The general visceral efferent axons in the canine oculomotor nerve are located superficially on the medial side of the nerve, where they are especially susceptible to disturbance caused by compression of the nerve from midbrain swelling or displacement.[19] The nerve passes through the orbital fissure into the periorbita. At the rostral end of the oculomotor nerve, ventral to the optic nerve, the ciliary ganglion is located. The preganglionic general visceral

efferent axons of the oculomotor nerve synapse here with the dendritic zone and cell bodies of the postganglionic axons. The postganglionic axons pass by way of short ciliary nerves along the optic nerve to the eyeball to innervate primarily the ciliary muscle and the constrictor of the pupil.[7]

This system is sensitive to the amount of light received by the retinas of each eyeball. In diminished light its activity is decreased and the pupils dilate. In bright light the system is activated and pupillary constriction (miosis) occurs.

The function of this GVE lower motor neuron can be tested by the pupillary light reflex. Stimulation of the retina of one eyeball with a bright source of light causes constriction of the pupils of both eyeballs. The central area of each retina is the most sensitive to this light stimulus. It is lateral to the optic disk in carnivores. The constriction in the eyeball being stimulated is the direct response. That in the opposite eyeball is the indirect or consensual response. The afferent pathway to the parasympathetic oculomotor nucleus is through the optic nerve to the optic chiasm, where the majority of the axons cross, through both optic tracts over the lateral geniculate nuclei without synapse, and ventrally into the region between the thalamus and the rostral colliculus called the pretectal area. Synapse takes place in the pretectal nuclei (Plate 13).

It has been reported that the majority of the cell bodies in each pretectal nucleus have axons that cross in the caudal commissure to terminate in the contralateral parasympathetic portion of the oculomotor nucleus.[42] Some cell bodies project axons to the ipsilateral parasympathetic oculomotor nucleus. Therefore, light directed into one eye will predominantly influence the pretectal nucleus of the opposite side (because of crossing in the optic chiasm) and the ipsilateral oculomotor nucleus (because of crossing of the pretectal neurons in the caudal commissure). This results in the direct pupillary response. Either the impulses in the axons from the retina that do not cross in the optic chiasm or the axons from the pretectal nucleus that do not cross in the caudal commissure result in activation of the contralateral parasympathetic oculomotor nucleus, producing the indirect or consensual pupillary response in the opposite eye. The predominant crossing in the optic chiasm and caudal commissure accounts for the more rapid and complete response observed in the eye being stimulated in some animals.

Clinical Signs

Lesions restricted to the visual pathways in the cerebral hemispheres can cause blindness, but pupillary responses remain normal. With a lesion in the right GVE oculomotor neuron, the right pupil is dilated widely (mydriasis) and stimulation with light in either eyeball induces constriction only in the left eyeball. A lesion in the right optic nerve causes the pupil to be partially dilated on that side or no difference in resting pupil size occurs. Stimulation with light in the left eyeball induces constriction of both pupils. Light stimulation of the right eyeball produces no change in either pupil because of the interference with the sensory limb of the reflex at the level of the optic nerve. For evalution of the pupillary light reflex, a strong light source should be directed at the lateral aspect of the retina at the site of the area centralis, and the patient should be as relaxed as possible. Circulating epinephrine may interfere with the rapidity and degree of the response.

The reason why the pupil on the side with the optic nerve lesion may be the same size as the pupil in the normal eye is that enough light enters the normal eye and activates both GVE oculomotor nuclei. If the normal eye is covered, the pupil on the affected side will immediately dilate. As a bright light source is swung back and forth from one eye to the other, bilateral pupillary constriction occurs when the normal eye is stimulated. As the light swings to the abnormal eye, both pupils partially dilate.

It has been my experience that only severe retinal or optic nerve lesions will abolish the pupillary light reflex. Dogs that are functionally blind from retinal atrophy or optic neuritis may have pupils that still respond to a bright light source. On careful examination their pupils usually are more dilated in normal room light than are pupils of normal dogs in the same light. This is an important observation to make in localizing lesions of the visual system.

A lesion confined to one optic tract may not produce any abnormality with pupillary light response because of the crossing in the optic chiasm. If there is any interference with the pupillary light pathway there may be a slight resting pupil dilation in the eye contralateral to the optic tract lesion. At all times during the stimulation of either eye with light, the pupil in the eye ipsilateral to the optic tract lesion will respond more. This is explained by the predominance of crossing in the optic chiasm and from the pretectal nucleus to the opposite parasympathetic oculomotor nucleus.

Complete oculomotor nerve dysfunction will cause a widely dilated pupil that is unresponsive to light directed into either eyeball (general visceral efferent deficit) and a lateral and ventral strabismus (general somatic efferent deficit). Compression of the oculomotor nerve directly by an encroaching neoplasm or indirectly by herniation of the occipital lobe with pressure on the adjacent midbrain will usually compromise GVE function before GSE function. An expanding cerebral space-occupying lesion may cause a contralateral visual defect and contralateral postural reaction deficits with an ipsilateral dilated pupil that is unresponsive to light directed into either eye. The expanding cerebral lesion usually compresses the oculomotor nerve on the same side.

Pharmacologic testing to localize the lower motor neuron lesion in the first or second neuron is based on the same concepts as described for the sympathetic system.[42] Indirect-acting parasympathomimetic drugs require an intact second neuron innervating the pupillary constrictor for release of endogenous neurotransmitter. One drop of 0.5 per cent physostigmine causes rapid pupil constriction with UMN or first neuron (preganglionic) lesions and no constriction with second neuron lesions. The normal eye constricts 40 to 60 minutes after the eye with a UMN or preganglionic lesion. A direct-acting parasympathomimetic, such as 2 per cent pilocarpine, will produce a more rapid, more complete, and longer constriction in a denervated pupil than in a normal pupil. The normal pupil will respond in about 20 minutes. This drug does not differentiate between first or second neuron lesions. Any LMN lesion results in supersensitivity to pilocarpine.

If the normal pupil responds but the dilated pupil does not, this suggests either that the dilated pupil is the result of previously administered atropine or that there is iris disease present.

Diseases Associated with Anisocoria

Anisocoria is the occurrence of unequal or asymmetric pupils. Some of the causes include the following:

1. A unilateral oculomotor nerve lesion produces ipsilateral severe mydriasis, unresponsive to light directed into either eyeball.

2. A unilateral lesion of GVE sympathetic innervation of the pupil causes ipsilateral miosis that dilates slightly in reduced light.

3. Unilateral ocular disorders causing pain,

such as keratitis, cause activation of the oculopupillary reflex (V–III) and ipsilateral miosis.

4. Unilateral severe retinal or optic nerve lesions may result in partial ipsilateral mydriasis that responds only to light directed into the opposite eyeball. No miosis occurs in either eyeball from light directed into the affected eyeball.

5. Iritis causes ipsilateral miosis.

6. Iris degeneration with atrophy brings about ipsilateral mydriasis with a variable response to light, sometimes none. It is more common in older dogs.

7. Glaucoma is increased intraocular pressure created by abnormal circulation of aqueous. It may cause ipsilateral mydriasis that is unresponsive to light.

8. Anisocoria is occasionally observed with cerebellar lesions that are asymmetric. Usually the pupil on the side opposite to the lesion is partly dilated but will respond to light in either eye.

Pupils in Acute Brain Disease

Pupillary abnormalities are common following intracranial trauma, and often accompany severe acute brain lesions such as polioencephalomalacia or lead poisoning in ruminants. These may not necessarily reflect destruction of the general visceral efferent oculomotor neurons, or the origin of the lateral tectotegmentospinal system. Severe bilateral miosis is a sign of acute extensive brain disturbance that in itself is not necessarily of any localizing value. The return of the pupils to normal size and response to light is a favorable prognostic sign and indicates recovery from the brain disturbance, especially following trauma. In patients with intracranial trauma, progression from bilaterally miotic to bilaterally mydriatic fixed pupils unresponsive to light indicates that the brain disturbance is advancing and the general visceral efferent oculomotor neurons associated with the midbrain are nonfunctional. This often accompanies severe contusion of the midbrain with hemorrhage, usually along the midline. This may follow brain swelling and herniation of the occipital lobes ventral to the tentorium cerebelli accompanied by compression and displacement of the midbrain, or oculomotor nerve, or both.

The cause of unilateral or bilateral miotic pupils in acute brain disease is not understood clearly. It probably represents facilitation of the oculomotor general visceral efferent neurons that have been released from higher center (prosencephalon) inhibition owing to its functional disturbance. It may represent direct disturbance along the origin of the lateral tectotegmentospinal system, causing lack of facilitation of the sympathetic general visceral efferent lower motor neuron. However, the usual absence of the other signs of Horner's syndrome is evidence against this theory. The rapid recovery of the pupils that follows intracranial injury in patients with only cerebral signs supports the first hypothesis. Pupillary changes may take place hourly following head trauma. Unilateral mydriasis that in some cases may be accompanied by miosis of the opposite pupil is probably brought about by compression of the ipsilateral oculomotor nerve.

Experimental studies in dogs have shown that mild compression of the brain stem tectum at the level of the rostral colliculus causes miosis.[19] Compression of the third cranial nerve produces mydriasis. Acute cerebral swelling from a unilateral cerebral space-occupying lesion may result in compression of the ipsilateral midbrain and oculomotor nerve and an associated ipsilateral mydriasis. Bilateral herniation of the occipital lobes may compress the midbrain and initially produce miosis followed by mydriasis as the oculomotor neurons lose their function. A diagram of pupil size and prognosis in intracranial injury follows.

Protrusion of the Third Eyelid

The third eyelid (membrana nictitans) may protrude for a number of reasons. In all animals except for the cat, this protrusion is a passive event. The third eyelid passively protrudes when the eyeball is retracted actively by the retractor bulbi (VI) and other extraocular muscles (III, IV, and VI). In the cat, slips of striated muscle from the lateral rectus and levator palpebrae superiorus attach to the two extremities of the eyelid and may contract and contribute actively to this protrusion.

A constant partial protrusion of the third eyelid occurs in Horner's syndrome because of loss of the sympathetic innervation of the smooth muscle that normally keeps it retracted.

Brief, rapid, passive protrusions (flashing of the third eyelid) occur in tetanus owing to the effect of the tetanus toxin on the neurons that innervate the extraocular muscles. This causes brief contractions of these muscles, especially if the animal is startled. This is most noticeable in the horse with tetanus.

In facial paralysis the eyelids cannot close to blink when the animal is threatened. However, the eyeball is retracted, which causes a brief rapid protrusion of the third eyelid.

Cats with severe systemic disease and

PUPIL SIZE   PROGNOSIS

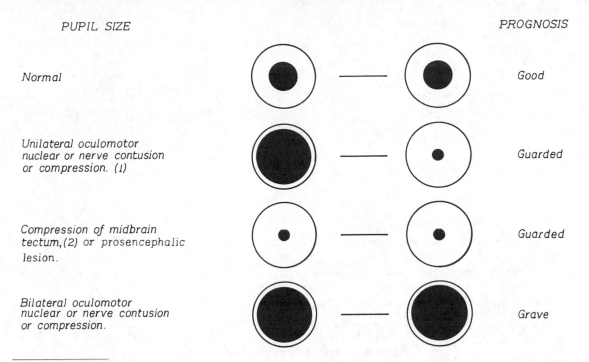

Normal		Good
Unilateral oculomotor nuclear or nerve contusion or compression. (1)		Guarded
Compression of midbrain tectum,(2) or prosencephalic lesion.		Guarded
Bilateral oculomotor nuclear or nerve contusion or compression.		Grave

1. Asymmetric interference with cerebral control of oculomotor neurons and/or the sympathetic upper motor neuron system.

2. Bilateral sympathetic upper motor neuron deficiency or loss of facilitation, bilateral release of oculomotor GVE neurons from cerebral inhibition.

depression often have a persistent bilateral protrusion of the third eyelid. This may result from dehydration and depression, with slight sinking of the eyeballs in their orbits resulting in third eyelid protrusion, or there may be a generalized decreased sympathetic tone resulting in the same signs. Sympathomimetic drugs will increase the smooth muscle tone in the eyelids and cause normal third eyelid retraction in these cats.

Severe atrophy of the muscles of mastication from myositis or trigeminal nerve lesions causes enophthalmos and secondarily a protruded third eyelid.

SACRAL PARASYMPATHETIC GVE LOWER MOTOR NEURON

The sacral part of the parasympathetic division of the GVE lower motor neuron has the cell bodies of its preganglionic neurons located in the intermediate grey column of the sacral spinal cord segments (the second and third sacral segments in the dog).[5, 11, 24, 26, 27, 35] The axons course with the ventral roots to the spinal nerves, where they leave as ventral branches that unite ventral to the sacral vertebrae to form the pelvic nerve on each side. The preganglionic neurons of the pelvic nerve to the bladder synapse in ganglia in the pelvic plexus or in the bladder wall. The pelvic nerve is distributed by way of the pelvic plexus to the urogenital organs, rectum, and descending colon.

CONTROL OF MICTURITION[11]

Micturition is a reflex function that primarily involves the sacral spinal cord segments and the pelvic and pudendal nerves. It is under the control of centers in the caudal brain stem that are influenced by the cerebrum and cerebellum (Fig. 6–2). The smooth muscle of the bladder wall that is responsible for contracting to evacuate the urine is called the detrusor muscle and is innervated by parasympathetic neurons from the sacral segments of the spinal cord. Preganglionic cell bodies are in the intermediate grey column of all three sacral segments.[24, 35] Their axons pass through the ventral roots into the sacral spinal nerves and then leave these nerves by branches that join to

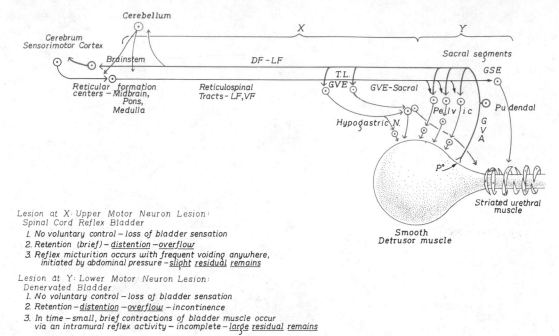

Lesion at X: Upper Motor Neuron Lesion:
Spinal Cord Reflex Bladder
1. No voluntary control – loss of bladder sensation
2. Retention (brief) – distention – overflow
3. Reflex micturition occurs with frequent voiding anywhere,
   initiated by abdominal pressure – slight residual remains

Lesion at Y: Lower Motor Neuron Lesion:
Denervated Bladder
1. No voluntary control – loss of bladder sensation
2. Retention – distention – overflow – incontinence
3. In time – small, brief contractions of bladder muscle occur
   via an intramural reflex activity – incomplete – large residual remains

Figure 6–2. Neuroanatomy of bladder function.

form the pelvic nerve. The pelvic nerve forms a pelvic plexus with the hypogastric nerve and is distributed to the bladder wall closely associated with the branches of the vaginal/prostatic artery. Cell bodies of postganglionic axons are located in the pelvic plexus or more commonly in the bladder wall. Stimulation of these neurons results in contraction of the detrusor muscle and evacuation of the bladder. The smooth muscle fibers of the bladder are oriented in an oblique fashion around the neck, which causes dilation of the opening of the bladder into the urethra when the detrusor muscle contracts to empty the bladder.

Sensory neurons responsive to stretch and/or pressure in the bladder wall have axons in the pelvic nerve and sacral spinal nerves and cell bodies in the sacral spinal ganglia.[44, 45] Axons of these general visceral afferent neurons enter the sacral segments over the sacral dorsal roots. Some of these axons terminate on interneurons that complete the reflex arc with preganglionic parasympathetic neurons. Others are concerned with projection pathways to the brain. As the detrusor muscle contracts, visceral afferents in the bladder wall are stimulated and project to the sacral segments, where they reflexly inhibit the activity of the general somatic efferent neurons to the striated urethral muscle, allowing this urethral muscle to relax and the urethra to expand. Other sacral afferents ascend the spinal cord to inhibit the

lumbar preganglionic sympathetic neurons. Inhibition of the alpha-adrenergic sympathetic neurons contributes to the urethral relaxation.

Urine retention is a function primarily of the striated urethral muscle that forms an external sphincter around the pelvic urethra. A smooth muscle internal sphincter has not been defined anatomically, but alpha-adrenergic sympathetic neurons increase the tone at the neck of the bladder, restricting outflow. The striated urethral muscle is primarily innervated by general somatic efferent neurons with cell bodies in the ventral grey column of usually the first two sacral segments.[28, 35] Axons pass through the sacral ventral roots, spinal nerves, and ventral branches to the sacral plexus and pudendal nerve, which innervate the urethral muscle. Afferents from the pelvic urethra and urethral muscle enter the sacral spinal cord via the pudendal nerve and sacral plexus.

Reflex micturition requires facilitation of the sacral parasympathetic neurons and inhibition of the sacral somatic neurons to the striated urethral muscle and lumbar sympathetic neurons to urethral musculature.

The sympathetic system has two functions in bladder innervation.[25] Preganglionic cell bodies are predominantly located in the spinal cord segments L1 to L4. Axons pass through rami communicantes, the sympathetic trunk, and lumbar splanchnic nerves to terminate in the caudal mesenteric ganglion. The postganglionic axons course through the hypogastric nerve and pelvic plexus to the body and neck of the bladder and the urethra. Some axons do not synapse in the caudal mesenteric ganglion but follow the same course and terminate on cell bodies of the second neurons in the wall of the bladder.[34] Those sympathetic postganglionic axons in the bladder neck and proximal urethra terminate on alpha receptors in smooth muscle and facilitate muscle contraction. Some may terminate in the urethral muscle to increase its tone. Sympathetic postganglionic axons that terminate on smooth muscle of the body of the bladder end on beta receptors and are inhibitory to the smooth muscle. Their activity permits the bladder wall to expand further and accommodate greater volume of urine. Sensory neurons responsive to stretch pressure enter the sacral spinal cord over the pelvic nerves and synapse in the dorsal grey column.[44, 45] These neurons project cranially to the L1 to L4 spinal cord segments to terminate on interneurons that activate the beta-adrenergic preganglionic sympathetic neurons, which in turn through their postganglionic axons will inhibit the bladder smooth muscle, allowing it to stretch and contain more urine. Stimulation studies show that the beta receptor activity predominates over that of the alpha receptors.[37]

These reflex centers are under the control of centers in the reticular formation of the midbrain, pons, and medulla concerned with the normal storage and evacuation of urine. Cortical influence on these centers initiates voluntary micturition. Ascending sensory pathways inform the cerebral cortex of the distended bladder. The cerebellum exerts an inhibitory modulating effect on this activity.

Sensory neurons (general visceral afferent, general proprioception) have stretch receptors in the bladder wall, axons in the pelvic nerves, and cell bodies in the sacral spinal ganglia. Some terminate in the dorsal grey column of the sacral segments on a second group of neurons that enter the lateral funiculus and ascend the spinal cord, primarily with the spinothalamic system. Other primary afferents enter the dorsal funiculus without interruption and ascend in the fasciculus gracilis to the medulla, where they synapse in the nucleus gracilis. Both of these pathways relay through the thalamus to reach the somesthetic cortex. By means of these pathways, bladder sensation reaches conscious perception. Collaterals of axons of these pathways project to the cerebellar cortex.

Voluntary micturition is mediated from the caudal brain stem by tectospinal and reticulospinal components of the upper motor neuron that project through lateral and ventral funiculi. These are facilitatory to sacral parasympathetic preganglionic neurons and inhibitory to sacral somatic efferent neurons to the urethral muscle and inhibitory to the cranial lumbar sympathetic preganglionic neurons. Facilitation of general somatic efferent neurons that innervate the abdominal muscles is an important part of normal micturition. Other pontomedullary reticulospinal neurons function in urine storage and maintaining continence.[9, 20]

Summary

NORMAL FILLING

A. Facilitation of sacral GSE—pudendal nerve to urethral muscle (contraction).
B. Facilitation of L1 to L4—sympathetics to alpha receptors—urethral smooth muscle (contraction).
C. Inhibition of sacral GVE—pelvic nerve—detrusor muscle (relaxation).
D. As bladder fills, pressure stimulates GVA in pelvic nerve to sacral segments—reflex to L1 to L4 GVE sympathetics—beta receptors in detrusor muscle—relaxation—retain more urine.
E. Brain stem pontomedullary centers concerned with urine storage are involved in facilitating and modulating these activities.

NORMAL MICTURITION

A. Activity of GVA—pelvic nerve to sacral segments—ascending pathways to brain stem, cerebellum, cerebrum; activation of micturition—upper motor neuron pathways in pons and medulla—reticulospinal tracts descend spinal cord.
B. Inhibition of L1 to L4 GVE sympathetics—beta receptors on detrusor muscle, alpha receptors on urethral musculature.
C. Inhibition of sacral GSE—pudendal nerve—striated urethral muscle (relaxation).
D. Facilitation of sacral GVE—parasympathetics—pelvic nerve to detrusor muscle (contraction).
E. Part of inhibition of sacral GSE and lumbar sympathetic GVE is mediated reflexly within the sacral segments and from sacral to lumbar segments.

NEUROLOGIC DISORDERS[23, 30, 38]

A. Upper Motor Neuron Bladder Paralysis: severe spinal cord disease cranial to sacral segments (most common with transverse spinal cord lesion in thoracolumbar area, less common with cervical spinal cord lesions because transverse lesions are not compatible with life).

1. No voluntary micturition—bladder distention—increased urethral resistance from uninhibited GSE activity to striated urethral muscle. May cause resistance to manual evacuation of bladder. This resistance may be augmented in severe spinal cord lesions between L4 and sacral segments in which GVE sympathetics maintain alpha-receptor tone in urethral musculature; these spinal cord neurons are not inhibited by ascending pathways from sacral segments that occur during normal micturition. Inconstant overflow incontinence may occur.

2. Reflex bladder may develop in one to a few weeks. Follows decrease in sacral GSE resting activity, results from stimulation of GVA in bladder as urine fills the bladder, reflexly activates sacral GVE parasympathetics with inhibition of sacral GSE. Mild abdominal wall pressure may activate this reflex. Slight residual urine remains in bladder.

3. Therapy for use prior to development of a functional reflex arc mechanism and when there is resistance to manual evacuation of bladder: Phenoxybenzamine to block alpha-receptor activity in urethral musculature. Bethanechol to stimulate detrusor activity in the bladder wall. Diazepam or dantrolene may help relax striated urethral muscle.

B. Lower Motor Neuron Bladder Paralysis: severe sacral spinal cord disease/sacral plexus disease.
1. No voluntary micturition—atonic distended bladder—urethral relaxation. Urine overflow—incontinence—is common and often continuous. Usually little resistance to manual evacuation of bladder. Any resistance results from activity of GVE alpha-adrenergic sympathetic neurons to urethral musculature. Note relaxation of anal sphincter.

2. Reflex micturition may occur in time if the bladder wall is healthy. This is intrinsic in the wall of the bladder, and detrusor contraction occurs as the pressure of urine collecting in the bladder increases. This is very incomplete and large residual urine is common.

3. Therapy: Phenoxybenzamine to block alpha-receptor activity in urethral musculature to overcome any urethral resistance and enhance bladder evacuation. Bethanechol to stimulate detrusor activity in bladder wall. If the lesion is in the peripheral nerve, regeneration may occur after a few months.

4. For reflex bladder contraction to occur, whether by way of the sacral spinal cord segments or the reflexes in the wall of the bladder, it requires healthy bladder smooth muscle. Excessive prolonged bladder distention eventually causes irreversible atonia of the muscle. Urea breaks down into ammonia in retained urine, and this is irritating to the bladder mucosa, causing inflammation. Opportunist bacteria often proliferate and augment the cystitis. Severe prolonged cystitis damages the bladder musculature. For these reasons overdistention and infection must be prevented by continual observation, manual evacuation or catheterization, and urinary antiseptic therapy if necessary.

C. Pelvic Nerve Destruction
1. Paralysis of detrusor muscle in bladder wall—atonic distended bladder—lack of conscious sensation of bladder filling. Urethral resistance maintained through sacral GSE—pudendal nerve. Note normal anal tone and perineal reflex. L1 to L4 alpha-adrenergic sympathetic neurons to alpha receptors in urethral musculature intact and maintain resistance.

2. Therapy: Phenoxybenzamine to block alpha receptors. Bethanechol to stimulate detrusor activity. Diazepam or dantrolene to relax striated urethral muscle.

D. Functional Outflow Obstruction: detrusor urethral ataxia/dyssynergia.
1. Failure of urethral relaxation during attempts to urinate from presumed overdischarge of GVE alpha-adrenergic sympathetics to alpha receptors on urethral musculature. Manual evacuation of the bladder causes increased resistance.

2. Therapy: Phenoxybenzamine to block alpha receptors. If the functional obstruction involves failure of urethral muscle to relax, use diazepam or dantrolene to attempt relaxation.

E. Brain stem lesions may result in the same signs that are observed with upper motor neuron spinal cord disease.

F. Cerebellar disease may rarely result in increased frequency of voluntary urination. Normally the cerebellum exerts an inhibitory effect on micturition.

G. Cerebral disease may result in loss of learned habits for micturition, and it may occur voluntarily without regard to where it is performed.

EXAMINATION

1. Examination for disorders of micturition should include an observation of the animal's attempts to urinate, bladder palpation, and ability to manually evacuate the bladder. Because the anal sphincter and bulbospongiosus muscles are innervated by branches of the pudendal nerve, their activity may reflect the activity of the striated urethral muscle. During normal micturition, when the urethral muscle relaxes, anal sphincter relaxation occurs. In lower motor neuron bladder paralysis from sacral spinal cord segment lesions, the urethral muscle as well as the anal sphincter will be atonic. Perineal and bulbospongiosus reflexes will be absent.

2. Other ancillary procedures that may help in

defining the disorder of micturition include anal sphincter electromyography, a cystometrogram, and a urethral pressure profile.[31, 40, 41]

CONTROL OF DEFECATION

Defecation is dependent on similar brain stem centers, spinal cord tracts and the same sacral spinal cord segments, and the pelvic nerve to the descending colon and rectum. Clinically, spinal cord lesions cranial to the first sacral segment that cause a loss of voluntary control over defecation usually do not result in obstruction to flow of bowel contents.[29] Although some retention may take place, evacuation usually follows involuntarily. Even with lower motor neuron lesions of the pelvic nerve neurons, although retention may be more of a problem, evacuation usually occurs. Occasionally, enemas are necessary to relieve retention. If retention persists and is not attended to, a chronic megacolon may result. Failure to defecate with these lower motor neuron lesions is more of a problem in the horse than in the dog.

Diseases

Any severe spinal cord or caudal brain stem lesion can result in a disorder of micturition. These spinal cord diseases are described elsewhere. Some examples follow.

Severe spinal cord contusion from an extruded intervertebral disk at the T13–L1 articulation interferes with the ascending and descending pathways to and from the brain for micturition, leading to an upper motor neuron paralysis accompanied by incontinence. Spinal reflex bladder results. A fracture and subluxation at the L7–S1 articulation destroys the sacral nerves, resulting in bladder paralysis and incontinence, followed by the development of a bladder with intrinsic reflex activity. Neuritis of the cauda equina in horses often destroys all sacral nerves, bringing about bladder and rectal paralysis. Daily manual evacuation of the rectum and bladder may be necessary.

PARASYMPATHETIC GVE LOWER MOTOR NEURON OF THE MEDULLA (CRANIAL NERVES VII, IX, X, AND XI —FACIAL, GLOSSOPHARYNGEAL, VAGUS, AND ACCESSORY NEURONS)

The nuclear column containing the cell bodies of these general visceral efferent preganglionic neurons is located dorsolateral to the general somatic efferent column, medial to the solitary tract and nucleus, and ventral to the floor of the fourth ventricle from about the level of the special visceral efferent facial nucleus in the rostral medulla to the obex (Fig. 6–3).

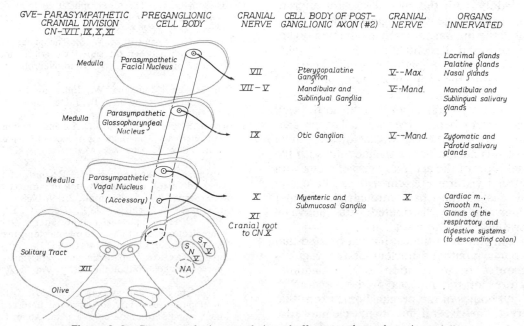

Figure 6–3. Parasympathetic general visceral efferent nuclear column in medulla.

Preganglionic GVE axons in the facial nerve synapse in the pterygopalatine ganglion, whose postganglionic axons innervate the lacrimal, palatine, and nasal glands. Other facial nerve preganglionic axons synapse in the mandibular and sublingual ganglia. The postganglionic axons innervate the mandibular and sublingual salivary glands. Preganglionic GVE axons in the glossopharyngeal nerve synapse in the otic ganglion. Postganglionic axons innervate the zygomatic and parotid salivary glands. All of these postganglionic axons pass to the glands to be innervated in branches of the trigeminal nerve.

The facial nerve contains parasympathetic preganglionic neurons that produce lacrimal gland secretion. These leave the facial nerve as it courses through the middle ear. Facial nerve lesions between the medulla and the middle ear that involve these fibers will cause decreased tear formation, which can be determined by the Schirmer tear test or by pressing on the closed eyelids for one minute and observing the amount of reflex lacrimation that occurs. Facial nerve lesions distal to the facial canal in the temporal bone will not affect these neurons.

The parasympathetic vagal nucleus comprises the majority of this nuclear column.[5] It is dorsolateral to the hypoglossal nucleus and slightly longer. It is medial to the solitary tract and nucleus that is part of the general visceral afferent system (Plates 3 and 4). The general visceral efferent axons leave the lateral side of the medulla with the special visceral efferent axons from nucleus ambiguus. They course through the jugular foramen and tympanoocipital fissure and descend the neck in the vagal part of the vagosympathetic trunk. They are distributed to the esophagus and organs in the thorax and abdomen, where they synapse on cell bodies of postganglionic axons in the wall of the viscera being innervated. The preganglionic axons of the cell bodies in the caudal part of this nucleus leave the medulla with the cranial roots of the accessory nerve, along with its special visceral efferent axons. These join the vagus as they pass through the jugular foramen and are distributed with the vagal general visceral efferent axons.

Investigations in the cat have suggested that this parasympathetic nucleus of the vagus is the source of innervation to the glandular structures of the mucosa of the viscera.[17, 18] The cell bodies of the preganglionic axons that innervate the visceral smooth muscle may arise from a nucleus located ventrolateral in the medulla between nucleus ambiguus and the spinal nucleus of the trigeminal nerve. However, it has also been reported that electrolytic lesions of the parasympathetic nucleus of the vagus in the cat caused paralysis of the esophagus. In the dog this dysfunction required bilateral lesions of nucleus ambiguus.

Some consider the general visceral efferent vagal neurons to be interneurons because they may not be necessary for direct initiation of smooth muscle activity in the digestive tract, but instead modulate the intrinsic reflex activity of the enteric plexus. The gastrointestinal tract can carry out its major functions without its extrinsic innervation. This is accomplished by (1) the intrinsic neural mechanism in the wall of the bowel, which can maintain small intestinal peristalsis and colonic mass movement, and (2) the ability of the smooth muscle cell to contract rhythmically. This intrinsic capability is more apparent in primates and carnivores than ruminants.

Unilateral vagus nerve lesions or vagotomy is not associated with clinical signs in dogs. Bilateral cervical vagal disease or vagotomy causes paralysis of the larynx with inspiratory dyspnea and cyanosis, and abnormal esophageal swallowing with regurgitation and megaesophagus.[15, 16] These signs are the result of loss of SVE function of the vagus nerve.

REFERENCES

1. Acheson, G. H.: The topographical anatomy of the smooth muscle of the cat's nictitating membrane. Anat. Rec., 71:297, 1938.
2. Barlow, C. M., and Root, W. S.: The ocular sympathetic path between the superior cervical ganglion and the orbit in the cat. J. Comp. Neurol., 91:195, 1949.
3. Bell, M., and Montagna, W.: Innervation of sweat glands in horses and dogs. Br. J. Dermatol., 86:160, 1972.
4. Bistner, S., Rubin, L., Cox, T. A., and Condon, W. E.: Pharmacologic diagnosis of Horner's syndrome in the dog. J. Am. Vet. Med. Assoc., 157:1220, 1970.
5. Carlsson, C-A., and Sundin, T.: Reconstruction of severed ventral roots innervating the urinary bladder. Scand. J. Urol. Nephrol., 2:199, 1968.
6. Carveth, S. W., Schlegel, J. F., Code, C. F., and Ellis, F. H.: Esophageal motility after vagotomy, phrenicotomy, myotomy, and myomectomy in dogs. Surg. Gynecol. Obstet., 114:31, 1962.
7. Christensen, K.: Sympathetic and parasympathetic nerves in the orbit of the cat. J. Anat., 70:225, 1936.
8. de Lahunta, A., and Alexander, J. W.: Ischemic myelopathy secondary to presumed fibrocartilaginous embolism in nine dogs. J. Am. Anim. Hosp. Assoc. 12:37, 1976.

9. Edvardsen, P.: Nervous control of urinary bladder in cats. I. The collecting phase. Acta Physiol. Scand., *72*:157, 1968.
10. Firth, E. C.: Horner's syndrome in the horse: Experimental induction and case report. Equine Vet. J. *10*:9, 1978.
11. Fletcher, T. F., and Bradley, W. E.: Neuroanatomy of the bladder-urethra. J. Urol., *119*:153, 1978.
12. Fox, J. G., and Gutnick, M. J.: Horner's syndrome and brachial paralysis due to lymphosarcoma in a cat. J. Am. Vet. Med. Assoc., *160*:977, 1972.
13. Greene, C. E., and Higgins, R. J.: Fibrocartilaginous emboli as the cause of ischemic myelopathy in a dog. Cornell Vet., *66*:131, 1976.
14. Harding, R., and Leek, B. F.: The locations and activities of medullary neurons associated with ruminant forestomach motility. J. Physiol., *219*:587, 1971.
15. Higgs, B., and Ellis, F. H.: The effect of bilateral supranodosal vagotomy on canine esophageal function. Surgery, *58*:828, 1965.
16. Huang, K., Essex, H., Essex, E., and Mann, F. C.: A study of certain problems resulting from vagotomy in dogs with special reference to emesis. Am. J. Physiol., *149*:429, 1947.
17. Kerr, F. W. L.: Function of the dorsal motor nucleus of the vagus. Science, *157*:451, 1967.
18. Kerr, F. W. L., Hendler, H., and Bowren, P.: Viscerotopic organization of the vagus. J. Comp. Neurol., *138*:279, 1970.
19. Kerr, F. W. L., and Hollowell, O. W.: Location of pupillomotor and accommodation fibres in the oculomotor nerve: Experimental observations on paralytic mydriasis. J. Neurol. Neurosurg. Psychiatry, *27*:473, 1964.
20. Kuru, M., and Iwanaga, T.: Ponto-sacral connections in the medial reticulospinal tract subserving storage of urine. J. Comp. Neurol., *127*:241, 1966.
21. Mayhew, I. G.: Horner's syndrome and lesions involving the sympathetic nervous system. Equine Pract., *2*:44, 1980.
22. McGrath, J. T.: Neurologic Examination of the Dog. 2nd. ed. Philadelphia, Lea and Febiger, 1960.
23. Moreau, P. M.: Neurogenic disorders of micturition in the dog and cat. Compend. Contin. Ed., *12*:12, 1982.
24. Morgan, C., Nadelhaft, I., and de Groat, W. C.: Location of bladder preganglionic neurons within the sacral parasympathetic nucleus of the cat. Neurosci. Letters, *14*:189, 1979.
25. Nergardh, A.: Autonomic receptor functions in the lower urinary tract: A survey of recent experimental results. J. Urol., *113*:180, 1975.
26. Oliver, J. E., Jr., Bradley, W. E., and Fletcher, T. F.: Identification of preganglionic parasympathetic neurons in the sacral spinal cord of the cat. J. Comp. Neurol., *137*:321, 1969.
27. Oliver, J. E., Jr., Bradley, W. E., and Fletcher, T. F.: Spinal cord representation of the micturition reflex. J. Comp. Neurol., *137*:329, 1969.
28. Oliver, J., Bradley, W., and Fletcher, T.: Spinal cord distribution of the somatic innervation of the external urethral sphincter of the cat. J. Neurol. Sci., *10*:11, 1970.
29. Oliver, J. E., and Selcer, R. R.: Neurogenic disorders of the rectum and anal sphincter. Vet. Clin. North Am., *4*:551, 1974.
30. Oliver, J. E., and Selcer, R. R.: Neurogenic causes of abnormal micturition in the dog and cat. Vet. Clin. North Am., *4*:517, 1974.
31. Oliver, J. E., and Young, W. O.: Air cystometry in dogs under xylazine-induced restraint. Am. J. Vet. Res., 34:1433, 1973.
32. Osborne, C. A., Clifford, D. H., and Jessen, C.: Hereditary esophageal achalasia in dogs. J. Am. Vet. Med. Assoc., *141*:572, 1967.
33. Owen, R. ap R.: Epistaxis prevented by ligation of the internal carotid artery in the guttural pouch. Equine Vet. J., *6*:143, 1974.
34. Petras, J. M., and Cummings, J. F.: Sympathetic and parasympathetic innervation of the urinary bladder and urethra. Brain Res., *153*:363, 1978.
35. Purington, P. T., and Oliver, J. E.: Spinal cord origin of innervation to the bladder and urethra of the dog. Exp. Neurol., *65*:422, 1979.
36. Purohit, R. C., McCoy, M. D., and Bergfield, W. A., III: Thermographic diagnosis of Horner's syndrome in the horse. Am. J. Vet. Res., *41*:1180, 1980.
37. Rohner, T. J., Rezar, D. M., Wein, A. J., and Schoenberg, H. W.: Contractile responses of dog bladder neck muscle to adrenergic drugs. J. Urol., *105*:657, 1971.
38. Rosen, A. H., and Ross, L.: Diagnosis and pharmacological management of disorders of urinary continence in the dog. Compend. Contin. Ed., *3*:601, 1981.
39. Rosenblueth, A., and Bard, P.: The innervation and function of the nictitating membrane in the cat. Am. J. Physiol., *100*:537, 1932.
40. Rosin, A. E., and Barsanti, J. A.: Diagnosis of urinary incontinence in dogs: Role of the urethral pressure profile. J. Am. Vet. Med. Assoc., *178*:814, 1981.
41. Rosin, A., Rosin, E., and Oliver, J.: Canine urethral pressure profile. Am. J. Vet. Res., *41*:1113, 1980.
42. Scagliotti, R. H.: Current concepts in veterinary neuro-ophthalmology. Vet. Clin. North Am., *10*:417, 1980.
43. Smith, J. S., and Mayhew, I. G.: Horner's syndrome in large animals. Cornell Vet., *67*:529, 1977.
44. Sundin, T., and Carlsson, C-A.: Reconstruction of severed dorsal roots innervating the urinary bladder: An experimental study in cats. I. Studies on the normal afferent pathways in the pelvic and pudendal nerves. Scand. J. Urol. Nephrol., *6*:176, 1972.
45. Sundin, T., and Carlsson, C-A.: Reconstruction of severed dorsal roots innervating the urinary bladder: An experimental study in cats. II. Regeneration studies. Scand. J. Urol. Nephrol., *6*:185, 1972.
46. Thompson, J. W.: The nerve supply to the nictitating membrane of the cat. J. Anat., *95*:371, 1961.

ing the pyramid on the ventral surface of the medulla. Their telodendron is in the grey matter of the spinal cord. This is an uninterrupted, monosynaptic, corticospinal pathway from the cerebrum to the spinal cord by way of the pyramids of the medulla.

In contrast, the extrapyramidal system consists of neurons that originate in the cerebral cortex, including the motor area, and descend into the brain stem directly or by way of subcortical nuclei. Synapse occurs with additional neurons in the subcortical nuclei and brain stem nuclei. Axons course from specific brain stem nuclei caudally through the spinal cord, without traversing the pyramids of the medulla. The telodendron of the final neuron is in the grey matter of the spinal cord. This is a multineuronal, multisynaptic, corticospinal pathway. These two systems overlap anatomically and function together. The extrapyramidal system is of much greater importance in the domestic animal. They will be considered together as the upper motor neuron in clinical discussions.

PYRAMIDAL SYSTEM

The development of the pyramidal system is related directly to the capacity of the animal to perform finely skilled movements. In primates its termination in the spinal cord is most dense in the areas of the lateral portion of the ventral grey column, in which the cell bodies of the general somatic efferent lower motor neuron to muscles of the digits are located. Here it may synapse directly on the dendritic zone of the alpha motor neuron (GSE). Such development has been observed in the primate and the raccoon, two unrelated species that possess considerable manipulative ability in their thoracic limb digits.[1] This system is developed poorly to the spinal cord in domestic animals, especially in the horse, the ox, and the sheep. In the horse, this system makes a sizable contribution to the facial muscles for lip movement, suggesting that these muscles perform the most highly skilled activity of this species. In the larger species of domestic ani-

The upper motor neuron (UMN) is the motor system confined to the central nervous system that is responsible for the initiation of voluntary movement, the maintenance of tone for support of the body against gravity, and the regulation of posture to provide a stable background upon which to initiate the voluntary activity. Traditionally, it is divided into pyramidal and extrapyramidal components. This separation is more significant in the primate, in whom the pyramidal system is more highly developed and has a more important function than has been observed in domestic animals.

The pyramidal system consists of those neurons whose cell bodies are located predominantly in the motor area of the cerebral cortex, and whose axons descend through the white matter of the cerebrum and brain stem, includ-

mals, it also terminates in the spinal cord dorsal grey column, where it influences ascending sensory systems.

The cell body of the neuron of the pyramidal system is located in the cerebral cortex. Although these are found throughout the cerebrum, the majority are located in the motor area in the frontal lobe or adjacent parietal lobe (Fig. 7–1). In primates, this mostly involves the precruciate gyrus. In carnivores, it overlaps on the sensory area and is limited to the postcruciate gyrus and rostral suprasylvian gyrus.[23, 26, 53] In ungulates, it is located medially along the frontal lobe in the region of the precruciate gyrus.[21] Stimulation studies have shown that these motor areas can be subdivided into regions of the body that are innervated by lower motor neurons receiving impulses from the pyramidal system neurons that originate in these specific parts of the motor area. This is referred to as a somatotopic organization. The various portions of the body are represented topographically on specific areas of cerebral gyri. The homunculus drawn for the human brain depicts this phenomenon. Regions involved in more highly skilled functions have a larger representation in the motor area. Muscles with small motor units have a larger area of representation. The primary motor area of one cerebral hemisphere serves the musculature on the opposite side of the body. In the carnivore the postcruciate gyrus is related to the innervation of the appendicular musculature.[23, 24] The suprasylvian gyrus is related to the motor function of the cervical muscles and the muscles of specific areas of the head. Many of these cell bodies are large and are referred to as giant pyramidal cells or Betz's cells.[53] They are located in lamina V of the cerebral cortex of the gyri in the motor area.

The axons of these cells descend through the white matter of the brain, which includes, in this order: the corona radiata of the motor cortex, the internal capsule of telencephalon and diencephalon, the crus cerebri of the mesencephalon (in which they occupy the central portion), the longitudinal fibers of pons, and the pyramid of medulla. Caudal to the obex of the medulla, approximately 75 per cent or more of these axons cross in the pyramidal decussation located adjacent to the ventral median fissure, and pass through the grey matter to the dorsal part of the lateral funiculus (Plate 2). Here they descend as the lateral corticospinal tract medial to the ascending spinocerebellar tracts.[124] In the dog, approximately 50 per cent of these axons terminate in the cervical spinal cord grey matter, 20 per cent in the thoracic grey matter, and 30 per cent in the lumbosacral grey matter.[69] Most influence the general somatic efferent lower motor neuron by way of synapse with interneurons.[90, 102] The remaining 25 per cent or less descend without crossing in the ventral funiculus adjacent to the ventral median fissure as the ventral corticospinal tract. This tract is not as well defined as the lateral tract. The axons of the ventral corticospinal tract descend the spinal cord as far as the midthoracic level and the majority cross at their termination. In ungulates, the entire pyramidal system is confined to the cervical spinal cord.[10] A few axons have been found caudal to the cervical segments in the horse.[20, 21] In cats the pyramid has been mapped according to the muscle groups affected by its neurons.[28]

In addition to influencing the spinal nerve lower motor neuron, this system also affects the cranial nerve lower motor neuron. This is mediated by axons that leave the descending pathway as it moves through the brain stem. These axons synapse on or near the general somatic efferent and special visceral effer-

1. POSTCRUCIATE GYRUS
   A. Pelvic limb
   B. Thoracic limb
2. ROSTRAL SUPRASYLVIAN GYRUS
   C. Ear
   D. Eyelid
   E. Masseter, temporal mm.
   F. Lateral cervical mm.

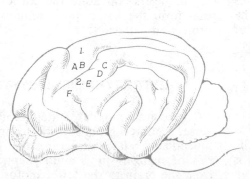

Figure 7–1. Topography of the cerebral motor cortex.

ent lower motor neurons and are called corticonuclear (corticobulbar) fibers. The pyramidal system axons are organized regionally in the central white matter. In the crus cerebri the pyramidal system is in the center, with the axons to the pelvic limb lateral, those to the thoracic limb in the middle, and those to the muscles of the head medial.

Disturbances in the pyramidal system demonstrate the different role this system plays in primates as compared with domestic animals. Lesions in the cerebral origin of this system in humans cause a paralysis of contralateral voluntary muscle activity. In dogs examined a few days after experimental removal of the motor area there is no defect in the gait, but there is a deficiency in the response to postural reaction testing in the contralateral limbs.[136] Numerous kinds of lesions in this same area in all domesticated animals present a similar clinical syndrome of gait preservation and deficiency of contralateral postural reactions. Section of the canine pyramidal system in the crus cerebri or pyramid also does not affect the gait.[59]

HISTOLOGY OF THE CEREBRAL CORTEX

The cerebral cortex is made up of an elaborate organization of neural structures with innumerable interconnections that form the basis for the numerous functions allotted to it. These include consciousness, intellect, emotion, behavior, perception, and control of somatic and visceral motor functions. These are performed by the reciprocal relationship of the cortex with the rest of the central and the peripheral nervous systems.

The cerebral cortex varies from 1.5 to 4 mm in thickness and is situated between the pia mater and the underlying white matter of the corona radiata, which it covers. It contains neuronal cell bodies of many different sizes and shapes: axons, telodendria, the processes of the dendritic zone, and neuroglial cells. The neurons in the cortex constitute a system of chains of interrelated neurons. It is a laminated structure based either on the organization of the processes, the study of which is called myeloarchitectonics, or on the arrangement of the cell bodies, the study of which is termed cytoarchitectonics. When viewed according to the organization of the cell bodies, as many as six layers can be recognized (Fig. 7–2). The extent to which each of these six laminae is developed varies throughout the cerebrum. In

general, the neopallium has six layers, and the archipallium and paleopallium each have less than six. Some functional significance has been attached to the variation in lamination in the different regions of the cerebrum. Various maps have been prepared showing the laminar variations that occur throughout the cerebrum. Some include over 100 different areas based on cytoarchitectonic studies. The cortical laminations of the archipallium and paleopallium are different from the lamination of the neopallium and of each other. Specific characteristics of each permit their identification.

In general, the neuronal cell bodies are of two types. The stellate or granule cell has a round cell body and short processes, which usually are confined to the cortex. The pyramidal cell has a pyramid-shaped cell body that varies in size and has long processes. The axon of the pyramidal cell projects from the cortex into the white matter of the corona radiata as an association axon to another cortical area in the same hemisphere, or as a commissural axon that crosses to a cortical area in the opposite hemisphere, or as a projection axon that projects to nuclear areas in the brain stem or spinal cord. The corticospinal neuron is an example of the latter type. Each cortical area receives axons from other cortical areas in the same hemisphere (association), from the opposite hemisphere (commissural), and from the brain stem, especially the thalamus (projection). The study of the arrangement of these processes in the cortex, and of the processes of the granule cells, is referred to as myeloarchitectonics.

In the neocortex, the six layers from external to internal consist of the molecular layer, external granular layer, pyramidal cell layer, internal granular layer, ganglion cell layer, and multiformic cell layer. The processes of the molecular and external and internal granular layers are confined mostly to the cortex. Axons from the pyramidal, ganglionic, and multiformic layers constitute the cortical efferents that form the association, commissural, and projection pathways.

EXTRAPYRAMIDAL SYSTEM

The extrapyramidal system embraces diverse, scattered groups of interconnected and functionally related structures that form a series of neurons in a multisynaptic pathway from the brain to the lower motor neuron of

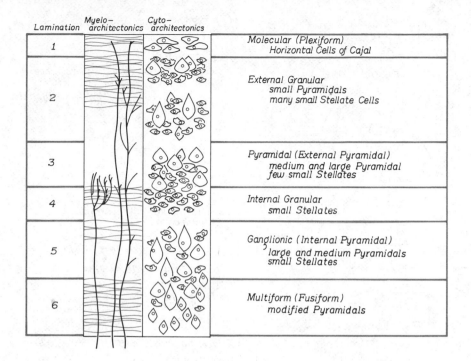

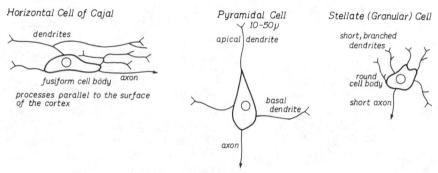

Figure 7–2. Histology of the cerebral cortex.

the brain stem and spinal cord (Fig. 7–3). These pathways do not traverse the pyramids of the medulla, but function with the pyramidal system in providing tonic mechanisms for the support of the body against gravity and in the recruitment of spinal reflexes for the initiation of voluntary movement. These functions are performed ultimately by the influence of this system (UMN) on the alpha and gamma motor neurons (LMN) in motor nuclei in the brain stem and in the ventral grey column of the spinal cord.

The cell bodies of neurons in the extrapyramidal system are located in nuclei in all divisions of the brain. The more important of these will be described for each of the divisions, along with the course of the axons. Only the extrapyramidal nuclei in the mesencephalon and rhombencephalon have axons that descend the spinal cord to influence the activity of the lower motor neuron.

Telencephalon

Neuronal cell bodies in the telencephalon are located either on the surface in laminae of the cerebral cortex or deep to the surface in subcortical collections known as basal nuclei. (Basal nuclei in the past have also been referred to as basal ganglia.[40, 125])

1. Extrapyramidal neurons are located in the cerebral cortex throughout the cerebrum, but mostly in the frontal and parietal lobes, in which they occur in the cortex of the motor area and adjacent gyri. These project to basal nuclei and other extrapyramidal nuclei in the brain stem (Fig. 7–4).

2. The basal nuclei are subcortical collec-

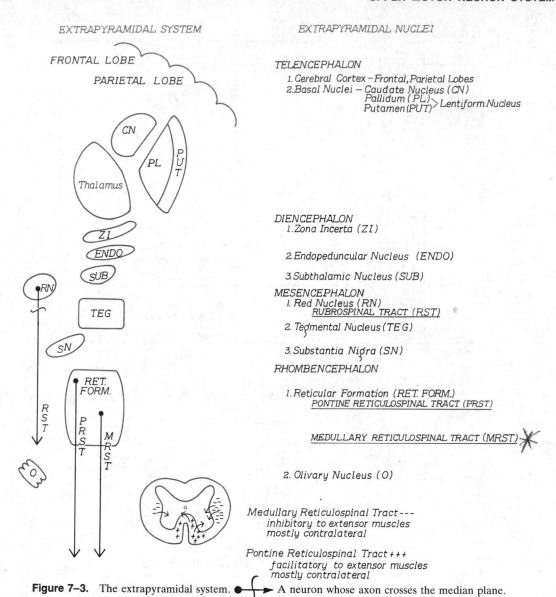

Figure 7–3. The extrapyramidal system. ●⟍→ A neuron whose axon crosses the median plane.

tions of neuronal cell bodies. These include the septal nuclei, amygdala and claustrum, which function in the limbic system. The caudate nucleus, putamen, and pallidum are extrapyramidal basal nuclei. The putamen and pallidum are referred to as the lentiform nucleus because of their overall shape on transverse or dorsal section. The corpus striatum refers to all three of these extrapyramidal basal nuclei and the intervening internal capsule that is traversed by their processes.

The caudate nucleus is located primarily in the floor of the lateral ventricle, medial to the internal capsule (Plate 16). The large head and most of the body are rostral to the diencephalon. The body extends caudally dorsolateral to the diencephalon, medial to the internal capsule, and is continued by a small tail into the temporal lobe of the cerebrum, in which it is lateral to the internal capsule (Plate 15). It receives afferents from extrapyramidal neurons in the cerebral cortex and projects mostly to the adjacent pallidum.[131]

The lentiform nucleus comprises the pallidum (globus pallidus) medially and the putamen laterally, separated by a layer of white matter. It is bounded medially by the internal capsule and laterally by the thin external capsule (Plates 16, 15). This nucleus begins rostrally in the frontal lobe, in which it is separated from the head and body of the caudate nucleus by the internal capsule. It extends

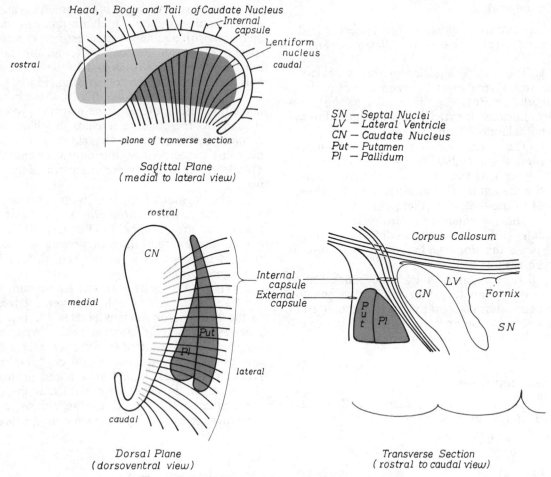

Figure 7–4. Extrapyramidal nuclei of the telencephalon.

caudally through the parietal and into the temporal lobe to a level caudal to the amygdala in the pyriform lobe, in which the lateral ventricle and hippocampus are located. It is dorsal to the amygdaloid nucleus and lateral to the optic tract and internal capsule.

A feedback circuit is provided by a multi-synaptic pathway from cortical extrapyramidal neurons to caudate nucleus, to pallidum, to ventral rostral nucleus of thalamus, to cerebral cortex. At the time of cortical initiation of voluntary movement such a circuit provides a modifying control mechanism. Certain thalamic nuclei serve to project information from the brain stem to the cerebrum. The ventral rostral thalamic nucleus is an example of such a projection nucleus for the extrapyramidal system.

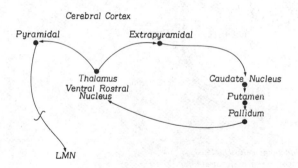

Diencephalon

The extrapyramidal nuclei are located in the ventrolateral region of the thalamus (Fig. 7–5).

1. The endopeduncular nucleus is located in the rostral thalamus between the optic tract and the internal capsule medial to the lentiform nucleus. It extends caudally lateral to the hypothalamus (Plate 15).

2. The zona incerta is a narrow nucleus located dorsomedial to the internal capsule and lateral to the external medullary lamina of the thalamus. This nucleus extends through most of the thalamus (Plate 14).

3. The subthalamic nucleus is in the caudal thalamus, caudal to the endopeduncular nucleus on the dorsomedial surface of the crus cerebri (Plate 14).

All three of these nuclei are connected to the extrapyramidal nuclei in the telencephalon and caudal brain stem by afferent and efferent axons, but none projects directly to the spinal cord lower motor neuron.

Mesencephalon

There are three extrapyramidal nuclear areas in the midbrain (Fig. 7–6).

1. The substantia nigra is so named because its cell bodies contain a melanin pigment that increases with age and is macroscopic in some species.[75] This nucleus can be found throughout the mesencephalon dorsal to the crus cerebri and ventral to the tegmentum (Plates 13, 12, 11). It is bounded rostrally by the subthalamic nucleus. Some of these neurons project rostrally to the caudate nucleus in which dopamine, synthesized in the substantia nigra neurons, is secreted as the neurotransmitter. This is referred to as the nigrostriatal pathway.[122]

2. The tegmental nucleus is an ill-defined area in the reticular formation of the tegmentum of the mesencephalon (Plates 11, 10). It extends the length of the mesencephalon. Rostrally it is dorsolateral to the red nucleus in the tegmentum.

3. The red nucleus is in the tegmentum at the level of the rostral colliculus ventrolateral to the oculomotor nucleus (Plates 12, 11). It receives a group of afferent axons from the ipsilateral motor area of the cerebral cortex by way of the internal capsule and crus cerebri. Axons of the cell bodies in the red nucleus decussate at the level of the nucleus in the tegmentum and descend as the rubrospinal tract through the ventrolateral mesencephalon,

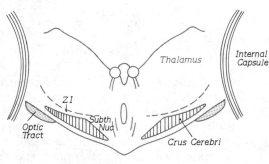

ZI: Zona Incerta
Subth Nuc: Subthalamic Nucleus

Figure 7–5. Extrapyramidal nuclei of the diencephalon.

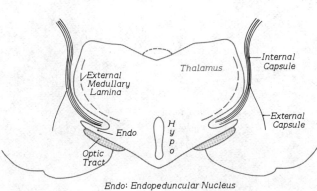

Endo: Endopeduncular Nucleus
Hypo: Hypothalamus

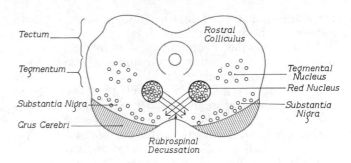

Figure 7–6. Extrapyramidal nuclei of the mesencephalon.

pons, medulla, and lateral funiculus of the spinal cord. Here the tract is associated closely with the lateral corticospinal tract deep to the superficially positioned ascending spinocerebellar tracts in the dorsal portion of the lateral funiculus. This tract descends through the entire spinal cord. Its axons terminate on interneurons in the ventral grey column of the spinal cord that influence the activity of the lower motor neurons. This corticorubrospinal system is organized somatotopically.[58, 106] The neurons in the thoracic limb area of the motor cortex project on the dorsal part of the red nucleus, whose neurons project on the spinal cord grey matter that innervates the thoracic limb. Corticorubral neurons from the pelvic limb region of the motor cortex synapse in the ventral portion of the red nucleus, whose neurons descend in the rubrospinal tract to influence the pelvic limb lower motor neuron. Neurons in the rubrospinal tract are predominantly facilitatory to motoneurons of flexor muscles.[61]

Rubrobulbar neurons course with the rubrospinal neurons; and at various levels leave the rubrospinal tract as it courses through the caudal brain stem. The rubrobulbar neurons synapse in the cranial nerve nuclei for general somatic efferent and special visceral efferent function.

The red nucleus also receives a group of afferent axons from the contralateral lateral (dentate) nucleus of the cerebellum. These axons enter the mesencephalic tegmentum, and synapse on neurons in the red nucleus. These cell bodies of the red nucleus project rostrally to the ventral rostral nucleus of the thalamus, in which synapse occurs, and these thalamic neurons project to the cerebral cortex. The red nucleus in this instance is part of a cerebellorubrothalamic system that is part of a feedback circuit to the cerebral cortex. The cerebellum receives cortical projections by way of the pontine nucleus and middle cerebellar peduncle. The complete circuit involves the corticopontocerebellar and cerebellorubrothalamic pathways.

In addition, there are afferent and efferent connections of the red nucleus with the telencephalic basal nuclei.

Rhombencephalon

1. The reticular formation is located in the core of the medulla, the pons, the tegmentum of the midbrain, and the caudal diencephalon. It is an ill-defined meshwork of a variety of cell types engulfed in a diffuse network of neuronal processes. Anatomic studies have defined nuclear areas within the reticular formation. It receives projections primarily from the cerebellum, spinal cord, and higher levels of the brain, including extrapyramidal nuclei. The reticular formation, in turn, projects to these three areas. A large projection serves the spinal cord.[10, 11, 89]

Many functions have been attributed to the reticular formation. These include activation of the cerebral cortex for awake state (ascending reticular activating system—ARAS), sleep mechanisms, control of vital functions such as respiratory and cardiac functions, control over voluntary excretion, control over vomiting and swallowing, and control over muscle tone and motor function. Some authors divide the reticular formation into an ascending portion that functions in the activation of the higher brain structures, and a descending portion that influences ventral grey column internuncial activity and the alpha and gamma efferent neurons affecting motor tone and motor activity. The descending portion includes its participation in the extrapyramidal system.

Studies in the cat have defined an area of the reticular formation in the pons that exerts facilitatory influence on motoneurons of extensor muscles by way of a descending reticulospinal tract (Plates 9, 8).[102] This pontine reticulospinal tract courses mostly in the ipsilateral ventral funiculus. Similarly, an area of the medullary reticular formation has inhibitory influence on the motoneurons of extensor muscles in the spinal cord by way of a medullary reticulospinal tract that course in the lateral funiculus in a medial intermediate position, mostly on the ipsilateral side (Plates 7, 6, 5, 4). The axons that course in these two tracts terminate in the ventral grey column of the spinal cord on the same side.

2. The olivary nucleus is located ventrally in the medulla, from a level caudal to the facial nucleus to a level caudal to the obex and rostral to the pyramidal decussation. It is dorsolateral to the pyramids and medial lemniscus, medial to the descending hypoglossal axons (Plates 4, 3). It comprises three nuclear groups that at some levels have the appearance of fingers directed ventrolaterally. This extrapyramidal nucleus receives afferents from many of the extrapyramidal nuclei in the telencephalon, diencephalon, and mesencephalon. Its efferents project primarily to the contralateral portion of the cerebellum. This is a primary source of extrapyramidal system projection to the cerebellum. The axons cross the midline dorsal to the pyramids, intermingle with the medial lemniscus, and continue in an arc dorsolaterally to enter the caudal cerebellar peduncle, where they are distributed to the cerebellum.

A feedback circuit exists to the cerebral cortex by way of the cerebellum through this nucleus.

In this presentation of the extrapyramidal portion of the upper motor neuron, the final efferent pathways by which this system exerts influence over the lower motor neuron are rubrospinal, medullary, and pontine reticulospinal tracts. Other descending tracts influence motor tone and motor activity by their connections with the ventral grey column of the spinal cord. These include the vestibulospinal tract, the medial longitudinal fasciculus, and the tectospinal tract. These sometimes are included in descriptions of the extrapyramidal

descending projections. In this book they are considered together with the different systems that have their own anatomic components and functional attributes, separate from but interrelated with the extrapyramidal system. Most of these descending tracts influence the lower motor neuron through interneurons in the grey matter where these extrapyramidal neurons terminate. In addition there are long spinal interneurons that descend the spinal cord and may be a component of this UMN influence over the LMN.[79]

A comparison of the development of the upper motor neuron tracts in the cranial cervical spinal cord of man, the cat, and the horse reveals the decrease in importance of the pyramidal system (corticospinal tract) and the increase in the contribution of the extrapyramidal system (rubrospinal tract) in the domestic animal (Fig. 7–7).

FUNCTION

The functions of the upper motor neuron can be summarized as: (1) the initiation of voluntary activity of the motor system, (2) the maintenance of muscle tone to support the body against gravity and to establish the posture upon which the voluntary activity can be performed, and (3) the control of muscular activity associated with visceral functions (respiration, cardiovascular, urination).[32]

The extrapyramidal system exerts its functions by influencing the activity of the alpha and gamma motor neurons in the ventral grey column of the spinal cord. Its activity in modulating muscle tone involves its control over the myotatic reflex. The sensory receptor organ for this reflex is the neuromuscular spindle located in the belly of the skeletal muscles

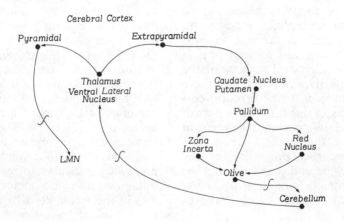

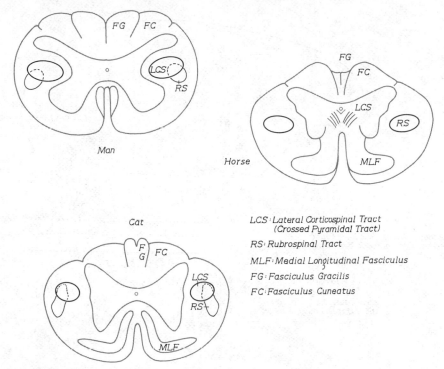

Figure·7–7. Comparison of first cervical spinal cord segment in man, the cat, and the horse.

(Fig. 7–8). These spindle-shaped structures are composed of intrafusal fibers, which are modified small striated muscle cells. The intrafusal fibers are parallel to the extrafusal fibers, which are the larger striated skeletal muscle cells. A connective tissue capsule encloses the group of intrafusal fibers and is attached to the endomysium of the adjacent extrafusal fibers. Within the spindle there are two types of intrafusal fibers. One type (nuclear bag) is interrupted near its middle by a nonstriated dilation containing many cell nuclei. The second type (nuclear chain) has no central dilation, although its nuclei are accumulated in the middle of the fiber. These features create for the neuromuscular spindle a central distended nuclear bag region augmented by a lymph space that envelops the middle portion of the intrafusal fibers. The poles of the spindle are tapered and contain the contractile striated portion of the intrafusal fibers.

The intrafusal fibers are innervated in the polar regions by small myelinated neurons whose cell bodies are in the ventral grey column of the spinal cord, intermingled with the larger general somatic efferent neurons. These small neurons are called gamma neurons or efferents, while the larger GSE neurons are referred to as alpha neurons or efferents.

There are two types of gamma efferent neurons, depending on the form of their termination on the intrafusal muscle fiber. The gamma plate neurons terminate on the nuclear bag intrafusal fibers in the neuromuscular spindle. The nuclear bag region is surrounded by the processes of a sensory neuron whose axon is large and classified as Ia. These Ia afferents, with their annulospiral endings on the nuclear bag, have their cell bodies in spinal ganglia, and the axon courses through the dorsal root and the doral grey column, into the ventral grey column, to synapse directly on an alpha motor neuron of an extensor muscle. This is described as the tonic gamma loop mechanism, which is responsible for normal muscle tone. Impulses are stimulated in the dendritic zone (annulospiral ending) of the Ia afferent by any action that stretches the nuclear bag region of the spindle, including passive stretch of the skeletal muscle by gravity, tapping the tendon of the muscle with a blunt instrument, or active stretch by contraction of the intrafusal fibers mediated by the gamma efferent neuron.

The gamma trail neurons terminate on the nuclear chain fibers in the neuromuscular spindle. Group II sensory neurons innervate the central nuclear region of these fibers, and their dendritic zones respond to contraction of these

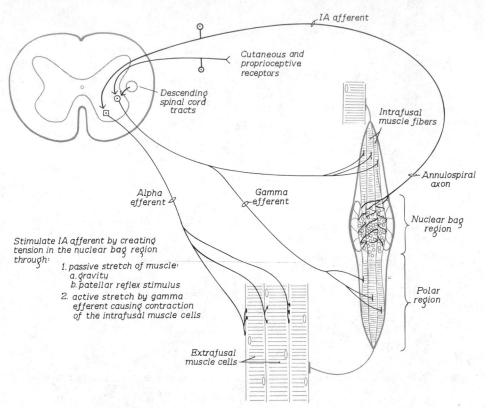

Figure 7–8. Neuromuscular spindle—function and anatomy.

nuclear chain muscle cells. These sensory neurons terminate on interneurons in the spinal cord grey matter that are inhibitory to alpha motoneurons to extensor muscles and facilitatory to alpha motoneurons to flexor muscles. Referred to as the phasic gamma loop or flexor reflex gamma loop, this functions with the UMN to initiate flexor reflexes in the generation of gait.

Posture is maintained against the steady force of gravity by this mechanism. The force of gravity stretches extensor muscles and the nuclear bag region of the spindles. The Ia afferent is stimulated. In turn, the Ia afferent stimulates the alpha motor neuron (GSE), causing contraction of the extrafusal fibers of the extensor muscle. Collaterals of the Ia afferent stimulate interneurons in the ventral grey column that are inhibitory to the GSE neurons innervating the muscles antagonistic to the action of the extensor muscle. The activity of this myotatic reflex maintains the constant low-level state of contraction known as muscle tone. Other collateral axons of the Ia afferent are involved in ascending proprioceptive pathways to the cerebellum and sen-

sory cortex, providing higher centers with information on the state of muscle contraction to be used in the proper coordination of motor activity. The gamma efferent is subject to influence by descending spinal cord tracts of the extrapyramidal system.

Golgi tendon organs are the receptors (dendritic zone) of Ib sensory neurons that are located in tendons. They have a higher threshold to the stimulus of stretching muscles than Ia annulospiral afferents, and are stimulated when the tendon is stretched by contraction of the extrafusal fibers of the muscle. Within the ventral grey column of the spinal cord, the Ib afferent projects on interneurons that are inhibitory to the alpha motor neuron innervating the contracting muscle, and that are facilitatory to the alpha motor neuron innervating the antagonist of this muscle, thus lowering its threshold to stimulus. This inverse myotatic reflex provides for smooth coordination of skeletal muscle activity and protects against overstretching of tendons.

The classic example used by the physiologist to demonstrate the role of the extrapyramidal system in the control of motor tone is the phenomenon of decerebrate rigidity. When the brain stem is transected between the colliculi of the midbrain, an uninhibited extensor tonus of all the antigravity muscles is produced. The head and neck are extended markedly in a posture of opisthotonos, and all four limbs in the quadriped are extended rigidly. This is explained as a release mechanism. The tonic mechanism or myotatic reflex involving the lower motor neuron has been released from the effects of the descending inhibitory upper motor neuron pathways. The facilitatory centers in the pontomedullary reticular formation for motor tone can function autonomously (pontine reticulospinal tract). The inhibitory centers in the pontomedullary reticular formation require continual input from the cerebral cortex, basal nuclei, and cerebellum to function (medullary reticulospinal tract). This input is sacrificed by the lesion, causing the imbalance in function observed as a release phenomenon. In decerebrate rigidity there is a release of the alpha and gamma efferent neurons of extensor motoneurons from the influence of the inhibitory descending upper motor neuron spinal cord tracts. The vestibulospinal tract contributes its facilitatory influence to that of the pontine reticulospinal tract. These same clinical signs may occur with acquired lesions in this part of the brain stem.

The myotatic reflex and normal tonic mechanisms also can be influenced by disturbances in the spinal cord segments. As a result of the intoxication caused by the growth of *Clostridium tetani* in the tissues and the production of the tetanus toxin, or by the absorption of ingested strychnine, a similar release phenomenon occurs, consisting of opisthotonos and persistent rigid extension of all four limbs.[80, 132, 134] These toxins are inhibitory to the activity of interneurons in the ventral grey column of the spinal cord which are known as Renshaw cells. These interneurons normally are inhibitory to the alpha motor neuron and are stimulated by recurrent collaterals of the alpha motor neurons. They function to limit the duration, intensity, and distribution of the motor neuron discharge. These toxins interfere with postsynaptic inhibition at the telodendron of the Renshaw cells. The clinical signs reflect the released alpha motor neuron activity from this source of inhibition.

Tetanus. Tetanus occurs in all domestic animals and humans.[12, 43, 51, 65, 76, 140] *Clostridium tetani* produces spores that are very resistant and can persist for long periods in the environment. When spores gain entrance to an anaer-obic environment in an animal's tissues, they will convert to the vegetative form and produce toxin in 4 to 8 hours. An area of tissue damage is ideal for this. The toxin binds to the gangliosides in axons of peripheral neurons and ascends to the spinal cord within a few hours.[112, 117] The toxin passes from the neuronal cell bodies to the inhibitory interneurons (Renshaw cells) in the adjacent grey matter, where the toxin binds to the interneuron and blocks the release of inhibitory neurotransmitter. The toxin will remain bound to the interneuron for 3 or more weeks. Blood and cerebrospinal fluid distribution of toxin may also occur. The toxin can also bind at the neuromuscular ending and on other neurons in the brain, but in domestic animals the bulk of toxin binds on spinal cord inhibitory interneurons and the signs reflect their functional deficit. These inhibitory interneurons predominate on alpha motor neurons to antigravity (extensor) muscles, and the signs reflect the overactivity of these extensor muscles.

Most signs occur 5 to 10 days after a wound becomes infected. In the most severe form of tetanus, the animal will be recumbent, with extensor rigidity of all limbs, opisthotonos, rigid facial muscles, inability to open the jaw, and possibly seizures. Death occurs from failure to respire adequately. Milder effects include a stiff gait, elevated tail, erect ears, retracted lips, elevated upper eyelid, and a spasmodically protruding third eyelid (mostly in horses), which is secondary to extraocular muscle spasms. Bloat may occur in cattle. The unique facial expression due to the severe contraction of all the facial muscles is most pronounced in dogs and cats, and in humans is referred to as risus sardonicus. The ears may be elevated so much that they nearly touch on the median plane.

The signs may be most pronounced in the area of the body innervated by the spinal cord where the toxin first reaches the spinal cord. A cat with an infected hock lesion had the worse signs in the pelvic limbs. A dog with an infected lesion on the side of its neck had the most extensive rigidity in the thoracic limbs and a severe lateral flexion of the neck on that side. Both of these animals also had severe contraction of the facial muscles.

All of these signs are exacerbated by activity or excitement, and the rate of axonal transport of toxin may be increased by neuronal activity. Treatment should consist of rest and a quiet environment, wound debridement, penicillin, and immediate administration of antitoxin (horse: 300 IU per lb intravenously every 12 hours for three times; cats and dogs: *one* dose of 50 to 250 IU per lb intravenously).[87] The antitoxin has little effect on the toxin already bound to the interneurons but should prevent further axonal ascent and binding. Local injection of antitoxin around and proximal to the wound site may be beneficial. Acepromazine, or promazine and barbiturates, or chloral hydrate in horses is useful to relax the patient.[130] Xylazine is useful in cattle, and diazepam may be helpful in the dog and cat. Be patient; it takes weeks for the patient to recover if you can avoid respiratory arrest and keep the patient nourished. The latter may be enhanced by a rumen fistula in cattle, pharyngostomy tube in dogs and cats, and leaving a nasogastric tube in place and hitched to the halter or bandaged to the neck in horses. Rarely, tracheostomy may be necessary to help respiration.

The site of infection and source of toxin are not always evident. Severe enteritis or metritis can provide an anaerobic environment and alter the mucosa to permit toxin to reach the telodendria of neurons.

Gait.   A recent review of the neural control of locomotion has attempted to apply a model for normal voluntary locomotor function to clinical problems in animals.[70] The basic assumption is that two systems control skeletal muscle movement. The postural control system maintains posture by controlling trunk muscles and the antigravity (extensor) muscles of the proximal limbs. The vestibulospinal and reticulospinal tracts from the medulla and pons facilitate these postural muscles and inhibit most flexor muscles. The voluntary control system initiates voluntary locomotor movement and emanates from the cerebral cortex, extrapyramidal basal nuclei, and red nuclei. It influences spinal motoneurons by way of the corticospinal and rubrospinal tracts. Their function is opposed to that of the postural system, and is facilitatory to flexor muscles and all distal limb muscles, while simultaneously inhibiting antigravity muscles.

Basic locomotor activity may involve recruitment of reflexes by these control mechanisms, alternating between the voluntary and postural systems. The voluntary system recruits flexor reflexes (muscles) to initiate the protraction phase of the gait, and the postural system recruits extensor reflexes for the supporting

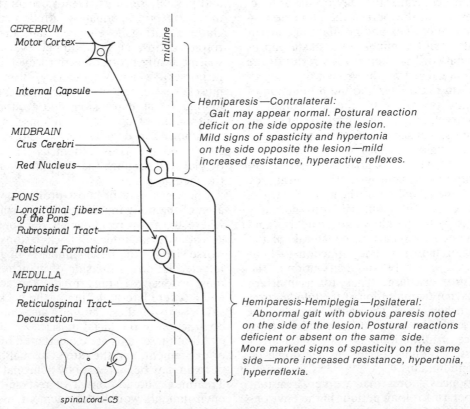

Figure 7–9.   Diagram of upper motor neuron pathways for voluntary movement.

and propulsive phases of the gait. This hypothesis is attractive and is supported by physiologic studies, but it oversimplifies the voluntary control system. The components that are described can be absent, and other components that presumably are brain stem mechanisms can function in the voluntary initiation of locomotion.

Clinical and experimental lesions that destroy the motor cortex or lentiform and caudate nuclei in the domestic animal provide evidence that these anatomic structures are not necessary for the initiation of voluntary movement.[40, 125] Progressing caudally, evidence of paresis of voluntary movement only first occurs with lesions in the midbrain, but experimental destruction of the red nucleus does not induce paresis. Postural reactions are deficient, possibly due to some loss of voluntary facilitation of flexor muscles necessary to initiate the motor phase of most of these reactions. Whereas experimental lesions that destroy the lateral corticospinal and rubrospinal tracts do not produce a gait deficiency, clinical disease (infarction) that destroys all of the lateral funiculus but spares the other funiculi produces an ipsilateral hemiplegia. The loss of other descending motor systems in this funiculus, presumably reticulospinal, must be responsible for the inability to initiate movement. Although the voluntary initiation of locomotion in domestic animals is assumed to be a brain stem function, it has not been defined specifically in anatomic terms.

CLINICAL SIGNS: UPPER MOTOR NEURON DISEASE

Paresis. Disturbance to the mechanism for initiating voluntary motor function causes paresis (weakness) or paralysis, depending on the severity and location of the lesion. The severity of the paresis increases as the location of the lesion descends in the upper motor neuron to involve more of the pathways (Fig. 7–9).

Unilateral lesions of the upper motor neuron rostral to the red nucleus cause contralateral hemiparesis that is so mild that it usually is not apparent in the gait. However, the response to postural reaction testing is deficient. This is exemplified by experimental removal of the motor area of the cerebrum or complete removal of the cortex of one hemisphere. Chronic lesions confined to one cerebrum or its internal capsule involving the upper motor neuron present a similar clinical syndrome.

Lesions that involve the upper motor neuron in the motor cortex or internal capsule also involve the ascending cerebral pathway for general proprioception. The contralateral deficit that is observed in the postural reaction is designated hemiparesis but in reality is also a reflection of this proprioceptive deficit. Unilateral lesions in the midbrain tegmentum, substantia nigra, and crus cerebri produce a contralateral hemiparesis that usually is observed as a mild deficiency in gait and in postural reactions. The degree of paresis may depend on the acuteness of the lesion.

Unilateral lesions in the pons and medulla usually produce an ipsilateral hemiparesis of the gait and a postural reaction deficiency. The gait dysfunction is more obvious if the unilateral lesion is further caudal in the medulla or cranial cervical spinal cord.

Apparently the anatomic landmark for focal lesions that produce an ipsilateral hemiparesis apparent in the gait is in the region of the caudal mesencephalon and rostral pons. When the lesion occurs rostral to this area, the hemiparesis is contralateral and less profound.

A lesion that destroys only the lateral funiculus of the cervical spinal cord causes complete paralysis of the ipsilateral limbs. This is a hemiplegia. Lesions that involve both sides of the caudal brain stem or cervical spinal cord cranial to the second thoracic spinal cord segment cause tetraparesis or tetraplegia (quadriplegia). Lesions of the spinal cord caudal to the second thoracic spinal cord segment cause loss of voluntary movement in the pelvic limbs or paraparesis if partial, paraplegia if complete.

If the lesion that disturbs the upper motor neuron pathways does not interfere with the grey matter or roots of the spinal cord in the cervical or lumbosacral intumescence, no loss of the reflex arcs occurs and no lower motor neuron clinical signs appear.

Spasticity.[9, 139] Usually UMN lesions show the effects of loss of inhibition of myotatic reflexes which results in spasticity or hypertonia and hyperactive reflexes. Spasticity is observed in the gait as stiffness. In mild lesions spasticity may be the only evidence in the gait of a UMN lesion. Paresis may not be evident under the usual conditions of the neurologic examination. With more extensive lesions a spastic paresis is observed.

This spasticity is particularly prominent in horses with mild focal cervical or diffuse spinal cord disease affecting the white matter. The pelvic limb strides will be stiff and the hoof will often slap the ground surface sharply. The length of the stride will usually depend on the degree of general proprioceptive deficit which may cause a longer stride. The thoracic limbs will appear stiff and show a slight delay in the termination of the protraction phase of the gait, causing a slight floating motion before the hoof strikes the ground surface. This spasticity in the thoracic limbs will cause dogs and horses to appear to throw their limbs forward from the shoulder, with decreased flexion of the joints as the limb is protracted.

Myotatic Reflexes. The disturbance to the descending upper motor neuron pathways involved in the maintenance of muscle tone ususally causes signs of myotatic reflexes released from the effects of the inhibitory UMN pathways.[72] All spinal reflexes are intact. Myotatic reflexes—patellar, biceps, triceps—may be intact, or hyperactive (hyperreflexia), or clonus may be observed. Hypertonia is manifested by increased resistance to passive manipulation of the limbs, and represents exaggerated contraction of muscles subjected to stretch due to the released myotatic reflex. Flexor reflexes may show a prolonged afterdischarge, which is observed as repetitive flexion of the limb in the absence of repeated stimuli. The crossed extensor reflex is an example of this release phenomenon when exhibited in a recumbent animal that exerts no voluntary effort to remove itself from the stimulus. In most cases of focal spinal cord lesions that disturb the descending upper motor neuron pathways, one or more of these signs of a released lower motor neuron are observed. Occasionally, hypotonia instead of hypertonia is seen. However, reflexes are still intact because of the lack of direct disturbance of the lower motor neuron. Whether this represents a greater disturbance to the descending facilitatory pathways is not known.

Upper motor neuron disease with spinal cord lesions is described in Chapter 10. The degree of upper motor neuron disturbance with cerebral lesions is considered next.

CLINICAL SYNDROMES

Cerebral Vascular Disease in Cats. A naturally occurring disease syndrome in cats causes acute destruction of the cerebral portions of this upper motor neuron and demonstrates its limited effect on locomotion. A neurologic syndrome has been recognized in cats which consists of a peracute onset of signs of a cerebral disturbance that most often are unilateral. These signs are caused by an extensive ischemic necrosis of cerebral tissue.

The disease affects adult cats of all ages and both sexes. Although it tends to occur more commonly in the summer months, a few cases have been seen in the fall and winter.

The onset is always peracute but the signs are variable. Some cats show only severe depression with mild ataxia, or circling, or both. Some animals circle continuously. Others begin with seizures, and the seizure activity may be unilateral and consist of tonic or clonic activity of the muscles on one side of the head, trunk, and limbs. Changes in attitude and behavior are common and may involve severe aggression. Pupils often are dilated, and blindness may be apparent. For the first 1 to 2 days there may be an observable hemiparesis in the gait.

These acute signs usually resolve in a few days to residual signs of a nonprogressive unilateral cerebral lesion. Destruction of the sensorimotor cortex or its cerebral pathway causes an obvious deficit in the contralateral postural reactions, but there is little interference with the gait. The loss of the visual cerebral cortex or optic radiation results in a contralateral failure to respond to a menacing gesture, but pupillary responses to light are normal. Unilateral cerebral lesions often cause an animal to pace slowly, usually in a circle toward the side of the abnormal cerebrum. These lesions are usually in the frontal lobe or rostral thalamus, and the head turning and circling toward the diseased cerebrum sometimes are referred to as part of the adversive syndrome. The specific cause is unknown, but these are fairly reliable signs. Occasionally, a cat continues to have seizures. These may be generalized or partial motor seizures in which the seizure activity is observed in the muscles on the side of the head and body opposite to the diseased cerebrum. This shows the influence of the cerebral upper motor neuron on the lower motor neuron to the opposite side of the head and body. Involvement of limbic system structures such as the amygdala and hippocampus may be the cause of the behavioral change, which is often permanent.

Occasionally, bilateral blindness persists along with dilated unresponsive pupils, because of ischemic necrosis of the optic chiasm. Careful examination may reveal a unilateral facial hypalgesia, contralateral to the cerebral lesion. No other cranial nerve deficits have been observed. Spinal flexor reflexes are normal, as is pain perception from the limbs.

There may be mild hypertonia and hyperreflexia of tendon reflexes that are more pronounced on the side on which the postural reactions are deficient.

The lesion consists of a variable degree of ischemic necrosis of the cerebral hemisphere, usually unilateral but occasionally bilateral. Most of the necrosis is entirely ischemic. Occasionally, hemorrhages occur in the parenchyma or in the leptomeninges. The necrosis may be multifocal or the infarction may involve up to two thirds of one entire cerebrum. Frequently the major infarction lesion has been in the distribution of the middle cerebral artery. In chronic cases, gross atrophy is most marked in the vicinity of this vessel on the lateral side of the infarcted cerebrum. As a rule the distribution of the lesion reflects multiple vessel involvement. Neutrophils are abundant in the degenerate tissue of an acute ischemic lesion if the blood supply remains. These soon are replaced by mononuclear cells that phagocytize the dead debris.

Vascular lesions have been found in only a few cats. These have consisted of a large thrombus in the middle cerebral artery, venous thrombosis, and vasculitis consisting of mononuclear cells in old cases and neutrophils in early cases. In one case autopsied 3 months after the onset, a dead nematode was found in the thalamus. Its significance remains to be proved. No lesions have been found in other organs, including the heart. There has been no evidence of cardiomyopathy to date. Up to the present time tissue culture studies for viral isolation have been unrewarding.

Hematologic studies and urinalysis have been normal in these subjects. CSF often has a mildly elevated protein level, with little to no cell accumulation. Scintigraphy and electroencephalography sometimes have indicated the location of the lesion.

The prognosis for life is good after the first 48 hours since this is not a progressive disorder. However, the behavioral changes often have interfered with the relationship of the patient with its owner. In a few instances persistent uncontrollable seizures have been a problem.

Similar clinical observations and cerebral infarction have been reported in cats in the Northeast.[3] In some of these cats vascular lesions were found which consisted of emboli from endocardial thrombosis, carcinomatous emboli, heartworms in cerebral vessels, and cerebral arterial thrombi with heartworm microfilaria in the lungs.

There are many examples of lesions that occur in one cerebral hemisphere that present the mild signs of upper motor neuron disturbance similar to those in these cats. These include injury, malformation, abscess, chronic inflammation, and neoplasia, some of which will be discussed in other chapters. Numerous examples of lesions of the upper motor neuron in the spinal cord will be discussed in Chaper 10.

Involuntary Adventitious Movements. In primates disturbances to the extrapyramidal system in the brain sometimes result in the production of repetitive, involuntary, adventitious movements. These diseases usually affect areas of cerebral cortex or specific extrapyramidal nuclei in the telencephalon or rostral brain stem. Examples of these adventitious movements are postural tremor, athetosis, dystonia, ballism, chorea, and myoclonus.[33] The presence of one of these signs is not pathognomonic for any one specific disease or deficiency of any one nuclear area.

A postural tremor is produced by small, rapid, alternating contractions of opposed muscle groups. It is observed at rest and often disappears with activity. It is evident especially in the hands and fingers and is characteristic of the patient with Parkinsonism. These patients also may develop rigidity of joints from incapacitating relentless muscle hypertonia. In the past, therapy for this has included surgical destruction of a specific anatomic site in the extrapyramidal system that is responsible for initiating the tremor and hypertonia. More recently, therapy has involved the replacement of a deficient neurotransmitter substance, dopamine.

Athetosis is slow, writhing movements of the extremities. Dystonia is the same phenomenon in the axial musculoskeletal system. Ballism is violent flailing of a limb. Chorea is continual but irregular jerky rapid movements of different muscle groups. Myoclonus is repetitive, rhythmic contractions of the same group of muscles that may persist during sleep and under light anesthesia. Comparable diseases and signs in domestic animals are rare.

Experimental lesions in these extrapyramidal nuclei of dogs and cats do not produce overt signs of paresis or adventitious movements.[50] In some instances dogs with such lesions may tend to circle or turn the head to one side.

Experimental removal of caudate nuclei from cats bilaterally resulted in no obvious disturbance of motor function after the postoperative recovery.[125-127, 129] Behavioral changes were noted. A compulsory approaching syndrome was described consisting of stereotyped and prolonged approaching and following of persons, cats, or objects. Visual stimuli were the most effective in eliciting this behavior. Other changes included a marked passivity, rooting and purring, exaggerated forelimb treading, hyperactivity, and hyperreactivity. Lesions of the cortex of the frontal lobes did not produce these changes. However, removal of the sensorimotor cortex resulted in loss of contact-placing reactions. These were lost contralateral to unilateral lesions. Recovery of these reactions began 3 to 4 months after the surgery and was complete by 6 to 9 months.[128] No recovery occurred if a complete cerebral hemisphere was removed. In experiments in which cats are trained to press a lever with their paw to obtain a milk reward, they usually do not use the paw contralateral to a unilateral caudatectomy.[92]

A hereditary disease occurs in Kerry blue terriers in which a bilateral symmetric degeneration occurs in the substantia nigra and caudate nucleus, along with the cerebellar cortex. The clinical signs of severe spastic dysmetric ataxia reflect the cerebellar lesion that precedes the extrapyramidal lesion.[37]

For comparative purposes, two syndromes are described that emphasize the role of extrapyramidal nuclear lesions in animals and the basis for an involuntary adventitious movement. One involves a specific bilaterally symmetric extrapyramidal nuclear lesion in horses. The other concerns the development of involuntary adventitious movements in dogs.

EQUINE NIGROPALLIDAL ENCEPHALOMALACIA. A disease is found in horses that causes an acute destruction of extrapyramidal nuclei, with signs of muscle rigidity. Nigropallidal encephalomalacia occurs in horses that consume a specific plant over a prolonged period.[34, 47, 82, 137] The plant usually involved is *Centaurea solstitialis,* yellow star thistle, found mostly in California and Oregon, or *Centaurea repens,* Russian knapweed, found in Colorado. Signs of intoxication appear suddenly after weeks of grazing on these plants, with marked hypertonia, rigidity of the muscles of the head causing facial immobility, retraction of the lips and nose, protrusion of the tongue, inability to prehend food, and mild dysphagia. Death results from starvation. Continual purposeless chewing movements may occur. There is no other evidence of involuntary adventitious movement. Limb hypertonia is less evident.

The patients are depressed. The major lesion is a bilateral symmetric necrosis of the substantia nigra and pallidum related to the chronic consumption of this plant. The lesion occurs suddenly and is ischemic in nature. It is found only in horses and can be produced experimentally. The pathogenesis is unknown.

These signs are similar to the hypertonia and rigidity seen in some of the diseases of the extrapyramidal nuclei in humans, and reflect the role of this system in the maintenance of normal muscle tone and motor activity. It is of interest that the muscles most obviously affected in the horse have the largest representation in the motor area of the cerebral cortex.

CANINE MYOCLONUS. Involuntary adventitious movements are common only in one clinical disease of domestic animals, canine myoclonus. Its pathogenesis differs from that usually observed in humans. Myoclonus occurs in dogs and usually is related to a previous or concurrent nonsuppurative encephalitis or myelitis caused by the canine distemper virus.[19, 77, 80, 119, 120, 133] Many synonyms for this disease exist in the literature, including canine chorea, flexor spasm, and tremor syndrome. Most veterinarians call it distemper chorea. Using human medical terminology for involuntary adventitious movements, it is not chorea but myoclonus, a repetitive, rhythmic contraction of the same group of muscles, up to 60 per minute. Repetitive flexion of one limb, thoracic or pelvic, or both limbs on one side, or contractions of the muscles of mastication, are examples of the groups involved. The muscle groups involved may change as the disease progresses. There may be mild paresis of these muscles. The movements usually persist during sleep and at times under light anesthesia. These signs usually follow the overt signs of encephalitis. Occasionally, myoclonus precedes the signs of encephalitis or it may appear with no other signs of encephalomyelitis. The pathogenesis of the myoclonus is unknown. Experimental studies have shown that once the myoclonus has been established, the segments of the spinal cord that contain the lower motor neuron of the muscles involved in the myoclonus can be cut off from the brain by transection of the spinal cord cranial to their level, and the myoclonus still persists. It even continues following section of the dorsal roots of these spinal cord segments. Ventral root section abolishes the myoclonus. It is hypothesized that a pacemaker is established in the spinal cord motor neuron pool that causes a spontaneous depolarization and discharge of the alpha motor neurons. When repetitive involuntary myoclonus is the only or most significant clinical sign, lesions may be absent or minimal at autopsy. These mild lesions may consist of gliosis with or without nonsuppurative inflammation in and around the involved ventral grey column motor neuron pool. It is not known if the myoclonus is initiated by a brain stem extrapyramidal nuclear lesion and maintained by a local pacemaker mechanism. There is no specific treatment, and the accompanying signs of encephalomyelitis may progress. Occasionally, the encephalitic signs regress or stabilize and the myoclonus persists. In a few cases the myoclonus has resolved spontaneously after months to years.

In patients in which the only clinical sign is myoclonus, this may be alleviated by continuous oral therapy with procainamide.[118] The effective dose varies with each patient. The initial dose can be 125 to 250 mg 2 to 4 times per day. Larger amounts may be required. If the treatment lapses, the signs will return. The specific effect of this drug is unknown. Intravenous administration of 1 to 2 per cent procaine will similarly alleviate these signs. In humans tetrabenazine and clonazepam are used for myoclonus.[57] Antiparkinsonism drugs have not been effective in human spinal myoclonus.

Although this rhythmically repetitive myoclonus is most commonly associated with canine distemper encephalomyelitis, other focal spinal cord lesions can produce these signs. In humans, spinal myoclonus has been observed with inflammations, injuries, neoplasia, and degenerative processes. It has been described in a dog with lead poisoning.[91] I have observed a cat with a repetitive myoclonus predominantly of the thoracic axial muscles that caused rhythmic trunk flexion and an associated limb flexion. At autopsy a mild nonsuppurative myelitis was present in the thoracic segments, with areas of gliosis throughout the grey matter of these segments. The cause was not determined.

Spasticity Syndromes. A number of syndromes occur in domestic animals that presumably involve a disturbance of the myotatic reflex mechanism, resulting in excessive muscle contraction usually producing spasticity. No lesions are associated with these syndromes and a neurochemical disturbance is postulated. These include spastic paresis, spastic syndrome, shivering, and scotty cramp.

SPASTIC PARESIS. This disease in young cattle occurs most commonly in Europe, where it is also called Elso heel and is considered to be a polygenic disorder of low heritability. Many breeds are affected. Holsteins and Angus are reported to be the most commonly affected in the United States. It is a rare disease in my experience. The disease involves the function of one or both pelvic limbs, beginning from a few weeks to six months of age as a rule. Rarely the onset occurs in adult cattle.[18] The earliest sign is a stiff gait in the pelvic limbs, with the most affected limb assuming a straight extended posture as attempts are made to use the limb. The signs are usually asymmetric and slowly progress. They are evident only when the limbs are used. As it worsens, the affected limb may extend caudally during attempts to walk and swing like a pendulum. Every time the hoof touches the ground the limb extends caudally. The signs can be severe enough to keep an animal from getting up and walking.

This is an idiopathic disease with no observable lesions. The pathogenesis is thought to involve uncontrolled or excessive activity of the neuromuscular spindle reflex arc mechanism, primarily in the caudal leg muscles.[14] Selective procaine anesthesia of the small neurons in the ventral roots, the gamma efferents, will stop the clinical signs.[39] Similarly, section of the doral roots of L5 and L6 that contain the IA efferents from neuromuscular spindles will alleviate the signs.[38] On the initiation of voluntary movement, hyperactivity of the gamma efferents to the caudal leg muscles induces impulses in the IA afferents, which in turn synapse on the alpha-motor neurons to cause the extrafusal fibers to contract, extending the tarsus. The reciprocal mechanism through the peroneus tertius causes extension of the stifle.

The disease can be treated by cutting the branches of the tibial nerve to the medial and lateral gastrocnemius muscles.[17] This will permit these cattle to keep up with the other feeder cattle and grow adequately to a marketable age. Affected cattle should not be used for breeding.

This same clinical syndrome has been observed in an Alpine goat.[111]

SPASTIC SYNDROME. Spastic syndrome, crampiness, or stretches occurs most commonly in the Holstein and Guernsey breeds, commencing between 3 and 7 years of age.[109, 110] The signs are most evident in confined cattle and are associated with rising to stand or a sudden movement after a period of relaxation. The signs are characterized by episodes of marked extension of the pelvic limbs. The spasms may be prolonged and may be evident in the extensor muscles of the lumbar vertebrae. These signs disappear when the animal lies down, may be aggravated by stress or excitement, and may progress to prevent an animal from standing. In most cattle the signs are mild, with the episodes lasting from a few seconds to several minutes or occasionally longer. These signs persist for the duration of the animal's life but can slowly progress and be debilitating to the animal. This syndrome is thought to be inherited as a single recessive factor with incomplete penetrance. The pathogenesis is unknown. It may represent a primary disturbance of the myotatic reflex, similar to spastic paresis, or may be a defect in the postural reflex mechanism.

SHIVERING. Shivering is a rare syndrome in horses mostly of the heavy draft breeds that are used regularly for strenuous work.[25] It can occur at any age. The signs of shivering consist of spasms of the muscles in the pelvic region, pelvic limbs, and tail. Mildly affected horses show a tenseness or trembling of the hindlimbs and sudden jerky extensor movements of the tail that cause it to elevate. The signs may occur only when the animal is backed. Upon backing suddenly, more severely affected animals flex a limb and abduct it, holding the hoof in the air. The limb trembles, and the tail is elevated and trembles. In a few seconds the limb and tail stop trembling and return to a normal position. However, the signs will recur if the animal is made to back up again. Forelimb signs are rare and consist of elevation and abduction of the limb with flexion of the carpus. The signs may remain unchanged for long periods or may slowly progress. There is no treatment. Occasionally the signs regress after long periods of rest. No lesions have been described and the cause is unknown.

"SCOTTY CRAMP." Hyperkinetic episodes occur predominantly in Scottish terrier dogs and often are called "Scotty cramp."[31, 83, 84, 86] The syndrome also has been reported in 2 dalmatians.[135] The signs, which are variable with each case, commence between 6 weeks and 18 months of age, and are stimulated by exercise or excitement. The dogs are normal at rest and initially walk normally when they start to exercise. Signs follow continued excitement and exercise. Increased "stiffness" and hyperflexion followed by hyperextension of the limbs are observed. The hyperflexion will appear as a "goose-stepping" gait. Rapid extension of the

pelvic limbs may cause the animal to lose its balance. The back may arch (flex) and occasionally the pelvic limbs become resistant to flexion and act like pillars, so that the dog is unable to walk. The spasms may affect the cervical and facial musculature. Severely affected dogs may curl up and respiration may be impaired. These episodes are not accompanied by any disturbance in consciousness. A short period of rest usually alleviates the signs. These episodes are closely related to environmental, psychological, and health factors that affect the patient.

Treatment with diazepam (Valium), a muscle relaxant that functions in the CNS, stops the signs and continual daily therapy decreases their incidence. Vitamin E has also been found effective in elevating the threshold for eliciting clinical signs. Physiologic studies suggest that the muscle hypertonicity is the result of a spinal cord disturbance and is not due to a muscle disorder. The disturbance may involve the myotatic reflex mechanism. Pharmacologic studies have suggested that this may be a disorder of serotonergic neurons that normally inhibit motor activity.[101] The syndrome is inherited as an autosomal recessive disease.[85]

Tetany-Tremors. Because tetany and tremors represent a neuromuscular disturbance that in some instances may have its genesis in the extrapyramidal system, a differential diagnosis is briefly described here.

TETANY. Tetany is a disorder marked by *intermittent* tonic muscular contractions, as opposed to tetanus, which is a sustained muscular contraction usually manifested in the antigravity muscles. In some instances tetany may accompany the tetanus that occurs in the disease tetanus or in strychnine poisoning. Tetany may accompany other signs of diffuse brain disease, such as encephalitis caused by a variety of agents, polioencephalomalacia from abnormal thiamine metabolism and lead intoxication, and acute organophosphate intoxication.

Transport tetany has been described in lambs shortly after arrival at a feedlot. Ewes and cows, especially late in gestation, are susceptible to a similar syndrome of tetany following prolonged transport.[16, 68, 104] Mortality is high, with death following a period of coma. The pathogenesis is unknown beyond the obvious involvement of severe physical stress, but hypocalcemia and hypomagnesemia often accompany the tetany. A similar syndrome occasionally is seen in horses, especially in lactating mares, that have been feeding on lush pasture and suddenly become severely stressed. Hypocalcemia is a constant finding, and the response to calcium therapy may be dramatic.

Grass tetany occurs in lactating cattle that recently have been exposed to fresh lush pasture, and often is accompanied by hypomagnesemia and hypocalcemia. Calves may show tetany with an electrolyte imbalance associated with profuse diarrhea, or tetany with hypomagnesemia, hypocalcemia, and occasionally diarrhea when fed solely on a whole milk diet. Hypomagnesemic tetany and sudden death have been observed in beef calves nursing on cows that were fed on a natural diet low in magnesium. No other clinical signs were apparent in these calves.[54]

Tetany also may occur in white muscle disease of calves and lambs.

Tetany is found most commonly in dogs in association with parturition, and usually hypocalcemia and occasionally hypoglycemia are present. It also may occur in chronic kidney disease accompanied by uremia, especially when of a congenital nature. These dogs also may be hypocalcemic. Inadvertent removal of both parathyroid glands causes hypocalcemia and tetany. Hypocalcemia associated with hypoparathyroidism may produce generalized seizures, tremor, or tetany. Some of these dogs have a lymphocytic parathyroiditis.[67, 113]

Hereditary Neuraxial Edema. This is an autosomal recessive inherited disease of polled Herefords.[15, 27] These calves are unable to stand at birth and usually lie in lateral recumbency. The stimulus of a sudden touch or loud noise induces a severe contraction (tetanic spasm) of trunk and limb muscles, resulting in extensor rigidity of the limbs and a rigid vertebral column without opisthotonos. Each tetanic episode lasts a few seconds to 2 minutes, and brief apnea usually occurs. These spasms occasionally occur spontaneously. The calves can be placed in a standing position during the tetany, and the rigidly extended limbs and trunk will support them but no movement occurs. They are alert and responsive and have normal cranial nerve function.

These signs usually persist unchanged. Occasionally slight improvement has been observed. At autopsy there may be widespread myelin edema of the terminal portions of central neurons, or no lesions may be evident.

Similar signs of coarse tonic muscle spasms have been observed in inbred horned Hereford calves.[63] In these calves there was widespread edema of grey and white matter and a spongy degeneration of myelin.

TREMORS. Tremors, trembling, repetitive diffuse myoclonus, or shaking also can occur as the only clinical sign or as one of a group of clinical signs associated with a diffuse disturbance of central nervous system function.

Congenital Tremors: Hypomyelinogenesis-Dysmyelinogenesis. Constant tremors present at birth—congenital myoclonia—have been observed in lambs, calves, and pigs with congenital abnormality of myelin formation.[46, 74] The tremors are associated with voluntary movement and worsen with increased motor activity. They nearly disappear in the relaxed, recumbent animal.

The biochemical nature of the myelin defect has been studied most extensively in pigs.[95-97] Two causes have been defined in pigs. In utero viral infection of the developing central nervous system with the swine fever virus or with another unidentified virus can result in a hypomyelinogenesis and congenital tremors.[56, 73] A hereditary basis has also been established for the myelin defect in pigs. In British saddleback pigs it is due to an autosomal recessive gene; in Landrace pigs in England it is due to a sex-linked recessive gene. The disease is observed sporadically in the United States without knowledge of its specific pathogenesis. Some of the pigs, if hand-fed and protected from the sow, will slowly grow out of the clinical problem. Presumably, as the myelin formation develops, the tremor disappears.

The degree of myelin abnormality is not always closely correlated with the degree of myoclonic activity. Ablation studies implicate a spinal cord mechanism in the genesis of the myoclonus.[45] Although dorsal root sectioning will alter the myoclonus, only ventral root sectioning will abolish it.

In Border disease of sheep, a similar tremor syndrome, along with an abnormally hairy fleece, is observed in newborn lambs.[2, 6, 7, 29, 62, 74, 93, 99] These have been referred to as "hairy shaker" lambs. Neurochemical studies have defined a generalized deficiency of myelin lipids with abnormal quantities of esterified cholesterol.[4, 95, 98, 99] There is evidence of an in utero viral infection of the developing nervous system with subsequent interference with myelin formation. An agent closely related to the bovine mucosal disease virus has been implicated.[5, 8, 41, 55, 105] These lambs may sometimes recover spontaneously during the first few weeks.

Hereditary hypomyelinogenesis with significant cerebellar involvement and signs of cerebellar ataxia has been reported in Jersey, Hereford, Shorthorn, and Angus-Shorthorn breeds of cattle.[60, 111, 138] A spastic dysmetric gait is evident if the calf can stand to walk. A head and whole-body rapid tremor occurs and is exacerbated by attempts to move.

In dogs a congenital, diffuse tremor syndrome associated with abnormal myelination has been observed in puppies. These signs may not be evident until the puppies are first observed to walk. It has been reported as an isolated event in a dalmatian puppy whose signs were severe.[52] Autopsy revealed a myelin deficiency with no evidence of abnormal myelin degradation. An autosomal recessive inherited hypomyelinogenesis is proposed for a similar syndrome in chow chows.[123] Pathologic studies revealed a severe myelin deficiency in the central nervous system. Clinical recovery occurs in 8 to 12 months. A sex-linked recessive inheritance is thought to be the cause of a myelin abnormality in male springer spaniels.[42, 144, 145] In Australia a congenital spongy degeneration of the central nervous system myelin in the Australian silky terrier has been associated with severe, coarse tremors associated with voluntary movement.[107] These tremors caused the dog to jerk and bounce violently as it tried to walk. A similar lesion and generalized tremor were reported in 4 of a litter of 9 Samoyed puppies.[78] I have observed the clinical signs in 2 of a litter of 6 miniature schnauzers. Complete recovery occurred by 3 months of age.

Acquired Tremors: Large Animals. Mycotoxins: In animals that graze, a number of diseases of suspected mycotoxic origin have been recognized.[36, 66, 81, 100, 115] Paspalum staggers or dallis grass poisoning affects cattle, sheep, and horses that graze on grasses of the genus *Paspalum,* which support the growth of the fungus *Claviceps paspali.* Tremors, hyperexcitability, and ataxia occur. Similarly, animals grazing on plants or soils infected by various species of *Penicillium* may show a tremor that is exacerbated by forced movement or excitement. This produces a spastic ataxia that may cause them to fall, and convulsions may occur. A number of tremorgenic toxins have been isolated from these fungi. Similar signs have occurred in cattle following the ingestion of feed contaminated with *Aspergillus clavatus.*[64]

Poisonous Plants: Some plants may produce a toxin at various stages of their growth that on ingestion produces tremors, staggering, and ataxia, with occasional falling. Probably the best example of this is phalaris staggers, which is seen commonly in sheep in Australia and New Zealand that graze on Harding grass (*Phalaris tuberosa*).[48, 49] Some sheep collapse suddenly and die after an acute course, whereas others show signs of a chronic neurologic disturbance consisting of tremors, ataxia, and occasionally convulsions. A tryptamine alkaloid is being investigated as the possible toxic substance that may interfere with serotonin metabolism in these animals.[71] Cobalt may be protective for the chronic neurologic form.

An outbreak of possibly similar phalaris staggers has been reported in cattle in California grazing on canary grass (*Phalaris minor*). Only the chronic signs of intoxication were seen, with a spastic (stiff-legged) ataxia accompanied by falling, trembling, difficulty in prehension, and licking movements of the tongue. All signs were exacerbated by excitement. Organophosphate poisoning could not be excluded completely from this report as a cause.

Rye grass staggers may occur in grazing sheep, cattle, and horses.[13, 30] It is less fatal than the type caused by the phalaris grasses. Clinical signs vary in severity, from slight spasms and stiffness of the limbs after running to total tetany, causing immobility and often lateral recumbency. The signs are aggravated by excitement and forced locomotion. Recovery usually follows removal of the animal from the rye grass pasture. The toxic principle is unknown. There is some evidence that toxins of soil fungi are ingested with this grass and account for the clinical signs.[114]

A toxic alcohol, tremetol, present in white snakeroot (*Eupatorium rugosum*) causes severe muscle tremors, salivation, vomiting, and dyspnea, which progress to recumbency, coma, and death.

Acquired Tremors: Small Animals. In dogs, tremors are associated most often with other signs of diffuse brain disease frequently caused by an intoxication. Metaldehyde (snail bait), organophosphates, chlorinated hydrocarbons, and fluoroacetate are the most common causes of these signs. Occasionally, tremors occur with varying degrees of diffuse nonsuppurative encephalitis. Tremors also may accompany the tetany of hypocalcemia and sometimes appear in hypoglycemic animals. Refrigerated cottage cheese infected with *Penicillium crustosum* was the source of the mycotoxin penitrem A that caused diffuse tremors and generalized seizures in a dog.

Shaker Dogs: In young mature dogs often of small breeds (Maltese, West Highland white, beagle), a syndrome occurs of unknown pathogenesis characterized by a sudden onset of constant tremors all over the body, including the head and eyeballs. It is exaggerated by handling, forced locomotion, and exitement. It decreases but may not completely disappear with total relaxation. The dogs are alert and responsive and have no deficiency in cranial nerve function. The tremors may be severe enough to cause an ataxic gait, but strength remains normal. Postural reactions are usually normal. Occasionally one of these dogs convulses.

These signs require a diffuse disturbance of the central nervous system. Their direct association with voluntary movement would tend to implicate the cerebellum, which may be involved but cannot be the sole source of the signs. In the many well-described lesions limited to the cerebellum, there is no description of tremors of this nature. Truncal swaying and a mild head tremor associated with a voluntary movement occur with cerebellar disease, but a severe whole body tremor does not. Similar signs occur in newborn animals with abnormal myelination. This lesion is diffuse throughout the central nervous system, interfering with the normal flow and pattern of impulse transmission. A similar diffuse structural, metabolic, or neurochemical disorder is hypothesized for this disease.

All laboratory studies for blood cytology and chemistry, including electrolytes, are normal. CSF determinations may be normal or reveal a mild increase in lymphocytes. No history or evidence of intoxication can be found. Anticonvulsive therapy with primidone, phenobarbital, diphenylhydantoin, and diazepam has not proved obviously efficacious.

If treated early in the course of the disease many of these dogs will respond in a few days to immunosuppressive levels of corticosteroids. Some dogs may have to be maintained on low dose alternate-day therapy to control the signs. If untreated these signs will persist for the life of many dogs, although the severity may decrease. In a few dogs spontaneous recovery will occur in a few weeks. It is rare for the disease to progress to other signs of brain disease. Autopsy has revealed no lesion in a few dogs, but in most there is a very mild diffuse nonsuppurative encephalomyelitis. The lesion consists of an occasional small lymphoid perivascular cuff in each section of tissue studied. There is no associated parenchymal lesion evident. The choroid plexus may contain a few lymphocytes and plasma cells. Serologic and viral isolation studies have not revealed a cause. The disease has been observed in most parts of the United States[116] and in Australia.[44]

Hypothesis: Because of the high incidence of this disease in the white breeds (Maltese terrier, West Highland white terrier), the presence of lymphocytes around blood vessels in the nervous system and in the cerebrospinal fluid of some patients, and the clinical response to immunosuppressive levels of corticosteroids, the following hypothesis is offered. These white dogs have an acquired immunologic disease that is directed at cells that metabolize tryosine to produce neurotransmitters. This includes one or more of the catecholamine neurotransmitters—dopamine, epinephrine, and norepinephrine. The neurotransmitter abnormality accounts for the diffuse nature of the clinical signs. A possible pathogenetic relationship may be made to a syndrome described in humans. It has been suggested that the Vogt-Koyanagi-Harada syndrome in humans,[142] which probably also occurs in dogs,[143] is an immunologic disease directed aginst melanin-producing cells.[141] This may account for the vitiligo, poliosis, uveitis, and leptomeningitis that occur. Tyrosine is metabolized to produce melanin in melanocytes. The common denominator of the cells affected in this disease may be their origin from neural crest. This hypothesis remains to be proved or refuted as more information is obtained on this unique disease.

REFERENCES

1. Amann, J. F.: The organization of spinal motoneurons and their relationship to corticospinal fibers in the raccoon (*Procyon lotor*). Ph.D. thesis, Cornell University, 1971.
2. Ames, T. R., Robinson, R. A., Johnson, D. W., O'Leary, T. P., and Fahrmann, J. W.: Border disease in a flock of Minnesota sheep. J. Am. Vet. Med. Assoc., *180*:619, 1982.
3. Averill, D. A., Jr.: The nervous system. *In* Holzworth, J. (ed.): Diseases of the Cat. Philadelphia, W. B. Saunders Company, in preparation.
4. Barlow, R. M., and Dickinson, A. G.: On the pathology and histochemistry of the central nervous system in border disease of sheep. Res. Vet. Sci., *6*:230, 1965.
5. Barlow, R. M., Rennie, J. C., Gardiner, A. C., and Vantsis, J. T.: Infection of pregnant sheep with the NADL strain of bovine virus diarrhea virus and their subsequent challenge with Border disease IIB pool. J. Comp. Pathol., *90*:67, 1980.
6. Barlow, R. M., and Storey, I. J.: Myelination of the ovine CNS with special reference to Border disease. I. Qualitative aspects. II. Quantitative aspects. Neuropathol. Appl. Neurobiol., *3*:237, 255, 1977.
7. Barlow, R. M., Vantsis, J. T., Gardner, A. C., and Linklater, K. A.: The definition of Border disease: Problems for the diagnostician. Vet. Rec. *104*:334, 1979.
8. Barlow, R. M., Vantsis, J. T., Gardiner, A. C., Rennie, J. C., Herring, J. A., and Scott, F. M. M.: Mechanisms of natural transmission of Border disease. J. Comp. Pathol., *90*:57, 1980.
9. Barnes, C. D., and Shadt, J. C.: Release of function in the spinal cord. Prog. Neurobiol., *12*:1, 1979.

10. Barone, R.: Les voies descendantes dans le névraxe des Equidés. Bull. Acad. Vet. Fr., 39:137, 1966.
11. Belmusto, L., Waldring, S., and Owens, G.: Localization and patterns of potentials of the respiratory pathway in the cervical spinal cord in the dog. J. Neurosurg., 22:277, 1965.
12. Beroza, G. A.: Tetanus in the horse. J. Am. Vet. Med. Assoc., 177:1152, 1980.
13. Berry, P. H., Howell, J. McC., Cook, R. D., Richards, R. B., and Peet, R. L.: Central nervous system changes in sheep and cattle affected with natural or experimental annual rye grass toxicity. Aust. Vet. J., 56:402, 1980.
14. Bijleveld, K., and Hartman, W.: Electromyographic studies in calves with spastic paresis. Tijdschr. Diergeneesk., 101:805, 1976.
15. Blood, D. C., and Gay, C. C.: Hereditary neuraxial edema of calves. Aust. Vet. J., 47:520, 1971.
16. Blood, D. C., and Henderson, J. A.: Veterinary Medicine. 4th ed. Baltimore, Williams & Wilkins, 1974.
17. Bouckaert, J. H., and DeMoor, A.: Treatment of spastic paralysis in cattle: Improved denervation technique of gastrocnemius muscle and postoperative course. Vet. Rec., 79:226, 1966.
18. Bradley, R., and Wijeratne, W. V. S.: A locomotor disorder clinically similar to spastic paresis in an adult Friesian bull. Vet. Pathol., 17:305, 1980.
19. Breazile, J. E., Blaugh, B. S., and Nail, N.: Experimental study of canine distemper myoclonus. Am. J. Vet. Res., 27:1375, 1966.
20. Breazile, J. E., Jennings, D. P., and Swafford, B. C.: Conduction velocities in the corticospinal tract of the horse. Exp. Neurol., 17:357, 1967.
21. Breazile, J. E., Swafford, B. C., and Biles, A. R.: Motor cortex of the horse. Am. J. Vet. Res., 27:1605, 1966.
22. Breazile, J. E., Swafford, B. C., and Thompson, W. D.: Study of the motor cortex of the domestic pig. Am. J. Vet. Res., 27:1369, 1966.
23. Breazile, J. E., and Thompson, W. D.: Motor cortex of the dog. Am. J. Vet. Res., 28:1483, 1967.
24. Buxton, D. F., and Goodman, D. C.: Motor function and the corticospinal tracts in the dog and raccoon. J. Comp. Neurol., 129:341, 1967.
25. Catcott, E. J., and Smithcors, J. F.: Equine Medicine and Surgery. 2nd ed. Wheaton, Ill., American Veterinary Publications, Inc., 1972.
26. Chambers, W. W., and Liu, C. N.: Corticospinal tract in the cat. J. Comp. Neurol., 108:23, 1957.
27. Cho, D. Y., and Leipold, H. W.: Hereditary neuraxial edema in polled Hereford calves. Pathol. Res. Pract., 163:158, 1978.
28. Cioni, M., Perciavalle, V., Santangelo, F., Sapienza, S., and Urbano, A.: Motor responses to microstimulation of the medullary pyramidal tract in the cat. Exp. Neurol., 61:664, 1978.
29. Clarke, G. L., and Osburn, B. I.: Transmissible congenital demyelinating encephalopathy of lambs. Vet. Pathol., 15:68, 1978.
30. Clegg, F. G., and Watson, W. A.: Rye grass staggers in sheep. Vet. Rec., 72:731, 1960.
31. Clemmons, R. M., Peters, R. I., and Meyers, K. M.: Scotty cramp: A review of cause, characteristics, diagnosis and treatment. Compend. Contin. Ed., 2:385, 1980.
32. Cohen, F. L.: Effects of various lesions on crossed and uncrossed descending inspiratory pathways in the cervical spinal cord of the cat. J. Neurosurg., 39:589, 1973.
33. Cooper, I. S., Samra, K., and Bermann, L.: The thalamic lesion which abolishes tremor and rigidity of Parkinsonism. A radiologic-clinico-anatomic correlation study. J. Neurol. Sci., 8:69, 1969.
34. Cordy, D. R.: Nigropallidal encephalomalacia in horses associated with ingestion of yellow star thistle. J. Neuropathol. Exp. Neurol., 13:330, 1954.
35. Cordy, D. R., Richards, W. P. C., and Stormont, C.: Hereditary neuraxial edema in Hereford calves. Pathol. Vet., 6:487, 1969.
36. Cysewski, S. J.: Paspalum staggers and tremergen intoxication in animals. J. Am. Vet. Med. Assoc., 163:1291, 1973.
37. de Lahunta, A., and Averill, D. R., Jr.: Hereditary cerebellar cortical and extrapyramidal nuclear abiotrophy in Kerry Blue Terriers. J. Am. Vet. Med. Assoc., 168:1119, 1976.
38. DeLey, G., and DeMoor, A.: Bovine spastic paralysis: Results of surgical desafferentation of the gastrocnemius muscle by means of spinal dorsal root resection. Am. J. Vet. Res., 38:1899, 1977.
39. DeLey, G., and DeMoor, A.: Bovine spastic paralysis: Results of selective gamma efferent suppression with dilute procaine. Vet. Sci. Comm., 3:289, 1979/1980.
40. Denny-Brown, D., and Yanagisawa, N.: The role of the basal ganglia in the initiation of movement. In Yahr, M. D. (ed.): Basal Ganglia. New York, Raven Press, 1976.
41. Dickinson, A. G., and Barlow, R. M.: The demonstration of the transmissibility of Border disease of sheep. Vet. Rec., 81:114, 1967.
42. Duncan, I.: Personal communication, 1982.
43. English, P. B., and Carlisle, C. H.: Tetanus in the dog. Aust. Vet. J., 37:62, 1961.
44. Farrow, B.: Personal communication, 1982.
45. Fletcher, T. F.: Ablation and histopathologic studies on myoclonia congenita in swine. Am. J. Vet. Res., 29:2255, 1968.
46. Foulkes, J. A.: Myelin and dysmyelination in domestic animals. Vet. Bull., 44:441, 1974.
47. Fowler, M. E.: Nigropallidal encephalomalacia in the horse. J. Am. Vet. Med. Assoc., 147:607, 1965.
48. Gallagher, C. H., Koch, J. H., and Hoffman, H.: Diseases of sheep due to ingestion of Phalaris tuberosa. Aust. Vet. J., 42:279, 1966.
49. Gallagher, C. H., Koch, J. H., Moore, R. M., and Steel, J. D.: Toxicity of Phalaris tuberosa for sheep. Nature, 204:542, 1964.
50. Ganes, T., Kaada, B. R., and Nyberg-Hansen, R.: Failure to produce postural tremor by mesencephalic lesions in cats. J. Comp. Neurol., 128:127, 1969.
51. Greene, C. E.: Tetanus. In Kirk, R. W. (ed.): Current Veterinary Therapy VIII: Small Animal Practice. Philadelphia, W. B. Saunders Co., 1983.
52. Greene, C. E., Vandevelde, M., and Hoff, E. J.: Cerebrospinal hypomyelinogenesis in a dog. J. Am. Vet. Med. Assoc., 171:534, 1977.
53. Groos, W. P., Ewing, L. K., Carter, C. M., and Coulter, J. D.: Organization of corticospinal neurons in the cat. Brain Res., 143:393, 1978.
54. Haggard, D. L., Whitehair, C. K., and Langham, R. F.: Tetany associated with magnesium defi-

ciency in suckling beef calves. J. Am. Vet. Med. Assoc., *172*:495, 1978.

55. Hamilton, A. F., and Timoney, P. J.: Bovine virus diarrhea-mucosal disease virus and Border disease. Res. Vet. Sci., *15*:265, 1973.

56. Harding, J. D. J., Done, J. T., Harbourne, J. F., Randall, C. J., and Gilbert, F. R.: Congenital tremor type A III in pigs and hereditary sex-linked cerebrospinal hypomyelinogenesis. Vet. Rec., *92*:527, 1973.

57. Hoehn, M. M., and Cherington, M.: Spinal myoclonus. Neurology, *27*:942, 1977.

58. Hongo, T., Jankowska, E., and Lundberg, A.: The rubrospinal tract. 1. Effects on alpha-motor neurons innervating hind limb muscles in cat. Exp. Brain Res., *7*:334, 1969.

59. Hukuda, S., Jameson, H. D., and Wilson, C. B.: Experimental cervical myelopathy. III. The canine corticospinal tract. Anatomy and function. Surg. Neurol., *1*:107, 1973.

60. Hulland, T. J.: Cerebellar ataxia in calves. Can. J. Comp. Med. Vet. Sci., *21*:72, 1957.

61. Ingram, W. R., and Ranson, S. W.: Effects of lesions in the red nuclei in cats. Arch. Neurol. Psychiatry, *28*:483, 1932.

62. Innes, J. R. M., and Saunders, L. Z.: Comparative Neuropathology. New York, Academic Press, 1962.

63. Jolly, R. D.: Congenital brain edema of Hereford calves. J. Pathol., *114*:199, 1974.

64. Kellerman, T. S., Pienaar, J. G., Van der Westhuizen, G. C. A., Anderson, L. A. P., and Naude, T. W.: A highly fatal tremorgenic mycotoxicosis of cattle caused by *Aspergillus clavatus*. Onderstepoort J. Vet. Res., *43*:147, 1976.

65. Killingsworth, C., Chiapella, A., Veralli, P., and de Lahunta, A.: Feline tetanus. J. Am. Anim. Hosp. Assoc., *13*:209, 1977.

66. Koehne, G.: Neurologic disease of fungal origin in three herds of cattle. J. Am. Vet. Med. Assoc., *179*:480, 1981.

67. Kornegay, J. N., Greene, C. E., Martin, C., Gorgacz, E. J., and Melcon, D. K.: Idiopathic hypocalcemia in four dogs. J. Am. Anim. Hosp. Assoc., *16*:723, 1980.

68. Kronfeld, D. S., and Hammel, E. P.: Differential diagnosis, treatment, and prevention of tetany in cattle. Am. Assoc. Bovine Pract. Proc., 1974.

69. Lassek, A. M., Dowd, L. W., and Weil, A.: The quantitative distribution of the pyramidal tract in the dog. J. Comp. Neurol., *51*:153, 1930.

70. Latshaw, W. K.: A model for the neural control of locomotion. J. Am. Anim. Hosp. Assoc., *10*:598, 1974.

71. Lee, H. J., Kuchel, R. E., Good, B. F., and Trowbridge, R. F.: The etiology of phalaris staggers in sheep. IV. The site of preventive action and its specificity to cobalt. Aust. J. Agri. Res., *8*:502, 1957.

72. Magoun, H. N., and Rhines, R.: Spasticity, the Stretch Reflex, and Extrapyramidal Systems. Springfield, Ill., Charles C Thomas, 1948.

73. Mare, C. J., and Kluge, J. P.: Pseudorabies virus and myoclonia congenita in pigs. J. Am. Vet. Med. Assoc., *164*:309, 1974.

74. Markson, L. M., Terlicki, S., Shand, A., Sellers, K. C., and Woods, A. J.: Hypomyelinogenesis congenita in sheep. Vet. Rec., *71*:269, 1959.

75. Marsden, C. D.: The development of pigmentation and enzyme activity in the nucleus substantiae nigrae of the cat. J. Anat. (Lond.), *99*:175, 1965.

76. Mason, J. H.: Tetanus in the dog and cat. J. S. Africa Vet. Med. Assoc., *35*:209, 1964.

77. Mason, M. M.: Rhythmic myoclonic convulsions in dogs. Vet. Rec., *58*:247, 1946.

78. Mason, R. W., Hartley, W. J., and Randall, M.: Spongiform degeneration of the white matter in a Samoyed pup. Aust. Vet. Pract., *9*:11, 1979.

79. Matsushita, M., Ikeda, M., and Hosoya, Y.: The location of spinal neurons with long descending axons (long descending propriospinal tract neurons) in the cat: A study with the horseradish peroxidase technique. J. Comp. Neurol., *184*:63, 1979.

80. McGovern, V. J., Steel, J. D., Wyke, B. D., and Dobson, M. E.: Canine encephalitis causing a syndrome characterized by tremor. Aust. J. Exp. Biol. Med. Sci., *28*:433, 1950.

81. Mendel, V. E., Crenshaw, D. L., Baker, N. F., and Muniz, R.: Staggers in pastured cattle. J. Am. Vet. Med. Assoc., *154*:769, 1969.

82. Mettler, F. A., and Stern, G. M.: Observations on the toxic effects of yellow star thistle. J. Neuropathol. Exp. Neurol., *22*:164, 1963.

83. Meyers, K. M., and Clemmons, R. C.: Scotty cramp. *In* Kirk, R. W. (ed.): Current Veterinary Therapy VIII: Small Animal Practice. Philadelphia, W. B. Saunders Co., 1983.

84. Meyers, K. M., Dickson, W. M., and Schaub, R. G.: Serotonin involvement in a motor disorder of Scottish terrier dogs. Life Sci., *13*:1261, 1973.

85. Meyers, K. M., Padgett, G. A., and Dickson, W. M.: The genetic basis of a kinetic disorder of Scottish terrier dogs. J. Hered., *61*:189, 1970.

86. Meyers, K. M., Lund, J. E., Padgett, G., and Dickson, W. M.: Hyperkinetic episodes in Scottish terrier dogs. J. Am. Vet. Med. Assoc., *155*:129, 1969.

87. Muylle, E., Oyaert, W., Ooms, L., and Decraemere, H.: Treatment of tetanus in the horse by injections of tetanus antitoxin into the subarachnoid space. J. Am. Vet. Med. Assoc., *167*:47, 1975.

89. Nyberg-Hansen, R.: Sites and mode of termination of reticulospinal fibers in the cat. J. Comp. Neurol., *124*:71, 1965.

90. Nyberg-Hansen, R., and Brodal, A.: Sites of termination of corticospinal fibers in the cat. An experimental study with silver impregnation methods. J. Comp. Neurol., *120*:369, 1963.

91. O'Brien, D. P.: Lead toxicity in a dog. J. Am. Anim. Hosp. Assoc., *17*:845, 1981.

92. Olmstead, C. E., Villablanca, J. R., Marcus, R. J., and Avery, D. L.: Effects of caudate nuclei on frontal cortical ablations in cats. IV. Bar pressing, maze learning, and performance. Exp. Neurol., *53*:670, 1976.

93. Osborne, B. I., Clarke, G. L., Stewart, W. C., and Sawyer, M.: Border disease-like syndrome in lambs: Antibodies to hog cholera and bovine viral diarrhea viruses. J. Am. Vet. Med. Assoc., *163*:1165, 1973.

94. Patterson, D. S. P., and Done, J. T.: Neurochemistry as a diagnostic aid in the congenital tremor syndrome of piglets. Br. Vet. J., *133*:11, 1977.

95. Patterson, D. S. P., and Sineasey, D.: Lipid hexose:phosphorus ratio as an aid to the diagnosis of

congenital myelin defects in lambs and piglets. Acta Neuropathol., *15*:318, 1970.

96. Patterson, D. S. P., Sweasey, D., Brush, P. J., and Harding, J. D. J.: Neurochemistry of the spinal cord in British Saddleback Piglets affected with congenital tremor, type A-IV, a second form of hereditary cerebrospinal hypomyelinogenesis. J. Neurochem., *21*:397, 1973.

97. Patterson, D. S. P., Sweasey, D., and Harding, J. D. J.: Lipid deficiency in the central nervous system of Landrace piglets affected with congenital tremor A-III, a form of cerebrospinal hypomyelinogenesis. J. Neurochem., *19*:2797, 1972.

98. Patterson, D. S. P., Sweasey, D., and Herbert, C. N.: Changes occurring in the chemical composition of the CNS during fetal and postnatal development of the sheep. J. Neurochem., *18*:2027, 1971.

99. Patterson, D. S. P., Terlecki, S., Done, J. T., Sweasey, D., and Herbert, C. N.: Neurochemistry of the spinal cord in experimental Border disease (hypomyelinogenesis congenita) of lambs. J. Neurochem., *18*:883, 1971.

100. Penny, R. H. C., O'Sullivan, B. M., Mantle, P. G., and Shaw, B. I.: Clinical studies of tremorgenic mycotoxicoses in sheep. Vet. Rec., *105*:392, 1979.

101. Peters, R. I., Jr., and Meyers, K. M.: Precursor regulation of serotonergic neuronal function in Scottish terrier dogs. J. Neurochem., *29*:753, 1977.

102. Petras, J. M.: Afferent fibers to the spinal cord. The terminal distribution of dorsal root and encephalospinal axons. Med. Serv. J. Can., *22*:668, 1966.

103. Petras, J. M.: Cortical, tectal, and tegmental fiber connections in the spinal cord of the cat. Brain Res., *6*:275, 1967.

104. Pierson, R. E., and Jensen, R.: Transport tetany of feedlot lambs. J. Am. Vet. Med. Assoc., *166*:260, 1975.

105. Plant, J. W., Gard, G. P., and Acland, H. M.: A mucosal disease virus infection of the pregnant ewe as a cause of a Border disease-like condition. Aust. Vet. J., *52*:247, 1976.

106. Pompeiano, O., and Brodal, A.: Experimental demonstration of a somatotopical origin of rubrospinal fibers in the cat. J. Comp. Neurol., *108*:225, 1957.

107. Richards, R. B., and Kakulas, B. A.: Spongiform leucoencephalopathy associated with congenital myoclonia syndrome in the dog. J. Comp. Pathol., *88*:317, 1978.

108. Rinvick, E., and Walberg, F.: Demonstration of a somatotopically arranged corticorubral projection in the cat: An experimental study with silver methods. J. Comp. Neurol., *120*:393, 1963.

109. Roberts, S. J.: A spastic syndrome in cattle. Cornell Vet., *43*:380, 1953.

110. Roberts, S. J.: Hereditary spastic disease affecting cattle in New York State. Cornell Vet., *55*:637, 1965.

111. Saunders, L. Z., Sweet, J. D., Martin, S. M., Fox, F. H., and Fincher, M. G.: Hereditary congenital ataxia in Jersey calves. Cornell Vet., *42*:559, 1952.

112. Schwab, M. E., and Thornen, H.: Electron microscopic evidence for a transsynaptic migration of tetanus toxin in spinal cord motoneurons: An autoradiographic and morphometric study. Brain Res., *105*:213, 1976.

113. Sherding, R. G., Meuten, D. J., Chew, D. J., Knaack, K. E., and Houpt, K. H.: Primary hypoparathyroidism in the dog. J. Am. Vet. Med. Assoc., *176*:440, 1980.

114. Shreeve, B. J., Patterson, D. S. P., Roberts, B. A., MacDonald, S. M., and Wood, E. N.: Isolation of potentially tremorgenic fungi from pasture associated with a condition resembling rye grass staggers. Vet. Rec., *103*:209, 1978.

115. Shreeve, B. J., Patterson, D. S. P., Roberts, B. A., and MacDonald, S. W.: The occurrence of soil-borne tremorgenic fungi in England and Wales. Vet. Rec., *104*:509, 1979.

116. Smith, L.: Personal communication, 1982.

117. Spring-Mills, E., and Elias, J. J.: Tetanus toxin: Direct evidence for retrograde intraaxonal transport. Science, *188*:945, 1975.

118. Steinberg, S. A.: Personal communication, 1982.

119. Turbes, C.: Studies on involuntary movements at rest in the dog. Anat. Rec., *118*:362, 1954.

120. Turbes, C. C., Abreau, B., and Richards, A.: Experimental studies of involuntary motor activity. Neurology, *13*:351, 1963.

121. Udall, D. H.: The Practice of Veterinary Medicine. Ithaca, N.Y., 1954.

122. Usunoff, K. G., Hassler, R., Romansky, K., and Usunova, R. P.: The nigrostriatal projection in the cat. Part 1. Silver impregnation study. J. Neurol. Sci., *28*:265, 1976.

123. Vandevelde, M., Braund, K. G., Walker, T. L., and Kornegay, J. N.: Dysmyelination of the central nervous system in the Chow Chow dog. Acta Neuropathol., *42*:211, 1978.

124. Verhaart, W. J. C.: The pyramidal tract—its structure and function in man and animals. World Neurol., *3*:43, 1962.

125. Villablanca, J. R., and Marcus, J. R.: The basal ganglia: A brief review and interpretation. Acta Neurol. Latinoam., *21*:157, 1975.

126. Villablanca, J. R., Marcus, R. J., and Olmstead, C. E.: Effects of caudate nuclei on frontal cortical ablations in cats 1. Neurology and gross behavior. Exp. Neurol., *52*:389, 1976.

127. Villablanca, J. R., Marcus, R. J., and Olmstead, C. E.: Effects of caudate nuclei on frontal cortical ablations in cats. II. Sleep-wakefulness, EEG, and motor activity. Exp. Neurol., *53*:31, 1976.

128. Villablanca, J. R., Marcus, R. J., Olmstead, C. E., and Avery, D. L.: Effects of caudate nuclei on frontal cortical ablations in cats. III. Recovery of limb placing reactions, including observations in hemispherectomized animals. Exp. Neurol., *53*:289, 1976.

129. Villablanca, J. R., Olmstead, C. E., Levine, M. S., and Marcus, R. J.: Effects of caudate nuclei on frontal cortical ablations in kittens: Neurology and gross behavior. Exp. Neurol., *61*:615, 1978.

130. Webster, R. A.: Centrally acting muscle relaxants in tetanus. Br. J. Pharmacol., *17*:507, 1961.

131. Webster, K. E.: The cortico-striatal projection in the cat. J. Anat., *99*:329, 1965.

132. Weinstein, L.: Tetanus—current concepts. N. Engl. J. Med., *289*:1293, 1973.

133. Whittier, J. R.: Flexor spasm syndrome in the carnivore. Am. J. Vet. Res., *17*:720, 1956.

134. Wilson, V. J.: Inhibition in the central nervous system. Sci. Am., *214*:102, 1966.

135. Woods, C. B.: Hyperkinetic episodes in two Dalmatian dogs. J. Am. Anim. Hosp. Assoc., *13*:255, 1977.

136. Woosley, C. N.: Postural relations of the frontal and motor cortex of the dog. Brain, *56*:353, 1933.

137. Young, S., Brown, W. W., and Klinger, H.: Nigro-

pallidal encephalomalacia in horses caused by ingestion of weeds of the genus *Centaurea*. J. Am. Vet. Med. Assoc., *157*:1602, 1970.

138. Young, S.: Hypomyelinogenesis congenita (cerebellar ataxia) in Angus-Shorthorn calves. Cornell Vet., *52*:84, 1962.

139. Young, R. R., and Delwaide, P. J.: Spasticity. N. Engl. J. Med., *304*:28, 1981.

140. Zontine, W. J., and Uno, T.: Tetanus in a dog. VM/SAC, *63*:341, 1968.

141. Snyder, D. A., and Tessler, H. H.: Vogt-Koyanagi-Harada syndrome. Am. J. Ophthalmol., *90*:69, 1980.

142. Lubin, J. R., Loewenstein, J. I., and Frederick, A. R., Jr.: Vogt-Koyanagi-Harada syndrome with focal neurologic signs. Am. J. Ophthalmol., *91*:332, 1981.

143. Baussanich, M. N., Rootman, J., and Dolman, C. L.: Granulomatous panuveitis and dermal depigmentation in dogs. J. Am. Anim. Hosp. Assoc., *18*:131, 1982.

144. Griffiths, I. R., Duncan, I. D., McCulloch, M., and Harvey, M. J. A.: Shaking pups: A disorder of central myelination in the spaniel dog. Part 1. Clinical, genetic and light microscopical observations. J. Neurol. Sci., *50*:423, 1981.

145. Griffiths, I. R., Duncan, I. D., and McCulloch, M.: Shaking pups: A disorder of central myelination in the spaniel dog. II. Ultrastructural observations on the white matter of the cervical spinal cord. J. Neurocytol., *10*:847, 1981.

8 GENERAL PROPRIOCEPTION SYSTEM—GP

SENSORY SYSTEMS

Sensory systems are characterized by a peripheral afferent neuron with a dendritic zone (modified in many neurons to form a receptor organ), an axon that courses into the grey matter of the central nervous system, a cell body in a ganglion of the peripheral nervous system, and centrally located relay nuclei and tracts primarily passing to a specific thalamic projection nucleus, which relays to a sensory area of the cerebral cortex. Each type of sensation is known as a modality, a form of energy converted by the receptor organ into a neuronal impulse. These include touch, temperature, movement, light, sound, chemicals, and pressure, and they inform the nervous system of the features of the external and internal environments of the body. In some instances there is a specific neuroanatomic structural pathway for certain modalities. Most receptor organs have a low threshold for a certain modality, but still can be stimulated by other modalities. This form of energy to which a receptor organ is most sensitive is referred to as the adequate stimulus. Anatomically, there are encapsulated and nonencapsulated receptor organs. The neuronal terminal of the encapsulated receptor (dendritic zone) is associated with a well-developed connective tissue capsule, of which there are many varieties. In the nonencapsulated forms there is no connective tissue modification of the dendritic zone. Although the connective tissue modification of the encapsulated endings may provide the structural features necessary for that receptor to be sensitive to one specific modality or energy form, the sensitivity is not limited necessarily to that one modality. Several forms of energy may excite that receptor. Even without obvious connective tissue modification, the nonencapsulated receptors exhibit low thresholds of sensitivity to one specific modality. The histologic characteristics of the receptor do not necessarily restrict the receptor to sensitivity to one specific modality. Nevertheless, they are classified as thermoreceptors, mechanoreceptors, chemoreceptors, and photoreceptors, based on their adequate stimulus.

Receptors have been classified according to their location in the body. Exteroceptors are located on the surface of the body, and are sensitive to changes in the external environment affecting the body surface. These include general somatic afferent (GSA) neurons for touch, temperature, pressure, and noxious stimuli, and special somatic afferent (SSA) neurons for light and sound. Proprioceptors are sensitive to movement, and are located in the internal mass of the body in muscles, tendons, and joints (general proprioception—GP), and in the labyrinth of the inner ear (special proprioception—SP). Interoceptors are located within the body viscera, and are sensitive to changes in the internal environment. These include general visceral afferent (GVA) neurons for body temperature, blood pressure, gas concentration, pressure and movement in viscera, and special visceral afferent (SVA) neurons for chemical energy (smell and taste).

The sensation of pain is a cerebral interpretation, a subjective response to the stimulation of various receptors called nociceptors. This group of receptors is nonselective in the form of energy that elicits its maximal response, but the stimulus threshold for these modalities is high. The intensity of stimulation necessary to evoke an impulse from these receptors is at a level that is potentially destructive to tissue; for example, high-intensity excitation by mechanical, electrical, thermal, or chemical stimuli.

GENERAL PROPRIOCEPTION—GP

General proprioceptive neurons constitute a sensory system to detect the state of position or movement in muscles, tendons, and joints. Two basic pathways will be described for this system. One involves the pathway for segmental reflex activity and for transmitting proprioceptive information to the cerebellum. The other involves the transmission of proprioceptive information to the sensory somesthetic cerebral cortex. These pathways will be considered separately for spinal nerves and cranial nerves.

SPINAL NERVES

The general proprioceptive (GP) afferent has its dendritic zone (receptor organ) in a muscle, a tendon, or a joint (Fig. 8–2). The Ia afferent in neuromuscular spindles and the Golgi tendon organs are examples of such receptors. The axons course proximally in peripheral nerves to the spinal nerve and through the spinal ganglion associated with the dorsal root of that spinal nerve. The cell body of the GP afferent is in the segmental spinal ganglion. The axon continues in the dorsal root and enters the spinal cord along the dorsolateral sulcus.

Proprioceptive Pathway for Reflex Activity and Cerebellar Transmission[26, 27, 32, 38]

REFLEX. The axons enter the dorsal grey column of the spinal cord. Some axons (Ia) synapse directly on alpha motor neurons (general somatic efferent) in the ventral grey column to complete a reflex arc. Others (Golgi tendon organ) indirectly influence an alpha motor neuron and complete the reflex arc by synapsing on an interneuron. Activity of some interneurons influences alpha motor neurons in other segments of the spinal cord by passing cranial and caudal in the fasciculus proprius of the lateral funiculus, which is the white matter immediately adjacent to the grey matter. This also is referred to as the propriospinal fiber system, which connects adjoining and distant segments of the spinal cord. This provides a means of interrelating neural activity within the spinal cord.

CEREBELLAR PATHWAY: FROM TRUNK AND PELVIC LIMBS (Figs. 8–1 to 8–3)

Dorsal Spinocerebellar Tract. The GP axon enters the dorsal grey column and synapses on a cell body medially at the base of the dorsal grey column. This is in the nucleus of the dorsal spinocerebellar tract (nucleus thoracicus, Clarke's nucleus).[10, 32] The axon of this cell body enters the lateral funiculus of the same side and passes cranially on the surface of the dorsal portion of the lateral funiculus in the dorsal spinocerebellar tract. Here it is lateral to the lateral corticospinal and rubrospinal tracts (Fig. 8–2). The nucleus thoracicus extends from approximately C8 to L4 in the cat. Pelvic limb GP afferents must course cranially to the cranial lumbar segments to synapse in this nucleus. The dorsal spinocerebellar tract passes cranially through the entire spinal cord and joins the caudal cerebellar peduncle by way of the superficial arcuate fibers on the

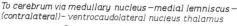

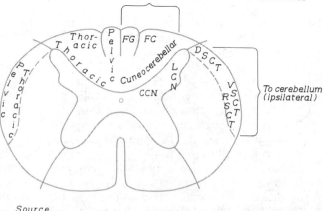

Figure 8–1. General proprioceptive pathways at the second cervical segment.

CCN: Central Cervical Nucleus
FC: Fasciculus Cuneatus
LCN: Lateral Cervical Nucleus
DSCT: Dorsal Spinocerebellar Tract
VSCT: Ventral Spinocerebellar Tract
RSCT: Rostral Spinocerebellar Tract

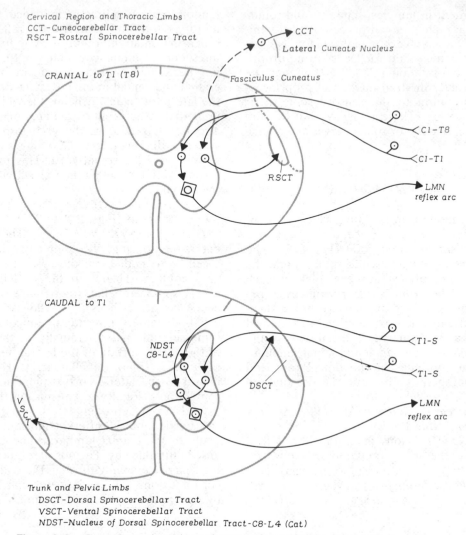

Figure 8–2. General proprioceptive pathways to the cerebellum–spinocerebellar pathways.

surface of the medulla (Plates 3–5).[9, 17] It is distributed primarily to the cerebellar cortex of the vermal and paravermal lobules.

Ventral Spinocerebellar Tract. The GP axon enters the dorsal grey column and synapses on cell bodies near its base laterally.[11, 19] These form a continuous column from the cranial thoracic segments caudally throughout the lumbar and sacral segments. Most axons of these cell bodies cross to the opposite lateral funiculus by way of the ventral white commissure. In the contralateral lateral funiculus they form the ventral spinocerebellar tract on the surface of the lateral funiculus ventral to the dorsal spinocerebellar tract.

This tract courses cranially throughout the spinal cord, through the medulla and pons on the lateral side to reach the rostral cerebellar

peduncle, which it joins, and then courses caudally into the cerebellum, mostly to the vermal and paravermal lobules of the contralateral side.[9, 17] Many of these ventral spinocerebellar tract axons recross in the cerebellum before terminating, thus influencing the cerebellum on the same side as the stimulus to the cell bodies of these axons.

CEREBELLAR PATHWAY: FROM CERVICAL REGION AND THORACIC LIMBS (FIGS. 8–1 TO 8–3)

Cuneocerebellar Pathway. This thoracic limb pathway is homologous to the dorsal spinocerebellar tract from the pelvic limbs.[18, 30] The GP dorsal root axons pass dorsal to the dorsal grey column and enter the lateral portion of the dorsal funiculus, which is the fasciculus cuneatus. They pass cranially in the fasciculus cuneatus to the caudal medulla, where they terminate in the lateral cuneate nucleus (Fig. 8–2; Plates 3 and 4). This nucleus is located dorsally in the medulla, dorsolateral to the parasympathetic nucleus of the vagus. It is ventromedial to the caudal cerebellar peduncle, rostral to the obex and medial cuneate nucleus, and caudal to the spinal vestibular nucleus. It contains afferents from the dorsal roots of spinal nerves C1 to T8.

Axons of the cell bodies in the lateral cuneate nucleus enter the adjacent caudal cerebellar peduncle and pass into the cerebellum.

Cranial (Rostral) Spinocerebellar Tract. This thoracic limb pathway is homologous to the ventral spinocerebellar tract from the trunk and pelvic limbs. The GP dorsal root axons enter the dorsal grey column and synapse on cell bodies near its base in the centrobasilar nucleus.[32] The axons of these cell bodies enter the ipsilateral lateral funiculus and course cranially medial and ventral to the ventral spinocerebellar tract (Fig. 8–2). They enter the cerebellum through both the caudal and rostral cerebellar peduncles. *(only read dif)*

Cervicospinocerebellar Pathway.[8, 15, 25] The central cervical nucleus is located in the intermediate grey column of the first four cervical spinal cord segments. It receives direct innervation from cervical spinal ganglion cells that are thought to be mostly concerned with general proprioception from the neck. This nu-

cleus predominantly projects through the contralateral caudal cerebellar peduncle to the cerebellum. These neurons terminate in the vermis of the rostral lobe of the cerebellum. Therefore, this central cervical nucleus serves as a direct link between neck afferents and the cerebellum via a crossed cervicospinocerebellar pathway.

In summary, these spinocerebellar pathways provide the cerebellum, predominantly ipsilaterally, with information about where the trunk and limbs are in space, both during movement and during a fixed posture. This information aids the cerebellum in its role of regulating posture, tone, locomotion, and equilibrium.[32]

Proprioceptive Pathway to the Somesthetic Cortex for Conscious Perception (Figs. 8–1, 8–4, 8–6)

Fasciculus Gracilis and Fasciculus Cuneatus. The GP axons are in the dorsal roots of all the spinal nerves. Each enters the spinal cord at the dorsolateral sulcus, passes dorsal to the dorsal grey column, and enters the dorsal funiculus and courses cranially. GP *(w/o synapse)* axons from the pelvic limbs and caudal trunk (caudal to T6) course in the medial portion of the dorsal funiculus in the fasciculus gracilis (Fig. 8–4).[13] Cranial to T6 the GP axons are situated more laterally in the fasciculus cuneatus. The dorsal funiculus is organized somatotopically so that the GP axons from the more caudal levels are situated medially in the dorsal

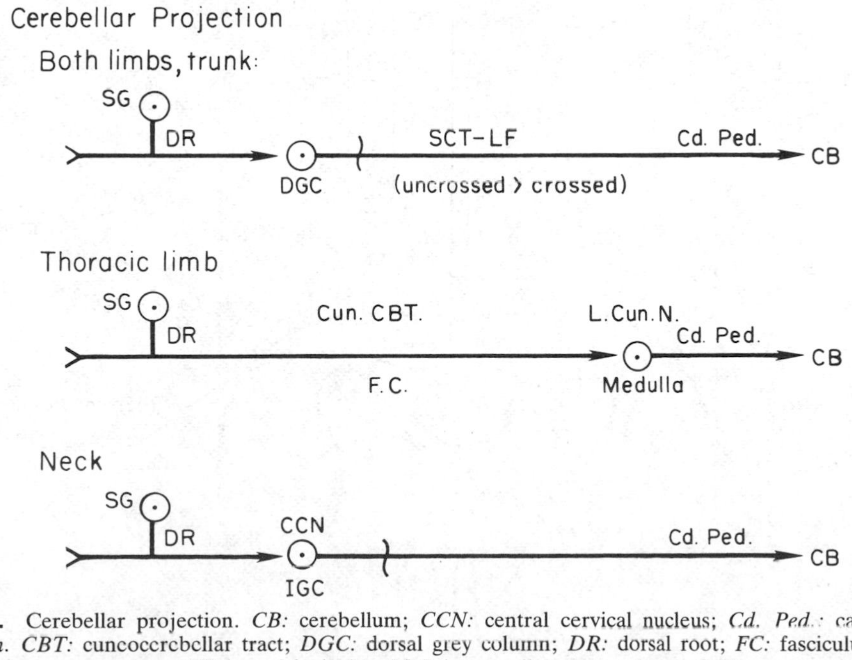

Cerebellar Projection

Both limbs, trunk:

Thoracic limb

Neck

Figure 8–3. Cerebellar projection. *CB:* cerebellum; *CCN:* central cervical nucleus; *Cd. Ped.:* caudal cerebellar peduncle; *Cun. CBT:* cuneocerebellar tract; *DGC:* dorsal grey column; *DR:* dorsal root; *FC:* fasciculus cuneatus; *L. Cun. N.:* lateral cuneate nucleus; *LF:* lateral funiculus; *IGC:* intermediate grey column; *SCT:* spinocerebellar tract; *SG:* spinal ganglion; ₹ : crossed pathway.

funiculus. As the funiculus passes cranially, the GP axons are contributed to the lateral aspect. Thus cervical GP axons are the most lateral in the funiculus. As these axons course cranially, many leave this pathway to terminate in the spinal cord grey matter (Plate 1).

NUCLEUS GRACILIS AND MEDIAL CUNEATE NUCLEUS.[14]   The GP axons that reach the medulla in the fasciculus gracilis terminate in the nucleus gracilis in the dorsal part of the caudal medulla (Figs. 8–4, 8–5). This nucleus begins in the fasciculus gracilis caudal to the

obex at the level of the pyramidal decussation. It is lateral to the dorsal median sulcus and extends rostrally to the level of the obex, where it is dorsal to the parasympathetic nucleus of the vagus and medial to the medial cuneate nucleus (Plates 2, 3).

The GP axons in the fasciculus cuneatus (exclusive of those in the cuneocerebellar pathway) terminate in the medial cuneate nucleus in the dorsal part of the caudal medulla. This nucleus extends caudally in the fasciculus cuneatus to the level of the pyramidal decussa-

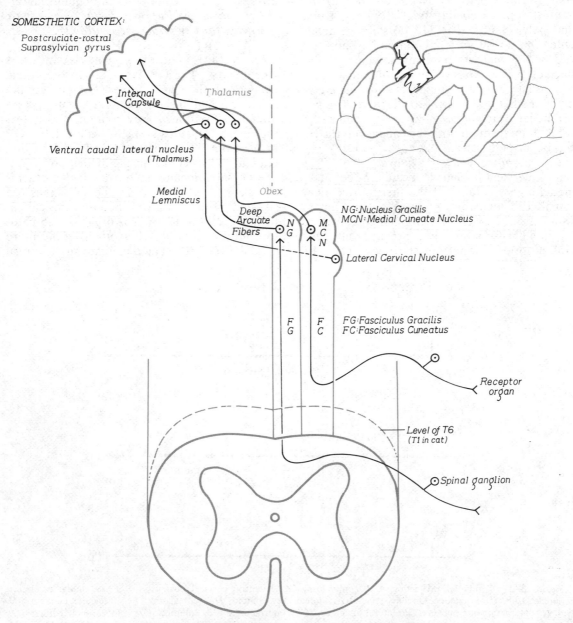

Figure 8–4.   General proprioception, spinal nerve, conscious pathway to somesthetic cortex.

Figure 8–5. Dorsal view of brain stem. *1:* Stria habenularis thalami; *2:* dorsal aspect of thalamus; *3:* habenular commissure; *4:* lateral geniculate nucleus; *5:* medial geniculate nucleus; *6:* rostral colliculus; *7:* commissure of caudal colliculi; *8:* caudal colliculus; *9:* crossing of trochlear nerve fibers in rostral medullary velum; *10:* middle cerebellar peduncle; *11:* caudal cerebellar peduncle; *12:* rostral cerebellar peduncle; *13:* acoustic stria; *14:* dorsal median sulcus in fourth ventricle; *15:* lateral cuneate nucleus; *16:* fasciculus cuneatus; *17:* nucleus gracilis; *18:* spinal tract of trigeminal nerve; *19:* superficial arcuate fibers; *20:* left ventral cochlear nucleus; *21:* brachium of caudal colliculus; *22:* optic tract; *23:* brachium of rostral colliculus; *24:* cut surface between cerebrum and brain stem; *25:* pineal body or epiphysis; *II:* optic nerves; *IV:* trochlear nerve; *V:* trigeminal nerve; *VIII:* vestibulocochlear nerve.

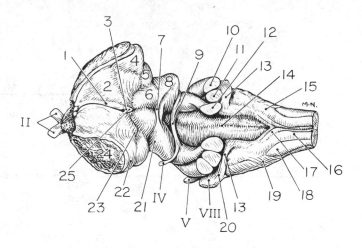

tion. It is lateral to the nucleus gracilis and extends rostrally beyond the obex. Its rostral portion is medial to the caudal portion of the lateral cuneate nucleus (cuneocerebellar pathway) (Plates 2, 3).

MEDIAL LEMNISCUS—VENTRAL CAUDAL LATERAL NUCLEUS, THALAMUS. Axons from the nucleus gracilis and medial cuneate nucleus course ventrally and transversely through the medulla as the deep arcuate fibers to the opposite side of the midline (Plates 3, 4). Here they form the medial lemniscus dorsal to the contralateral pyramid and ventromedial to the olive (Fig. 8–4).[28]

The medial lemniscus, oriented in a dorsal plane, courses rostrally through the medulla dorsal to the pyramid (Plates 3, 4, 5). As it passes through the dorsal part of the trapezoid body, it is medial to the dorsal nucleus of the trapezoid body (Plates 6, 7). In the pons it is located dorsal to the longitudinal fibers (Plates 8, 9). In the mesencephalon it is ventral in the caudal tegmentum, dorsal to the substantia nigra, and shifts laterally as it courses through the tegmentum of the rostral mesencephalon and into the caudal diencephalon (Plates 10–13). The medial lemniscus terminates in a specific projection nucleus of the thalamus, the ventral caudal lateral nucleus. This nucleus is ill defined; it is located ventral in the thalamus, dorsal to its external medullary lamina. The axons of this nucleus project to the sensory, somesthetic cortex of the cerebrum by way of the internal capsule.

The somesthetic cortex is described classically as located in the parietal lobe of the cerebrum caudal to the cruciate sulcus.[1,2] In the dog it overlaps with the motor cortex, being located in the caudal part of the postcruciate gyrus and the rostral suprasylvian gyrus.

There is a somatotopic organization of the medial lemniscus, the ventral caudal lateral nucleus of the thalamus, and the somesthetic cortex.[20]

All sensory systems project to localized regions of the cerebral cortex called primary sensory areas. Five of these are well established: auditory, visual, olfactory, gustatory, and somesthetic. The somatotopic organization of the somesthetic cerebral cortex reflects the density of receptor organs in the different regions of the body. For example, the prehensile organs of an animal (the lips of a pig, a horse, and a dog, and the forepaws or hands of a raccoon, a cat, a monkey, and a human being) have an abundance of receptor organs for this function, and a correspondingly large representation in the somesthetic cortex.[1, 2, 21, 36, 37]

Lateral Cervical Nucleus. An additional somesthetic pathway for general proprioception occurs by way of the lateral cervical nucleus.[3, 7, 12, 33, 35] This nucleus projects from the lateral side of the dorsal grey column in the dorsolateral funiculus in the first three cervical spinal cord segments. It receives afferents from the spinocervical tract in the ipsilateral lateral funiculus. The cell bodies of this tract are located predominantly in the ipsilateral lamina IV of the dorsal grey column along the entire spinal cord.[5, 6] In addition this nucleus receives axons from the dorsal column nuclei and the trigeminal nucleus in the medulla.

The axons of the cell bodies in the lateral cervical nucleus pass cranially and cross to the opposite side of the caudal medulla to join the contralateral medial lemniscus. Their course in the medial lemniscus to the ventral caudal lateral nucleus of the thalamus and the somesthetic cortex is similar to that of the deep

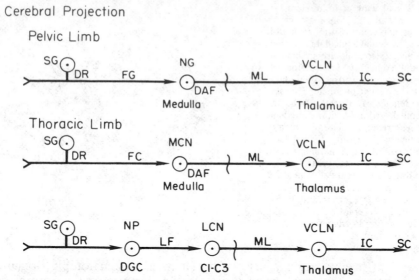

Figure 8–6. Cerebral projection. *C1-C3:* Cervical spinal cord segments 1–3; *DAF:* deep arcuate fibers; *DGC:* dorsal grey column; *DR:* dorsal root; *FC:* fasciculus cuneatus; *FG:* fasciculus gracilis; *IC:* internal capsule; *LCN:* lateral cuneate nucleus; *LF:* lateral funiculus; *MCN:* medial cuneate nucleus; *ML:* medial lemniscus; *NG:* nucleus gracilis; *NP:* nucleus proprius; *SC:* Somesthetic cortex; *SG:* spinal ganglion; *VCLN:* ventral caudal lateral nucleus of thalamus; ⟩: crossed pathway.

arcuate fibers that make up the medial lemniscus. The lateral cervical nucleus is somatotopically organized. Hindlimb afferents terminate in the dorsolateral part of the lateral cervical nucleus and forelimb afferents in the ventromedial portion. In the dog and cat this nucleus serves mainly as a relay for tactile sensation (Fig. 8–6).

CRANIAL NERVES

The majority of the GP axons in the head have been considered to arise from receptor organs in muscles of mastication, facial and extraocular muscles, and the temporomandibular joint. They course in the nerve branches from the trigeminal nerve (cranial nerve V). These GP axons in the ophthalmic, maxillary, and mandibular nerves course through the trigeminal ganglion and enter the pons with the trigeminal nerve. The axons course rostrally along the lateral border of the central grey substance of the fourth ventricle and mesencephalic aqueduct in the mesencephalic tract of the trigeminal nerve.

Although cell bodies of peripheral afferent neurons normally are located in ganglia of the peripheral nervous system, the cell bodies of these neurons are an exception to this rule. The cell bodies of these GP axons are located in the nucleus of the mesencephalic tract of the trigeminal nerve in a narrow band on the

lateral border of the central grey substance throughout the mesencephalon.

Reflex. For reflex function the axons may pass from the nucleus directly to the adjacent general somatic efferent and special visceral efferent nuclei of cranial nerves to synapse on the alpha motor neuron (Fig. 8–7). These alpha motor neurons may also be influenced indirectly by neurons in the pontine sensory nucleus of the trigeminal nerve, which are stimulated by the GP axons from the nucleus of the mesencephalic tract.

Conscious Perception. Other GP axons from the nucleus of the mesencephalic tract course caudolaterally to terminate in the pontine sensory nucleus of the trigeminal nerve. This nucleus is located in the caudal pons and rostral medulla, where it is situated between the entrance of the trigeminal nerve and its motor nucleus, ventromedial to the middle and rostral cerebellar peduncles. The axons of these cell bodies cross through the ventral reticular formation to the opposite side to form the trigeminal lemniscus (quintothalamic tract), which joins the medial lemniscus and courses rostrally to the caudal thalamus. They terminate in the ventral caudal medial nucleus of the thalamus adjacent to the ventral caudal lateral nucleus. Axons of these cell bodies course through the internal capsule to the somesthetic cortex.

The predominant role of this mesencephalic nucleus in all cranial nerve GP has been dis-

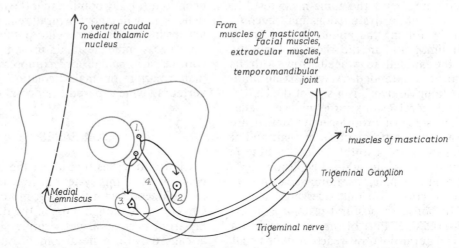

Level of Metencephalon–Mesencephalon

Figure 8–7. Trigeminal proprioceptive pathways. *1:* Nucleus of the mesencephalic tract of the trigeminal nerve; *2:* pontine sensory nucleus of the trigeminal nerve; *3:* motor nucleus of the trigeminal nerve; *4:* mesencephalic tract of the trigeminal nerve.

puted. Recent horseradish peroxidase studies of the afferent neurons of the canine tongue showed no evidence of cell bodies in the mesencephalic nucleus of the trigeminal nerve.[4] The cell bodies of the intramuscular neurons of both intrinsic and extrinsic tongue muscles were located in the first cervical spinal ganglion, the distal vagal ganglion, and the trigeminal ganglion. None was found in hypoglossal ganglia. Other studies in the sheep and pig demonstrated cell bodies of afferent neurons of extraocular muscles in the trigeminal ganglion.[24]

CLINICAL SIGNS

Ataxia (incoordination) is the principal sign observed with lesions in the general proprioceptive system. This sometimes is referred to as sensory ataxia as opposed to motor ataxia of cerebellar cortical disease. Ataxia is a result of lack of kinesthesia, a lack of the sense of motion or of the position of the body or limbs in space.

The animal may show a standing posture with the distal portion of the extremities placed more lateral than normal, a basewide stance. On moving, the limbs may swing to the side and circumduct or abduct more than normal, or cross beneath the trunk, or adduct more than normal, sometimes interfering with the opposite limb. There may be a delay in initiating protraction of the limb on getting up or on walking, causing a longer stride than normal and a tendency for the hindquarters to appear slightly lower (crouched) than usual. This may contribute to the wobbly appearance of the pelvic limb gait. The animal may walk on the dorsal surface of its distal extremity, or "knuckle over." Occasionally, a degree of overresponse is seen during flexion of the limb when the animal is in movement. This uninhibited flexion causes the limb to be lifted higher than usual. This may be combined with excessive abduction. The excessive flexion is often called hypermetria, and also occurs in a more severe form in cerebellar disease.

This hypermetria with general proprioceptive deficit may be explained by the lack of spinocerebellar input to the cerebellar cortex. Spinocerebellar neurons terminate in the cerebellar cortex, in which Purkinje neurons are activated. These are inhibitory neurons that indirectly affect brain stem neurons through their effect on neurons in the cerebellar nuclei. Thus spinocerebellar activation of the cerebellar cortex typically results in inhibition of the brain stem mechanism that induces voluntary locomotion, so that once limb flexion is induced for the protraction phase of locomotion, it is inhibited in turn in time for the appropriate extensor support phase to occur. A deficiency in this inhibition induced by the spinocerebellar deficit results in a prolonged flexor phase of the gait observed as hyperflexion or hypermetria.[16, 23]

Defects may be observed in the response of

the patient to testing postural reactions such as placing, hopping, hemiwalking, proprioceptive positioning, and the tonic neck test. In mild lesions subtle dysfunctions may become apparent by forcing the animal to hop slowly on each limb, and in the thoracic limbs by forcing the animal to wheelbarrow with its head and neck extended. An occasional tendency to "knuckle over" is a sign of deficit.

With unilateral lesions in the spinocerebellar system the signs of proprioceptive deficit are ipsilateral and are observed in the gait and/or in the response to postural reaction testing in the limbs on the same side as the lesion.

Lesions in the thalamus, internal capsule, or somesthetic cortex on one side cause an abnormal response to postural reactions on the contralateral side. Part of the explanation for the contralateral postural reaction deficit may be related to the disruption of the thalamocortical pathway of the GP system, in addition to the disruption of the telencephalic portion of the upper motor neuron. The gait is usually normal with lesions that are not acute. Occasionally, as an animal turns slowly, there is a delay in the onset of protraction of the affected thoracic limb.

It may be difficult to separate paresis from proprioceptive deficiency on clinical examination of the patient, but this usually does not interfere with the interpretation of the gross location of the lesion. The upper motor neuron and GP systems accompany each other through most of the neuraxis. Mild compression of the spinal cord at the thirteenth thoracic segment causes paraparesis and ataxia in the pelvic limbs because of interference with the upper motor neuron in the ventral and lateral funiculi and the GP system in the lateral (and dorsal) funiculi. Thoracic limb function is normal.

A unilateral midcervical spinal cord lesion produces a profound upper motor neuron and GP deficit in the gait and postural reactions in the ipsilateral thoracic and pelvic limbs, with only a mild dysfunction in postural reactions in the contralateral pelvic limb.

Clinicopathologic and experimental studies indicate that lesions of the spinocerebellar system have a more profound influence on gait than do lesions of the dorsal columns.[22] Experimental section of the dorsal column bilaterally at C4 in the dog initially produced a high stepping gait in the thoracic limbs, but after 2 to 3 weeks it was nearly completely compensated.[34] The same results have been found in cats and monkeys.[29] In my clinical experience I have not been able to clearly differentiate between lesions of the cerebral and cerebellar pathways for general proprioception. It is my opinion that the more serious deficits in gait and postural reactions reflect lesions in the spinocerebellar pathways. I have observed significant ataxia in dogs and horses with cervical spinal cord compression from a malformation or malarticulation of cervical vertebrae which spared the dorsal columns.

DISEASES

Clinical diseases that affect the spinal nerve component of this system have been discussed in conjunction with the lower motor neuron in Chapter 4. Although most of the deficit resulting from peripheral nerve injury is described as caused by the general somatic efferent lower motor neuron loss, some may be due to loss of the general proprioceptive system. I have observed 2 dogs with a slowly progressive ataxic gait from a general proprioceptive deficit that had a diffuse spinal ganglionitis. No cause was determined. One of these had a diffuse facial hypalgesia from general somatic afferent neuron dysfunction of the trigeminal ganglion.

If the peroneal nerves are compressed for a prolonged period of time by ropes placed just above the tarsus to tie the dog to a surgery table, a transient neurologic deficit may be observed after recovery from anesthesia. At this level the nerve is compromised distal to its muscle innervation to the flexors of the tarsus and extensors of the digits. Nevertheless, the dog can stand and walk on the dorsum of the paw. There is no evidence of paresis. The dysfunction is presumably due to the loss of function of the GP and general somatic afferent neurons present in the nerve at the site of the compression. Hypalgesia or analgesia may accompany the proprioceptive deficit.

Spinal cord diseases are described in Chapters 10 and 11. No clinical signs have been associated with diseases that affect the cranial nerve component of this system.

REFERENCES

1. Adrian, E. D.: Afferent areas in brain of ungulates. Brain, 66:89, 1943.
2. Adrian, E. D.: The somatic receiving area in the brain of the Shetland pony. Brain, 69:1, 1946.
3. Brodal, A., and Rexed, B.: Spinal afferents to the lateral cervical nucleus in the cat. An experimental study. J. Comp. Neurol., 98:179, 1953.

4. Chibuzo, G. A., and Cummings, J. C.: The origins of the afferent fibers to the lingual muscles of the dog: A retrograde labeling study with horseradish peroxidase. Anat. Rec., *200*:95, 1981.

5. Craig, A. D.: Spinocervical tract cells in cat and dog, labeled by the retrograde transport of horseradish peroxidase. Neurosci. Let., *3*:173, 1976.

6. Craig, A. D., Jr.: Spinal and medullary input to the lateral cervical nucleus. J. Comp. Neurol., *181*:729, 1978.

7. Craig, A. D., Jr., and Burton, H.: The lateral cervical nucleus in the cat: Anatomic organization of the cervicothalamic neurons. J. Comp. Neurol., *185*:329, 1979.

8. Cummings, J. C., and Petras, J. M.: The origin of spinocerebellar pathways. 1. The nucleus cervicalis centralis of the cranial cervical spinal cord. J. Comp. Neurol., *173*:655, 1977.

9. Grant, G.: Spinal course and somatotopically localized termination of the spinocerebellar tracts. An experimental study in the cat. Acta Physiol. Scand., *56*[Suppl.]:193, 1962.

10. Grant, G., and Rexed, B.: Dorsal spinal root afferents to Clarke's column. Brain, *81*:567, 1958.

11. Ha, H., and Liu, C.-N.: Cell origin of the ventral spinocerebellar tract. J. Comp. Neurol., *133*:185, 1968.

12. Ha, H., and Liu, C.-N.: Organization of the spinocervico-thalamic system. J. Comp. Neurol., *127*:445, 1966.

13. Hand, P. J.: Lumbosacral dorsal root terminations in the nucleus gracilis of the cat. Some observations on the terminal degeneration in other medullary sensory nuclei. J. Comp. Neurol., *126*:137, 1966.

14. Hand, P. J., and Van Winkle, T.: The efferent connections of the feline nucleus cuneatus. J. Comp. Neurol., *171*:83, 1977.

15. Hirai, N., Hongo, T., and Sasaki, S.: Cerebellar projection and input organizations of the spinocerebellar tract arising from the central cervical nucleus in the cat. Brain Res., *157*:341, 1978.

16. Hartley, W. J., and Palmer, A. C.: Ataxia in Jack Russell terriers. Acta Neuropathol., *26*:71, 1973.

17. Holmquist, B., and Oscarsson, O.: Location, course, and characteristics of uncrossed and crossed ascending spinal tracts in the cat. Acta Physiol. Scand., *58*:57, 1963.

18. Holmquist, B., Oscarsson, O., and Rosen, I.: Functional organization of the cuneocerebellar tract in the cat. Acta Physiol. Scand., *58*:216, 1963.

19. Hubbard, J. I., and Oscarsson, O.: Localization of the cell bodies of the ventral spinocerebellar tract in lumbar segments of the cat. J. Comp. Neurol., *118*:199, 1962.

20. Johnson, J. I., Jr., Welker, W. I., and Pubols, B. H., Jr.: Somatotopic organization of raccoon dorsal column nuclei. J. Comp. Neurol., *132*:1, 1968.

21. Landgren, S., and Silfvenius, H.: Projection to cerebral cortex of group I and muscle afferents from the cat's hindlimb. J. Physiol., *200*:353, 1969.

22. Lassek, A. M.: Motor deficits produced by posterior rhizotomy versus section of the dorsal funiculus. Neurology, *4*:120, 1954.

23. Latshaw, W. K.: A model for the neural control of locomotion. J. Am. Anim. Hosp. Assoc., *10*:598, 1974.

24. Manni, E., Bartolani, R., and Desole, C.: Peripheral pathway of eye muscle proprioception. Exp. Neurol., *22*:1, 1968.

25. Matsushita, M., and Ikeda, M.: The central cervical nucleus as cell origin of a spinocerebellar tract arising from the cervical cord: A study in the cat using horseradish peroxidase. Brain Res., *100*:412, 1975.

26. Matsushita, M., and Ikeda, M.: Spinocerebellar projection to the vermis of the posterior lobe and the paramedian lobule in the cat, as studied by retrograde transport of horseradish peroxidase. J. Comp. Neurol., *192*:143, 1980.

27. Matsushita, M., Hosoya, Y., and Ikeda, M.: Anatomical organization of the spinocerebellar system in the cat, as studied by retrograde transport of horseradish peroxidase. J. Comp. Neurol., *184*:81, 1979.

28. Matzke, H. A.: The course of the fibers arising from the nucleus gracilis and nucleus cuneatus of the cat. J. Comp. Neurol., *94*:439, 1951.

29. McCormack, M., and Dubrovsky, B.: Impairment in limb action after dorsal funiculi section in cats. Exp. Brain Res., *37*:31, 1979.

30. Oscarsson, O.: Functional organization of the spino- and cuneocerebellar tracts. Physiol. Rev., *45*:495, 1965.

32. Petras, J. M., and Cummings, J. F.: The origin of spinocerebellar pathways. II. The nucleus centrobasalis of the cervical enlargement and the nucleus dorsalis of the thoracolumbar spinal cord. J. Comp. Neurol., *173*:693, 1977.

33. Rexed, B., and Brodal, A.: The nucleus cervicalis lateralis—a spinocerebellar relay nucleus. J. Neurophysiol., *14*:399, 1951.

34. Reynolds, P. J., Talbott, R. E., and Brookhart, J. M.: Control of postural reactions in the dog: The role of the dorsal column feedback pathway. Brain Res., *40*:159, 1972.

35. Truex, R. C., Taylor, M. J., Smyth, M. Q., and Glidenberg, P. L.: The lateral cervical nucleus of cat, dog and man. J. Comp. Neurol., *139*:93, 1970.

36. Welker, W. I., and Campos, G. B.: Physiological significance of sulci in somatic sensory cerebral cortex in mammals of the family Procyonidae. J. Comp. Neurol., *120*:19, 1963.

37. Welker, W. I., and Seidenstein, S.: Somatic sensory representation in the cerebral cortex of the raccoon *(Procyon lotor)*. J. Comp. Neurol., *111*:469, 1959.

38. Yezierski, R. P., Culberson, J. L., and Brown, P. B.: Cells of origin of propriospinal connections to cat lumbosacral gray as determined with horseradish peroxidase. Exp. Neurol., *69*:493, 1980.

Chapter

9

GENERAL SOMATIC AFFERENT SYSTEM—GSA

The general somatic afferent system is referred to as the "pain, temperature, touch" system. The receptor organs, both encapsulated and nonencapsulated, are classified as exteroceptors, being stimulated by physical contact with the external environment. These exteroceptors are classified further physiologically as mechanoreceptors, thermoreceptors, and nociceptors on the basis of the form of energy that is their adequate stimulus.

Although the neurons in this system are concerned with the perception of temperature, crude and discriminating touch, and pain, it is often difficult to interpret the animal's response to testing these modalities. Therefore, the clinical neurologist is most concerned with pain perception. The ability to assess the patient's perception of touch and various degrees of mechanical stimuli is extremely variable. In some normal patients a very slight stimulus will elicit a recognizable response, whereas in others even closing hemostats on the skin may not elicit a response.

SPINAL NERVE

The axons course from the receptor organ on the surface of the body through peripheral nerves, spinal nerves, and through the segmental spinal ganglion related to the dorsal root. These GSA neurons are unipolar, and the cell body is in the spinal ganglion. The axon continues proximally through the dorsal rootlet to the dorsolateral sulcus, where it enters the spinal cord. The axon branches dorsal to the dorsal grey column and courses cranially and caudally through the adjacent two or three segments. The pathway formed by these axons at the apex of the dorsal grey column is referred to as the dorsolateral fasciculus (Lissauer's tract). Collaterals of these axonal branches enter the dorsal grey column all along the segments that are traversed. They pass into the middle of the dorsal grey column, giving off collaterals to interneurons located at the apex of the dorsal grey column in an area called substantia gelatinosa (Fig. 9–1).

Reflex GSA Pathway. The GSA axons synapse on interneurons in the grey matter of the spinal cord, which in turn influence the alpha motor neurons. Interneurons with axons passing in the fasciculus proprius can influence the alpha motor neurons of adjacent segments to stimulate the complete general somatic efferent system of the lower motor neuron of the reflex arc. This is the reflex pathway for the flexor reflex, limb withdrawal phenomenon. It requires only the peripheral nerves to the area stimulated, the muscles that contract, and the segments of the spinal cord from which the peripheral nerves originate.

The surface of the body can be mapped according to the distribution of general somatic afferent receptor organs either associated with peripheral nerves, or associated with specific dorsal roots (dermatomes).[10, 15] The latter is referred to as dermatomal mapping, and represents the distribution of a dorsal root's axons (receptor organs) over the body surface. This demonstrates the embryonic fate of the dorsal root axons that innervated the dermatomal portion of the somite. As the dermatome contributed to the body surface, its dorsal root innervation extended with it by way of branches of spinal or peripheral nerves.

Studies in the dog have shown that each dermatome of the trunk extends from the dorsal to the ventral midline, and there is a craniocaudal overlap of up to three dorsal roots in the lumbosacral region.[10] The cutaneous zone is the surface of the body innervated with GSA neurons in one peripheral

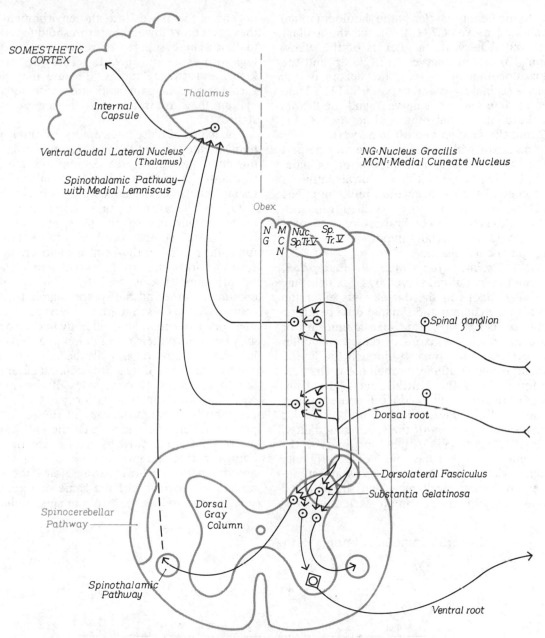

Figure 9–1. Spinal cord reflex and conscious perception GSA pathways.

nerve. There is considerable overlap in the cutaneous zones of adjacent peripheral nerves. The autonomous zone is the skin area that is innervated by GSA neurons from only one peripheral nerve. An awareness of these autonomous zones is most important to the clinical neurologist.[25]

Sensory deficit, like motor deficit, is more obvious with disrupted peripheral nerves than with a disrupted spinal nerve or its roots.

A noxious stimulus (a pin or forceps) applied to the skin in the center of the medial side of the antebrachium causes withdrawal of the limb by flexion of the shoulder, elbow, carpus, and digits. The axons of the nociceptors course proximally in the medial cutaneous antebrachial nerve, the musculocutaneous nerve, and the sixth, seventh, and eighth cervical spinal nerves and their dorsal rootlets. Collaterals of these axons terminate on interneurons in the grey matter of these and the adjacent spinal cord segments. These interneurons synapse on alpha motor neurons of the same segments and those caudal to this site that have axons coursing to the flexor muscles of the shoulder (spinal roots and nerves C7, C8, T1 and the axillary and radial nerves), the flexors of the elbow (spinal roots and nerves C6, C7, C8 and the musculocutaneous nerve), the flexors of the carpus (spinal roots and nerves C8, T1, T2 and the median and ulnar nerves), and the flexors of the digits (spinal roots and nerves C8, T1, T2 and the median and ulnar nerves).

The flexor withdrawal response may be part of an animal's conscious perception of pain, but this requires additional central pathways not needed for the segmental reflex arc. The two responses must be distinguished from each other. Ascertaining cerebral response to noxious stimuli is especially important in evaluating spinal cord disease.

GSA Pathway for Conscious Perception. For all the modalities served by GSA neurons, the GSA axons in the dorsal roots enter the dorsal grey column and synapse on a dendritic zone or cell body in a specific nucleus or laminar zone. The axons of these cell bodies project cranially primarily through the lateral funiculus and continue through the brain stem to terminate in the ventral caudal lateral nucleus of the thalamus. These cell bodies project axons to the somesthetic cerebral cortex for conscious perception of the specific modality.

PAIN PATHWAY. About one half of the afferent axons in cutaneous nerves originate from nociceptors. These receptors are stimulated by strong mechanical and thermal and occasionally chemical stimuli. Release of en-

dogenous substances into the environment of these receptors lowers their threshold for stimulation. These substances result from pathologic processes and include serotonin, bradykinin, and prostaglandins. Because they play a causal role in pain associated with inflammation they are referred to as algesic substances.

The axons of these nociceptors are small and unmyelinated or lightly myelinated. These axons enter the dorsal grey column through the substantia gelatinosa and synapse on cell bodies at the base of the dorsal grey column (Fig. 9–1).[19, 22] The axons of these dorsal grey column neurons course to the ipsilateral and contralateral ventral portions of the lateral funiculus medial to the ventral spinocerebellar tract and form the lateral spinothalamic tract. In primates this is essentially an entirely crossed system, and the spinothalamic tract is composed of axons that are uninterrupted from their place of origin at a cell body in the dorsal grey column to their termination in a thalamic nucleus. In domestic animals the axons leaving cell bodies in one dorsal grey column enter the lateral funiculus of both sides of the spinal cord. The spinothalamic pathway in the lateral funiculus is dorsal in the cat and ventral in the pig.[1-4, 13] There is evidence that the pathway is interrupted frequently by axons leaving the path, entering the grey matter to synapse on another neuron whose axon rejoins the spinothalamic pathway of the same or opposite side. Thus, in contrast to humans, animals

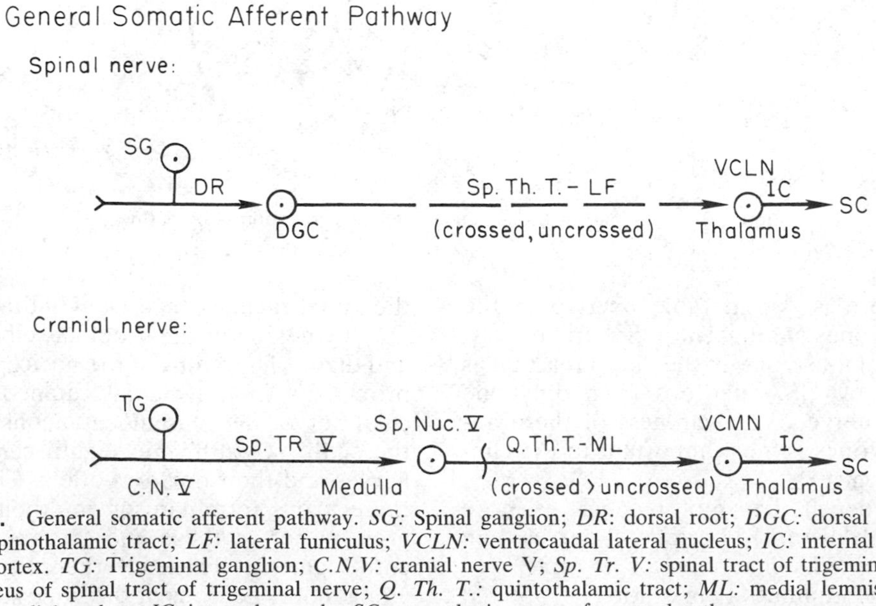

Figure 9–2. General somatic afferent pathway. *SG:* Spinal ganglion; *DR:* dorsal root; *DGC:* dorsal grey column; *Sp. Th. T.:* spinothalamic tract; *LF:* lateral funiculus; *VCLN:* ventrocaudal lateral nucleus; *IC:* internal capsule; *SC:* somesthetic cortex. *TG:* Trigeminal ganglion; *C.N.V:* cranial nerve V; *Sp. Tr. V:* spinal tract of trigeminal nerve; *Sp. Nuc. V:* nucleus of spinal tract of trigeminal nerve; *Q. Th. T.:* quintothalamic tract; *ML:* medial lemniscus; *VCMN:* ventrocaudal medial nucleus; *IC:* internal capsule; *SC:* somesthetic cortex; *ʃ:* crossed pathway.

have a diffuse, bilaterally represented multi-synaptic pathway for the conduction of impulses stimulated by noxious stimuli (Fig. 9–2).

In primates hemisection of the spinal cord causes ipsilateral motor deficit (upper motor neuron) and contralateral sensory deficit (general somatic afferent) caudal to the lesion. This syndrome, called Brown-Séquard, is explained by the level of crossing being at the origin of these systems, which is the brain stem for the upper motor neuron and approximate site of entrance to the spinal cord for the general somatic afferent system. The contralateral hypalgesia is not as evident in the domestic animal because of the bilateral spinal cord pathways for the GSA system. Nevertheless, clinical experience with a few unilateral lesions in the spinal cord and rostral brain stem occasionally has demonstrated a contralateral hypalgesia. Lesions of the somesthetic area of the cerebral cortex or the pathway from the thalamic relay nucleus to that cortex will cause a mild hypalgesia in the contralateral limbs in cooperative sensitive patients. This is best determined by the patient's response to a mild pin prick to the skin. It cannot be observed in a stoic animal. This would suggest that a contralateral pathway may predominate.

Experimental evidence indicates that in addition to the spinothalamic pathway, other tracts in the lateral funiculus, such as spinoreticular and fasciculus proprius pathways, also may conduct the modality of "pain." The proprioceptive pathways that project to the thalamus and cerebrum also serve mechanoreceptor function and may play a role in the perception of pain.

In the standard description of the conscious pathway for the general somatic afferent system, the axons in the spinothalamic tract pass cranially through the entire spinal cord, and through the medulla, pons, and midbrain associated with the lateral aspect of the medial lemniscus. In the caudal thalamus these axons synapse in the specific projection nucleus for the general somatic afferent system in spinal nerves, the ventral caudal lateral nucleus of the thalamus. Axons of these cell bodies enter the internal capsule and are distributed to the somesthetic cortex.[12] Conscious perception of pain may occur at both the thalamic and cortical levels of this pathway. As an example of thalamic perception of pain, I have observed a newborn calf that had complete absence of both cerebral hemispheres show a painful response to noxious stimuli applied to the digits.

As these spinothalamic axons traverse the brain stem, collaterals terminate in the reticular formation in its ascending division. These are afferents to the ascending reticular activating system (ARAS) concerned with the arousal of the cerebral cortex, the maintenance of the state of consciousness.

For pain to be perceived there must be a sensation spatially and temporally of nociceptor impulses in the central nervous system. This is influenced by a number of neuroanatomic and neurochemical factors.[23, 24] There is evidence that considerable modulation of pain occurs at the termination of primary afferents in the dorsal grey column. Interneurons in the substantia gelatinosa are inhibitory to the dorsal grey column neurons that project into the spinothalamic "pain" pathway. Most nociceptive afferents are small axons that terminate mostly on the spinothalamic projection neurons. Large diameter myelinated non-nociceptive axons terminate on other projection neurons in the dorsal grey column and on large numbers of substantia gelatinosa interneurons. By this mechanism these inhibit the "pain" pathway by modulating the activity of the nociceptive afferents.

Descending pathways from the periaqueductal grey area of the mesencephalon, locus ceruleus of the pons, and raphe nuclei of the medulla are inhibitory to the dorsal grey column neurons of the pain projection pathway. Some of the inhibition is mediated by serotonin in the dorsal grey column.

The cell bodies of nociceptor neurons in spinal ganglia contain substance P, which is a neurotransmitter that upon stimulation is released at the telodendron in the dorsal grey column.[23] This pain pathway neurotransmitter is inhibited by the local action of morphine and enkephalin. One of the sites of inhibition of pain by opiate mechanisms is in the spinal cord dorsal grey column.

CRANIAL NERVE

The general somatic afferent axons course from the receptor organ on the surface of the head through the branches of the ophthalmic, maxillary, and mandibular nerves, and the trigeminal nerve and ganglion. The cell bodies of these unipolar GSA neurons are in the trigeminal ganglion, which is located in the canal for the trigeminal nerve in the rostral part of the petrosal bone. The trigeminal nerve enters the pons through the caudolateral portion of the transverse fibers of the pons as they form the middle cerebellar peduncle. This is rostral to the origin of the facial and vestibulocochlear nerves (Fig. 9–3, Plate 8).

The GSA axons of the trigeminal nerve course caudally on the lateral side of the medulla in the spinal tract of the trigeminal nerve. This tract is shaped like a quarter circle, with the concave surface medial (Plates 1 thru 7). As it passes from rostral to caudal, it is medial to the cochlear nuclei in the vestibulocochlear nerve, and to the dorsal spinocerebellar tract as it enters the caudal cerebellar peduncle in the superficial arcuate fibers. At the obex it becomes superficial on the lateral side of the medulla between the fasciculus cuneatus dorsally and the dorsal spinocerebellar tract ventrally. The tract continues caudally into the first cervical spinal cord segment, in which it is continued by the dorsolateral fasciculus (Lissauer's tract) (Plates 1, 2). Throughout this course a nuclear column is located medial to this tract. In the pons, it is the pontine sensory nucleus of the trigeminal nerve (Plate 7). Throughout the medulla and into the first cervical segment, it is the nucleus of the spinal tract of the trigeminal nerve (Plates 1 thru 6). This nuclear column is similar in shape to the spinal tract of the trigeminal nerve. In the

cervical spinal cord it is continuous with the substantia gelatinosa. General somatic afferent axons in the spinal tract of the trigeminal nerve terminate in the nuclear column medial to it, the pontine sensory nucleus and nucleus of the spinal tract of the trigeminal nerve. The pontine sensory nucleus is thought to be primarily concerned with mechanoreception. The rostral part of the spinal nucleus primarily projects face and head somatic sensation to the cerebellum. The majority of the spinal nucleus is concerned with nociception.

Reflex GSA Pathway. Axons of the cell bodies in this nuclear column project to the lower motor neuron nuclei of cranial nerves to complete reflex arcs. The closure of the eyelids on stimulation of the cornea (ophthalmic nerve) and the eyelids (ophthalmic and maxillary nerves) is evidence of the termination of these trigeminal neurons on cell bodies in the pontine and spinal tract nuclei whose axons terminate on the special visceral efferent neurons of the facial nucleus. These are the corneal and palpebral reflexes.

GSA Pathway for Conscious Projection. Other axons from cell bodies in the pontine sensory nucleus and nucleus of the spinal tract of the trigeminal nerve predominantly cross to

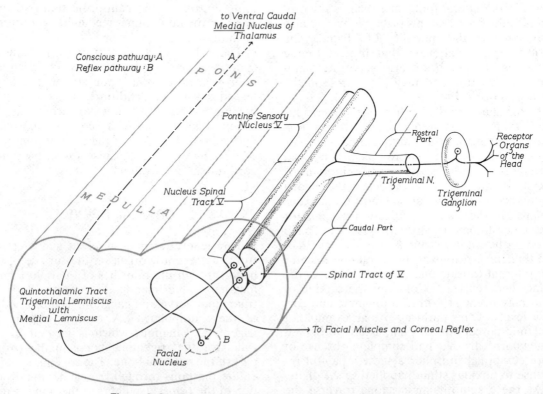

Figure 9–3. Trigeminal nerve, general somatic afferent pathways.

the opposite side, become associated with the medial lemniscus, and course rostrally with this bundle. These are sometimes referred to as the trigeminal lemniscus or the quintothalamic tract. In the caudal thalamus these axons synapse in the specific projection nucleus of the thalamus for the GSA system in cranial nerves, the ventral caudal medial nucleus. Axons of these cell bodies enter the internal capsule and are distributed to the head region of the somesthetic cortex (Figs. 9–2, 9–3). There is clinical evidence for a predominantly contralateral projection of this trigeminal pain pathway. Unilateral lesions of the somesthetic cortex, internal capsule, or ventral caudal medial nucleus of the thalamus cause a contralateral facial hypalgesia.

CLINICAL SIGNS

In the neurologic examination of animals, the most reliable modality for testing the GSA system is that of nociception—pain. Analgesia means complete absence of pain perception. Hypalgesia means decreased pain perception.

Pain is not just an exteroceptive modality, but is the subjective interpretation of nerve impulses produced peripherally by a stimulus that is actually or potentially harmful to tissue. This interpretation of pain varies with each individual.[2, 16, 17] The interpretation of these impulses is modified and conditioned by past experiences and memories, by an understanding of the cause of the impulses, and by the consequence expected. The degree of attention and emotional state of the individual also modifies the response. The response often is related more to the significance of an injury than to its size. Even in animals a considerable variation occurs in the cerebral response to stimuli considered by the investigator to be noxious or painful. This often makes interpretation of dysfunction of the spinothalamic pathway difficult. A stimulus that elicits a "pain" response in the normal small animal in most cases is the

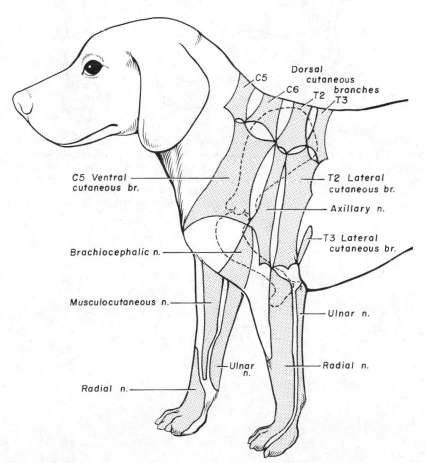

Figure 9–4. Autonomous zones of the cutaneous innervation of the thoracic limb.[25]

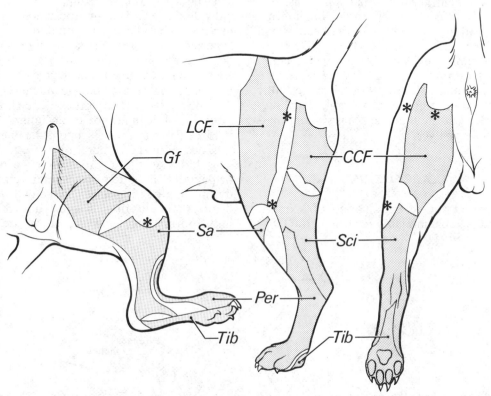

Figure 9–5. Autonomous zones of the cutaneous innervation of the canine pelvic limb. Caudal cutaneous femoral (CCF), genitofemoral (GF), lateral cutaneous femoral (LCF), peroneal (Per), Saphenous (Sa), sciatic (Sci), tibial (Tib). Asterisks indicate palpable bony landmarks—medial and lateral tibial condyles, greater trochanter, and lateral end of tuber ischiadicum (From R. L. Kitchell, to be published). The sciatic nerve autonomous zone is for lesions proximal to the greater trochanter and includes the zones for the peroneal and tibial nerves. For sciatic nerve lesions caudal to the femur, the autonomous zone varies, depending on how many of its cutaneous branches are affected.

application of pressure to the base of the toenails with forceps. Response to pin pricking is often unreliable, because many normal patients show no cerebral response. In large animals for whom a pin or forceps may not be adequate, an electric prod may be used. The horse often responds well to a pin or closed forceps. The area most sensitive to a noxious stimulus in the head of domestic animals is the nasal mucosa. If an area of hypalgesia or analgesia is suspected, this region should be tested.

Interpretation of an intact or interrupted spinothalamic pathway is most important in the evaluation of the degree of nervous tissue damage following injury. Injuries to the spinal cord that cause complete motor paralysis and complete analgesia or lack of sensation to noxious stimuli caudal to the lesion have a poor prognosis and require prompt surgical intervention if it is warranted. Patients with complete motor paralysis but with hypalgesia or depressed response to noxious stimuli caudal to the lesion have a better prognosis. The presence of a cerebral response to noxious stimuli indicates that some pathways in the spinal cord are intact at the site of the lesion. With peripheral nerve lesions, the same signs of paralysis but accompanied by hypalgesia in the area of distribution of the involved peripheral nerves indicate that the nerve is still intact, and the prognosis is not as grave as it would be with paralysis and analgesia. In evaluating the cutaneous innervation of peripheral nerves, it is important to test only the autonomous zone, that area of skin innervated only by that specific nerve (Figs. 9–4, 9–5).

DISEASES

Some of the clinical diseases that affect the spinal and peripheral nerve components of this system were considered in conjunction with the lower motor neuron in Chapter 4. In these diseases the predominant clinical sign was paresis due to lower motor neuron disease. Sensory neuropathy is less common but has been described.

Canine Sensory Neuropathy. Self-mutilation of the digits (acral mutilation) and nociceptive loss were observed in 3 of a litter of 9 English pointers.[6] A similar clinical syndrome with autosomal recessive inheritance has been described in short-haired pointers.[18, 20] Around 3 months of age the affected English pointers began to constantly lick or bite at their paws. Severe acral mutilation resulted, sometimes accompanied by complete loss of pain sensa-

tion in the digits of the hind paws. Gait, postural reactions, and spinal reflexes remained normal. There were no electrophysiologic abnormalities detected in the peripheral nerves.

Necropsy of one dog revealed a decrease in size of the spinal ganglia from a deficiency of ganglionic neurons. Small-sized neurons predominated. There was reduced fiber density in the dorsolateral fasciculus and mild degeneration in spinal roots, ganglia, and peripheral nerves. A developmental hypoplasia and slowly progressive postnatal degeneration were hypothesized.

Two young long-haired dachshunds were studied for a slowly progressive pelvic limb ataxia, urinary incontinence, episodes of gastrointestinal disturbance, and a peripheral nociceptive deficit.[7, 8] The pelvic limbs would abduct and overflex on protraction, producing a bouncy type of hypermetric gait. There was complete loss of proprioception. One dog constantly chewed on its penis. All four paws were analgesic on one dog and hypalgesic on another. Loss of or decrease in pain perception occurred all over the body including the face. The patellar reflex was normal, but flexor reflexes were usually absent owing to the nociceptive deficit.

These signs began shortly after these dogs could first walk and were obvious by 12 weeks of age. After months of slow progression, the signs remained unchanged.

Motor nerve conduction was normal but sensory nerve conduction was decreased or absent. Autopsy revealed a distal axonopathy of sensory neurons with loss or degeneration of large myelinated axons and unmyelinated axons.[9] A history of similar affected littermates suggested that this may be a familial disorder.

Feline Chronic Relapsing Polyneuritis. A chronic relapsing polyneuritis has been described in an 18-month-old cat with a 6-month history of muscle twitching, hypermetric ataxia, and biting at its hind paws. Patellar reflexes were exaggerated, but pin prick response was absent in the hind paws. Transient remissions occurred during the clinical course.

At autopsy an extensive neuritis was found in the dorsal and ventral rootlets of spinal nerves and in cranial nerves. Extensive demyelination and remyelination were evident. The cause is unknown.

Ganglioradiculitis. We have observed three adult dogs with a nonsuppurative cranial and spinal ganglioradiculitis. Clinical signs included facial hypalgesia, gagging, regurgitation, megaesophagus, atrophy of masticatory muscles, mild ataxia and paresis, scapular muscle atrophy, and depressed or absent patellar reflexes. Signs and lesions may be asymmetric. Cell bodies were lost from inflamed ganglia, and dorsal root degeneration was extensive. The cause is unknown but a viral or immune pathogenesis is suspected.

Facial Hypalgesia-Analgesia. Hypalgesia or analgesia of the face is caused by lesions that interfere with the trigeminal nerve, its ganglion, or its tract in the pons and medulla. The most common causes are injuries, neoplasms, and granulomas. The presence of facial analgesia in an animal with intracranial injury is a poor prognostic sign, because it suggests contusion of the caudal brain stem. Facial hypalgesia (cranial nerve V) on the same side as a facial muscle paresis (cranial nerve VII) and vestibular ataxia (cranial nerve VIII) suggests an intracranial and usually medullary location of the lesion and a more cautious prognosis. Otitis media-interna can affect only cranial nerves VII and VIII, not V. The bilateral nonsuppurative trigeminal neuritis in the dog that causes paralysis of the muscles of mastication also may produce a hypalgesia, but it is difficult to detect.

A bilateral trigeminal sensory neuropathy was described in a 2-year-old female collie.[5] There was bilateral sensory loss over the entire distribution of both trigeminal nerves. Motor function of the trigeminal nerves was normal. There was extensive loss of cell bodies in the trigeminal ganglia with Wallerian degeneration throughout the branches of the trigeminal nerves and the spinal tracts in the medulla. No cause was found.

When the eyeball is denervated of its sensory nerves (trigeminal-ophthalmic nerve), degenerative changes occur in the cornea.[21] This is referred to as neurotrophic keratitis and consists of edema and erosion of epithelial cells. The relationship of the cellular metabolism of the cornea to its sensory nerve supply is not clearly understood.

Lesions that destroy the ventral caudal medial thalamic nucleus or its projection pathway in the internal capsule or the somesthetic cortex may produce a hypalgesia of the contralateral face. This may best be determined by palpation of the nasal mucosa with a blunt instrument.

Spinal cord diseases that affect this system will be discussed in Chapter 10.

REFERENCES

1. Anderson, F. D., and Berry, C. M.: Degeneration studies of long ascending fiber systems in the cat brain stem. J. Comp. Neurol., *111*:195, 1959.
2. Breazile, J. E., and Kitchell, R. L.: Pain perception in animals. Fed. Proc., *28*:1379, 1969.
3. Breazile, J. E., and Kitchell, R. L.: A study of fiber systems within the spinal cord of the domestic pig that subserve pain. J. Comp. Neurol., *133*:373, 1968.
4. Breazile, J. E., and Kitchell, R. L.: Ventrolateral spinal cord afferents to the brain stem in the domestic pig. J. Comp. Neurol., *133*:363, 1968.
5. Carmichael, S., and Griffiths, I. R.: Case of isolated sensory trigeminal neuropathy in a dog. Vet. Rec., *107*:280, 1981.
6. Cummings, J. C., de Lahunta, A., and Winn, S. S.: Acral mutilation and nociceptive loss in English Pointer dogs. Acta Neuropathol., *53*:119, 1981.
7. Duncan, I. D., and Griffiths, I. R.: A new canine sensory neuropathy. *In* Proceedings of the Peripheral Nerve Study Group, Lexington, Ky, 1981.
8. Duncan, I. D., and Griffiths, I. R.: A sensory neuropathy affecting long-haired Dachshund dogs. J. Small Anim. Pract., *23*:381, 1982.
9. Duncan, I. D., Griffiths, I. R., and Munz, M.: The pathology of sensory neuropathy affecting long-haired Dachshund dogs. Acta Neuropathol., *58*:141, 1982.
10. Fletcher, T. F., and Kitchell, R. L.: The lumbar, sacral and coccygeal tactile dermatomes of the dog. J. Comp. Neurol., *128*:171, 1966.
11. Halliwell, R. E. W.: Pathogenesis and treatment of pruritus. J. Am. Vet. Med. Assoc., *164*:793, 1974.
12. Hamey, T., Bromley, R. B., and Woosley, C. N.: Somatic afferent area I and II of dog's cerebral cortex. J. Neurophysiol., *19*:485, 1956.
13. Kennard, M. A.: The course of ascending fibers in the spinal cord of the cat essential to the recognition of painful stimuli. J. Comp. Neurol., *100*:511, 1954.
14. Kerr, F. W. L.: Pain—A central inhibitory balance theory. Mayo Clin. Proc., *50*:658, 1975.
15. Kirk, E. J.: The dermatomes of the sheep. J. Comp. Neurol., *134*:353, 1968.
16. Melzack, R.: The perception of pain. Sci. Am., *204*:41, 1961.
17. Melzack, R., and Wall, P. D.: Pain mechanisms. A new theory. Science, *150*:971, 1965.
18. Pivnik, L.: Zur vergleichenden Problematik einiger akrodystrophischer Neuropathien bei Menschen und Hund. Schweiz. Arch. Neurol. Neurochir. Psychiatr., *112*:365, 1973.
19. Ralston, H. J.: The organization of the substantia gelatinosa Rolandi in the cat lumbosacral spinal cord. Z. Zellforsch. Mikrosk. Anat., *67*:1, 1965.
20. Sanda, A., and Pivnik, L.: Die Zehennehrose bei kurzhaarigen Vorstehhunden. Kleintierpraxis, *9*:76, 1964.
21. Scott, D. W., and Bistner, S. I.: Neurotrophic keratitis in a dog. Vet. Med. Small Anim. Clin., *68*:1120, 1973.
22. Szentágothai, J.: Neuronal and synaptic arrangement in the substantia gelatinosa Rolandi. J. Comp. Neurol., *122*:219, 1964.
23. Terenius, L.: Biomechanical mediators in pain. Triangle, *20*:19, 1980.
24. Zimmerman, M.: Physiologic mechanisms of pain and pain therapy. Triangle, *20*:7, 1981.
25. Kitchell, R. L., Whalen, L. R., Bailey, C. S., and Lohse, C. L. Electrophysiologic studies of cutaneous nerves of the thoracic limb of the dog. Am. J. Vet. Res., *41*:61, 1980.

SMALL ANIMAL SPINAL CORD DISEASE

The objective of this chapter is first to review the method and interpretation of the neurologic examination, which determines the location of the lesion in the spinal cord. Following that, the different kinds of lesions that affect the spinal cord are discussed on a regional basis in general.

NEUROLOGIC EXAMINATION

The complete neurologic examination is described in chapter 21. The components referable to spinal cord function are reviewed here.

There are five parts to the neurologic examination: examination of gait and posture, postural reactions, spinal reflexes, and cranial nerves and sensorium. All are necessary to determine whether a lesion is confined to the spinal cord, and at what level. As indicated in Chapter 4, spinal reflexes require only specific peripheral nerves and the spinal cord segments with which they connect. A postural reaction depends on the same components as the reflex, in addition to the ascending pathways through the white matter of the spinal cord and brain stem to the cerebellum and somesthetic cortex of the cerebrum, and the descending upper motor neuron pathways that return from the cerebrum and the brain stem and comprise spinal cord white matter (lateral and ventral funiculi). These postural reactions test the integrity of nearly the entire peripheral and central nervous systems. By themselves they are relatively nonlocalizing for lesions.

GAIT

In most spinal cord disease the abnormality of the gait and the postural reactions reflect the degree of involvement of the ascending general proprioceptive tract (ataxia) and the descending upper motor neuron tracts (paresis). Determination of the site and degree of hypalgesia or analgesia helps to localize the lesion and to indicate its severity.

The degree of paresis is shown by the ability of the patient to stand, support itself, and walk. With upper motor neuron disease, the earliest sign in the gait may be spasticity, a stiffness in the limbs as the patient walks. Be aware that an animal with severe upper motor neuron paresis with spasticity may be unable to stand, but if placed in a supporting position may extend its limbs and support its weight in a reflex response, although it is unable to move voluntarily. This reflex extensor thrust does not indicate voluntary movement and strength. Ataxia is manifested by a tendency to cross the limbs so that they interfere with one another, to walk on the dorsal surface of the paw, to have a longer stride with a prolonged supporting phase before protraction, to abduct the limb, especially on turns, or to appear mildly hypermetric.

The gait should be examined in a place in which the patient can move freely, unleashed, and the ground surface is not slippery. The floor of many examining rooms is too slippery for adequate evaluation of gait. In some patients with vertebral column injury with spinal cord contusion resulting in paresis and ataxia, moving the patient on a slippery floor may cause it to fall, and further injury may result.

The degree of functional deficit dictates the need for further examination of the animal's strength and coordination. In a patient that is severely tetraparetic, is recumbent and unable to support its weight or move its limbs when weight is borne on them, there is no need for further tests to be performed for postural reactions. A paraplegic patient does not have to be examined for postural reactions in the pelvic limbs, but the thoracic limbs should be examined carefully. Occasionally, a patient with progressive myelitis may present as paraplegic because of an extensive thoracolumbar spinal cord location of the lesion, and also may have an asymmetric thoracic limb gait because of a less severe focus of the lesion in the cervical spinal cord. An early sign in dogs with ascending myelomalacia associated with an acute intervertebral disk extrusion may be a hesitant, stumbling, awkward gait in the thoracic limbs. The severity of pelvic limb weakness is evaluated best by holding the patient suspended at the base of the tail and observing its gait. The degree of pelvic limb strength from thoracolumbar spinal cord lesions in small animals may be graded according to the scheme below.[168]

POSTURAL REACTIONS

Following observation of the gait for strength and coordination the postural reactions can be tested, especially to determine if there are less obvious deficiencies in strength and coordination when the gait appears to be normal.

Wheelbarrowing. The thoracic limbs may be tested by supporting the patient under the abdomen so that the pelvic limbs are off the ground surface, and forcing the patient to walk on its thoracic limbs. The normal animal walks with symmetric movements of both thoracic limbs and the head extended in normal position. Patients with lesions of the peripheral nerves of the thoracic limbs, cervical spinal cord, or brain stem may have asymmetric movements, with stumbling or knuckling over on the dorsum of the paw of the affected limb. Hypermetria occasionally is observed. With more severe lesions in this area that involve the central nervous system, there is a tendency to carry the head flexed with the nose close to and occasionally reaching the ground surface for support. If no deficit is observed, extend the neck while the animal is wheelbarrowed. This sometimes reveals a mild deficit, a tendency to knuckle over on the dorsum of the paw, which was not observed before. This is often helpful in confirming a cervical spinal cord lesion in Great Danes or Doberman pinschers that have a cervical vertebral malformation and show mild pelvic limb paresis and ataxia, but no overt thoracic limb signs.

Hopping—Thoracic Limb. While still supporting the pelvic limbs, hop the animal laterally on one thoracic limb while holding the other off the ground surface so that the entire weight of the body is supported by the limb to be tested. Observe the strength and coordination of the limb. Repeat this on the other thoracic limb and compare the response. Asymmetry occurs with paresis or ataxia. There will be no response in severely affected animals and the animal will collapse on the limb. Abnormalities include a stiff-spastic, awkward response, a tendency to buckle over on the dorsum of the paw, or a delay in the onset of the response. The hopping response should occur as soon as the shoulder is moved over the distal extremity. Hypermetria may occur with general proprioceptive or cerebellar deficits. This is an effective way of determining minor deficits when the gait appears to be

Grade	Sign
0	Absence of purposeful movement—paraplegia
1	Unable to stand to support; slight movement when supported by the tail—severe paraparesis
2	Unable to stand to support; when assisted moves limbs readily but stumbles and falls frequently—moderate paraparesis and ataxia
3	Can stand to support but frequently stumbles and falls—mild paraparesis and ataxia
4	Can stand to support; minimal paraparesis and ataxia
5	Normal strength and coordination

normal, as is the case with contralateral cerebral sensorimotor cortex lesions.

Compare one forelimb response with the other. Do not compare the forelimb with the hindlimb on the same side. The normal pelvic limb response is more stiff and has a wider excursion than the forelimb.

If a dog presents with a grade 0 to 1 spastic paraplegia and a mild asymmetry in the hopping reaction of the thoracic limbs with no other abnormality of their function, this justifies the diagnosis of a multifocal lesion with a major lesion between T3 and L4 and a minor lesion cranial to C5. Canine distemper myelitis is a common cause of this kind of syndrome.

Extensor Postural Thrust. The same sequence of tests can be done on the pelvic limbs. The extensor postural thrust reaction is performed by holding the patient off the ground surface by supporting it caudal to the scapulae and lowering it to the ground surface, and observing the patient extend its pelvic limbs to support its weight. Moving the patient forward and backward in this position tests the symmetry of pelvic limb function, their strength and coordination.

Hopping—Pelvic Limb. Continuing to support the patient by the thorax so that the thoracic limbs are not in contact with the ground surface, one pelvic limb can be held up and the patient forced to hop laterally on the supporting limb. Both pelvic limbs should be tested in this way and the response compared.

Hemistanding and Hemiwalking. The patient's ability to stand and walk on the thoracic and pelvic limbs on one side can be tested by holding the opposite thoracic and pelvic limbs off the ground surface and forcing the patient to walk forward or to the side. These are referred to as the hemistanding and hemiwalking reactions. In animals that are too large to hop on one limb or are not cooperative, the forelimb and hindlimb hopping responses can be observed as the animal is hemiwalked.

A patient with a unilateral lesion of the sensorimotor cortex or internal capsule may have a normal gait, but show deficits in its postural reactions on the side opposite the lesion. Attempts to hemiwalk on the contralateral side are delayed, exaggerated (hypermetric), and spastic, and stumbling may occur. With unilateral cervical spinal cord lesions the limbs on the same side as the lesion show a deficiency in the gait, are unresponsive on postural reaction testing, and unable to support the animal in the hemiwalking reaction.

Placing. Other postural reactions that can be tested include placing with the thoracic limbs. The patient is supported off the ground surface, and its thoracic limbs are brought to the edge of a table or similar surface so that the dorsal surface of the paws makes contact. This test should be performed on both thoracic limbs simultaneously and individually, with and without blindfolding the patient. Vision can compensate for the lack of sense of position when the general proprioceptive system is abnormal. Before a response is considered abnormal, be certain it is deficient regardless of the side from which the animal is held.

Tonic Neck Reaction. The tonic neck reaction involves extension of the head and neck so that the nose is directed dorsally. The normal patient responds by extention of all the joints of both thoracic limbs. A patient with disease of the general proprioceptive system in the cervical spinal nerves, cervical spinal cord, or medulla fails to extend its carpus, or digits, or both, and these joints flex passively so that the weight is borne on the dorsal surface of the paw. The same response may occur if a patient is paretic either as a result of disease of the motor neurons that innervate the thoracic limb, or disease of the white matter of the spinal cord that influences these motor neurons.

Proprioceptive Positioning. Proprioceptive positioning tests this afferent system by determining the patient's ability to recognize when a paw has been flexed so that the weight is borne on its dorsal surface. The normal animal returns the paw to its usual position. In patients with severe paresis, response to this test may be deficient.

SPINAL REFLEXES

Muscle tone and spinal reflexes are evaluated best when the patient is in lateral recumbency and is as relaxed as possible. It is important to test muscle tone, tendon reflexes, and the flexor reflex to noxious stimuli in that order so as to maintain the cooperation of the patient.

Muscle Tone. Muscle tone is evaluated by passive manipulation of each limb individually. The degree of resistance is determined to be less than normal (hypotonic), normal, or greater than normal (hypertonic). The latter condition may be referred to as spasticity. The degree of spasticity varies from a mild increased resistance to passive manipulation to a marked increase that may be "clasp knife" in character. It is referred to as "clasp knife" because as attempts are made to flex a limb, the degree of extension of the limb increases, until suddenly it gives way to complete flexion of the limb without resistance.

Hypotonia usually occurs with lower motor neuron disease, whereas upper motor neuron disease is characterized by hypertonia or spasticity. The functional integrity of the lower motor neuron is necessary to cause muscle cell contraction and to maintain muscle tone. It is also necessary to maintain the normal health of the muscle cell it innervates. When denervated, these cells degenerate. This is observed clinically as neurogenic atrophy, and can be detected electromyographically by the production of abnormal potentials in resting muscle. The upper motor neuron influences the activity of the lower motor neuron to produce voluntary motor activity and to maintain muscle tone for support of the body against gravity. Although the upper motor neuron includes both facilitatory and inhibitory functions on the activity of the lower motor neuron, when the upper motor neuron is diseased the result usually seen is a release of the lower motor neuron to antigravity muscles from inhibition and overactivity of the facilitatory mechanism. This release is observed as hypertonia or spasticity.

Extensor Thrust. With the animal in a nonsupporting position of lateral recumbency, place the palm of the hand against the ventral surface of the paw and exert a sudden mild pressure against the paw. This is a reflex response that evaluates muscle tone, and the function of the femoral nerve and L4-L6 spinal cord segments. The normal animal extends the limb mildly against the hand of the examiner. In some patients with upper motor neuron disease it is extended vigorously against the hand. In patients with lower motor neuron disease there is no response.

Patellar Reflexes. The most reliable tendon reflex is the patellar reflex. It is obtained by lightly tapping the patellar ligament when the patient is in lateral recumbency and is as relaxed as possible for proper evaluation. A neurologic hammer used in pediatric examinations is the most useful instrument, but any hard object such as scissor handles can be used. The reflex can be elicited in all normal dogs, and is mediated by the femoral nerve through the fourth to sixth lumbar spinal cord segments. The degree of normal response varies with the breed. Large breeds of dogs have a brisker reflex than the short-legged breeds such as the dachshund. The response should be evaluated as absent (0), hyporeflexic (plus 1), normal (plus 2), hyperreflexic (plus 3,), or clonic (plus 4). An absent reflex or hyporeflexia occurs when a portion of the reflex arc is diseased. Hyperreflexia or clonus often is present in upper motor neuron disease.

The localizing value of this reflex can be demonstrated by the following example. Examination of an acutely paraplegic dachshund that had normal perineal and flexor reflexes but hypotonia and no patellar reflex suggested an L4 to L6 spinal cord lesion and possible midlumbar (L3-L4) location of an intervertebral disk extrusion.

Biceps and Triceps Reflex. In the thoracic limb the biceps and triceps reflexes can be elicited in many dogs that are relaxed and in lateral recumbency. Lightly tapping the tendon of insertion of the triceps proximal to the olecranon elicits a slight extension of the elbow. The reflex is mediated by the radial nerve through the seventh and eighth cervical and first and second thoracic spinal cord segments. The biceps reflex is elicited by placing a finger on the distal ends of the biceps and brachialis muscles at the level of the elbow. Tapping this finger with the hammer elicits a slight flexion of the elbow. The muscle contraction can be palpated in some instances when no movement of the joint is seen. The musculocutaneous nerve mediates this reflex through the sixth, seventh, and eighth cervical spinal cord segments. The normal patient has a mild reflex response to these stimuli. In some normal patients response is difficult to elicit and appears absent. These reflexes also are absent when there is disease in some portion of the reflex arc, and they may be hyperactive in some patients with disease of the upper motor neuron.

There are other tendon reflexes that can be tested, but similar to the biceps and triceps reflex they are not consistently present in the normal animal. Therefore, their absence is of no clinical significance. Their presence indicates the ability of the components of the reflex arc to function and their hyperactivity may relate to an UMN spinal cord lesion.

Flexor Reflex—Pelvic Limb. The flexor reflexes to painful stimuli determine the integrity of the reflex arc, as well as the pathway in the central nervous system that is concerned with the patient's response to painful stimuli. The most reliable stimulus is pressure exerted on the base of the toenail with hemostats.

Reflex	Nerve	Segments	Test—Response
Extensor carpi radialis	Radial	C7–T2	Tap muscle—extension of carpus
Cranial tibial—digital extensor	Peroneal	L6,L7(S1)	Tap muscle or plantar surface of calcaneus—flexion of tarsus
Common calcanean tendon	Tibial	(L6),L7,S1	Tap calcanean tendon—extension of tarsus

Many animals do not respond to the stimulus of a pin. In the pelvic limb, the flexor reflex is mediated by the sciatic nerve through the sixth and seventh lumbar spinal cord segments and the first sacral segment. Abnormality of the motor portion of the sciatic nerve distal to the pelvis causes paralysis, hypotonia, and atrophy of the flexors of the stifle, tarsus, and digits, as well as of the extensors of the hip, tarsus and digits. There is no resistance to flexion or extension of the paw. The patient can walk with a sciatic nerve paralysis because the hip will flex to advance the limb. On walking with a sciatic nerve paralysis, the tarsus will be lower on the affected side and the paw may be placed on its dorsal surface; however, the limb is able to support weight as long as the femoral nerve is intact.

Sensory branches of the peroneal nerves supply the dorsal surface of the paw (Fig. 9–5). The plantar surface is supplied by sensory branches of the tibial nerve. The medial side of the paw is supplied by the saphenous nerve, a branch of the femoral nerve at the femoral triangle. This enters the spinal cord through the fourth to sixth lumbar segments. A patient may have a contused sciatic nerve from a pelvic fracture and have no function of the muscles innervated by this nerve, and analgesia of the lateral, dorsal, and plantar surfaces of the paw. However, the intact saphenous nerve provides sensation to the medial surface of the paw. If this area is stimulated, the patient will flex the hip with the intact innervation of the iliopsoas muscle, but the stifle, tarsus, and digits will fail to flex. For this reason, both the medial and lateral surfaces of the paw should be tested for reflex response as well as for pain perception.

Pain Perception. The spinal reflex response should not be confused with the perception of pain. In addition to the sensory component of the peripheral nerves and their spinal cord segments, the pain pathway requires the ascending spinothalamic system in the lateral funiculus of the spinal cord, the brain stem, and the related thalamocortical

system. These all must be intact and functional for the normal perception of pain. A dog with a transverse spinal cord lesion at T13 has normal or hyperactive reflexes, but no perception of pain from the pelvic limbs or trunk caudal to the lesion. The patient shows signs of pain when the impulses generated by a noxious stimulus have entered the spinal cord over the peripheral nerves and dorsal roots and are relayed to tracts in the lateral funiculi of the spinal cord bilaterally. These tracts ascend the spinal cord in the lateral funiculi, and continue through the medulla, pons, and mesencephalon to specific nuclei in the thalamus for relay to the somatic sensory cerebral cortex. Pain may be evidenced when the impulses reach the thalamus or cerebrum.

Flexor Reflex—Thoracic Limb. In the thoracic limb the thoracodorsal, axillary, musculocutaneous, radial, median, and ulnar nerves primarily are responsible for flexion of the shoulder, elbow, carpus, and digits when a noxious stimulus is applied to the paw. These arise from the sixth cervical to the second thoracic spinal cord segments. The specific sensory nerve stimulated depends on the location of the stimulus (Fig. 9–4). The median and ulnar nerves innervate the skin of the palmar surface of the paw; the radial nerve supplies the dorsal surface. In the distal forelimb the radial nerve supplies the skin on the cranial and lateral surfaces. The ulnar nerve is the sole cutaneous nerve to a strip on the caudal surface, and the musculocutaneous nerve innervates a strip in the center of the medial surface.

Crossed Extensor Reflex. This reflex is a normal response in a standing animal. As an abnormal reflex it must be evaluated in the recumbent animal. In patients with upper motor neuron disease and release of the lower motor neuron, a crossed extensor reflex may be elicited in the recumbent animal when the flexor reflex is stimulated. This occurs in the limb opposite the one being tested for a flexor reflex. To avoid voluntary extension of the contralateral limb as a response to a noxious stimulus, the flexor reflex first should be elicited with a mild stimulus, and the opposite limb should be observed for extension. This reflex often is difficult to interpret in a patient that still has some voluntary movement of the limbs. It is an abnormal reflex, indicative of upper motor neuron disease when it is elicited in a patient in lateral recumbency. It has not proved useful in determining the prognosis of spinal cord lesions.

Perineal Reflex. The perineal reflex is elicited by stimulating the anus with a mild noxious stimulus, and observing contraction of the anal sphincter and flexion of the tail. It is mediated by branches of the sacral and caudal nerves through the sacral and caudal segments of the spinal cord.

Cutaneous Trunci Reflex. This reflex can be used to test the function of a considerable length of the spinal cord. Cutaneous stimulation along the thoracolumbar region will often elicit a twitching of the skin. The skin twitching is due to contraction of the cutaneous trunci, which is innervated by the lateral thoracic nerve from spinal cord segments C8 or T1. The sensory nerves involved are those that supply the specific segmental area of skin being stimulated. The impulses generated in these sensory neurons enter the spinal cord segment at the level of the stimulation. The impulses are transmitted cranially through the spinal cord white matter, probably via fasciculus proprius, to the C8 or T1 spinal cord segment, where synapse occurs on the lower motor neuron cell bodies of the lateral thoracic nerve. Stimulation of the skin on one side will elicit a bilateral response.

Two precautions are necessary. Some animals require numerous vigorous stimulations of the skin to elicit this response, and it may be absent in a few normal animals. In some animals it cannot be elicited from skin stimulation caudal to the L4 or L5 level of the vertebral column.

The reflex is most helpful in determining involvement of the grey matter or roots or spinal nerves of C8 and T1. In a complete brachial plexus avulsion this reflex will be absent on the side of the avulsion. Some very stoic dogs will not respond to noxious stimuli to allow you to determine a line of hypalgesia or analgesia associated with a serious thoracolumbar spinal cord lesion. The cutaneous trunci reflex will permit the same line to be determined because of the component of the reflex that must pass cranially through the spinal cord. In an animal with a transverse spinal cord lesion at T13, the cutaneous trunci reflex will be absent caudal to about the L1 to L2 vertebral level and will be intact cranial to this level.

CRANIAL NERVES

In evaluating spinal cord disease, the examination of cranial nerves is useful to exclude or implicate diffuse or multifocal lesions in an animal that presents with the signs of spinal cord disease. On examining the eyes, signs of a sympathetic paralysis (Horner's syndrome) may correlate directly with the location of a spinal cord lesion in the first three thoracic spinal cord segments, or with an unusually acute severe cervical spinal cord lesion that interferes with the lateral tectotegmentospinal system.

SUMMARY OF SIGNS WITH LESIONS AT SPECIFIC LOCATIONS IN THE SPINAL CORD (Fig. 10–1)

Lumbosacral: Fourth Lumbar to Fifth Caudal Segment

Complete malacia from fourth lumbar through fifth caudal segments:
Flaccid paraplegia: no support, gait, or movement of pelvic limbs and tail. Normal thoracic limbs.
No postural reactions in pelvic limbs.
Areflexia: flexor, patellar, perineal reflexes.
Atonia: soft muscles, no resistance to manipulation of pelvic limbs or tail.
Neurogenic atrophy: in chronic lesions.
Dilated anus.
Analgesia from pelvic limbs, tail, and perineum.
Partial malacia of gray and white matter between the fourth lumbar and fifth caudal segments:
Flaccid paraparesis and ataxia of pelvic limbs with normal thoracic limbs.
Postural reactions of pelvic limbs attempted, but poorly accomplished.
Hyporeflexia or areflexia: flexor and patellar reflexes.
Hypotonia: normal or weak resistance to manipulation of pelvic limbs.
Slight neurogenic atrophy: in chronic lesions.
Normal or depressed pain perception (hy-

REGIONAL NEUROLOGIC SIGNS IN SPINAL CORD DISEASE

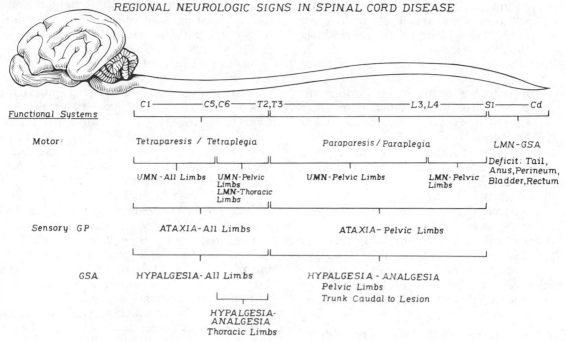

Figure 10–1.   Regional neurologic signs in spinal cord disease.

palgesia) from pelvic limbs, tail, and perineum.

Thoracolumbar: Third Thoracic to Third Lumbar Segment

Complete malacia—focal site between third thoracic and third lumbar segments:

Spastic paraplegia: no voluntary support, gait, or movement of pelvic limbs. Normal thoracic limbs. With acute lesions the thoracic limbs may be spastic (Schiff-Sherrington syndrome). With cranial thoracic lesions, there may be more difficulty in standing up on the thoracic limbs from a recumbent position, and loss of trunk support may also be observed when the patient is walked on the thoracic limbs with the pelvic limbs supported by the tail. The trunk may sway to the side abnormally.

No postural reactions in pelvic limbs.

Reflexes normal or hyperactive: flexor and patellar.

Crossed extensor reflex may occur.

Muscle tone normal or hypertonic, no atrophy.

Analgesia from area caudal to the lesion.

Partial malacia—focal site between third thoracic and third lumbar segments:

Spastic paraparesis and ataxia of pelvic limbs with normal thoracic limbs.

All postural reactions poorly performed in pelvic limbs.

Reflexes normal or hyperactive: flexor and patellar.

Crossed extensor reflex may occur.

Muscle tone normal or hypertonic, no atrophy.

Pain perception normal or depressed from area caudal to the lesion.

Note: Lesions confined to the white matter from L4 to L6 or L7 may produce the same signs.

Caudal Cervical: Fifth Cervical to Second Thoracic Segment

Partial malacia of gray and white matter between fifth cervical and second thoracic segments:

Tetraparesis and ataxia of all four limbs, with the thoracic limb deficit sometimes worse than that of the pelvic limb, or tetraplegia, with the patient in lateral recumbency. Lesions confined to the white matter at this level usually cause more abnormality in the pelvic limbs than thoracic limbs.

Thoracic limbs: hyporeflexic or areflexic; normal tone or hypotonic; neurogenic atrophy if a chronic lesion. Lesions confined to the white matter at this level cause hypertonia, hyperreflexia, and no atrophy.

Pelvic limbs: normal reflexes or hyperreflexia; normal tone or hypertonia; no atrophy.

Pain perception: normal or depressed from all four limbs, or depressed from thoracic limbs only.

All postural reactions poorly performed with the thoracic limb function sometimes worse than that of the pelvic limb.

Miosis, protruded third eyelid, ptosis, and enophthalmos (T1-T3 lesion).

Cranial Cervical: First Cervical to Fifth Cervical Segment

Partial malacia—focal site between first and fifth cervical segments:

Spastic tetraplegia with patient in lateral recumbency: (1) No postural reactions present. (2) Reflexes normal or hyperactive in all four limbs. (3) Crossed extensor reflexes may occur. (4) Muscle tone usually hypertonic, occasionally normal. (5) Hypalgesia from area caudal to the lesion.

Spastic tetraparesis and ataxia of all four limbs. The deficit in the pelvic limbs is often worse than in the thoracic limbs. Occasionally, the opposite is found. (1) Postural reactions poorly performed. (2) Reflexes normal or hyperactive. (3) Crossed extensor reflexes may occur. (4) Muscle tone usually hypertonic, occasionally normal. (5) Pain perception normal or depressed from area caudal to the lesion.

Dogs with cervical spinal cord disease that have a significantly worse abnormality in the forelimbs compared to the hind limbs usually have two possible locations for lesions. Extensive lesions in the cervical intumescence with grey matter involvement cause hypotonic hyporeflexic thoracic limbs and more severe thoracic limb deficit. An extramedullary lesion that compresses the central region of any segment of the cervical spinal cord from a ventral midline site has also been observed with this disparity in limb abnormality. Most commonly these are midline intervertebral disk extrusions, less commonly atlantoaxial subluxations

or neoplasms. The spinal cord is "tented" over the compressing mass which apparently interferes more with the medially situated upper motor neurons to the cervical intumescence.

Bladder dysfunction often accompanies severe spinal cord disease. Total lower motor neuron paralysis occurs with sacral spinal cord lesions. Severe or total focal thoracolumbar spinal cord lesions produce an upper motor neuron type of paralysis. Paralysis is less common with cervical spinal cord lesions, unless the lesion is severe. With both LMN and UMN paralysis, retention of urine occurs. Overflow takes place with both, but is more constant with lower motor neuron disease. It is less frequent in UMN disease because greater intraluminal pressure is required to overcome the tone in the striated urethral muscle. If the integrity of the bladder wall is retained, reflex urination may follow within a variable period of time. Reflex urination is more efficient in upper motor neuron disease, utilizing the intact peripheral nerves and sacral spinal cord segments. In lower motor neuron disease this must be mediated within the wall of the bladder and is very inefficient.

SPINAL CORD DISEASE IN SMALL ANIMALS

For each of the following regions of the spinal cord where lesions are located, the diseases are organized by the kind of lesions that occur in the spinal cord: injury, inflammation, degeneration, neoplasia, or malformation. This follows the procedure that should be adhered to in clinical neurology of first making an anatomic diagnosis and then considering the various kinds of lesions that could occur in that anatomic area. The selection of the kinds of lesions will be determined by the signalment of the patient and the history of the onset and course of the disease.

LUMBOSACRAL SPINAL CORD DISEASE (L4-Cd)

Some examples of lumbosacral spinal cord disease already have been considered in Chapter 4 on lower motor neuron disease.

Trauma

External Injury. Fracture with displacement of L7 is a common injury which usually produces total paralysis of the tail, anus, perineum, bladder, and rectum. The degree of pelvic limb paresis and ataxia depends on the degree of involvement of the lumbar roots and nerves. If both the L6 and L7 spinal nerves are compromised on the cranial and caudal aspects of the fractured vertebra, in addition to the S1 roots coursing through the L7 vertebral foramen, there is a complete sciatic nerve paralysis, unilateral or bilateral. The flexor reflex is absent from the stifle, tarsus, and digits, but hip flexion and the patellar reflex are preserved. There is analgesia of the dorsal, lateral, and plantar surfaces of the hind paw, but not of the medial surface (femoral, saphenous nerves, L4-L6 roots).

If the trauma from the accident is severe, hemorrhage and necrosis may occur in the spinal cord segments cranial to the site of the fracture and produce more extensive signs with paraplegia with atonia, areflexia, and analgesia of the pelvic limbs, perineum, anus, and tail.

There is a better prognosis for direct injury to the spinal roots and nerves than for injury to spinal cord segments. Spinal roots are more resistant to injury because of their structure, and they tend to recover more often following contusion, and even can regenerate if necessary. For these reasons, although vertebral canal displacement may be severe with an L7 fracture and luxation, the prospect for recovery is not hopeless. The most serious impediment to functional recovery of the house pet is the delay or lack of recovery of bladder function. Contusion of the sacral nerves in the L7 foramen produces LMN bladder paralysis with incontinence. Decompression should be considered as an aid to this recovery.

Internal Injury. Intervertebral disk extrusions in the middle and caudal lumbar vertebral column are not common but do occur. Their location is predicted by the nature of the lower motor neuron signs they produce and by the paresis, ataxia, or paralysis of the gait. An L3-L4 extrusion often produces a loss of the patellar reflex because of involvement of the adjacent L4 to L6 spinal cord segments. If L6 and L7 are spared, the flexor reflex is preserved. An L4-L5 or L5-L6 extrusion produces loss of the flexor reflex. At the L4-L5 articulation, the spinal cord segments L6, L7, and S1 are vulnerable. At the L5-L6 articulation the roots of these segments are vulnerable. Decreased or absent anal and tail tone and perineal reflex, along with lower motor neuron bladder paralysis, accompany extrusions at or caudal to the L5-L6 articulation.

Similarly, other forms of space-occupying lesions can be located in this region of the spinal cord. The following case report is a typical example.

Signalment. An 8-year old male Weimaraner.

Chief Complaint. The patient had lumbar pain and pelvic limb dysfunction.

History. Two and one-half weeks prior to referral, this dog was presented to a veterinarian with the complaint of an arched back and soreness in this area. The signs persisted without a definite diagnosis. One week prior to referral, soreness during examination was noticed in the right pelvic limb. Neurologic signs were first evident to the owner 3 days before presentation, and consisted of paresis, ataxia, or both, of the right pelvic limb. These signs had progressed by the time of the referral examination.

Physical Examination. The dog was an alert, aggressive patient with normal thoracic limb function. The pelvic limbs were paretic and ataxic, especially the right one. It frequently was placed on its dorsal surface, crossed under the body, or abducted widely. When bearing weight, the right tarsus was closer to the floor than the left tarsus. Occasionally, the limbs only partially supported the caudal trunk. If weight was added to the pelvis by manual pressure, the pelvic limbs could not support the body owing to paresis.

Postural reactions were most deficient in the right pelvic limb. Hopping and proprioceptive positioning were performed poorly on the right and showed a fair but not normal response on the left. Muscle tone was moderately hypotonic in the right pelvic limb, and slightly hypotonic to normal in the left pelvic limb. The tail was hypotonic. The anus showed only equivocal hypotonia. Atrophy was evident in the right caudal thigh muscles and all the right leg muscles. The right pelvic limb flexor reflex was depressed markedly. Pain was perceived and the hip flexed, but stifle, tarsal, and digital flexion were absent. On striking the patellar ligament some contraction was observed in the quadriceps muscle, but the only action seen was hip flexion. In the left pelvic limb the patellar reflex was plus 1 to 2. The flexor reflex was intact but slightly depressed. Pain perception was normal. Pressure applied to the spines of the vertebrae elicited pain from the caudal lumbar and sacral vertebrae. Brisk extension of the tail elicited pain.

Anatomic Diagnosis. The lesion predominantly involved the spinal cord segments, roots, or spinal nerves L6, L7, S1-S3, and caudal primarily on the right side. The site of pain on vertebral manipulation suggested a vertebral or root lesion.

Laboratory Findings: CSF. Cisternal CSF examination revealed 93 mg of protein per dl and no WBC. Plain radiography showed no lesion.

Myelography. It was not possible to enter the subarachnoid space between L5 and L6. Radiopaque dye was introduced between L4 and L5. The dye column caudal to the injection site stopped abruptly over the caudal end of the body of L5. CSF from the L4-L5 tapping site contained 430 mg of protein per dl and no WBC.

Surgery. A laminectomy at L5, L6, and L7 revealed an elongate mass in the epidural space between the laminae on the right side and the spinal cord, which was compressed dorsolaterally to the left. The right roots and spinal nerves from L5 caudally were compressed ventrally. The mass was dissected free of the neural structures and removed. It was not attached to the meninges of the spinal cord or the roots. It was diagnosed as a fibrosarcoma.

Outcome. The dog improved mildly in a few weeks, then remained stable for about 8 months, when the same signs appeared again. Euthanasia then was performed.

Inflammation (see Chapter 4)

Rabies encephalomyelitis in all species.
Canine distemper myelitis.
Toxoplasma myelitis in dogs and cats.
Feline infectious peritonitis focal myelitis in cats.

Degeneration (see Chapter 4)

Embolic myelopathy: fibrocartilaginous.
Diffuse myelomalacia.
Hereditary abiotrophy: Swedish Lapland dog.

Neoplasia

Intramedullary. Spinal cord gliomas or metastases to the parenchyma are uncommon. Diagnosis requires myelography.
Extramedullary. See trauma and case report in the preceding section.

Malformation (see Chapter 2)

Myelodysplasia and meningomyelocele commonly are associated with spina bifida of the caudal lumbar or sacral vertebrae. Segmental hypoplasia may isolate sacral and caudal segments, producing analgesia. As a rule, the malformation does not interfere enough with grey matter morphology to cause lower motor neuron signs. The pelvic limb gait may be ataxic and weak. Although all individuals are susceptible, this malformation is found more commonly in Manx cats and English bulldogs.[32]

THORACOLUMBAR SPINAL CORD DISEASE (T3-L3)

Trauma

External Injury. External injuries most often are caused by automobiles, gunshot wounds, and wounds acquired while fighting. Characteristically, such spinal cord trauma is sudden in onset, usually immediately related to the time of the accident, but occasionally it may follow the accident by a few hours. It generally is nonprogressive; however, it may progress within the first 24 hours post trauma, and only in the second 24 hours post trauma if there is continual bleeding or excessive movement at the site of the vertebral column injury with continued trauma to the spinal cord. Following this, the signs remain stable or improve.

Most fractures in this region occur at the thoracolumbar junction, but they can occur at any level. They vary in type and degree of subluxation. Be aware that the radiograph can determine only the degree of subluxation present at that time. It may have been far worse at the time of the injury, but immediately returned to a normal position. Always examine the radiograph for the size of the intervertebral disks. They often are extruded with external injury, and their normal location is reduced in size. In fact, a narrow space between two vertebrae may be the only evidence of an external injury, and be diagnostic for an acutely extruded intervertebral disk. Sometimes slight subluxation of an adjacent vertebra or a small chip fracture may accompany the intervertebral disk extrusion. Occasionally the external injury causes spinal cord contusion without vertebral column injury.

Be sure to evaluate radiographically all of the vertebral column where spinal cord injury could explain the clinical signs. There may be more than one fracture that could produce these signs. Remember that lower motor neuron signs will mask an associated upper motor neuron lesion. A caudal lumbar fracture could produce lower motor neuron signs which would not permit observation of an upper motor neuron lesion from another, more cranially located fracture and spinal cord injury.

Sudden complete compression of the thoracolumbar spinal cord causes paralysis of all the muscles caudal to the lesion and analgesia of the skin. Unlike incomplete, subacute, or chronic spinal cord lesions in this region, a specific syndrome of muscle tone and reflexes accompanies the paraplegia observed in these acute complete lesions. This is referred to as the Schiff-Sherrington syndrome. Although the lesion is caudal to T2, there is rigid extension of the thoracic limbs. However, they still function normally but with stiffness in the postural reactions and all efforts of voluntary movement. Despite the fact that the paralysis is caused by direct interference with the upper motor neuron, there is remarkable hypotonia of the pelvic limbs. However, all spinal reflexes caudal to the lesion are normal. The level of the lesion can be determined best by locating a line of analgesia, or the level of detection of the cutaneous trunci reflex, or both. This line usually is caudal to the spinal cord lesion by one to two spinal cord segments because of the caudal distribution of the cutaneous branches of the spinal nerves after they emerge from the intervertebral foramina.

The term Schiff-Sherrington syndrome has been applied to the clinical phenomenon of thoracic limb extensor hypertonia associated with paraplegia from acute thoracolumbar spinal cord lesions in dogs. It is rarely observed in other domestic animals.[146, 147] It is explained by the fact that there are neurons located in the lumbar spinal cord that are responsible for the tonic inhibition of extensor muscle alpha motoneurons in the cervical intumescence. These inhibitory neurons are called "border cells," and their cell bodies are located on the dorsolateral border of the ventral grey column from L1 through L7, with a maximal population from L2 through L4.[160] Their axons cross to the contralateral fasciculus proprius of the lateral funiculus, where they ascend to their termination in the cervical intumescence. Acute severe lesions cranial to these "border cell" neurons and caudal to the cervical intumescence that suddenly deprive the cervical intumescence neurons of this source of tonic inhibition cause a "release" of these latter neurons. This results in the extensor hypertonia observed in the thoracic limbs. There is no compromise of the descending upper motor neuron system to the cervical intumescence and therefore the thoracic limbs can function normally in the gait and postural reactions, except for the hypertonia.

In primates such acute spinal cord lesions cause spinal cord shock caudal to the lesion. This is a physiologic phenomenon that severely depresses lower motor neuron function of all the spinal cord segments caudal to the site of the morphologic lesion. It results in complete atonia and areflexia caudal to the lesion, which

persists for 2 to 3 weeks. This phenomenon may result from the functional disturbance caused by the sudden widespread disorganization that occurs on the dendritic zone and cell body of the general somatic efferent motor neuron.[82] This is produced by the degeneration of telodendria of the efferent spinal cord neurons that were interrupted by the lesion.

Spinal shock in domestic animals is of much less magnitude and is of little clinical significance. Spinal reflexes usually are present caudal to the lesion by the time the veterinarian observes the injured patient. They may be absent for 30 to 60 minutes after the injury. If you examine the patient that soon after an injury, be sure to reevaluate the patient 1 to 2 hours later before determining the location and extent of the lesion. Possibly, the hypotonia that persists in the pelvic limbs is attributable to spinal shock, but the degree of lower motor neuron depression is not sufficient to interfere with the spinal reflexes except transiently. This species difference in the phenomenon of spinal shock may be due to the fact that fewer spinal cord efferent neurons synapse directly on the GSE motoneuron in domestic animals, and thus less direct synaptic disorganization occurs. Pelvic limb hypotonia and thoracic limb hypertonia usually disappear in 10 to 14 days after the onset of neurologic signs. Normal to increased tone appears in the pelvic limbs, along with hyperreflexia.

Although the Schiff-Sherrington syndrome indicates severe spinal cord dysfunction and a cautious prognosis, it does not imply that no recovery can occur. It does not signify the degree of morphologic disturbance at the site of the spinal cord injury. Some recovery may follow the resolution of spinal cord hemorrhage and edema, and remyelination of intact axons.

Whenever the possibility exists that a patient has a vertebral column injury, the area should not be handled more than necessary. As a rule, the location of these injuries can be found with minimal manipulation of the patient. The entire examination can be performed with the animal in lateral recumbency. To determine whether the thoracic limb hypertonia represents the Schiff-Sherrington phenomenon or is due to a cervical spinal cord injury, minimal stimulation of the forepaws with a pin or mild pressure with forceps readily determines if pain and voluntary movement are present. In the Schiff-Sherrington syndrome they are present in the thoracic limbs but absent in the pelvic limbs. With cervical spinal cord injuries, there is more equal tone and deficit in pain and voluntary movement in all four limbs.

Therapy should be prompt and vigorous (see Chapter 20).[112, 148] Corticosteroids and the hypertonic solution mannitol are usually used to reduce spinal cord edema. Intravenous dimethyl sulfoxide (40 per cent, 1 gm per kg) has been proposed for treatment of these injuries because of its membrane-stabilizing and oxygen-sparing effects on tissues.[36] The results of experimental studies have been variable.[136] It may be most effective when combined with surgical decompression and myelotomy. No clinical trials are available. Surgery usually involves decompression, normothermic or hypothermic lavage, occasionally myelotomy, vertebral reduction, and immobilization. There may be a discrepancy between the degree of vertebral column and spinal cord injuries. In most instances it is not possible to judge the severity of the spinal cord injury by the degree of displacement of the vertebrae, and it is dangerous to give a prognosis based solely on the degree of subluxation observed on radiographs. Some patients that appeared hopeless radiographically have made some recovery.

Currently extensive research is being performed on the pathophysiology of spinal cord injury.[122, 188] A posttraumatic progressive hemorrhagic necrosis has been recognized that is related to local hypoxia from direct vascular injury, or the accumulation of toxic amounts of neurotransmitter amines that cause further vasoconstriction and tissue damage, or both. Surgical and medical treatments for this condition are being studied.

Progression of neurologic signs following an external injury may relate to this progressive autodestruction of the spinal cord. This is usually limited to the segments immediately adjacent to the vertebral injury. Rarely does this progress into extensive ascending-descending myelomalacia.

Progression beyond 24 hours may be due to continual bleeding from an internal vertebral venous plexus producing an expanding compressive extradural hematoma. An excessively active patient may continually contuse the spinal cord at the site of the injury where vertebral stability may be compromised.

Internal Injury. Numerous lesions can slowly or suddenly occupy space in the vertebral canal and injure the spinal cord by compression. These are referred to as internal injuries, and usually are not associated with any source of external trauma.

INTERVERTEBRAL DISK DISEASE.[45, 61, 67, 76, 137, 169] Intervertebral disk protrusion-extrusion occurs in all breeds of dogs. It is most common in the chondrodystrophic breeds (dachshund, Pekingese, French bulldog, beagle), and it can occur in these breeds at a young age.[14, 141] This is related to the early spontaneous degeneration of the intervertebral disks that takes place in these breeds. The incidence of this disease in dachshunds is estimated at 19 per cent. Within this breed a higher incidence occurs in lines in which a hereditary basis is proposed.[7] This genetic model involves the cumulative effect of several genes with no sex linkage and is subject to environmental modification. The average age of clinically affected dogs is 5 years. However, the occurrence of this neurologic syndrome at 3 years of age is common, and occasionally it appears at 2 years. If the dog is less than 1 year old with thoracolumbar signs, you should look for another cause. The incidence is also high in the Welsh corgi, Lhasa apso, Shih Tzu, miniature poodles, and cocker spaniels. It is found occasionally in other breeds (nonchondrodystrophic) associated with aging, and therefore generally is not observed before about 4 to 5 years of age.

The nature and the time of onset of the intervertebral disk degeneration differs between the chondrodystrophic and nonchondrodystrophic breeds.[59] A chondroid metamorphosis occurs in chondrodystrophic breeds with replacement of the nucleus pulposus with hyalin cartilage. This often begins prior to 1 year-of-age, which accounts for the earlier age of onset of extrusions in these breeds. This chondroid change precedes calcification. A fibroid metamorphosis occurs in nonchondrodystrophic breeds with gradual replacement of the nucleus pulposus by collagenous tissue. This starts at a later age, 4 to 5 years or older, and progresses slowly.

Although intervertebral disk protrusions are fairly common in the older adult cat, compressive myelopathy with clinical signs is rare.[87, 156] In one necropsy study, dorsal protrusions were most common in the cervical region and especially at C2-C3. The thoracolumbar junction was not commonly involved.

Studies have shown that about 80 per cent of thoracolumbar intervertebral disk protrusions-extrusions in dogs occur between T11 and L3. On radiographs these may be evident on the floor of the vertebral canal if they are calcified, or their protrusion-extrusion may be indicated by the narrowing of the intervertebral disk space that prolapsed its nuclear contents. It may be necessary to use myelography to demonstrate the lesion.[118] Intervertebral disk protrusions and extrusions are rare in thoracic vertebrae cranial to T10, probably because of the intercapital ligament that passes between rib heads dorsal to the anulus fibrosus. One study on vertebral mobility in the dog showed that the most movement occurred at the lumbosacral articulation followed by the L6-L7 articulation.[15] No differences were found between chondrodystrophic and nonchondrodystrophic breeds.

Intervertebral disk protrusion is defined as dorsal bulging of the anulus fibrosus and dorsal longitudinal ligament without rupture and release of degenerate nuclear material on the floor of the vertebral canal (Hansen's type II). Extrusion of the intervertebral disk involves rupture of the anulus fibrosus and release of degenerate nucleus pulposus in the vertebral canal (Hansen's type I). Extrusions are more commonly associated with focal myelopathy and clinical signs.

These protrusions or extrusions produce varying degrees of an ischemic myelopathy in the spinal cord by interfering with the circulation of blood through the parenchyma. Most slow or mild compressions result in some degree of demyelination and axonal degeneration. Sudden large extrusions may produce focal hemorrhage and necrosis in the grey and white matter. There is no evidence of a myelitis other than the normal vascular response to the tissue damage..

The signs caused by the extrusion vary from pain without neurologic deficit, to mild paraparesis and ataxia, to severe paraparesis and ataxia, to paraplegia with pain response intact, to paraplegia with pain response absent. The pain associated with these intervertebral disk lesions may not represent direct meningeal involvement, but may result from the disruption of the periosteum, anulus fibrosus and dorsal longitudinal ligament associated with the protrusion or extrusion. These structures are innervated by general somatic afferent neurons. Additionally lateral extrusions that entrap spinal nerves may be a common cause of pain without other signs of parenchymal involvement.

In mildly affected patients it may be impossible to distinguish between paresis and ataxia, but this is not important in establishing the location of the lesion and providing a prognosis. In all patients spinal reflexes are intact. In most patients they are hyperactive, and

hypertonia is evident on manipulation of the limbs. These are the classic signs of upper motor neuron disease. Occasionally, hypotonia occurs without other signs of lower motor neuron disease. Pain sensation (general somatic afferent-spinothalamic pathway) is almost always intact in paraparetic patients. Paraplegic animals with pain sensation have a better prognosis than those in whom there is no cerebral response to an unequivocal noxious stimulus, such as forceps pressed on the base of the toenail. In the latter patients, it is helpful to establish the line of analgesia by pinching the skin with forceps along the ventral abdomen and along the dorsum of the vertebral column. Keep in mind the caudoventral course of the caudal thoracic and lumbar nerves across the abdomen. The dorsal branches of the thoracolumbar spinal nerves also course caudally, which accounts for the line of analgesia being caudal to the site of the lesion by one to two segments. The level of detection of the cutaneous trunci reflex may be interpreted similarly.

It is the responsiblity of the examiner to establish the degree of paresis, spinal reflex function, and cerebral response to pain in order to establish a prognosis and select a course of therapy.

In some instances lumbar intervertebral disk extrusions cause a necrosis in a number of segments without developing into progressive myelomalacia. When the examiner can establish from indications of loss of lower motor neuron function that extensive grey matter necrosis has occurred, the prognosis is poor and surgery usually is not warranted.

The degree of paraparesis and ataxia should be graded according to a scheme such as the one described in the examination portion of this chapter. This permits the clinician to follow the course of the patient to greater advantage.

Therapeutic procedures are varied and include rest with and without administration of corticosteroids and muscle relaxants, fenestration (surgical removal of degenerate nucleus pulposus), and a procedure for removal of the vertebral arches to decompress the spinal cord with removal of the extruded intervertebral disk material. The latter is called a dorsal decompressive laminectomy or hemilaminectomy. A ventral decompressive procedure may be used on cervical intervertebral disk protrusions-extrusions. The therapeutic procedure selected depends on the duration and the extent of the clinical signs, the past medical and surgical history of the patient, and the experience and expertise of the examining clinician.[17, 46, 53, 75, 138, 158, 159, 164, 189] Decompressive laminectomy is indicated in the paraplegic patient. The shorter the duration of signs before surgery, the better is the prognosis. If pain sensation is still intact in the paraplegic patient, the prognosis is better. However, in some patients improvement has occurred following delayed decompression of dogs with paraplegia and analgesia. There are numerous descriptions of the surgical procedures applicable to this disease.[47-50, 102, 169, 170] Each surgeon has established guidelines for the selection of the form of therapy, if any, to be employed. Considerable variation exists in these guidelines, although in many cases the experimental work of Tarlov has served as a basis.[164]

The following patient description exemplifies the value of a thorough neurologic evaluation of the patient prior to the recommendation of therapy.

Signalment. A 4-year-old female dachshund.

History. Four days prior to admission, the owner noticed that the dog's gait in the hindlimbs was stiff and the dog appeared to be in pain. One day later, the patient became paralyzed completely in the hindlimbs. Hyperesthesia was evident over the caudal thoracic vertebrae.

Physical Examination. On the day of examination the animal was alert and responsive. The patient lay in lateral recumbency and attempted to bite anyone who handled it. It seemed to be in severe pain. When placed on the ground in a supporting position, it showed no voluntary movement of the pelvic limbs (grade 0 paraplegia). It readily wheelbarrowed, but the gait with the thoracic limbs was asymmetric. There was some awkwardness in the use of the thoracic limbs; there was a short stride in the left forelimb, and occasionally the dog had difficulty keeping the head elevated and the nose dropped toward the floor.

Spinal Reflexes. The flexor, patellar, and perineal reflexes all were intact. The patellar reflex was hyperactive (plus 3). There was a slightly increased resistance to passive manipulation of the pelvic limbs. No atrophy was evident. No pain was elicited when the digits were compressed.

The thoracic limbs evidenced marked increased resistance to manipulation. Flexor reflexes were intact and pain was perceived.

Postural Reactions. No postural reactions were present in the pelvic limbs. There was a variable response in the thoracic limbs, but often abnormal, to placing, hopping, and the tonic neck tests.

The abdominal muscles were completely flaccid. No intercostal muscle activity was evident. Respirations were predominantly diaphragmatic. Analgesia was apparent in the tail, anus, pelvic limbs, abdomen, and thorax up to the thoracic inlet. In the thoracic limbs and cranial to the thoracic inlet, pain was perceived. There was no cutaneous trunci reflex or local mass reflex along the thoracic and lumbar epaxial region.

Cranial Nerves. Cranial nerve examination was unremarkable except for the pupils. Considering the excited state of the dog, they both seemed smaller than normal. The third eyelids were prominent but not fully protruded.

Anatomic Diagnosis: This is a diffuse lesion from the cranial lumbar through the cranial thoracic spinal cord segments. The grade 0 paraplegia with functional thoracic limbs, despite their mild abnormality, must be explained by an extensive spinal cord lesion caudal to T2. The increased tone and reflexes in the pelvic limbs places the lesion cranial to L4. The line of analgesia indicated that the transverse spinal cord dysfunction was located in the cranial thoracic area.

The abnormal gait and postural reactions in the thoracic limbs suggested a lesion of mild nature in the cervical spinal cord. The partial bilateral Horner's syndrome indicated involvement of the cranial thoracic segments. The lack of intercostal muscle activity and obvious diaphragmatic respirations suggested that these muscles were denervated by a diffuse thoracic spinal cord grey matter lesion, leaving only the phrenic nerves (cervical spinal cord segments 5, 6, and 7) for the control of respirations. The abdominal muscle atonia indicated denervation of these muscles by a caudal thoracic and cranial lumbar spinal cord grey matter lesion. The denervation of intercostal and abdominal muscles thus suggested a diffuse lower motor neuron lesion in the thoracic spinal cord.

Differential Diagnosis. Diffuse myelomalacia from the cranial lumbar segments to the cranial thoracic segments. In this instance, the progressive myelomalacia spared the lumbosacral intumescence. These extensive lesions are most often related to an acute intervertebral disk extrusion.

Ancillary Procedures. Radiographs demonstrated a narrow intervertebral disk between disk segments T12 and T13. Cerebrospinal fluid from the cerebellomedullary cistern contained 60 mg of protein per dl, many neutrophils, and some mononuclear cells and erythrocytes.

Prognosis. There is no therapy available for a spinal cord lesion of this nature as extensive as these signs suggest.[62] Euthanasia was recommended.

Necropsy. At necropsy there was extrusion of the T12-T13 intervertebral disk. The spinal cord was discolored grossly and soft from L3 to C8. On transverse section, total malacia of the segments from L3 to T3 was found, with partial sparing of the first two thoracic and caudal cervical segments. The segments caudal to L3 were normal.

NEOPLASIA. Extradural and intradural extramedullary neoplasms compress the spinal cord and produce an ischemic myelopathy.[2, 13, 27, 30, 70, 73, 113, 120, 129, 165, 172, 173, 178, 181, 183] An intradural extramedullary neoplasm is one that is contained within the dura, but is primarily outside the spinal cord parenchyma. In this position it usually displaces and compresses the spinal cord parenchyma, and only occasionally does it infiltrate the spinal cord.

In dogs neurofibromas commonly are intradural, but occasionally they are found in the epidural space. Meningiomas and metastatic choroid plexus carcinomas usually are intradural. A neuroepithelioma occurs intradurally in young dogs. In cats of all ages the most common spinal cord neoplasm is lymphosarcoma.[119, 151] It usually is extradural in the epidural space and rarely invades the vertebra.[119] Occasionally, it is found intradurally. The same neoplasm occurs extradurally in dogs, but is less common. Meningiomas also occur intradurally in cats. Most metastatic neoplasms are extradural.[21, 106]

These extramedullary neoplasms typically produce a progressive neurologic disability. Although sometimes slow in onset and progression, it is common for the clinical signs to come on fairly suddenly and progress rapidly. From retrospective study of necropsied cases it would appear that some of these masses may grow slowly for a considerable period of time, with the spinal cord adapting to the compression. The onset of neurologic signs may represent the critical point when the compression interferes with the spinal cord circulation, rapidly resulting in lesions and clinical signs. It is astounding to observe at necropsy how severe a compression there is in an animal that was still ambulatory. The adaptation of the spinal cord to compression that is produced slowly appears to be phenomenal, whereas sudden compression produces a devastating effect on spinal cord structure and function. The general anesthesia used to obtain radiographs and for myelography may be responsible for a sudden deterioration in spinal cord function that may occasionally accompany this procedure. This could be explained by the temporary decrease in cardiac outflow, preventing sufficient blood supply to the critical area of the spinal cord that is under compression.

Neoplasms often are located laterally, and therefore it is common for the neurologic signs to be asymmetric, at least at the onset of the observed disability. The paresis and ataxia are more pronounced on the side of the lesion.

Plain radiographs are normal, unless the neoplasm has invaded or originated from a vertebra. A myelogram usually demonstrates the location of the neoplasm, and careful comparison of ventrodorsal and lateral views should differentiate extradural from intradural lesions.[18, 55, 161]

A thorough physical examination and thoracic radiographs should be made to diagnose metastatic neoplasia.

Canine Neuroepithelioma. An intradural mostly extramedullary neoplasm occurs in the thoracolumbar region of young dogs.[152, 166] The age at the time of examination for neurologic deficit ranges from 6 months to 3 years. The patients have included both sexes and numerous breeds. German shepherds have predominated in our experience, and this is more than would be expected from our hospital population of this breed. This neoplasm is solitary and has always been located between T10 and L2 spinal cord segments in the leptomeninges. The signs often are fairly rapid in onset and progression. Occasionally, temporary improvement is observed with steroid therapy, but this is followed by continued progression of signs. Myelography is necessary for diagnosis. In one patient surgical removal was followed by improvement, which did not deteriorate over the next 8 months in which the animal was followed.

Examination of the neoplasm microscopically by numerous pathologists has resulted in mixed opinions. The general consensus is that this may represent a neuroepithelioma arising on the spinal cord surface from undifferentiated neuroepithelial cells. The clinician must be aware of this disease when examining young dogs with signs of progressive thoracolumbar spinal cord disease.

In the literature there are a number of reports of this same neoplasm at the same location and all in young dogs.[104, 152, 166, 182] All of these publications call the neoplasm an ependymoma despite its extramedullary location and the lack of cilia on the cells that surround a lumen as a rosette. The gross and microscopic descriptions are identical to the neoplasm I have described here and named a neuroepithelioma.

Multiple Cartilaginous Exostoses. Although not a neoplastic disease, multiple cartilaginous exostoses occur in young dogs and cats and may invade the vertebral canal as a space-occupying lesion.[8, 25, 38, 54, 57] These exostoses represent a benign proliferation of cartilage and bone associated with an epiphyseal plate in bones, and grow by endochondral formation. These growths are covered by hyalin cartilage and undergo normal endochondral ossification similar to that at the epiphyseal plate. They are common in long bones, ribs, and vertebrae. They form large, easily palpable masses at these sites. Those that grow from a vertebral arch into the canal cause extradural spinal cord compression and progressive neurologic signs. Most occur in the thoracic or lumbar vertebrae. These growths cease spontaneously when normal bone growth stops at the epiphyseal plates under the control of the endocrine system. There is no sex or breed predilection, but a familial basis is suspected. It is considered an hereditary disease in humans. The onset of neurologic signs occurs prior to 1 year of age unless the compression is caused by subsequent development of a neoplasm from multiple cartilaginous exostoses. Surgical excision is necessary only for cosmetic purposes, if abrasions occur over a mass, or if signs of spinal cord compression occur.

Vertebral osteomas may occur in young dogs and produce excessive pain with or without signs of spinal cord compression. The pain is similar to that observed with osteomyelitis but leukocytosis, fever, and response to antibiotics do not occur.

VERTEBRAL MALFORMATION. Vertebral column malformation should be considered in young dogs less than 1 year old that have signs of a progressive thoracolumbar spinal cord lesion, usually beginning between 3 and 9 months of age.[5, 55, 88, 116] The disease is *not* restricted to the brachycephalic breeds. Careful physical examination usually discloses the malformation because of the deviation of the vertebral column. There may be an associated line of hypalgesia. The neurologic deficit usually is symmetric.

Radiographs generally reveal a marked dorsal deviation of the thoracic vertebral column, kyphosis, with one or more wedge-shaped vertebral bodies and ventrally deviated spines at the most dorsal point of the kyphosis. At this point the vertebral canal is smaller than normal. A myelogram shows compression of the subarachnoid space by a symmetric decrease in diameter of the vertebral canal over one or more of the wedge-shaped vertebral bodies.

These dogs are born with this vertebral column malformation, which often is referred to as "hemivertebra" because of the wedge-shaped appearance of one or more of the vertebrae at the dorsal aspect of the kyphosis. Hemivertebra is a misnomer, however, because more than one half of the vertebra is formed, and it is fallacious to propose that this resulted from a failure of the two vertebral body ossification centers to develop and fuse. There is only one such ossification center in the normal dog.

Since there is no spinal cord malformation, neurologic signs do not appear until the spinal cord is compressed. Presumably, the onset of neurologic signs, that is, spinal cord compression, is delayed for one of two reasons, or both. Either the kyphosis is progressive as the dog grows, ultimately resulting in compression, or as the dog grows the vertebral canal at the site of the malformation does not grow sufficiently by resorption and remodeling to accommodate the growth of the spinal cord, and compression results.

If surgical decompression is to be performed, be aware that the vertebral column may be quite unstable at the site of the malformation and some immobilization should be performed prior to completion of the laminectomy.

VERTEBRAL OSTEOMYELITIS–DISKOSPONDYLITIS. Diskospondylitis is an inflammation of the vertebral bodies and associated intervertebral disk.[50, 74, 81, 92, 94-96] Diskospondylitis is more common in large breeds and usually in middle-aged adults. Some patients have a history of previous vertebral column trauma, but this is not consistent. It is usually a septic condition from a hematogenous source, but occasionally is associated with an adjacent tissue infection or foreign body migration. *Staphylococcus aureus* is the most common organism cultured from the lesion, blood, or urine. Others include *Corynebacterium diphtheroides*, *Streptococcus canis*, *Brucella canis*, and *Nocardia*. Concurrent bacteremia and urinary tract infection may occur. Cultures occasionally are negative and even biopsy may not reveal the cause of the sepsis.

The most diagnostic clinical sign is severe vertebral column pain associated with a progressive paraparesis and ataxia. The neurologic deficit results from the bone proliferation associated with the lesion that encroaches on the vertebral canal and compresses the spinal cord. Fever is common but leukocytosis is inconsistent. CSF is usually normal because the infection and compressive mass are extradural. Protein elevation may reflect a more severe myelopathy.

Radiographs reveal an irregular bone proliferation of the vertebral bodies adjacent to an intervertebral disk, which is usually narrow. Lytic lesions often are present in the vertebrae at this site. The reactive sclerotic bone proliferation extends outward in all directions. The part that invades the vertebral canal causes extradural spinal cord compression. Occasionally clinical signs precede radiographic changes.

Treatment should include long-term antibiotic therapy specific for the organism that is cultured. Spinal cord decompression and vertebral immobilization to allow arthrodesis of the involved vertebrae[50] may be used when neurologic deficits are significant and do not respond to antibiotic therapy.

SPONDYLOSIS DEFORMANS AND DURAL OSSIFICATION. Although spondylosis deformans and dural ossification frequently are incriminated as causes of spinal cord compression, they rarely cause this condition. The proliferative bone lesion of spondylosis deformans produces ventral and lateral exostosis on the vertebral bodies, but rarely enters the vertebral canal to compress the spinal cord.[98, 114, 115] A myelogram is required to confirm whether this bone lesion actually has compressed the spinal cord. These are more common in the older dogs of large breeds. The lumbosacral articulation and the vertebrae at the thoracolumbar junction are more commonly affected.

Dural ossification, erroneously called pachymeningitis, is a common finding, especially in the larger breeds of dogs.[117, 150, 177] It is a metaplasia of the inner surface of the dura resulting in the production of bony plaques containing marrow. It occurs at an early age (1 to 2 years), but its development is more extensive in the older dog. Although it can occur at all levels of the spinal cord dura mater, it is found most commonly ventrally in the cranial and caudal cervical areas and the lumbar area. It also may occur laterally and dorsally, and almost surround the spinal cord at some levels. Despite the massive development of this condition, associated spinal cord lesions are rare.

Inflammation

Canine Distemper Myelitis. Dogs of any age are susceptible to the canine distemper virus. Its effect on the nervous system is variable, and may be dependent on the strain or properties of the virus. Some dogs with this disease present with signs caused by the pre-

dominant action of this virus on the spinal cord, with or without a history of previous systemic illness. If the nonsuppurative myelitis that occurs is most developed between segments T3 and L3, there are signs of a spastic paraparesis and ataxia that is often asymmetric, or spastic paraplegia.

This disease is especially suspect in dogs that are less than 1 year old. The history should indicate that the neurologic signs have been progressive.

Clinical information that contributes to this etiologic diagnosis is the finding of other neurologic deficits that cannot be explained by a focal thoracolumbar spinal cord lesion alone. It is unusual for the signs of myelitis to be confined to the pelvic limbs. Mild thoracic limb deficit in a paraplegic dog can be explained best by two lesions—one mild cervical spinal cord lesion and one severe thoracolumbar lesion. A head tilt, abnormal nystagmus, and/or head tremor suggest cerebellovestibular dysfunction. Visual deficit in a dog with normal eyes and pupillary light reflexes suggests central visual pathway disease. Typically, the inflammatory demyelinating lesion in this disease is most prominent in the white matter of the optic tracts, cerebellar peduncles, and the spinal cord, although no part of the brain is immune to it. The diffuse distribution of lesions, as well as their progressive nature, should suggest an inflammatory disease.

A mild increase in mononuclear cells, or protein, or both in the cerebrospinal fluid may be observed in patients with canine distemper encephalomyelitis. The presence of lesions of chorioretinitis observed with the ophthalmoscope also suggests exposure to this virus.

To date, there is no specific therapy for this central nervous system viral disease, and the prognosis is poor. In most patients the lesions continue to progress. In a few instances they have ceased spontaneously and some improvement has occurred, either as a result of compensatory mechanisms, or possibly owing to relief of the inflammation and remyelination of intact axons.

Toxoplasmosis. *Toxoplasma gondii,* the protozoan that causes toxoplasmosis, may affect the CNS of dogs and cats, but is much less common than canine distemper. It may be focal or diffuse in distribution, and usually alters the CSF more remarkably than the canine distemper virus. In some instances neutrophils may appear in the CSF.[1]

Cryptococcosis. *Cryptococcus neoformans* produces a severe diffuse meningitis with ependymitis and some associated encephalomyelitis in dogs and cats. Although pelvic limb paresis and ataxia may be the most obvious clinical signs, the diffuse nature of the lesion usually causes signs of cervical spinal cord and brain involvement as well. The CSF generally contains large complements of inflammatory cells and protein, and consistently contains the organism, which can be identified readily. Wright's stain or India ink can enhance the identification. Both toxoplasmosis and cryptococcosis may produce a characteristic granulomatous chorioretinitis that can be observed with the ophthalmoscope.

Feline Infectious Peritonitis. The coronavirus that causes feline infectious peritonitis (FIP) frequently affects the central nervous system. Usually this is a diffuse involvement of the ependymal surfaces of the choroid plexuses and ventricles with variable involvement of the leptomeninges.[91] As a result, the clinical signs often reflect a diffuse distribution of lesions. Rarely a focal granulomatous lesion results from this agent.[101] If this focal parenchymal involvement occurs in the thoracolumbar spinal cord, a progressive paresis and ataxia of the pelvic limbs results. Usually the CSF is very abnormal with occasionally up to hundreds of leukocytes per cubic millimeter and up to 500 mg of protein per deciliter. These leukocytes are usually lymphocytes and monocytes. Occasionally neutrophils predominate. Increased serum gamma globulin is common in this disease. A significantly elevated serum FIP antibody titer is usually consistent with clinical disease.[153] This agent can also affect the uvea of the eye and produce focal areas of chorioretinitis.

Degeneration

Degenerative Myelopathy in German Shepherds. A degenerative myelopathy occurs predominantly in the aging German shepherd, and is characterized by a slowly progressive paraparesis and ataxia of the pelvic limbs.[3, 16, 65, 66, 89] It occasionally occurs in older dogs of other breeds. It is rare in cats.[192] Most patients are over 5 years old. A history of a progressive course over 5 to 6 months is common. Its onset is insidious, and loss of position sense is often the first indication of the disease. Paw-dragging, crossing the limbs, and incomplete extension of the limbs for full support usually is accompanied by hypertonia and increased reflexes in the pelvic limbs. Occasionally, hypotonia and hyporeflexia have been observed. This may include loss of the patellar reflex in one limb without obvious neurogenic atrophy. The signs may be asymmetric. There often occurs a general wasting (disuse atrophy) of the muscles in the caudal thoracic and lumbosacral region. Postural reactions often are poorly performed in the pelvic limbs, especially the response to proprioceptive positioning. Although the dog eventually may be unable to get up on the pelvic limbs, grade 0 paraplegia or analgesia have not been observed. Thoracic limb function appears normal.

The lesion consists of a diffuse degeneration of white matter in both the ascending and descending spinal cord tracts in all funiculi in all the segments of the spinal cord. It is referred to as a multisystem degeneration. The lesion is most extensive in the thoracic regions. This is a degeneration of individual neurons and not groups of neurons in specific regions of these funiculi. Both the myelin sheaths and the axons degenerate. The lesion also may involve peripheral nerves, which may account for those patients with loss of spinal reflexes. Although mild lesions may occur in the cervical spinal cord, no thoracic limb deficits have been observed. One study did not support a dying-back of axons as the basis for this lesion.[16]

Immunologic studies have shown a relationship between German shepherds with this clinical disease and impaired blood leukocyte response to thymus-dependent mitogens.[175, 176] It has been suggested that this disease is either an immunodeficiency or autoimmune disease that may be genetically determined. A typical patient report follows.

Signalment. The patient was an 8-year-old male German shepherd.

History. Four months prior to admission, the owner noticed a slight ataxia in the hindlimbs. In time, weakness became obvious and the ataxia more pronounced, and both progressed slowly until the animal became severely paraparetic 10 to 12 weeks following the onset of the signs.

Physical Examination. On admission the dog was alert and responsive. The animal was unable to use the pelvic limbs unaided. When wheelbarrowed, the head was held erect and the gait of the thoracic limbs was normal. When supported, a very slight swinging motion of the pelvic limbs was evident (grade 1 paraparesis).

Spinal Reflexes. The flexor, patellar, and perineal reflexes were intact. The patellar reflex was of normal amplitude (plus 2). There was moderate increased resistance to passive manipulation of the pelvic limbs. Pain was perceived when the digits were compressed. All reflexes, tone, and resistance were normal in the thoracic limbs.

Postural Reactions. No postural reactions were present in the pelvic limbs. They were normal in the thoracic limbs.

Cranial Nerves. There were no abnormalities noticed.

Anatomic Diagnosis. These signs indicate an extensive focal or diffuse symmetric lesion of the spinal cord white matter between T3 and L3 segments.

Ancillary Procedures. Radiographs revealed minor spurring of the vertebral bodies ventrally, indicative of spondylosis. There was no lesion seen involving the vertebral canal. A myelogram also did not reveal any significant lesion within the vertebral canal. Cerebrospinal fluid contained 1 white blood cell per cmm and 30 mg of protein per dl.

Although radiographs often may demonstrate dural ossification or spondylosis deformans in a dog of this age, these lesions rarely affect the spinal cord. Significant geriatric intervertebral disk protrusion can be eliminated by plain radiography as well as by myelography. Small prominences of the anulus fibrosus are common and may compress the spinal cord, but do not produce lesions or clinical signs. In degenerative myelopathy, myelograms demonstrate a normal subarachnoid space not compromised by a space-occupying mass (neoplasm or intervertebral disk). CSF usually shows no abnormality unless the protein level is increased slightly.

Hereditary Myelopathy with Myelinolysis in Afghan Hounds. A primary myelin degeneration occurs in young Afghan hounds of both sexes, starting usually between 3 and 13 months of age, and progressing in 7 to 10 days from mild paraparesis and pelvic limb ataxia to paraplegia.[4, 28, 31, 84] As the disease progresses, the thoracic limbs often are affected and tetraplegia may ensue within 2 to 3 weeks of the onset of clinical signs. As the paraparesis worsens, paresis of the axial musculature of the middle to caudal trunk is evident.

Owing to the severity of the lesion in the cranial thoracic segments, there is loss of upper motor neuron to the thoracolumbar axial muscles. These dogs have difficulty supporting their trunks to rise on their forelimbs or to walk when supported by the tail without the trunk swaying to the side.

Usually the pelvic and thoracic limbs have normal to increased muscle tone and reflexes and no neurogenic atrophy is apparent. Occasionally the lesion affects the stability of the ventral grey column of the cervical and lumbar intumescence, and tone and spinal reflexes are lost. This occurs only in the most severely affected patients that are tetraplegic.

In the paraplegic dog hypalgesia is found in the pelvic limbs and trunk caudal to a cranial thoracic level. There will be hypalgesia in all limbs of the tetraplegic dog.

The lesion consists of an extensive destruction of myelin with sparing of the axons in a bilaterally symmetric pattern in ventral, lateral, and sometimes dorsal funiculi. The fasciculus proprius adjacent to the grey matter is often spared. The lesions are most extensive throughout the thoracic segments and usually gradually decrease as you progress caudally in the lumbar segments or cranially into the cervical segments. There is an extensive macrophage response to the lesion but minimal astrocytic reaction. The only brain lesion observed is a similar destruction of myelin in the neurons surrounding the dorsal nucleus of the trapezoid body in the medulla. Despite the extensive necrosis, cisternal CSF may be normal or have a mild elevation of protein.

The specific cause of the myelin dissolution or the explanation for the topography of the lesion is unknown. The cause of the presumed metabolic or enzymatic defect involving the myelin is genetic. Breeding studies and evaluation of pedigrees of clinically affected dogs support an autosomal recessive inheritance for this disease.

Demyelinating Myelopathy in Miniature Poodles. A rare idiopathic demyelination of the brain stem and spinal cord has been reported in miniature poodle puppies, with the onset of signs usually between 2 and 4 months of age.[39] The signs are those of progressive, diffuse spinal cord white matter disease. Spastic paraparesis is followed rapidly by paraplegia and tetraplegia. Hypertonia and hyperreflexia are marked. When tetraplegic, the patient lies in lateral recumbency with the thoracic limbs rigidly extended. The patient remains alert and responsive, and has no demonstrable cranial nerve deficit. Pain perception is retained. The lesion is restricted to white matter, in which the destruction is extensive. In general, the axons are spared. The myelin degeneration occurs symmetrically in all funiculi of all segments of the spinal cord, especially in the cervical segments, and may affect the reticular formation of the medulla and cerebellar peduncles in a patchy or diffuse manner. The pathogenesis is unknown, but a familial (hereditary) basis is suspect.

Embolic Myelopathy. Embolic myelopathy caused by vascular emboli presumed to be fibrocartilage can occur at any level of the spinal cord in dogs and cats.[34, 58, 63, 64, 71, 93, 185] If it occurs in the thoracolumbar region, a *sudden* spastic paraparesis with ataxia or paraplegia results. The signs are ipsilateral or bilateral, with or without symmetry, depending on the location and degree of ischemic myelopathy. These lesions usually do not produce pain on vertebral manipulation, and affected dogs do not have a history of pain at the onset. The signs are always sudden in onset and usually nonprogressive after 24 hours. Radiographs are normal. A myelogram may suggest slight spinal cord swelling at the site of the lesion. CSF may contain more protein than normal.

Recovery may be spontaneous if the ischemic episode is mild. Some evidence of improvement should be apparent during the first week of the disease. If the ischemia is severe, an infarct or focal myelomalacia results, with permanent neurologic deficit. See Chapter 4 for further discussion of this disease.[184, 187]

Dogs have been observed with a nontraumatic sudden onset of complete spastic paralysis of one pelvic limb. The dog will walk on three limbs with the affected pelvic limb rigidly extended caudally and dragged on the dorsal surface of the paw. Muscle tone and reflexes are all increased in the affected limb. Pain perception is usually normal. Careful observation of the opposite pelvic limb will reveal that although the dog walks with that limb, it sinks on turns and is slow on postural reactions. These signs are explained by an extensive lesion of one side of the spinal cord between T3 and L3. This lesion is on the same side as the paralyzed pelvic limb. The two primary causes of this clinical syndrome, which is sudden in onset, nonprogressive, and occurs in the absence of external trauma, are embolic myelopathy and a unilateral intervertebral disk extrusion. The latter may be associated with a history of pain at onset or demonstrate pain on vertebral manipulation. Radiography with myelography is essential to differentiate these two causes, for a disk extrusion with these severe signs should be treated surgically and embolic myelopathy should be treated medically as any other spinal cord injury. Prompt treatment of either condition should result in significant recovery of function.

Although embolic myelopathy has been observed in cats with fibrocartilaginous emboli in the spinal vasculature, other cats have been observed with spinal cord infarcts in the absence of fibrocartilaginous emboli. Some of these cats have had evidence of cardiomyopathy at necropsy, and this may be the basis for the vascular thromboembolism or compromise and spinal cord infarction.[167]

Neoplasia—Intramedullary

Intramedullary neoplasia of the spinal cord is less common than the extramedullary form. Gliomas are the most common form of intramedullary neoplasia. There is no clear clinical feature that differentiates these two forms of neoplasia. Parenchymal destruction may be greater with the intramedullary form, and clinical signs appear earlier and are more severe when comparing neoplasms of similar size. Much depends on the rate of growth of the neoplasm.

Diagnosis can be confirmed only by myelography, and in some cases exploratory laminectomy may be necessary to distinguish the intramedullary from extramedullary form of neoplasia. Intramedullary neoplasms are much less amenable to surgical removal because of their intimate relationship with the parenchyma that has been infiltrated with the neoplastic cells.

Malformation

Canine Myelodysplasia. The myelodysplasia referred to as spinal dysraphism usually produces symmetric pelvic limb ataxia that can be observed by 4 to 6 weeks of age.[40, 111] It was described in Chapter 2 and is the most common spinal cord malformation in the dog.

The disease is most prevalent in the Weimaraner breed, in which it is considered to be inherited as a codominant gene. It has been reported in many other breeds. Breeding clinically affected Weimaraners to normal German shepherds or Norwegian elkhounds produces some clinically affected puppies. Breeding the normal offspring of these matings also produces some affected puppies.

The classic clinical sign observed is a symmetric simultaneous use of both pelvic limbs, referred to as "bunny hopping." This is associated with a variable degree of proprioceptive deficit, with a tendency to overextend a limb on getting up or walking and standing or walking on the dorsal surface of the paw. Paresis is observed only occasionally. Patellar reflexes are normal. The pelvic limb flexor reflex stimulated in one limb usually elicits a simultaneous flexion of both limbs. Postural reactions are performed poorly in these limbs.

In dogs that are affected severely by the spinal cord malformation, there also may be abnormalities of the musculoskeletal system accompanied by scoliosis, spondylosis, koilosternia, kinked tails, and decreased pelvic muscle mass. In litters with affected offspring, some pups may be born dead or die shortly after birth.

Occasionally, a remarkable abnormality of vestibular system function is observed for a few weeks in puppies with clinical signs of the spinal cord malformation. This consists of a severe head tilt and a tendency to drift or fall to the same side. The pathogenesis of this disturbance has not been found, and it usually resolves spontaneously or is compensated.

Spinal cord lesions are described in Chapter 2. It should be remembered that any clinical signs related to these lesions are present at birth and do not progress. Signs of progressive pelvic limb ataxia in Weimaraners that were born with normal gait and posture are caused by some other acquired disease.

Other Malformations. Be aware of the association between vertebral column and spinal cord malformations. They can occur at any level, but more often are caudal thoracic and lumbar. Scoliosis or kyphosis may be associated with spinal cord aplasia, hypoplasia or a myelodysplasia with syringomyelia, hydromyelia, central canal abnormalities or hyperplasia of spinal cord tissue, or both. Neurologic signs are present at birth but usually are not apparent until 4 to 6 weeks of age in puppies and kittens, when they first become ambulatory. Ataxia most commonly accompanies the myelodysplasia, whereas paresis is more evident in hypoplasia, and paraplegia in cases of aplasia. The signs are nonprogressive. The cause of these isolated cases is unknown.

CERVICAL SPINAL CORD DISEASE

Cervical spinal cord lesions from C1 to C5 or those that predominantly affect the white matter at C6 or C7 cause a spastic paresis and ataxia of all four limbs or the ipsilateral forelimb and hindlimb if the lesion is unilateral (Fig. 10–2). With mild lesions, especially those that are circumferentially compressive around the spinal cord, the clinical signs are worse in the pelvic limbs but thoracic limb signs are

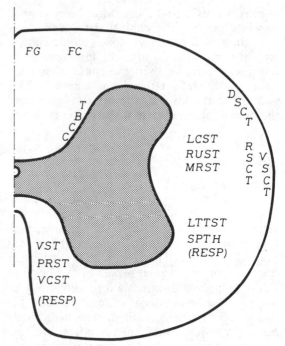

Figure 10–2. Schematic distribution of tracts in cervical spinal cord. *FG:* Fasciculus gracilis; *FC:* fasciculus cuneatus; *CCBT:* cuneocerebellar tract; *DSCT:* dorsal spinocerebellar tract; *VSCT:* ventral spinocerebellar tract; *RSCT:* rostral spinocerebellar tract; *LCST:* lateral corticospinal tract; *RUST:* rubrospinal tract; *MRST:* medullary reticulospinal tract; *LTTST:* lateral tectotegmentospinal tract; *SPTH:* spinothalamic tract; *(Resp):* respiratory upper motor neurons; *VST:* vestibulospinal tract; *PRST:* pontine reticulospinal tract; *VCST:* ventral corticospinal tract.

evident. The thoracic limb signs may be limited to a slight stiffness and tendency to "float" on protraction. The slight delay in returning the limb to the ground looks as if the limb "floats" briefly. Various explanations for this disparity in thoracic and pelvic limb signs include the more significant involvement of the superficial tracts in the lateral funiculi, which carry pelvic limb proprioceptive neurons, the evidence that some upper motor neuron systems have more endings in the cervical than in the lumbosacral intumescence, and the greater distance of the pelvic limbs from the center of gravity.

Animals with ventral median compressive lesions at any level of the cervical spinal cord that cause the spinal cord to "tent" over it may have more significant defects in the thoracic than in the pelvic limbs. This may reflect the more medial location of UMN tracts to the cervical intumescence.

Similarly, animals with involvement of the grey matter of the cervical intumescence may have more deficit in the thoracic limb(s). With lesions from C6 to T1 that affect grey as well as white matter, the clinical signs in the thoracic limbs will reflect the lower motor neuron and general somatic afferent involvement in the grey matter at that level; the pelvic limb signs will all reflect the disturbance of UMN and GP at the level of the cervical lesion and the spinothalamic tracts if the lesion is severe enough. *pain perception*

Trauma

External Injury. Fractures of cranial cervical vertebrae may produce considerable displacement, yet present with remarkably few signs of neurologic deficit. The attitude, posture, and gait all depict the severe neck pain that is present. This is especially true for fractures of the cranial aspect of the body of C2.[168] Following anesthesia for radiography or surgery, the instability is exacerbated and the dog is often worse, with obvious neurologic signs of cervical spinal cord compression.

Spinal cord concussion or contusion can occur with or without fractures of the cervical vertebrae and intervertebral disk extrusion.

The principles described for external injury of the thoracolumbar spinal cord also apply to the cervical spinal cord. Unlike the Schiff-Sherrington syndrome, the thoracic limb hypertonia in cervical spinal cord injury is associated with severe paresis of voluntary function of all the limbs and pelvic limb hypertonia.

The following patient report exemplifies unilateral cervical spinal cord injury.

Signalment. A 10-year-old male mongrel.

History. On the morning of examination, the patient was found with about 4 inches of skin torn over the midthoracic vertebral spines, and having difficulty with its gait. The animal had been normal when put outdoors the night before.

Physical Examination. The patient was a stoic but responsive and cooperative dog that walked with an obvious asymmetry to its gait. The toes of both the right thoracic and right pelvic limbs were dragged along the floor. This was not noted on the left side. Weight was supported more by the left limbs than the right, but occasionally the dog swayed slightly on the left limbs.

Spinal Reflexes. All flexor reflexes were normal. Crossed extension occurred in the right thoracic and pelvic limbs. Pain perception was normal from all limbs. The patellar reflex was hyperactive (plus 3) on the left side and a prolonged clonus (plus 5) was elicited on the right side. The perineal reflex was normal.

Passive manipulation of the limbs elicited a mild

increased resistance on the left side and marked resistance on the right side. Clonus could be elicited in the right pelvic limb merely by putting pressure on the plantar surface of the paw.

Postural Reactions. All these tests demonstrated a deficit on the right side. The left limbs responded normally to the tonic neck and eye test, proprioceptive positioning, placing, hopping, and extensor postural thrust. The right limbs responded poorly if at all to these tests. If the right limbs were held up, the patient could support itself and walk on the left limbs. If the left limbs were held up, the dog could support itself only momentarily on the right limbs before collapsing. Normal gait was not possible on the right limbs alone.

Anatomic Diagnosis. These clinical signs indicated a lesion on the right side of the cervical spinal cord cranial to C6.

Differential Diagnosis. The sudden onset suggested external or internal trauma or a vascular disturbance as the main mechanism for the lesion. The skin lacerations indicated some form of external trauma.

Radiography. Many lead pellets were found in the cervical region. One was located in the vertebral canal on the right side at C2.

Prognosis and Therapy. While surgery was under consideration for removal of this foreign body, the dog suddenly expired from a venous embolus that arose from an area of the femoral vein injured by the same gunshot accident. This embolus had occluded the conus arteriosus and pulmonic valve.

Internal Injury

INTERVERTEBRAL DISK EXTRUSION.[123, 149, 158, 159] Cervical pain is the sign most commonly associated with cervical intervertebral disk extrusion. Although any of the disks can be affected, the C2–C3 articulation has the highest incidence. If the spinal cord is compressed, signs of neurologic deficit appear, involving all four limbs. Pelvic limb paresis and ataxia usually exceed that of the thoracic limbs, but occasionally the reverse occurs, with marked hypertonia and loss of voluntary function of the thoracic limbs. Hypertonia and hyperreflexia are observed in all four limbs with lesions from C1 to C5 or limited to the white matter at C6 or C7.

In those patients with more severe thoracic limb deficit, the extrusion has been largest on the midline, compressing more of the central portion of the spinal cord. Perhaps this involves more of the upper motor neuron to these limbs, since they course more medially to reach the grey matter in which they terminate. Occasionally, more caudally located cervical intervertebral disk extrusions also cause more severe thoracic limb deficit with

LMN signs. Pain on manipulation of the cervical vertebrae does not always accompany the neurologic signs.

Sometimes the neurologic signs are asymmetric and an ipsilateral spastic hemiparesis occurs associated with a lateral intervertebral disk extrusion.

Occasionally a complete spastic hemiplegia occurs suddenly with an explosive unilateral intervertebral disk extrusion.[60] If the ipsilateral spinal cord dysfunction is severe there may be a sympathetic paralysis of the entire ipsilateral side of the head, body, and limbs. This follows compromise of the UMN sympathetic pathway, the lateral tectotegmentospinal tract, which is facilitatory to the entire column of preganglionic cell bodies in the intermediate grey column. The signs are most evident in the eye and orbit as Horner's syndrome. If skin temperature is measured, it is increased on the paralyzed side from vasodilation. In addition there is a truncal postural asymmetry that is evident when the animal is placed in lateral recumbency on the normal side. Immediately it turns its head and neck into the ground surface to force its body to roll over to the paralyzed side. It will not or cannot flex its neck toward the paralyzed side. When placed in lateral recumbency on the paralyzed side, the patient lies comfortably or flexes its neck to the normal side with no postural dystonia. This is thought to be due to compromise of the vestibulospinal tract in the ventral funiculus on the side of the lesion. The truncal postural dystonia results from the imbalance in vestibulospinal tract function.

In some patients there are continual irregular contractions or spasms of the cervical muscles usually associated with neck pain, with or without mild signs of ataxia and paresis. In others, one forelimb may be held in partial flexion and the dog is reluctant to use the limb or walks lame on that limb. These dogs often show considerable pain on manipulation of the neck or the affected limb. This forelimb flexion has been referred to as a "root signature" because of the presumed lateral intervertebral disk extrusion with entrapment of the spinal nerve near the intervertebral foramen. This may be the only sign of disk extrusion or it may accompany a hemiparesis and ataxia of the limbs on that side of the body.

NEOPLASIA—EXTRAMEDULLARY. Primary or metastatic neoplasms of the vertebral column, epidural space, or meninges can cause extramedullary compression of the cervical spinal cord. The kinds of neoplasms have been discussed in the section on thoracolumbar lesions. Meningiomas have been seen more commonly at the C1 or C2 levels in the dog. They cause varying degrees of progressive spastic tetraparesis and ultimately recumbency. If the lesion is unilateral, the signs may be asymmetric at their onset. Lymphosarcoma in the epidural space is the most common neoplasm in the vertebral column of cats. It is observed in cats of all ages but more commonly in young cats, and the onset of clinical signs is often sudden. Plain radiographs are normal unless there is a vertebral column neoplasm. Usually a myelogram is necessary to demonstrate the space-occupying lesion.

Neurofibroma. Neurofibromas of the first five cervical spinal nerves usually produce an ipsilateral spastic hemiparesis initially. The most common neoplasm that is found at the cervical intumescence in the dog is a neurofibroma of a spinal nerve or root that compresses the spinal cord at the intumescence.[121]

The signs vary with the rate of growth of the lesion and the awareness of the owner. Generally, it presents as a "lameness" in one thoracic limb with no radiographically demonstrable lesion. The "lameness" becomes a paresis and may be associated with diffuse muscle atrophy in the affected thoracic limb. As the paresis progresses in that limb, the ipsilateral pelvic limb develops a spastic paresis and ataxia caused by the compression of the spinal cord by the neoplasm growing through the intervertebral foramen and along the roots to the spinal cord. Continual spinal cord compression causes tetraparesis. Thoracic limb paresis is usually more conspicuous than the pelvic limb paresis.

In some patients with this disease, the unilateral thoracic limb atrophy is severe and associated with pain and lameness in that limb. Nevertheless, the limb is still functional. The only indication that the spinal cord is affected may be a slight tendency for the ipsilateral pelvic limb to slide out to the side on a slippery floor, and its postural reactions may be slightly slower.

When this lesion begins in a single spinal nerve or its roots, neurologic signs are not observed in the gait. Only when it applies pressure to the adjacent cervical intumescence is the neurologic deficit observed in the gait. If the lesion begins at the T1 or T2 spinal nerve and compresses the adjacent spinal cord and subsequently the intumescence, the ipsilateral upper motor neuron pelvic limb deficit may precede the lower motor neuron thoracic limb signs. Such a lesion may produce paraplegia and mild lower motor neuron thoracic limb signs.

Usually this neoplasm is intradural but extramedullary, and compresses the spinal cord at the site of origin of the rootlets. It is amenable to surgical removal, but the involved roots must be sacrificed. In some instances, it may not be possible to separate the mass from the adjacent spinal cord tissue. In this disease the spinal cord compression may be severe and yet the patient is still ambulatory. In a few patients the lesion is extradural to the spinal cord.

The following two patients are examples of this lesion at the cervical intumescence.

Signalment. A 7-year-old German shepherd.

History. Two weeks prior to examination, the owner first noticed some difficulty with the use of the left forelimb. During the next 10 days, the same difficulty involved the left hindlimb as well.

Physical Examination. The patient was in good physical condition, alert, and responsive. When standing, the left forepaw often was placed knuckled on its dorsal surface. When walking, the left forelimb was thrown forward more than the right so that it landed on the palmar surface of the paw. Otherwise it knuckled over on the dorsal surface of the paw. The left hind paw frequently was knuckled over on its dorsal surface. Atrophy was evident in the left supraspinatus, infraspinatus, and triceps muscles.

Spinal Reflexes. The flexor reflex of the left forelimb was weak compared to the right. The triceps reflex was present bilaterally and was symmetric. The flexor reflexes in the hindlimbs were intact and symmetric. Pain was perceived from all the limbs. The left patellar reflex was hyperactive, with transient clonus present (plus 4). The right patellar reflex was normal (plus 2). Increased resistance was noted in the left hindlimb on manipulation.

Postural Reactions. On tonic neck and eye testing, the left forelimb did not support weight properly and often knuckled. Pain was evident on neck manipulation. Proprioceptive positioning was performed poorly in the left forelimb, fairly in the left hindlimb, and normally on the right side. Hopping and placing were abnormal on the left side. On extensor thrust the left hindlimb was extended more than normal when compared to the right. When held by both left limbs, the patient supported its weight well on the right limbs and could walk on them. When held by the right limbs the left limbs could not support the weight of the dog and it collapsed.

Anatomic Diagnosis. The signs support a lesion on the left side of the cervical intumescence with LMN signs in the left thoracic limb and signs of UMN-GP deficit in the ipsilateral pelvic limb.

Radiography and Myelography. Plain radiographs revealed no lesion. A myelogram revealed a block to the flow of the dye at C6 with a deviation of the dye lines to the margins of the vertebral foramen on both views. Euthanasia was requested.

Presumptive Diagnosis. Intradural neoplasia.

Necropsy. The left intradural C6 rootlets were enlarged by a mass that pushed the spinal cord parenchyma to the right. It was diagnosed as a neurofibroma.

Signalment. A 10-year-old male springer spaniel.

Chief Complaint. The patient had neck pain and weakness.

History. Two weeks prior to admission, the dog suddenly developed cervical pain and the body was curved to the left (concave left). The pain persisted, and the dog became reluctant to move, or developed weakness that prevented normal freedom of movement. The gait difficulty progressed.

Physical Examination. The dog was mildly depressed and apprehensive. Paresis was pronounced in both thoracic limbs, with frequent collapse onto the carpus of the right limb. The pelvic limbs were paretic, but less so than the thoracic limbs. Postural reactions demonstrated that the right thoracic limb was the most paretic. Manipulation of the base of the neck occasionally elicited pain. The dog also continually moaned on being urged to move, as if the effort to walk caused pain. Muscle atrophy was pronounced in the thoracic limbs. The thoracic limbs were hypotonic and spinal reflexes were depressed markedly. Pain response was normal. The pelvic limbs were hypertonic and hyperreflexic (plus 3 patellar bilaterally). These signs progressed over a 7-day period of observation, and the thoracic limb atrophy increased. This atrophy occurred in all the muscles, but was pronounced in the scapular musculature.

Anatomic Diagnosis. A lesion involving the spinal cord grey matter or the associated roots that contribute to the brachial plexus and the white matter, with descending tracts to the lumbosacral segments.

Radiography. Intervertebral disks C5-C6 and C6-C7 were calcified markedly without obvious protrusion.

Radiopaque dye injected into the subarachnoid space at the L5-L6 level slowed to a narrow point at the level of the caudal end of the body of C5. There was no indentation of the dye column at the site of the intervertebral disks. An intradural mass was diagnosed.

Laboratory Findings. Examination of CSF revealed no abnormality.

Presumptive Diagnosis. Intradural neoplasia.

Surgery. Dorsal laminectomy was performed at C5 and C6. No epidural lesion was seen. The dura was opened longitudinally and a mass was found compressing the parenchyma on the right side. Because it was not amenable to removal, euthanasia was performed.

Necropsy. There was a mass in the right sixth cervical spinal nerve and its roots, which compressed the spinal cord at the origin of these roots. The mass was a neurofibroma.

VERTEBRAL MALFORMATION— MALARTICULATION

Atlantoaxial Subluxation. Atlantoaxial subluxation occurs most commonly in miniature or toy breeds of dogs as a result of fracture, degeneration, or malformation of the dens.[29, 55, 56, 97, 130] A fracture with subluxation is not limited to these small breeds. The pathogenesis of the absence of the dens in these small breeds is unknown. A degenerative process is suspected, causing dissolution of the bone and leaving only a remnant on the cranial articular surface of the axis. There is speculation that the mechanism is similar to the femoral head necrosis observed in Legg-Perthes disease, and possibly is related to the early development of the sex hormones in these breeds.[103] The main portion of the dens and the cranial articular surface of the axis constitute centrum 1, which has an ossification center that is seen first at 3 weeks and that fuses caudally with the ossification center of intercentrum 2 of the axis at 7 to 9 months of age. Intercentrum 2 is a narrow ossification center between the ossification center of the combined dens and cranial articular surface of the axis and centrum 2, which comprises most of the body of the axis. The apex of the dens is the centrum of the proatlas, which has an ossification center that fuses to the dens at 3 to 4 months.[174]

Luxation is found most commonly in the young dog 6 to 18 months old, but it is not limited by age. The loss of the dens may precede the subluxation by a considerable period of time if the dense connective tissue between the dorsal arch of the atlas and the spine of the axis resists the instability between the body of the axis and body of the atlas. This is the dorsal atlantoaxial ligament. Normally, the transverse ligament of the atlas helps maintain the dorsoventral alignment of the atlas and axis by holding the dens in the caudal articular fovea of the body of the atlas. Without a dens this supporting mechanism is lost, and the cranial aspect of the body of the axis rotates dorsally into the vertebral canal. When subluxation has occurred, the transverse ligament of the atlas may be forced cranially into a vertical position.

Radiographs demonstrate a narrowed vertebral canal over the cranial aspect of the body of the axis, where it has pivoted dorsally into the canal. The space between the arch of the atlas and the spine of the axis is widened. Usually, there is no dens evident on the axis. In a few cases a remnant may be apparent on the ventral aspect of the canal over the body of the atlas. There are many views that will permit you to see the dens or to notice its absence, but it is important not to manipulate a dog with a luxation any more than necessary. In a straight lateral view the wings of the atlas block your view of the dens. If the head is turned slightly, the wings of the atlas will no longer be superimposed on the dens and it can easily be observed on a lateral view.

The clinical signs vary from reluctance to have the head patted, to severe neck pain, to varying degrees of spastic tetraparesis and ataxia, and occasionally recumbency. Sometimes the thoracic limb paresis is more profound than the pelvic limb paresis. The dogs can stand and walk with their thoracic limbs positioned caudally under the thorax. They walk with a short, stiff stride and often place one paw in front of the other. Spasticity is severe in these limbs. The thoracic limb deficit may reflect the more pronounced midline rather than lateral spinal cord compression.

These patients should be handled with extreme care. The atlantoaxial region should not be manipulated. The signs may worsen after forced exercise. If the ataxia and paresis cause the dog to fall, the subluxation may be exacerbated, along with the spinal cord deficit. In one instance this was known to produce severe medullary edema leading to the death of the animal. Under anesthesia there is no muscle tone to support the alignment, and the danger of further subluxation is even more critical.

Rarely with an acute subluxation, hemorrhage or edema, or both, may ascend into the medulla, producing clinical signs of medullary deficiency—dysphagia, facial weakness, vestibular system deficits, opisthotonos, and death from respiratory paralysis.[6]

Surgery may be successful if spinal cord and medullary edema are prevented. The usual procedure is to wire the arch of the atlas to the spine of the axis. This requires passing a needle with wire beneath the arch of the atlas.

Because the dura usually adheres to this arch in C1, the needle passes through the dura as well. Extreme care must be taken so as not to injure the spinal cord. It must be remembered that by the time these dogs are presented with clinical signs, there already has been extensive damage to the spinal cord. Any further insult from the surgical procedure may readily precipitate signs of cervical or medullary edema with respiratory and cardiac arrest. Modifications of this wiring procedure have been described.[23, 79, 145] One utilizes the ligamentum nuchae in place of the wire.[100]

C5, C6, and C7: Great Danes, Doberman Pinschers. Cervical spinal cord compression caused by caudal cervical vertebral malformation-malarticulation occurs primarily in Great Danes and Doberman pinschers, producing clinical signs referred to as the wobbler syndrome.[22, 33, 37, 55, 107-109, 132, 133, 143, 157, 181, 190] The disease is not limited to these breeds.[142] The onset of clinical signs is extremely variable. They have been observed as early as 2 to 4 months of age and as late as 8 to 9 years of age. There is a higher incidence in younger Great Danes and older Doberman pinschers, but either breed can show clinical signs at any age.[143, 171]

The owner generally recognizes only an abnormality of the pelvic limbs, which is ataxia. The onset usually is insidious, with the owner assuming that the ataxia is normal for the rapid growth of the dog. In some dogs the onset is sudden. The signs usually are progressive, and often the thoracic limbs are abnormal by the time the dog is presented for examination.

Upon examination, there is obvious bilateral spasticity, paresis, and ataxia of the pelvic limbs and occasionally of the thoracic limbs. When the signs are mild, they may be most evident as the animal gets up. It may be unsteady and tend to overextend a pelvic limb. During walking and especially on turning, the pelvic limbs are stiff, may cross each other, abduct widely, or, in more severe cases, tend to collapse. The pelvic limb stride may be longer than usual and asymmetric, causing an awkward swaying movement of the hindquarters. Periodically, the animal may drag its toes or step with the dorsal surface of its paw on the ground. This often has caused the toenails to be worn dorsally. The signs are less obvious when the patient is gaited at faster speeds over a straight course. Abrupt change in speed or direction often exacerbates the deficit and frequently causes pelvic limb collapse. The animal

gives the impression of not knowing where its limbs are because of a proprioceptive deficit.

Thoracic limb signs, when present, are similar but often less remarkable than in the pelvic limbs. These include occasional stumbling with flexion of the carpus, so that the dorsal surface of the paw strikes the ground surface. The limbs may cross each other. Most commonly, the thoracic limbs have a restricted motion, appearing rigid. The dog will appear to throw the limbs forward from the shoulder as it walks. This spastic gait with limited joint flexion may give the appearance that the thoracic limbs tend to delay and "float" on protraction before striking the ground. This may appear as hypermetria.

The response to testing postural reactions usually is abnormal, especially in the more paretic and ataxic animals. Hopping and proprioceptive positioning demonstrate the greatest deficits. If there are signs of thoracic limb abnormality, the animal may flex the carpus and rest the dorsal surface of the paw on the ground, or collapse when the head and neck are extended fully. If the patient is forced to walk on its thoracic limbs with the pelvic limbs held off the ground, and the head and neck in full extension, it may drag its paws on their dorsal surfaces. This proprioceptive deficit sometimes has been the only sign of abnormality in the thoracic limb function. Manipulation of the neck usually does not elicit pain. Some neck pain may be evident in older dogs with significant intervertebral disk involvement in the lesion.

The degree of spastic tetraparesis and ataxia of all four limbs varies from mild to severe. The rate of progression is variable, depending on the nature of the vertebral lesion. Occasionally dogs become recumbent with a total spastic tetraplegia. Although some voluntary movement can be elicited in the dog in lateral recumbency when the flexor reflexes are tested with noxious stimuli, there is no response when the dog is held up. When supported in a standing position, the limbs are all rigidly extended and few to no attempts are made to move the limbs. These dogs can usually flex their necks to either side. Dogs that are tetraplegic from diffuse neuromuscular disease will have the same attitude and appearance when recumbent, but when held up in a supporting position, their flaccidity is a remarkable contrast to the spasticity of these dogs with cervical spinal cord disease.

In some dogs with a chronic compressive

myelopathy at C6 or C7, atrophy of the scapular muscles occurs usually bilaterally. This results from the chronic degeneration of the cell bodies in the region of the ventral grey column under compression and is the only evidence of LMN involvement in this lesion.

The signs described indicate a focal cervical spinal cord lesion. The spastic paresis is caused by the interference with the descending upper motor neuron tracts, and the ataxia is due to the lesion in the ascending proprioceptive tracts, especially the spinocerebellar tracts. Typically, pelvic limb signs are worse than those in the thoracic limbs. This may reflect the more superficial position of the pelvic limb spinocerebellar tracts in the spinal cord at the site of the injury, or the further distance of the pelvic limbs from the center of gravity of the animal, or both. The occasional mild scapular muscle atrophy reflects the chronicity of the lesion, with neuronal loss from the grey matter of the C6 and C7 segments.

In studying the gait disorder that occurs in this disease, it first must be determined that this is a neurologic disorder and not an abnormal gait caused by one or more of the several skeletal diseases that occur in the young, rapidly growing dogs of the giant breeds.

Coxofemoral dysplasia, osteochondrosis dissecans, hypertrophic osteodystrophy, and genu valgum are some of these diseases. On observing the gait, the examiner must keep in mind the question of whether the patient is unwilling to perform a function because of pain from skeletal disease, or is unable to perform it owing to neurologic dysfunction. In the skeletal diseases the stride usually is shortened, and the gait may appear choppy. There may be an asymmetric posture or function of the limbs, or both. In all instances, however, in the absence of neurologic disease the patient knows the position of its limbs at all times. The limbs are not crossed, or abducted excessively, nor do they appear to be positioned widely apart. If the patient responds to postural testing there is no failure to perform the tests. Careful palpation of the joints may reveal a lesion or cause pain. In some instances, the animal may have both a neurologic and a skeletal disease, but careful testing should reveal the neurologic deficit. The examiner must decide whether the dog will not or cannot carry out a function. The former indicates skeletal disease, the latter neurologic disease. The ataxic dog with a cervical spinal cord lesion does not have control over the position of its limbs. This accounts for the wide-based,

abducted gait with stumbling and flexing of the digits so that the dorsal surface of the paw is placed on the ground surface.

In the young dog the primary neurologic disease to differentiate is canine distemper myelitis. Occasionally a dog with encephalomyelitis caused by the canine distemper virus will present with signs of spinal cord disease. Careful neurologic examination of the patient with cervical spinal cord myelitis from canine distemper usually reveals other abnormalities that cannot be explained by a lesion that is localized solely in the cervical spinal cord. The distemper lesion in the nervous system usually is disseminated, and most of the time signs reflect the site of greatest damage. Paraplegia with mild thoracic limb deficit requires two lesions of different severity, one cervical and one thoracolumbar. Head tilts or tremor and abnormal nystagmus depend on a cerebellovestibular lesion. The cerebrospinal fluid is often abnormal.

Focal cervical spinal cord neoplasms must be ruled out, especially in the older dog. Neurofibroma, meningioma, and lymphosarcoma have been seen in young animals. These require myelography for diagnosis.

Intervertebral disk extrusions, not associated with caudal cervical vertebral malformation-malarticulation, usually occur in older dogs and most often can be identified readily by plain radiographs. Cervical pain, not usually observed in dogs with cervical vertebral malformation-malarticulation, is often the prominent sign in cervical disk disease. It is not clear if these diseases are separate entities or the malarticulation predisposes to the disk degeneration.

Ancillary studies include clinical laboratory studies, electromyography, and radiography. If there is ventral grey column involvement, electromyography of the scapular muscles may show denervation potentials. Laboratory studies of blood, urine, and CSF have revealed no abnormalities except for an occasional mild elevation of protein content of CSF.

Radiographs of the caudal cervical vertebrae of the normally fully extended and fully flexed neck in lateral view are the most helpful. In some patients the ventrodorsal view has revealed asymmetry of vertebral structures. The following observations may reflect the source of the spinal cord contusion:

1. Malarticulation: One of the caudal cervical vertebrae may be malarticulated so that the craniodorsal aspect of its vertebral body is displaced into the vertebral canal. This may

be stable and be evident on both flexed and extended neck views. It may be unstable and only be apparent on the flexed neck view. This unstable malarticulation is referred to as spondylolisthesis (spondylo = vertebra, listhesis = slipping).

2. Malformation: These changes may reflect the response of the vertebrae and adjacent soft tissues to the abnormal forces associated with or resulting in the malarticulation. The cranial orifice of the vertebral foramen may be stenotic, with or without deformity of the craniodorsal or cranioventral aspects of the vertebral body. Exostoses may occur, especially at the cranioventral aspect of the vertebral body. There may be degenerative changes in the associated intervertebral disks, which may culminate in complete collapse of the disk and ankylosis of the adjacent vertebrae. Chronic protrusion and enlargement of the intervertebral disk into the vertebral canal may occur in older dogs. Degenerative periarticular osteoarthropathy may be apparent at the synovial joints.

Ventrodorsal radiographs may reveal a stenotic caudal aspect of a vertebral foramen.[144] This is the result of too narrow a distance between the pedicles of the vertebral arch or medial encroachment by enlarged articular processes. This cannot be observed on a lateral radiograph. A ventrodorsal view of a cervical myelogram may be necessary to demonstrate this.

Most dogs have a combination of malarticulation and malformation. A few dogs have demonstrated the typical physical and neurologic signs, but no radiographic abnormality can be seen on plain radiographs. A myelogram may reveal soft tissue changes associated with the caudal cervical vertebrae. Proliferation of the interarcuate ligament (yellow ligament) or protrusion of the dorsal longitudinal ligament or the intervertebral disk may be identified. Patients with a protruded-extruded intervertebral disk may show more deviation of the myelogram in a lateral view of the neck in full flexion. If there is proliferation of the dorsal longitudinal ligament, this may fold and buckle on full extension of the neck and cause more deviation of the myelogram in this position.

In some dogs the stenosis of the cranial orifice of the vertebral foramen is associated with a deformation and elongation of the vertebral arch. This primarily compresses the spinal cord on neck extension and is best diagnosed with a myelogram performed in that position.[191] Be aware that excessive flexion or extension may exacerbate the compression.

In some patients there may be radiographic abnormalities at more than one cervical articulation. Therefore, a cervical myelogram is necessary to clearly define the location and nature of the spinal cord compression for surgical consideration.

At necropsy, disarticulation of cervical vertebrae often reveals a compressed spinal cord segment at the cranial orifice of one or more of the caudal cervical vertebrae. The vertebral foramen is often funnel-shaped, with the smaller orifice at the cranial end. Occasionally, an enlarged interarcuate ligament rests on the dorsal surface of the compressed spinal cord at the entrance to a vertebral foramen. If the stenosis is caudal in a vertebral foramen from too narrow an interpedicular distance, the spinal cord will be compressed from side to side.

Microscopy shows a focal spinal cord injury usually limited to the sixth and/or seventh cervical spinal cord segments. Occasionally, the fifth segment is involved. There is a variable degree of degeneration of the grey and white matter in these segments, involving almost all of the funiculi. Myelin degeneration is the most pronounced lesion in the white matter. Axonal degeneration is less prominent.

Sometimes there is a focal area of necrosis in one or more of the funiculi. At the site of the focal spinal cord lesion, there often is a paucity of neurons in the grey matter with an abundance of hypertrophied astrocytes.

In the spinal cord segments cranial to this focal lesion, the white matter degeneration is limited primarily to the ascending tracts in the dorsal funiculi and the superficial portions of the dorsolateral funiculi. Caudal to the focal lesion, the white matter degeneration is limited to the descending spinal cord tracts in the ventral funiculi and deep portions of the lateral funiculi. This pattern of noninflammatory degeneration of ascending neurons cranial to the injury and descending neurons caudal to the injury is explained by a Wallerian-type of degeneration of the axon and its myelin that occurs in the segment of the neuron which is separated from its cell body (Figs. 10–2, 10–3). In this disease, the neurons are destroyed at the site of the injury, usually the sixth, or seventh, or both cervical spinal cord segments.[78, 179, 180] For this Wallerian type of degeneration to occur, the focal lesion must be severe enough to destroy axons in the white matter. These will not repair. In milder lesions,

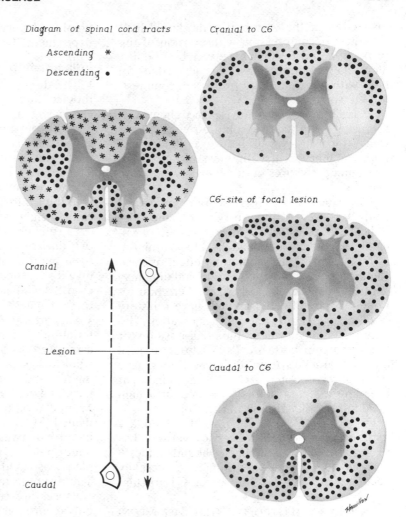

Diagram of spinal cord tracts

Ascending *

Descending •

Cranial to C6

C6 - site of focal lesion

Caudal to C6

Cranial

Lesion

Caudal

Figure 10–3. Pattern of spinal cord degeneration following a focal segmental lesion.

myelin may be lost at the focal lesion without axonal degeneration. This will interfere with function but the affected axonal segment can potentially be remyelinated. The latter lesion is part of the basis for surgical decompression.

Prognosis for recovery depends on the severity of the defect, the radiographic lesion, and the age of the patient. Some young dogs that are still ambulatory and have only slight radiographic lesions may respond spontaneously if their activity is restricted by confining them. Corticosteroids may help if the clinical signs suddenly exacerbate. These dogs may "grow out" of their problem by enlarging their vertebral canal sufficiently to accommodate the spinal cord.

Older dogs with a long, chronic course that are still ambulatory with mild radiographic lesions may respond to corticosteroid therapy and be maintained for months and treated when clinical signs exacerbate. Older dogs with an acute onset and even fairly severe signs and

mild radiographic lesions may respond to corticosteroid therapy. The response to corticosteroid therapy should be evaluated before a decision is made for surgery.

Surgery is advocated when the clinical signs and/or the radiographic lesions are severe or the response to corticosteroids is poor.[41, 52, 139, 162, 163] The chronically severely affected dog has the worst prognosis, for the spinal cord lesions may be permanent. The surgical procedure employed depends on the type of malarticulation/malformation that is present and the experience of the surgeon.[80] Three procedures are advocated.

Dorsal decompressive laminectomy (DDL) alone is advocated for a stenotic cranial orifice of a vertebral foramen, or a stable malarticulation. A DDL with arthrodesis of the articular processes is advocated for the unstable malarticulation without a deformity of the craniodorsal aspect of the vertebral body. Malarticulations with a prominent craniodorsal projection of the vertebral body should have a ventral decompression with excision of this projection and fusion of the vertebral bodies. Ventral decompressions are advocated for dogs with significant disk protrusion compressing the spinal cord.[24]

It is important to advise the client that following a dorsal decompressive laminectomy, most dogs will be worse before any improvement occurs. In most instances improvement requires a number of weeks to occur.

The cause of this disease is unknown. A study on overnutrition in Great Dane dogs indicated a possible role of excess dietary calcium, hypercalcemia, and hypercalcitoninism in this disease.[73] The inhibitory effect of calcitonin on bone resorption and remodeling may contribute to the stenosis of the vertebral foramen. Many affected animals have a history of excessive feeding and supplementation. Genetics may play a role in the predisposition for this disease in both breeds.[157] Closely related affected animals from different litters have been observed, and it has been found that breeding affected animals resulted in a high incidence of this disease in the progeny.

C3: Basset Hound. A possible hereditary malformation of the third cervical vertebra has been observed in male basset hounds under 6 months old.[125] Spinal cord compression usually occurs at either the C2-C3 or C3-C4 articulation.

VERTEBRAL OSTEOMYELITIS—DISKOSPONDYLITIS. (see discussion of Thoracolumbar Spinal Cord Disease, p. 190). In the cervical vertebrae this disease occurs more frequently in the caudal vertebrae. In areas of the country in which the parasite *Spirocerca lupi* exists, it may be the cause of such a caudal cervical lesion.

SPONDYLOSIS DEFORMANS—DURAL OSSIFICATION. (See discussion of Thoracolumbar Spinal Cord Disease.)

VERTEBRAL EXOSTOSIS—HYPERVITAMINOSIS A. Cats that are fed a diet with high levels of vitamin A such as raw liver develop extensive bone proliferation related to diarthrodial joints.[42, 154, 155] This exostosis becomes extensive and fuses cervical vertebrae, limb joints, and ultimately the entire vertebral column. Clinical signs of cervical pain and rigidity are common. Neurologic defects relate to cervical spinal nerve entrapment at intervertebral foramina and compression of the cervical spinal cord. The lesion is obvious on radio-

graphs. Hypervitaminosis A has been studied experimentally in dogs.[26]

Inflammation

The discussion of these diseases under the thoracolumbar spinal cord is referable to the cervical area, only the clinical signs indicate cervical spinal cord disease (see p. 191).

Canine distemper myelitis occasionally affects grey matter in a multifocal distribution. The sporozoan *Toxoplasma gondii* frequently affects grey matter. If a portion of the lesion is in the C6 to T1 segments of the spinal cord, clinical signs referable to this area are seen. As a rule, clinical signs also are found in these two diseases that are indicative of the multifocal nature of the lesion. Granulomatous myelitis (reticulosis) also must be considered.[45, 90] CSF studies are helpful in confirming these diagnoses.

Suppurative Meningitis and Myelitis. Bacterial-induced suppurative myelitis usually is associated with encephalitis and meningitis. Clinical signs mostly are referable to the meningitis, and consist of hyperesthesia, a stiff neck and gait, and severe pain induced by any manipulation of the patient. It often is accompanied by fever, anorexia, increased white blood cell count on hematologic study, and neutrophils in the CSF. The degree of CSF pleocytosis and protein elevation is variable. The response to antibiotic therapy is variable. Relapses are frequent and may be thwarted only by prolonged therapy. Whenever possible the infectious agent should be cultured and treatment based on antibiotic sensitivity testing.

Recently we have become more aware of a clinical syndrome that has the clinical and CSF features of a suppurative meningitis but without evidence of any infectious agent either in the neutrophils of the CSF or on extensive culture of blood and CSF. Some of these patients will respond only to corticosteroid therapy and may relapse if it is not continued. An immunologic pathogenesis is suspected.

Currently, this is the most common finding in patients that present with severe axial pain (especially in the neck region), depression, reluctance or inability to walk, high fever, and often a leukocytosis in the blood. CSF usually contains a significant elevation of neutrophils and protein. Occasionally a single sample of CSF will be normal. The procedure should be repeated before searching for a different cause for the signs.

An extremely severe form of meningitis and associated myclitis and encephalitis has been observed in young dogs of many breeds but predominantly in beagles.[68, 86] Most dogs are between 3 and 18 months of age, but a few older dogs have been affected. The signs are characterized by recurrent episodes of pain and fever that last 2 to 11 days, often followed by spontaneous improvement. Intervals between episodes range from a few days to months. Ultimately parenchymal involvement becomes too advanced for the dog to recover.

The pain is manifested by extreme reluctance to move, a short-strided, stiff gait when the patients move, a partly flexed and retracted neck, and screaming on being handled. As the parenchyma becomes involved the signs will reflect the segmental area most affected.

CSF pleocytosis is profound with hundreds to thousands of neutrophils per cmm. Xanthochromia is common owing to hemorrhage.

At necropsy an extensive suppurative leptomeningitis is found associated with severe arteritis with fibrinoid necrosis of the vessel wall. Hemorrhage is common. No infectious agents have been observed or cultured. An immunopathologic disorder is proposed for this disease.

Cerebrospinal Nematodiasis. Reports of cerebrospinal nematodiasis in dogs are rare. Two examples have been reported in Australia. One was a migration of the larval form of the rat lungworm, *Angiostrongylus cantonensis,* in the spinal cord and brain of puppies.[110] Clinical signs consisted of a progressive paralysis from the pelvic to the thoracic limbs. Paralysis of the tail, bladder, and rectum suggests significant involvement of the lumbosacral segments. Affected puppies were 6 to 14 weeks old.

In the second report, an adult *Ancylostoma caninum* was found in the cervical spinal cord of a 12-week-old puppy that had progressive neurologic disease including tetraplegia prior to death.[20]

The puppies in both reports were noted to show an excessive amount of pain on being handled.

Degeneration

Fibrocartilaginous Embolic Myelopathy. Spinal cord infarction from vascular emboli presumed to be fibrocartilage may occur in the cervical spinal cord and produce bilateral or unilateral clinical signs. Most cases have been unilateral, producing ipsilateral spastic hemi-

paresis or hemiplegia. The signs usually are sudden in onset, with full development in less than 12 hours. In one case that was an exception it took at least 48 hours for the complete development of the hemiplegia. In hemiplegic patients, varying degrees of Horner's syndrome have often been observed ipsilaterally, presumably from the sudden complete interruption of the lateral tectotegmentospinal system.

The CSF often has a mild elevation of its protein content, and for the first 24 hours or so may have an increased neutrophil population. A myclogram may reveal a swollen spinal cord at the site of the ischemic lesion.

Spontaneous recovery often has been observed, especially if some voluntary movement has been retained in the thoracic limb. Signs of improvement usually are evident during the first week after the onset of the signs. This improvement may be accounted for by the resolution of edema and hemorrhage, and collateral circulation to areas that were ischemic but not yet necrotic. In time, the dog may compensate for the permanent loss of a portion of its spinal cord parenchyma, and this also may contribute to its continued improvement. Prompt and vigorous corticosteroid therapy is advocated for this vascular insult.

At necropsy, the lesion often is limited to the lateral funiculus and adjacent grey matter on one side. A few hemorrhages may be present in the soft necrotic tissue. These lesions can be explained only by the occlusion of multiple vessels with emboli (see Fig. 10–4).

Occasionally a hemiplegic patient will show a remarkable tendency to force itself toward the paralyzed side. It will not lie on its normal side, but immediately attempts to roll itself to its paralyzed side. No neck or head disorientation is evident, and there is no abnormal nystagmus. This is evidence that the unilateral cervical spinal cord lesion involves the ventral funiculus with its vestibulospinal tract, which accounts for the torsion of the dog's trunk.

The following is a case report of a dog with this lesion in the right lateral funiculus of the cervical spinal cord.

Signalment. A 4-year-old female sheltie.

Chief Complaint. The patient was unable to get up.

History. Four days prior to examination, the patient was playing outside with another dog when it lay down and was unable to get up.

Physical Examination. The dog was reluctant to stand and walk. If supported, it moved the left limbs well but not the right limbs. Both right limbs

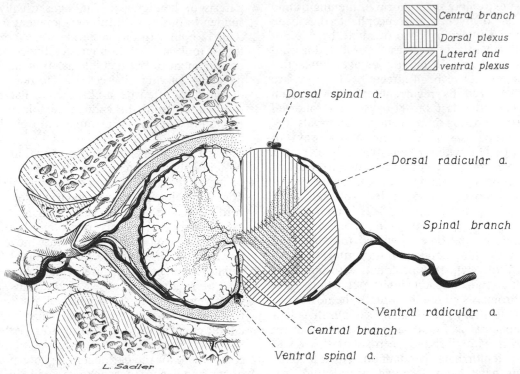

Central branch
Dorsal plexus
Lateral and
ventral plexus

Dorsal spinal a.

Dorsal radicular a.

Spinal branch

Ventral radicular a.

Central branch

Ventral spinal a.

L. Sadler

Figure 10–4. Arterial vasculature of the canine spinal cord. The lesion distribution following fibrocartilaginous emboli reflects multiple vascular occlusion. (From J. Am. Anim. Hosp. Assoc., *12*:37, 1976.)

were severely paretic, and hypertonic with no atrophy. The right patellar reflex was brisk. Flexor reflexes were intact and when elicited in the left limbs, crossed extension occurred in the right limbs. Postural reactions were absent in the right limbs. Most were performed adequately in the left limbs but the patient fell easily if pushed when hemiwalking on the left side. No neck pain was elicited.

Anatomic Diagnosis. The lesion was on the right side of the cervical spinal cord, probably cranial to the C6 segment.

Ancillary Procedures. Radiographs were normal. CSF contained 23 RBC and 12 mononuclear cells per cmm and 44 mg of protein per dl.

Differential Diagnosis. The sudden onset, non-progression of signs, lack of pain, normal radiographs, and elevated protein levels in the CSF with a few mononuclear cells suggest ischemic myelopathy.

Outcome. Over a period of 10 days in the hospital with no treatment, the dog slowly improved. At discharge, it could just stand and walk. After 3 months, the only residual deficit the owner noted was a slight tendency for the right thoracic limb to slide out on the slippery kitchen floor when the dog lowered its head to eat. Its gait was normal.

A common site for embolic-induced spinal cord infarction is the cervical intumescence. More often the lesion is unilateral. The disease

usually results in an acute onset of a very severe neurologic deficit. Usually, the more severe the degree of lower motor neuron deficit in the thoracic limb, the poorer are the chances for the patient's spontaneous improvement.

The following two case reports are concerned with this disease at this location.

Signalment. A 6-year-old male border collie.

Chief Complaint. The dog was unable to stand.

History. Five days prior to examination, in the evening, the dog suddenly was noted to have difficulty using the right thoracic limb. By the following morning, it could not use the right pelvic limb.

Physical Examination. The dog was alert and responsive. It could not stand up, but when given assistance readily moved the left limbs but not the right limbs. The right pelvic limb was hypertonic and supported weight in a reflex response. The left pelvic limb was not normal in its use, but was much better than the right pelvic limb. The right thoracic limb was atonic and could not support weight. The left thoracic limb was normal.

The right pupil was smaller than normal. The right third eyelid protruded, and the palpebral fissure was reduced slightly in size.

There was essentially no response to postural reaction testing in the right limbs. Occasionally, a slight attempt at hopping occurred in the right pelvic limb. The left pelvic limb was slow on hopping and proprioceptive positioning was abnormal. Hemiwalking was slightly weak on the left side, and the left thoracic limb occasionally knuckled when walking with the neck extended.

Muscle tone was reduced markedly in the right thoracic limb, and increased mildly in both pelvic limbs. There was a slight indication of atrophy in the right scapular muscles. Patellar reflexes were brisk bilaterally. The biceps and triceps reflexes were brisk in the left thoracic limb and absent in the right limb. The flexor reflexes were normal, except in the right thoracic limb, in which the reflex was absent. There was marked hypalgesia over most of the right thoracic limb distal to the elbow.

Anatomic Diagnosis. These signs indicate a severe lesion on the right side of the spinal cord from C6 to T1 or to T3 with involvement of the grey matter to account for the right forelimb LMN paralysis and hypalgesia and the white matter to account for the UMN paralysis of the right pelvic limb.

The Horner's syndrome can be explained by a grey matter lesion from T1 to T3 or a severe lateral funiculus lesion cranial to T1 involving the lateral tectotegmentospinal tract.

The mild left limb deficits can reflect mild swelling of the left side of the spinal cord at the site of the infarction or the involvement of GP tracts that cross at their origin in the spinal cord and UMN tracts that cross at their termination.

Radiography. Plain and contrast radiographs were normal.

Laboratory Findings. CSF contained 187 RBC and 4 mononuclear cells per cmm, and 57 mg of protein per dl.

Presumptive Diagnosis. The sudden onset without a history of trauma, the lack of progression, lack of neck pain, normal radiographs, and abnormal CSF suggest that spinal cord infarction is the kind of lesion present. Fibrocartilaginous embolic myelopathy is the most likely mechanism.

Outcome. No improvement occurred after 10 days of hospitalization. Euthanasia was performed.

Necropsy. There was ischemic and hemorrhagic infarction of the right side of the spinal cord from C6 to C8 in the dorsal and lateral funiculi and the grey matter on the right side. The ventral funiculus was spared. Fibrocartilaginous emboli were found in small arteries and veins associated with the parenchymal lesion.

The lack of lesion in the cranial thoracic segments indicated that the Horner's syndrome was caused by the destruction of the lateral tectotegmentospinal tract by the lateral funicular lesion.

Signalment. A 3-year-old male schnauzer.

Chief Complaint. The dog was unable to get up.

History. Four days prior to the referral examination, the owner noticed early in the morning that the dog was unable to use its right pelvic limb. By the time it was presented to the referring veterinarian later that morning, it could not use either right limb. These signs did not change in the interval prior to examination. There was no obvious source of injury, and no pain was associated with the problem.

Physical Examination. The dog was alert and responsive. There was no evidence of cerebral or cranial nerve involvement, but the right pupil and palpebral fissure were smaller than the left, and the right third eyelid was protruded.

The dog was in right lateral recumbency. Any attempts to put it in left lateral recumbency was met with strenuous resistance. The pelvic limbs extended caudally, and flailed along with the left thoracic limb until the dog righted itself to a sternal or right lateral recumbent position. The neck and head were well oriented, but the trunk frequently was curved. The disorientation stimulated on placing the dog in left lateral recumbency only seemed to involve the limbs and trunk caudal to the neck. On the animal's struggling to move out of left lateral recumbency, the body flexed, with the concavity to the right side. When in sternal recumbency the body often was twisted, mostly with the concavity to the right side. The left limbs seemed to be pushing the dog over to the right side during these periods of disorientation.

The dog could not stand to walk. If held up, the left limbs moved but were stiff or hypertonic. The right limbs did not move, except for an occasional attempt with the right thoracic limb. It was difficult to hold the dog straight to test this because of the tendency of the trunk to twist and fall to the right.

Postural reactions were intact on the left, but very brisk and spastic (hypertonic). The right thoracic limb made small, essentially useless attempts to hop; the right pelvic limb did not move. Placing, proprioceptive positioning, and hemiwalking were absent on the right side.

The pelvic limbs showed hypertonia, especially the right limb. The left thoracic limb was hypertonic, but the right thoracic limb was hypotonic. Patellar reflexes were brisk on the left, and the dog was too tense to adequately grade the reflex on the right. Flexor reflexes were intact except for the right thoracic limb, in which the reflex was depressed. There was a mild hypalgesia of the right thoracic limb.

Anatomic Diagnosis. These signs suggest a lesion of the caudal cervical and cranial thoracic spinal cord on the right side. The grey matter lesion accounts for the hypotonia and hyporeflexia of the right thoracic limb and Horner's syndrome, if the T1 through T3 segments were involved. The white matter lesion accounts for the spastic paralysis of the right pelvic limb and also possibly Horner's syndrome, by its interference with the descending lateral tectotegmentospinal tract in the lateral funiculus.

The tendency to lean, fall, and roll right with the trunk but without head, neck, or eye abnormalities suggests an ipsilateral (right) ventral funiculus lesion with loss of the vestibulospinal tract on that side.

Radiography. Plain radiographs were normal.

Laboratory Findings. CSF contained 9 RBC and 8 mononuclear cells per cmm, and 30 mg of protein per dl.

Presumptive Diagnosis. The sudden onset, without a history of trauma, and the lack of progression, lack of neck pain, normal radiographs, and abnormal CSF suggest spinal cord infarction with fibrocartilaginous emboli as the most likely cause.

Outcome. The dog improved over a period of 7 days' hospitalization. It could stand and walk at discharge. Five months later, examination only showed abnormality in proprioception of the right pelvic limb. It stood, walked, and ran freely without obvious abnormality.

Demyelinating Myelopathy in Miniature Poodles and Hereditary Myelopathy with Myelinolysis in Afghan Hounds. In these suspected familial diseases, pelvic limb deficits are the first to be observed. As the disease progresses, the cervical spinal cord and thoracic limb function become involved. (See discussion under Thoracolumbar Spinal Cord Disease, p. 193.)

Progressive Axonopathy of Boxer Dogs. Progressive axonopathy is a presumed autosomal recessive disease of Boxer dogs with an insidious onset of clinical signs usually prior to 6 months of age. The signs are slowly progressive and consist of an ataxia, swaying, hypermetric gait that is most pronounced in the pelvic limbs. Ataxia is much more evident than paresis. Forelimb signs follow the onset in the pelvic limbs and are less pronounced. In time the signs may become static.

Proprioceptive deficits are pronounced. Hypotonia and patellar areflexia develop, but flexor reflexes and pain perception remain normal. Muscle atrophy is minimal and cranial nerve function remains normal.

Motor nerve conduction velocity is decreased and the amplitude of motor and sensory action potentials decreases.

Lesions are most profound in the central nervous system and consist of large axonal spheroids and degenerating fibers in the spinal cord and brain. Symmetric degeneration occurs in the dorsolateral and ventral funiculi throughout the spinal cord with sparing of the dorsal funiculi. Spheroids are common in numerous brain stem nuclei and some tracts and the cerebellum. Peripheral nerve lesions are nonspecific with loss of myelinated fibers, axonal degeneration, primary and secondary demyelination, remyelination, and regenerating clusters of fibers.

Spinocerebellar Tract Degeneration. An hereditary autosomal recessive ataxia has been described in smooth-haired fox terriers[11, 12] and a similar ataxia was described in two Jack Russell terriers.[69] The onset of signs was between 10 and 16 weeks of age. These signs progressed rapidly at first then slowly and after a few months there was little change seen. The gait was described as consisting of "bouncy, dancing movements." The exaggerated limb movements and balance loss caused these dogs to fall frequently. The posture was basewide with a swaying trunk and head oscillations. Some animals became unable to stand and walk.

The pathology reports on both breeds of terriers describe a bilaterally symmetric spinal cord degeneration in the spinocerebellar tracts (dorsolateral funiculus) and the sulcomarginal tracts adjacent to the ventral median fissure. In the Jack Russell terriers a peripheral neuropathy was also observed as well as more extensive CNS tract degeneration.

Recent studies on human patients with Friedreich's ataxia have implicated a possible biochemical basis for the degenerative nervous system lesion.[9, 10, 85]

Neoplasia—Intramedullary (see Thoracolumbar Spinal Cord Disease, p. 194.)

Malformation

Myelodysplasia. Myelodysplasia usually is restricted to the thoracolumbar spinal cord. Cervical spinal cord malformations are rare but produce signs present at birth that are static and do not progress in severity.

Hydrocephalus-Hydromyelia. Dogs with noncommunicating hydrocephalus from failure of lateral apertures to develop may have cavitating lesions in the cervical spinal cord in addition to the extreme expansion of all the ventricles. Clinical signs may reflect involvement of the cerebral hemispheres, cerebellum, and cervical spinal cord. The hydrosyringomyelia in the cervical spinal cord is a rare lesion and probably results from the relentless intraventricular hypertension that is reflected in the central canal. Dogs with clinical signs referable to the cervical spinal cord lesion are usually a few months old. The signs are slowly progressive.

Swimmer Syndrome in Puppies. This is not a disorder of the cervical spinal cord, but is discussed here because of its consideration in a differential diagnosis of malformations.

Occasionally one or more of a litter of puppies is found with its limbs too abducted to stand and walk at a time when it normally should. These puppies make swimming motions with their abducted limbs in their attempts to move. There may be an associated severe dorsoventral compression of the thorax. They are alert, responsive, and strong. There is no detectable neurologic deficit. In time, permanent secondary joint deformities and ankylosis may occur in the limbs. The condition seems to represent a musculoskeletal growth abnormality. The pathogenesis is not well understood. There may be two mechanisms for this disease.

1. The disease has been reported in English bulldogs, Sealyham terriers, and Pekingese dogs with achondroplasia or osteochrondrodystrophy. This may be a metabolic or endocrine disease causing imperfect ossification of the long bones at the epiphyses, which may contribute to the development of the swimmer syndrome.

2. The disease also occurs in puppies of breeds with no detectable underlying skeletal disease. German shepherds, black and tan coonhounds, and miniature poodles have been involved. In these animals poor management may contribute to the syndrome. Puppies raised on a hard, slippery surface are unable to adduct their limbs to support themselves and walk, and the pressure of the body on the hard surface contributes to the deformity of the thorax.

In most necropsies of these dogs no discernible abnormality has been found in the nervous or musculoskeletal systems.

If the condition is recognized early, it may be reversed by management procedures. These include hobbling the puppies by tying their limbs in an adducted position and bedding them on deep, soft material such as a box of crumpled newspaper or on thick padding or blankets. Owners that have the most success attend these puppies continually.

REFERENCES

1. Averill, D. R., Jr., and de Lahunta, A.: Toxoplasmosis of the canine nervous system: Clinicopathologic findings in four cases. J. Am. Vet. Med. Assoc., 159:1134, 1971.
2. Alden, C. L., and Dickerson, T. V.: Osteochondromatosis of the cervical vertebrae in a dog. J. Am. Vet. Med. Assoc., 168:142, 1976.
3. Averill, D. R., Jr.: Degenerative myelopathy in the aging German shepherd dog: Clinical and pathologic findings. J. Am. Vet. Med. Assoc., 162:1045, 1973.
4. Averill, D. R., and Bronson, R. T.: Inherited necrotizing myelopathy of Afghan hounds. J. Neuropathol. Exp. Neurol., 36:734, 1977.
5. Bailey, C. S.: An embryological approach to the clinical significance of congenital vertebral and spinal cord abnormalities. J. Am. Anim. Hosp. Assoc., 11:426, 1975.
6. Bailey, C. S., and Holliday, T. A.: Diseases of the spinal cord. In Ettinger, S. J. (ed.): Textbook of Veterinary Internal Medicine. Philadelphia, W. B. Saunders Co., 1975.
7. Ball, M. U., McGuire, J. A., Swaim, S. F., and Hoerlein, B. F.: Patterns of occurrence of disk disease among registered Dachshunds. J. Am. Vet. Med. Assoc., 180:519, 1982.
8. Banks, W. C., and Bridges, C. H.: Multiple cartilaginous exostosis in a dog. J. Am. Vet. Med. Assoc., 129:131, 1956.
9. Barbeau, A.: Friedreich's ataxia 1979: An overview. J. Can. Sci. Neurol., 6:311, 1979.
10. Barbeau, A., Melancon, S., Butterworth, R. F., Filla, A., Izumi, K., and Ngo, T. T.: Pyruvate dehydrogenase complex in Friedreich's ataxia. Adv. Neurol., 21:203, 1978.
11. Bjorck, G., Dyrendahl, S., and Olsson, S. E.: Hereditary ataxia in smooth-haired fox terriers. Vet. Rec., 69:871, 1957.
12. Bjorck, G., Mair, W., Olsson, S. E., and Sourander, P.: Hereditary ataxia in fox terriers. Acta Neuropathol. [Suppl.]1:45, 1962.
13. Braund, K. G., Everett, R. M., Bartels, J. E., and DeBuysscher, E.: Neurologic complications of IgA multiple myeloma associated with cryoglobulinemia in a dog. J. Am. Vet. Med. Assoc., 174:1321, 1979.
14. Braund, K. G., Ghosh, P., Taylor, T. K. F., and Larsen, L. H.: Morphological studies of the canine intervertebral disc: The assignment of the Beagle to the achondroplastic classification. Res. Vet. Sci., 19:167, 1975.
15. Braund, K. G., Taylor, T. K. F., Ghosh, P., and Sherwood, A. A.: Spinal mobility in the dog: A study in chondrodystrophoid and nonchondrodystrophoid animals. Res. Vet. Sci., 22:78, 1977.
16. Braund, K. G., and Vandevelde, M.: German shepherd dog myelopathy—a morphologic and morphometric study. Am. J. Vet. Res., 39:1309, 1978.
17. Brown, N. O., Helphrey, M. L., and Prata, R. G.: Thoracolumbar disk disease in the dog: A retrospective analysis of 187 cases. J. Am. Anim. Hosp. Assoc., 13:665, 1977.
18. Bullock, L. P., and Zook, B. C.: Myelography in dogs using water-soluble contrast mediums. J. Am. Vet. Med. Assoc., 151:321, 1967.
19. Butler, H. C.: An investigation into the relationship of an aortic embolus to posterior paralysis in the cat. J. Small Anim. Pract., 12:141, 1971.
20. Bwick, T. D., Campbell, R. S. F., and Hutchinson, G. W.: Spinal nematodiasis of the dog associated with Ancylostoma caninum. Aust. Vet. J., 53:602, 1977.
21. Carlisle, C. H., Kelly, W. R., Samuel, J., and Robins, G. M.: Spinal cord compression caused by a metastatic lesion from an aortic body tumor. Aust. Vet. J., 54:311, 1978.
22. Chambers, J. N., and Betts, C. W.: Caudal cervical spondylopathy in the dog: A review of 20 clinical

cases and the literature. J. Am. Anim. Hosp. Assoc., *13*:571, 1977.

23. Chambers, J. N., Betts, C. W., and Oliver, J. E.: The use of nonmetallic suture material for stabilization of atlantoaxial subluxation. J. Am. Anim. Hosp. Assoc., *13*:602, 1977.

24. Chambers, J. N., Oliver, J. E., Jr., Kornegay, J. N., and Malnati, G. A.: Ventral decompression for caudal cervical disk herniation in large- and giant-breed dogs. J. Am. Vet. Med. Assoc., *180*:410, 1982.

25. Chester, D. K.: Multiple cartilaginous exostoses in two generations of dogs. J. Am. Vet. Med. Assoc., *159*:895, 1971.

26. Cho, D. Y., Frey, R. A., Guffy, M. M., and Leipold, H. W.: Hypervitaminosis A in the dog. Am. J. Vet. Res., *36*:1597, 1975.

27. Chrisman, C. L.: Electromyography in the localization of spinal cord and nerve root neoplasia in dogs and cats. J. Am. Vet. Med. Assoc., *166*:1074, 1975.

28. Cockrell, B. Y., Herigstad, R. R., Flo, G. L., and Legendre, A. M.: Myelomalacia in Afghan hounds. J. Am. Vet. Med. Assoc., *162*:362, 1973.

29. Cook, J. R., and Oliver, J. E., Jr.: Atlantoaxial luxation in the dog. Compend. Contin. Ed., *3*:242, 1981.

30. Cordy, D. R.: Vascular malformations and hemangiomas of the canine spinal cord. Vet. Pathol., *16*:275, 1979.

31. Cummings, J. F., and de Lahunta, A.: Hereditary myelopathy of Afghan hounds: A myelinolytic disease. Acta Neuropathol., *42*:173, 1978.

32. Deforest, M. E., and Basrur, P. K.: Malformations and the Manx syndrome in cats. Can. Vet. J., *20*:304, 1979.

33. de Lahunta, A.: Progressive cervical spinal cord compression in Great Dane and Doberman pinscher dogs (a wobbler syndrome). *In* Kirk, R. W. (ed.): Current Veterinary Therapy V. Small Animal Practice. Philadelphia, W. B. Saunders, 1974, 674–675.

34. deLahunta, A., and Alexander, J. W.: Ischemic myelopathy secondary to presumed fibrocartilaginous embolism in nine dogs. J. Am. Anim. Hosp. Assoc., *12*:37, 1976.

35. de La Torre, J. C., Johnson, C. M., Goode, D. J., and Mullan, S.: Pharmacologic treatment and evaluation of permanent experimental spinal cord trauma. Neurology, *25*:508, 1975.

36. de La Torre, J. C., Kawanaga, H. M., Rowed, D. W., Johnson, C. M., Goode, D. J., Kajihara, K., and Mullan, S.: Dimethylsulfoxide in central nervous system trauma. Ann. N.Y. Acad. Sci., *243*:362, 1975.

37. Denny, H. R., Gibbs, C., and Gaskell, C. J.: Cervical spondylopathy in the dog—a review of thirty-five cases. J. Small Anim. Pract., *18*:117, 1977.

38. Doige, C. E., Pharr, J. W., and Withrow, S. J.: Chondrosarcoma arising in multiple cartilaginous exostosis in a dog. J. Am. Anim. Hosp. Assoc., *14*:605, 1978.

39. Douglas, S. W., and Palmer, A. C.: Idiopathic demyelination of brain stem and cord in a miniature poodle puppy. J. Pathol. Bacteriol., *82*:67, 1961.

40. Draper, D. D., Kluge, J. P., and Miller, W. J.: Clinical and pathological aspects of spinal dysraphism in dogs. Proceedings of the 20th World Veterinary Congress. Thessaloniki, Greece, 1975.

41. Dueland, R., Furneau, R. W., and Kaye, M. M.: Spinal fusion and dorsal laminectomy for midcervical spondylolisthesis in a dog. J. Am. Vet. Med. Assoc., *162*:366, 1973.

42. English, P. B.: A case of hyperostosis due to hypervitaminosis A in a cat. J. Small Anim. Pract., *10*:207, 1969.

43. English, P. B.: Clinical communication: A case of hyperostosis due to hypervitaminosis A in a cat. J. Small Anim. Pract., *10*:207, 1969.

44. Fankhauser, R., Fatzer, R., Luginbuhl, H., and McGrath, J. T.: Reticulosis of the central nervous system in dogs. Adv. Vet. Sci. Comp. Med., *16*:35, 1972.

45. Funkquist, B.: Thoraco-lumbar disc protrusion with severe spinal cord compression in the dog. I. Clinical and patho-anatomic observations with special reference to the rate of development of symptoms of motor loss. Acta Vet. Scand., *3*:256, 1962.

46. Funkquist, B.: Thoraco-lumbar disc protrusion with severe spinal cord compression in the dog. II. Clinical observations with special reference to the prognosis in conservative therapy. Acta Vet. Scand., *3*:317, 1962.

47. Funkquist, B.: Thoraco-lumbar disc protrusion with severe spinal cord compression in the dog. III. Treatment by decompressive laminectomy. Acta Vet. Scand., *3*:344, 1962.

48. Funkquist, B.: Decompressive laminectomy in thoracolumbar disc protrusion with paraplegia in the dog. J. Small Anim. Pract., *11*:445, 1970.

49. Funkquist, B., and Schantz, B.: Influence of extensive laminectomy on the shape of the spinal cord. Acta Orthop. Scand. (Suppl.), *56*:1, 1962.

50. Gage, E. D.: Treatment of discospondylitis in the dog. J. Am. Vet. Med. Assoc., *166*:1164, 1975.

51. Gage, E. D., and Hoerlein, B. F.: Hemilaminectomy and dorsal laminectomy for relieving compressions of the spinal cord in the dog. J. Am. Vet. Med. Assoc., *152*:351, 1968.

52. Gage, E. D., and Hoerlein, B. F.: Surgical repair of cervical subluxation and spondylolisthesis in the dog. J. Sm. Anim. Hosp. Assoc., *9*:385, 1973.

53. Gambardella, P. C.: Dorsal decompressive laminectomy for treatment of thoracolumbar disc disease in dogs: A retrospective study of 98 cases. Vet. Surg., *9*:24, 1980.

54. Gambardella, P. C., Osborne, C. A., and Stevens, J. B.: Multiple cartilaginous exostoses in the dog. J. Am. Vet. Med. Assoc., *166*:761, 1975.

55. Geary, J. C.: Canine spinal lesions not involving discs. J. Am. Vet. Med. Assoc., *155*:2038, 1969.

56. Geary, J. C., Oliver, J. E., and Hoerlein, B. F.: Atlanto-axial subluxation in the canine. J. Small Anim. Pract., *8*:577, 1967.

57. Gee, B. R., and Doige, C. E.: Multiple cartilaginous exostoses in a litter of dogs. J. Am. Vet. Med. Assoc., *156*:53, 1970.

58. Greene, C. E., and Higgins, R. J.: Fibrocartilaginous emboli as the cause of ischemic myelopathy in a dog. Cornell Vet., *66*:131, 1976.

59. Ghosh, P., Taylor, T. K. F., Braund, K. G., and Larsen, L. H.: A comparative clinical and histochemical study of the chondrodystrophoid and nonchondrodystrophoid canine intervertebral disc. Vet. Pathol., *13*:414, 1976.

60. Griffiths, I. R.: A syndrome produced by dorsolateral "explosions" of the cervical intervertebral discs. Vet. Rec., *87*:737, 1970.

61. Griffiths, I. R.: Some aspects of the pathogenesis

and diagnosis of lumbar disc protrusion in the dog. J. Small Anim. Pract., *13*:439, 1972.

62. Griffiths, I. R.: The extensive myelopathy of intervertebral disc protrusions in dogs (the ascending syndrome). J. Small Anim. Pract., *13*:425, 1972.

63. Griffiths, I. R.: Spinal cord infarction due to emboli arising from the intervertebral discs in the dog. J. Comp. Pathol., *83*:225, 1973.

64. Griffiths, I. R., Barker, J., and Palmer, A. C.: Cholesterol masses in association with spinal cord infarction due to intervertebral disc emboli. Acta Neuropathol., *33*:85, 1975.

65. Griffiths, I. R., and Duncan, I. D.: Chronic degenerative radiculomyelopathy in the dog. J. Small Anim. Pract., *16*:461, 1975.

66. Griffiths, I. R., and Duncan, I. D.: Age changes in the dorsal and ventral lumbar nerve roots of dogs. Acta Neuropathol., *32*:75, 1975.

67. Hansen, H. J.: A pathologic-anatomical study on disc degeneration in the dog. Acta Orthop. Scand. [Suppl.], 11, 1952.

68. Harcourt, R. A.: Polyarteritis in a colony of Beagles. Vet. Rec., *102*:519, 1978.

69. Hartley, W. J., and Palmer, A. C.: Ataxia in Jack Russell terriers. Acta Neuropathol., *26*:71, 1973.

70. Hayes, K. C., and Schiefer, B.: Primary tumors in the CNS of carnivores. Pathol. Vet., *6*:94, 1969.

71. Hayes, M. A., Creighton, S. R., Boysen, B. G., and Holfeld, N.: Acute necrotizing myelopathy from nucleus pulposus embolism in dogs with intervertebral disk degeneration. J. Am. Vet. Med Assoc., *173*:289, 1978.

72. Hedhammer, A., Wu, F.-M., Krook, L., Schryver, H. F., de Lahunta, A., Whalen, J. P., Kallfelz, F. A., Nunez, E. A., Hintz, H. F., Sheffy, B. E., and Ryan, G. B.: Overnutrition and skeletal disease; An experimental study in growing Great Dane dogs. Cornell Vet. [Suppl. 5], *64*:1, 1974.

73. Helphrey, M., and Meierhenry, E. F.: Vulvar leiomyosarcoma metastatic to the spinal cord in a dog. J. Am. Vet. Med. Assoc., *172*:583, 1978.

74. Henderson, R. A., Hoerlein, B. F., Kramer, T. T., and Meyer, M. E.: Discospondylitis in three dogs infected with *Brucella canis*. J. Am. Vet. Med. Assoc., *165*:451, 1974.

75. Hoerlein, B. F.: The status of the various intervertebral disc surgeries for the dog in 1978. J. Am. Anim. Hosp. Assoc., *14*:563, 1978.

76. Hoerlein, B. F.: Comparative disk disease: Man and dog. J. Am. Anim. Hosp. Assoc., *15*:535, 1979.

77. Hopkins, A., and Rudge, P.: Hyperpathia in the central cervical cord syndrome. J. Neurol. Neurosurg. Psychiatry, *36*:637, 1973.

78. Hukuda, S., and Wilson, C. B.: Experimental cervical myelopathy: Effects of compression and ischemia on the canine cervical spinal cord. J. Neurosurg., *37*:631, 1972.

79. Hurov, L.: Congenital atlantoaxial malformation and acute subluxation in a mature Basset Hound: Surgical treatment by wire stabilization. J. Am. Anim. Hosp. Assoc., *15*:177, 1977.

80. Hurov, L. I.: Treatment of cervical vertebral instability in the dog. J. Am. Vet. Med. Assoc., *175*:278, 1979.

81. Hurov, L., Troy, G., and Turnwald, G.: Diskospondylitis in the dog: 27 cases. J. Am. Vet. Med. Assoc., *173*:275, 1978.

82. Illis, L. S.: The motor neuron surface and spinal shock. Mod. Trends Neurol., *4*:53, 1967.

83. Joshua, J. O., and Ishmael, J.: Pain syndrome associated with spinal hemorrhage in the dog. Vet. Rec., *83*:165, 1968.

84. Jones, B. R., and Richards, R. B.: Myelomalacia in Afghan hounds. Aust. Vet. J., *53*:Sept, 1977.

85. Kark, R. A. P., Rodriguez-Budelli, M., and Blass, J. P.: Evidence for a primary defect of lipoamide dehydrogenase in Friedreich's ataxia. Adv. Neurol., *21*:163, 1978.

86. Kelly, D. F., Grunsell, C. S. G., and Kenyon, C. J.: Polyarteritis in a dog: A case report. Vet. Rec., *92*:363, 1973.

87. King, A. S., and Smith, R. N.: Disc protrusions in the cat: Distribution of dorsal protrusions along the vertebral column. Vet. Rec., *72*:335, 1960.

88. Knecht, C. D., Blevins, W. E., and Raffe, M. R.: Stenosis of the thoracic spinal canal in English Bulldogs. J. Am. Anim. Hosp. Assoc., *15*:181, 1979.

89. Kneller, S. K., Oliver, J. E., and Lewis, R. E.: Differential diagnosis of progressive caudal paresis in an aged German Shepherd dog. J. Am. Anim. Hosp. Assoc., *11*:414, 1975.

90. Koestner, A., and Zeman, W.: Primary reticuloses of the central nervous system. Am. J. Vet. Res., *23*:381, 1962.

91. Kornegay, J. N.: Feline infectious peritonitis: The central nervous system form. J. Am. Anim. Hosp. Assoc., *14*:580, 1978.

92. Kornegay, J. N.: Canine diskospondylitis. Compend. Contin. Ed., *1*:930, 1979.

93. Kornegay, J. N.: Ischemic myelopathy due to fibrocartilaginous embolism. Compend. Contin. Ed., *2*:402, 1980.

94. Kornegay, J.: Diskospondylitis. *In* Kirk, R. W. (ed.): Current Veterinary Therapy VIII: Small Animal Practice. Philadelphia, W. B. Saunders Co., 1983.

95. Kornegay, J. N., and Barber, D. L.: Diskospondylitis in dogs. J. Am. Vet. Med. Assoc., *177*:337, 1980.

96. Kornegay, J. N., Barber, D. L., and Earley, T. D.: Cranial thoracic diskospondylitis in two dogs. J. Am. Vet. Med. Assoc., *174*:192, 1979.

97. Ladds, P., Guffy, M., Blauch, B., and Splitter, G.: Congenital odontoid process separation in two dogs. J. Small Anim. Pract., *12*:463, 1970.

98. Larsen, J. S., and Selby, L. A.: Spondylosis deformans in large dogs. Relative risk by breed, age, and sex. J. Am. Anim. Hosp. Assoc., *17*:623, 1981.

99. Lawson, D. D.: The diagnosis and prognosis of canine paraplegia. Vet. Rec., *89*:654, 1971.

100. LeCouteur, R. A., McKeown, D., Johnson, J., and Eger, C. E.: Stabilization of atlantoaxial subluxation in the dog using the nuchal ligament. J. Am. Vet. Med. Assoc., *177*:1011, 1980.

101. Legendre, A. M., and Whitenack, D. L.: Feline infectious peritonitis with spinal cord involvement in two cats. J. Am. Vet. Med. Assoc., *167*:931, 1975.

102. Leonard, E. P.: Orthopedic Surgery of the Dog and Cat. 2nd ed. Philadelphia, W. B. Saunders Co., 1971.

103. Ljunggren, G.: Legg-Perthes disease in the dog. Acta Orthop. Scand. [Suppl.], *95*:1, 1967.

104. Luttgen, P. J., and Bratton, G. R.: Spinal cord ependymoma: A case report. J. Am. Anim. Hosp. Assoc., *12*:788, 1976.

105. Luttgen, P. J., and Crawley, R. R.: Posterior paralysis caused by epidural dirofilariasis in a dog. J. Am. Anim. Hosp. Assoc., *17*:57, 1981.

106. MacCoy, D. M., Trotter, E. J., de Lahunta, A., and

MacDonald, J. M.: Pelvic limb paralysis in a young Miniature Pinscher due to a metastatic bronchogenic adenocarcinoma. J. Am. Anim. Hosp. Assoc., 12:774, 1976.

107. Mason, T. A.: Cervical vertebral instability (wobbler syndrome) in the Doberman. Aust. Vet. J., 53:440, 1977.

108. Mason, T. A.: Cervical vertebral instability in dogs. Vet. Annu., 18:194, 1978.

109. Mason, T. A.: Cervical vertebral instability in the dog. Vet. Rec., 104:142, 1979.

110. Mason, K. V., Prescott, C. W., Kelly, W. R., and Waddell, P. H.: Granulomatous encephalomyelitis of puppies due to Angiostrongylus cantonensis. Aust. Vet. J., 52:295, 1976.

111. McGrath, J.: Spinal dysraphism in the dog with comments on syringomyelia. Pathol. Vet. [Suppl.], 2:1, 1965.

112. Mendenhall, H. V., Litwak, P., Yturraspe, D. J., Ingram, J. T., and Lumb, W. V.: Aggressive pharmacologic and surgical treatment of spinal cord injuries in dogs and cats. J. Am. Vet. Med. Assoc., 168:1036, 1976.

113. Misdorp, W., and van der Heul, R. O.: Carcinosarcomas of uncertain origin in the lumbosacral region of three dogs. Vet. Pathol., 17:53, 1980.

114. Morgan, J. P.: Spondylosis deformans in the dog: Its radiographic appearance. J. Am. Vet. Radiol. Soc., 8:17, 1967.

115. Morgan, J. P.: Spondylosis deformans in the dog. Acta Orthop. Scand. [Suppl.]96:1, 1967.

116. Morgan, J. P.: Congenital anomalies of the vertebral column of the dog: A study of the incidence and significance based on a radiographic and morphologic study. J. Am. Vet. Radiol. Soc., 9:21, 1968.

117. Morgan, J. P.: Spinal dural ossification in the dog: Incidence and distribution based on radiographic study. J. Am. Vet. Radiol. Soc., 10:43, 1969.

118. Morgan, J. P., Suter, P. F., and Holliday, T. A.: Myelography with water-soluble contrast medium radiographic interpretation of disc herniation in dogs. Acta Radiol. [Suppl.], 319:217, 1972.

119. Northington, J. W., and Juliana, M. M.: Extradural lymphosarcoma in six cats. J. Small Anim. Pract., 19:409, 1978.

120. O'Brien, D., Parker, A. J., and Tarvin, G.: Osteosarcoma of the vertebra causing compression of the thoracic spinal cord in a cat. J. Am. Anim. Hosp. Assoc., 16:497, 1980.

121. Oliver, J. E., Eubank, N. J., and Geary, J. C.: Neurofibrosarcoma in a dog. J. Am. Vet. Med. Assoc., 146:965, 1964.

122. Osterholme, J. L.: The pathophysiological response to spinal cord injury: The current status of related research. J. Neurosurg., 40:5, 1974.

123. Palmer, A. C.: Clinical and pathologic aspects of cervical disc protrusion and primary tumors of the cervical spinal cord in the dog. J. Small. Anim. Pract., 11:63, 1970.

124. Palmer, A. C., Payne, J. E., and Wallace, M. E.: Hereditary quadriplegia and amblyopia in the Irish setter. J. Small Anim. Pract., 14:343, 1973.

125. Palmer, A. C., and Wallace, M. E.: Deformation of cervical vertebrae in basset hounds. Vet. Rec. 80:430, 1967.

126. Parker, A. J.: Canine spinal cord disease. Diagnosis and treatment of. Scope, 18:2, 1974:

127. Parker, A. J.: Diagnosing thoracolumbar cord disease. Ill. Vet., 13:12, 1970.

128. Parker, A. J.: Diagnosing cervical cord disease. Ill. Vet., 14:12, 1971.

129. Parker, A. J., Cusick, P. K., Park, R. D., and Henry, J. D.: Reticulum cell sarcoma producing spinal cord compression in a dog. J. Am. Anim. Hosp. Assoc., 10:21, 1974.

130. Parker, A. J., and Park, R. D.: Atlanto-axial subluxation in small breeds of dogs: Diagnosis and pathogenesis. Vet. Med., 68:1133, 1973.

131. Parker, A. J., and Park, R. D.: Occipital dysplasia in the dog. J. Am. Anim. Hosp. Assoc., 10:520, 1974.

132. Parker, A. J., Park, R. D., Cusick, P. K., Small, E., and Jeffers, C. B.: Cervical vertebral instability in the dog. J. Am. Vet. Med. Assoc., 163:71, 1973.

133. Parker, A. J., Park, R. D., and Gendreau, C.: Cervical disk prolapse in a Doberman pinscher. J. Am. Vet. Med. Assoc., 163:75, 1973.

134. Parker, A. J., Park, R. D., and Stowater, J. L.: Cervical kyphosis in an Afghan hound. J. Am. Vet. Med. Assoc., 162:953, 1973.

135. Parker, A. J., and Smith, G. W.: Meningeal cyst in a dog. J. Am. Anim. Hosp. Assoc., 10:595, 1974.

136. Parker, A. J., and Smith, C. W.: Lack of functional recovery from spinal cord trauma following dimethylsulphoxide and epsilon amino caproic acid therapy in dogs. Res. Vet. Sci., 27:253, 1979.

137. Pettit, C. D.: Intervertebral Disk Protrusion in the Dog. New York, Appleton-Century-Crofts, 1966.

138. Prata, R. G.: Neurosurgical treatment of thoracolumbar disks: The rationale and value of laminectomy with concomitant disk removal. J. Am. Anim. Hosp. Assoc., 17:17, 1981.

139. Prata, R. G., and Stoll, S. G.: Ventral decompression and fusion for the treatment of cervical disc disease in the dog. J. Am. Anim. Hosp. Assoc., 9:462, 1973.

140. Prata, R. G., Stoll, S. G., and Zaki, F. A.: Spinal cord compression caused by osteocartilaginous exostoses of the spine in two dogs. J. Am. Vet. Med. Assoc., 166:371, 1975.

141. Priester, W. A.: Canine intervertebral disc disease: Occurrence by age, breed, and sex among 8,117 cases. Theriogenology, 6:293, 1976.

142. Raffe, M. R., and Knecht, C. D.: Cervical vertebral malformation in Bull Mastiffs. J. Am. Anim. Hosp. Assoc., 14:593, 1978.

143. Raffe, M. R., and Knecht, C. D.: Cervical vertebral malformation: A review of 36 cases. J. Am. Anim. Hosp. Assoc., 16:881, 1980.

144. Rendano, V. T., Jr., and Smith, L. L.: Cervical vertebral malformation-malarticulation (wobbler syndrome): The value of the ventrodorsal view in defining lateral spinal cord compression in the dog. J. Am. Anim. Hosp. Assoc., 17:627, 1981.

145. Renegar, W. R., and Stoll, S. G.: The use of methylmethacrylate bone cement in the repair of atlantoaxial subluxation stabilization failures: case report and discussion. J. Am. Anim. Hosp. Assoc., 15:313, 1979.

146. Ruch, T. C.: Evidence of the nonsegmental character of spinal reflexes from an analysis of the cephalad effects of spinal transection (Schiff-Sherrington phenomenon). Am. J. Physiol., 114:457, 1936.

147. Ruch, T. C., and Watts, J. W.: Reciprocal changes in reflex activity of the forelimbs induced by postbrachial "cold block" of the spinal cord. Am. J. Physiol., 110:362, 1934.

148. Rucker, N. C., Lumb, W. V., and Scott, R. J.: Combined pharmacologic and surgical treatments for acute spinal cord trauma. Am. J. Vet. Res., *42*:1138, 1981.

149. Russell, S. W., and Griffiths, R. C.: Recurrence of cervical disc syndrome in surgically and conservatively treated dogs. J. Am. Vet. Med. Assoc., *153*:1412, 1968.

150. Sandersleben, J. von, and el Sergany, M. A.: Ein Beitrag zur sogenannten Pachymeningitis spinalis ossificans des Hundes unter Berücksichtigung pathogenetischer und ätiologischer Gesichtspunkte. Zbl. Veterinaermed. [A], *13*:526, 1966.

151. Schappert, H. R., and Geib, L. W.: Reticuloendothelial neoplasms involving the spinal cord of cats. J. Am. Vet. Med. Assoc., *150*:753, 1967.

152. Schiefer, B., and Dahme, E.: Primäre Geschwülste des ZNS bei Tieren. Acta Neuropathol., *2*:202, 1962.

153. Scott, F. W.: FIP Antibody test: Interpretations and recommendations. J. Am. Vet. Med. Assoc., *175*:1164, 1979.

154. Seawright, A. A., and English, P. B.: Deforming cervical spondylosis in the cat. J. Pathol. Bacteriol., *88*:503, 1964.

155. Seawright, A. A., English, P. B., and Gartner, R. J. W.: Hypervitaminosis A and deforming cervical spondylosis of the cat. J. Comp. Pathol., *77*:29, 1967.

156. Seim, H. B., and Nafe, L. A.: Spontaneous intervertebral disk extrusion with associated myelopathy in a cat. J. Am. Anim. Hosp. Assoc., *17*:201, 1981.

157. Selcer, R. R., and Oliver, J. E., Jr.: Cervical spondylopathy-wobbler syndrome in dogs. J. Am. Anim. Hosp. Assoc., *11*:175, 1975.

158. Shores, A.: Intervertebral disk syndrome in the dog. Part I. Pathophysiology and management. Compend. Contin. Ed., *3*:639, 1981.

159. Shores, A.: Intervertebral disk syndrome in the dog. Part II. Cervical disk surgery. Compend. Contin. Ed., *3*:805, 1981.

160. Sprague, J. M.: Spinal "border cells" and their role in postural mechanism (Schiff-Sherrington phenomenon). J. Neurophysiol., *16*:464, 1953.

161. Suter, P. F., Morgan, J. P., Holliday, T. A., and O'Brien, T. P.: Myelography in the dog: Diagnosis of tumors of the spinal cord and vertebrae. J. Am. Radiol. Soc., *12*:29, 1971.

162. Swaim, S. F.: Ventral decompression of the cervical spinal cord in the dog. J. Am. Vet. Med. Assoc., *162*:276, 1973.

163. Swaim, S. F.: Ventral decompression of the cervical spinal cord in the dog. J. Am. Vet. Med. Assoc., *164*:491, 1974.

164. Tarlov, I. M.: Spinal Cord Compression, Mechanism of Paralysis, and Treatment. Springfield, Ill., Charles C Thomas, 1957.

165. Teague, H. D., and Berg, J. A.: Myxoma of the spinal canal in a dog. J. Am. Vet. Med. Assoc., *173*:985, 1978.

166. Teuscher, E., and Cherrstrom, E. C.: Ependymoma of the spinal cord in a young dog. Schweiz. Arch. Tierheilk, *116*:461, 1974.

167. Tilley, L. P., and Liu, S. K.: Cardiomyopathy and thromboembolism in the cat. Feline Pract., *5*:32, 1975.

168. Trotter, E. J.: Surgical repair of fractured atlas in a dog. J. Am. Vet. Med. Assoc., *161*:303, 1972.

169. Trotter, E. J.: Canine intervertebral disk disease. *In* Kirk, R. W. (ed.): Current Veterinary Therapy V: Small Animal Practice. Philadelphia, W. B. Saunders Co., 1974.

170. Trotter, E. J., Brasmer, T. H., and de Lahunta, A.: Modified deep dorsal laminectomy in the dog. Cornell Vet., *65*:402, 1975.

171. Trotter, E. J., de Lahunta, A., Geary, J. C., and Brasmer, T. H.: Caudal cervical vertebral malformation-malarticulation in Great Danes and Doberman Pinschers. J. Am. Vet. Med. Assoc., *168*:917, 1976.

172. Troy, G. C., Hurov, L. I., and King, G. K.: Successful surgical removal of a cervical subdural neurofibrosarcoma. J. Am. Anim. Hosp. Assoc., *15*:477, 1979.

173. Vandevelde, M., Higgins, R. J., and Greene, C. E.: Neoplasms of mesenchymal origin in the spinal cord and nerve roots of three dogs. Vet. Pathol., *13*:47, 1976.

174. Watson, A. G., and Evans, H. E.: The development of the atlas-axis complex in the dog. Anat. Rec., *184*:558, 1976.

175. Waxman, F. J., Clemmons, R. M., and Henrichs, D. J.: Progressive myelopathy in older German Shepherd dogs. II. Presence of circulating suppressor cells. J. Immunol., *124*:1216, 1980.

176. Waxman, F. J., Clemmons, R. M., Johnson, G., Evermann, J. F., Johnson, M. I., Roberts, C., and Henrichs, D. J.: Progressive myelopathy in older German Shepherd dogs. I. Depressed response to thymus-dependent mitogens. J. Immunol., *124*:1209, 1980.

177. Wilson, J. W., Greene, H. J., and Leipold, H. W.: Osseous metaplasia of the spinal dura mater in a Great Dane. J. Am. Vet. Med. Assoc., *167*:75, 1975.

178. Withrow, S. J., and Doige, C. E.: Subperiosteal vertebral hematoma as a cause of acute paraplegia in two dogs. J. Am. Anim. Hosp. Assoc., *15*:295, 1979.

179. Wright, F., and Palmer, A. C.: Morphological changes caused by pressure on the spinal cord. Pathol. Vet., *6*:355, 1969.

180. Wright, E., Palmer, A. C., and Payne, J. E.: Pressure-induced lesions in the spinal cord of rabbits. Res. Vet. Sci., *17*:337, 1974.

181. Wright, F., Rest, J. R., and Palmer, A. C.: Ataxia of the Great Dane caused by stenosis of the cervical vertebral canal: Comparison with similar condition in the basset hound, Doberman pinscher, Ridgeback, and thoroughbred horse. Vet. Rec., *92*:1, 1973.

182. Zackary, J. F., O'Brien, D. P., and Ely, R. W.: Intramedullary spinal ependymoma in a dog. Vet. Pathol., *18*:697, 1981.

183. Zaki, F. A.: Vascular malformation (cavernous angioma) of the spinal cord in a dog. J. Small Anim. Pract., *20*:417, 1979.

184. Zaki, F., and Prata, R. G.: Necrotizing myelopathy secondary to embolization of herniated intervertebral disk material in the dog. J. Am. Vet. Med. Assoc., *169*:222, 1976.

185. Zaki, F., Prata, R. G., and Kay, W. J.: Necrotizing myelopathy in five Great Danes. J. Am. Vet. Med. Assoc., *165*:1080, 1974.

186. Zaki, F. A., Prata, R. G., Hurvitz, A. I., and Kay, W. J.: Primary tumors of the spinal cord and meninges in six dogs. J. Am. Vet. Med. Assoc., *166*:511, 1975.

187. Zaki, F., Prata, R. G., and Werner, L. L.: Necro-

tizing myelopathy in a cat. J. Am. Vet. Assoc., *169*:228, 1976.

188. Zivin, J. A., Doppman, J. L., Reid, J. L., Tappaz, M. L., Saavedra, J. M., Kopin, I. J., and Jacobowitz, D. M.: Biochemical and histochemical studies of biogenic amines in spinal cord trauma. Neurology, *26*:99, 1976.

189. Seim, H. B., and Prata, R. G.: Ventral decompression for the treatment of cervical disk disease in the dog: A review of 54 cases. J. Am. Anim. Hosp. Assoc., *18*:233, 1982.

190. Seim, H. B., and Withrow, S. J.: Pathophysiology and diagnosis of caudal cervical spondylo-myelopathy with emphasis on the Doberman Pinscher. J. Am. Anim. Hosp. Assoc., *18*:241, 1982.

191. Olsson, S.-E., Stavenborn, M., and Hoppe, F.: Dynamic compression of the cervical spinal cord: A myelographic and pathologic investigation in Great Dane dogs. Acta Vet. Scand., *23*:65, 1982.

192. Mesfin, G. M., Kusem, H. D., and Parker, A.: Degenerative myelopathy in a cat. J. Am. Vet. Med. Assoc., *176*:62, 1980.

LARGE ANIMAL SPINAL CORD DISEASE

This chapter covers the spinal cord diseases of horses, cattle, sheep, goats, and pigs.

NEUROLOGIC EXAMINATION

A complete neurologic examination should be performed on all patients with presumed neurologic disorders. This includes evaluation of the animal's sensorium, cranial nerves, gait and posture, postural reactions, and spinal nerves. The extent to which postural reactions and spinal nerves can be assessed will depend on the size of the animal and whether it is standing or recumbent.

The complete examination is described in Chapters 22 and 23. The components referable to spinal cord function are briefly reviewed here.

Gait. The animal's gait should be evaluated on a surface that is not slippery. Most deficits will be observed at the walk and during turning, but the trot should be evaluated in horses. Subtle deficits may be more obvious on a slope or if the animal is turned loose in a paddock.

As cervical spinal cord disease first occurs and progresses, the earliest signs are those of a mild pelvic limb ataxia, followed by spasticity and finally by paresis. Many mildly affected animals will show signs of ataxia and spasticity but weakness may not be apparent. The ataxia will usually be more obvious in the pelvic limbs. Spasticity is usually observed in all limbs and is the most significant sign in the thoracic limbs.

For small pigs, calves, foals, and most sheep and goats, the postural reactions can be tested as described for small animals. The hopping, hemistanding, hemiwalking, and proprioceptive positioning reactions are the most beneficial.

For the larger animals that are cooperative, there are some further manipulations that can be done which require normal spinal nerve and spinal cord function. They also require a normal brain stem and cerebellum. These include head elevation, swaying, circling, and backing.

HEAD ELEVATION. Cervical spinal cord lesions are common in horses, and when these are mild, the deficit in thoracic limb function may be subtle. Sometimes these deficits can be accentuated by walking the horse with the neck and head extended. This will accentuate a mild spasticity in the limbs with a tendency towards hypermetria, or floating, and sometimes the affected horse will scuff its toes and stumble. Possibly the neck extension alters the posture enough and initiates more neck proprioceptive neuronal activity to accentuate the clinical abnormality. Blindfolding usually does not significantly alter the gait of a horse with spinal cord disease.

SWAYING. If the standing or walking animal can easily be pulled to the side by the tail, this is an indication of possible weakness. This is most easily tested as the animal is walking and is pulled gently by the tail to each side. This will also accentuate an ataxic gait, for the animal may stumble as it adjusts to the change in posture on being pulled to the side.

CIRCLING. In the cooperative animal this is the most sensitive test for normal spinal nerve and spinal cord function. The animal should be walked slowly in a very tight circle for 8 to 10 times or more in one direction. The normal animal that knows where its feet are and is strong will step around very rapidly with short brisk strides and will not step on itself.

The animal with spinal cord disease will pivot on the inside limb, which is held in place and not protracted. If the lesion is severe, the animal will nearly collapse in the pelvic limbs with this maneuver. With mild lesions, there will be an obvious delay in the protraction of the limb. At the same time, the outside hindlimb may flex and abduct excessively as it is protracted. The outside forelimb may appear stiff and swing across in front of the still supporting inside limb as it attempts to circle. It may step on the supporting limb.

These deficits are common with spinal cord disease and reflect disturbances in the UMN and GP systems. It is not clear whether these clinical signs are a reflection of dysfunction of one or the other or both of these systems. It is probable that the hypermetric abduction of the pelvic limb is mostly a GP deficit. However, as previously stated, these systems run together through the spinal cord and it is not important in localizing a segmental spinal cord lesion to differentiate between them. What is important is to recognize the clinical signs of spinal cord disturbance.

BACKING. Cooperative animals with spinal cord disease will often have difficulty backing and will appear awkward or very slow to protract a limb. If the deficit is severe, they will not protract either pelvic limb and will collapse.

In animals with very mild lesions and questionable clinical signs, it may help to perform these maneuvers on a grassy slope where the footing is good. This may be enough alteration of posture to accentuate some clinical signs.

Spinal Nerves. Examination of spinal nerve function includes their components in specific segments of the spinal cord. Evaluation of muscle size, tone, spinal reflexes, and pain sensation should be included.

In the standing large animal, this examination will be limited to a careful examination by vision and palpation of muscle size, testing of the skin for normal sensation, the cutaneous trunci reflex, and tail and anal tone, reflex response, and sensation. In the recumbent animal, muscle tone can be assessed in the limbs as well as the patellar, flexor, and other tendon reflexes. These are most reliably tested on the nonrecumbent side. Muscle tone and reflexes may be depressed in the limbs that have been recumbent and immobile for any length of time.

MUSCLE ATROPHY. Muscles that are denervated will atrophy rapidly. Neurogenic atrophy occurs faster and is more complete than disuse atrophy, although these are not easy to differentiate in all patients. Neurogenic atrophy is a reflection of disease of the LMN in the ventral grey column of the spinal cord or in the ventral roots, spinal, and peripheral nerves specific to the muscle that is atrophied.

SKIN SENSATION. A focal loss of cutaneous pain sensation is rare except in the tail and perineal region. In the horse this is best evaluated with the blunt end of a pair of closed hemostats. It is easy to be misled by potential areas of decreased sensibility on a single testing. Before a region is considered to be hypalgesic or analgesic, this test should be repeated a number of times to be sure the observation is reliable. In the recumbent animal, this can be most difficult to evaluate reliably. The animal will often not respond to the same stimuli that it would if it were standing. Sometimes an electric prod is necessary to assess this.

A focal area of cutaneous hypalgesia or analgesia reflects a lesion in the GSA component of the specific peripheral nerve, spinal nerve, ganglion, dorsal roots, and segmental dorsal grey column of the spinal cord related to that cutaneous area.

CUTANEOUS TRUNCI REFLEX. Stimulation of the skin along most of the body through the thoracolumbar region will elicit a contraction of the cutaneous trunci muscle and a quick movement of the skin. The sensory components of this reflex are in the peripheral nerves that innervate the segmental dermatome that is stimulated. The impulses enter the spinal cord dorsal grey column at that segment and are passed cranially through the spinal cord, probably in the fasciculus proprius to the T1 and C8 segments where the LMN of the lateral thoracic nerve is stimulated, causing contraction of the cutaneous trunci muscle. In some animals this may require repeated stimulation of the skin of the trunk to elicit a response, and it may not occur caudal to the midlumbar region.

TAIL AND ANUS. A loss of tone in the tail implicates caudal nerves or spinal cord segments, and a loss of anal tone implicates sacral nerves or spinal cord segments. The perineal reflex tests both sacral and caudal components. Stimulation of the skin of the anus or adjacent area elicits impulses in the GSA components of nerves from the sacral plexus. These are conducted to the sacral segments of the spinal cord to stimulate the LMN of sacral segments (to cause closure of the anus) and LMN of caudal segments (to cause flexion of the tail).

PATELLAR REFLEX. Any blunt instrument can be used to test this tendon reflex. In horses and cattle, the side of the hand with digits extended can be used to strike the intermediate patellar ligament with the limb held relaxed in partial flexion. This tests the femoral nerve and the L4 and L5 segments of the spinal cord. With LMN disease the reflex is decreased or absent. With UMN disease it may be exaggerated. This is the only tendon reflex that can reliably be expected to be present in all normal animals.

There are other tendon reflexes that can be evaluated, but they are not always present in all normal animals. Their presence indicates that the components of the specific reflex are functioning; these reflexes may be exaggerated in UMN disease.

FLEXOR REFLEXES. In the normal animal, stimulation of the coronary region of the foot or the bulb of the heel with forceps or an electric prod (if necessary) will elicit flexion of all joints of the limbs, a withdrawal response. In the pelvic limb flexion of the stifle, tarsus, and digits is a function of the sciatic nerve and spinal cord segments L6, S1, and S2. Hip flexion is a function of the femoral and most of the lumbar nerves and segments.

In the thoracic limb, the flexor reflex involves a number of specific peripheral nerves and spinal cord segments from C6 to T2. The afferent neurons that are stimulated will depend on the site of the stimulus. The coronary or heel-bulb regions are innervated by the median and ulnar nerves. The withdrawal of the limb with flexion in all joints is mediated through almost all of the nerves of the brachial plexus—radial, axillary, musculocutaneous, median, and ulnar nerves.

Remember that these reflexes will be preserved with complete transverse spinal cord lesions cranial to the segments that mediate the reflex arc. Be aware that if an animal is recumbent on a limb for any length of time, the muscle may be temporarily or permanently affected by ischemia and may not function in the reflex.

PAIN PERCEPTION. With severe transverse thoracolumbar spinal cord lesions, there will be interruption of the ascending spinothalamic pathways concerned with pain perception. Detection of a line on the trunk caudal to which there is significant hypalgesia or analgesia implicates a transverse spinal cord lesion 1 to 2 segments cranial to that line. The same lesion interrupts the ascending pathway for the cutaneous trunci reflex, and this response will be absent behind the same line on the trunk established for the loss of pain perception.

Sympathetic Paralysis. The only spinal cord function reflected in the head is that of sympathetic innervation. Horner's syndrome may be observed with lesions in the intermediate grey column from T1 to T3 or with severe lesions in the lateral funiculus of the cervical spinal cord interfering with the UMN for the sympathetic system. Horses with UMN or LMN sympathetic paralysis will sweat abnormally. If a focal area of the LMN is destroyed, sweating may occur in a specific area of skin innervated by that focal LMN. This can occur anywhere along the trunk. With cervical spinal cord UMN lesions, the entire ipsilateral side of the head and body will sweat abnormally and Horner's syndrome will be evident in the eye.

Laryngeal Adduction. A test has been described for laryngeal adduction which requires the integrity of the cranial thoracic and cervical spinal cord as well as the LMN to the adductor muscles of the larynx.[54] With unilateral or bilateral cervical spinal cord lesions the test may be abnormal, as it is with recurrent lar-

Reflex	Nerve	Segments	Test—Response
Triceps	Radial	C7 to T1	Tap triceps tendon with limb held in flexion—observe elbow extension
Common calcanean tendon	Tibial	L6, S1, S2	Tap common calcanean tendon—observe hock extension or contraction of gastrocnemius

yngeal nerve disease. This is called the slap test for laryngeal adductory function and consists of observing the larynx through an endoscope while an attendant administers a series of 3 or 4 slaps of moderate intensity to the saddle area of the thorax. The laryngeal response is a slight brief adduction of the contralateral arytenoid cartilage associated with each slap. This laryngeal response is absent on the side of a recurrent laryngeal nerve lesion, on both sides with bilateral cervical spinal cord lesions from different causes, and on the same side as a unilateral cervical spinal cord lesion. The latter will be on the opposite side to the slap stimulus.

From limited observation it appears that the afferent impulses cross at the level of the dorsal root entrance to the spinal cord and ascend in the white matter on the opposite side to the contralateral nucleus ambiguus from the side of the stimulus.

It has been suggested that this test is particularly helpful in suggesting a cervical spinal cord lesion when the signs of ataxia are mild and observed only in the pelvic limbs. I have no personal experience with this test.

SUMMARY OF SIGNS WITH LESIONS AT SPECIFIC AREAS OF THE SPINAL CORD

Lumbosacral Intumescence (L4 through Caudal Segments)
1. Thoracic limbs normal.

2. Ataxic and paretic pelvic limbs, with decreased ability to support weight to paraplegia (total pelvic limb paralysis).

3. Decreased or absent tail, anal, and pelvic limb tone and reflexes. Atrophy of pelvic limb muscles.

4. Hypalgesia or analgesia of the same areas with a line at the cranial edge of the lesion.

5. Urinary incontinence and obstipation.

Thoracolumbar (T3-L3)
1. Thoracic limbs normal.

2. Pelvic limb ataxia spasticity and paresis to paraplegia.

3. Normal tail and anal tone and reflexes, and normal or exaggerated pelvic limb reflexes

with normal tone or hypertonia. No neurogenic atrophy.

4. Hypalgesia or analgesia caudal to the lesion.

5. In horses, focal area of sweating.

6. Urinary incontinence.

Cervical Intumescence (C6-T2)
1. Ataxia and paresis (tetraparesis) of all four limbs to tetraplegia. Spasticity of pelvic limbs.

2. Depressed to absent thoracic limb reflexes and tone with atrophy.

3. Normal or exaggerated pelvic limb reflexes and tone.

4. Hypalgesia or analgesia caudal to the cranial edge of the lesion. Hypalgesia may be more pronounced in the thoracic limbs.

5. In horses, sweating of entire side of head and body and Horner's syndrome.
   (intermediate grey column T₁-T₃)

Cervical Spinal Cord Cranial to the Intumescence (C1-C5)
1. Ataxia spasticity and paresis (tetraparesis) of all four limbs to tetraplegia. Ataxia and paresis may be more obvious in the pelvic limbs.

2. Normal or exaggerated reflexes and tone in all four limbs.

3. Hypalgesia caudal to the lesion.

4. In horses, sweating of the entire side of head and body and Horner's syndrome.
   (severe lesions to lateral funiculus)

In an attempt to quantify the neurologic signs for comparative diagnostic purposes and to follow the course of the disease with or without therapy, Mayhew has developed a grading system based on the degree of deficit present.[81] This differs from that used in small animals with thoracolumbar disease, primarily because the degree of spinal cord damage and resultant clinical signs and the basis for surgical selection and prognosis differ.

Grade 0—No deficit, normal function.

Grade 1—Deficit just detected at normal gait.

Grade 2—Deficit easily detected and exaggerated by backing, turning, swaying, loin pressure, and neck extension.

Grade 3—Deficit very prominent on walking gait, with a tendency to buckle or fall with backing, turning, loin pressure, neck extension.

Grade 4—Stumbling, tripping, falling spontaneously.

Grade 5—Recumbent, unable to rise.

SPINAL CORD DISEASE IN LARGE ANIMALS

A differential diagnosis for the entire spinal cord will be described according to the various kinds of lesions that occur. Those that are limited to a specific segment of the spinal cord will be indicated. If the assessment of the clinical signs and of the location of the lesion is accurate, then the consideration of the differential diagnosis can be more selective.

TRAUMA

External Injury. In fractures and subluxation, the clinical signs reflect a focal spinal cord contusion related to the site of the vertebral column injury. Horses are prone to sacral fractures on falling while backing off transport vans. Cattle are susceptible to caudal, sacral, or lumbar fractures from breeding accidents. The bones of foals, calves, or pigs with calcium deficiency may be more susceptible to fracture. These are usually thoracic or lumbar vertebral fractures. Vertebral body abscesses often result in a pathologic fracture and occur more commonly in cattle, sheep, and pigs. I have observed a horse cast itself in a stall and fracture its seventh cervical vertebra.

The Schiff-Sherrington syndrome has not been observed with thoracolumbar fracture in these species.

As a rule, the signs are sudden in onset and either remain static or improve. In one instance, an 11-month-old Appaloosa did not become recumbent for 48 hours following a fracture of the lamina of L5. When presented with a large animal that is recumbent and unable to get up, it often is necessary to sling the animal in order to evaluate the degree of function retained in the thoracic limbs and help locate the lesion to a cervical or thoracolumbar site.

An animal that is recumbent as a result of a caudal cervical spinal cord lesion usually still can flex the neck laterally on each side. The more cranial the location of the cervical spinal cord lesion, the less able is the animal to do this.

Careful palpation of the vertebral column may elicit pain at the site of the fracture. The level of the lesion may also be defined by determining a line of hypalgesia or analgesia with transverse thoracolumbar lesions or loss of the cutaneous trunci reflex.

Sometimes in cattle a line of hypalgesia or analgesia can be determined only by using an electric prod. Blunt-ended arterial forceps is usually sufficient in horses. It is especially important to locate the site of the spinal cord lesion accurately if radiography is to be performed.

Internal Injury

MALFORMATION-MALARTICULATION C1–C7: CERVICAL STENOTIC MYELOPATHY (CSM). Although many of the equine spinal cord and some brain lesions that do not produce recumbency cause the animal to wobble, the term "wobbler syndrome" has been used most often to refer to a specific disease syndrome. In this syndrome the cervical spinal cord is contused by a malarticulation or malformation between C1 and C7.[35, 37, 46, 63, 67, 79, 81, 85, 90, 97, 99, 102, 105-107, 111-113, 118, 122] The lesion in the spinal cord is a focal compressive myelopathy from a static or dynamic stenosis of the vertebral canal. Therefore, the more specific term "cervical stenotic myelopathy" has been applied to this disease. Although the vertebral abnormality may occur at any level in the cervical vertebrae, it is more common at the C3–C4 or C4–C5 articulations in the younger horses with a static or dynamic stenosis and in the C5 to C7 region of older horses that have stenosis related to degenerative osteoarthropathy of the synovial articulations.

Synonyms for this syndrome include wobbles and equine sensory ataxia. The latter refers to the pronounced signs of ataxia caused by the interference of the cervical spinal cord lesion with the general proprioception pathways. However, spasticity and paresis also occur and become evident as the deeper upper motor neuron pathways are compromised.

Horses often develop a wobbly gait, and because this "wobbler syndrome" has been recognized widely and published in the literature, it has been assumed that most wobbly horses have this syndrome of a focal cervical spinal cord contusion from a vertebral abnormality. Unfortunately, most of these horses have not been studied carefully at necropsy. When such a study is carried out, it is found that there are a significant number of these horses that do not have the expected lesions. Instead, primary degenerative spinal cord lesions and inflammatory lesions often are found.

Clinical Signs. Cervical vertebral malarticulation-malformation causes cervical spinal cord compression in many breeds of horses, including the draft horse, usually within the first year or two of life. Older horses may be affected, especially if degenerative osteoarthropathy has occurred. The incidence is highest in Thoroughbreds, particularly the young, rapidly growing, male Thoroughbred. Onset is most prevalent in the weanling or yearling periods. It may be gradual and insidious, but often is sudden. Occasionally it is associated with some form of trauma.

Typically, the signs of pelvic limb ataxia are the most pronounced. These are more evident at a slow walk or while turning in circles. The pelvic limb stride may be asymmetric, with one limb having a longer stride than the other. Occasionally, both pelvic limb strides are prolonged. In others the stride is shortened from spasticity and the hoof stabs sharply into the ground. One or both limbs may scuff the ground during the protraction phase of the gait. If the pelvis is pushed gently or the tail pulled as the horse walks, the ataxic-paretic horse may be pulled easily to the side, may stumble, cross one limb in front of the other, or step on itself. This test is called the sway response. The lack of resistance is a reflection of the paresis present.

When the horse walks in a wide or small circle, the outside pelvic limb often swings wide and high on protraction. This is referred to as abduction, circumduction, or hypermetria, and is assumed to be a sign of a general proprioceptive deficit. Turning the horse in a tight circle may cause it to pivot for a prolonged period on the inside pelvic limb, whereas the normal animal steps around briskly. This is a sign of a spinal cord lesion, but it has not been determined if it is a sign of general proprioception or upper motor neuron deficit. The latter is suspected.

Thoracic limb signs usually are less evident and may require careful observation to determine. In some animals there is quite remarkable spasticity, causing a stiff gait with less flexion of the joints on protraction. This may cause the limbs to delay slightly before reaching the ground and appear to float. This will appear as a slight hypermetria. Occasionally, a thoracic limb hoof scuffs on protraction. This may be elicited or accentuated by walking the horse with the neck extended and head held as high as possible. When signs are more severe, the horse often stumbles on the thoracic limbs and crosses one in front of the other. The stumbling may be exacerbated by moving the horse in a tight circle. During circling it may tend to pivot on the most affected thoracic limb, similar to the response of the pelvic limbs in this action.

The standing sway test with the thoracic or pelvic limbs is performed by gently pushing or pulling the horse by the withers or pelvic region, respectively. The normal horse resists this movement or steps sharply around. The ataxic, paretic horse may delay on protraction and then step on the opposite limb or abduct the opposite limb excessively.

Paresis may be detected by squeezing firmly so as to apply a downward pressure to the loin and withers regions separately. The horse may respond by extending its vertebral column, and if it is weak the thoracic or pelvic limbs, respectively, tend to flex and buckle. It is possible to cast the very weak horse in this manner.

On backing these horses, the severely affected horse may tend to collapse in the pelvic limbs, or be very slow to protract the limbs backward and sink toward the ground as this delay is prolonged. The mildly affected horse may back readily, but be slightly awkward (ataxic) in the placement of its hooves.

Most horses with this disease show little change in their signs on walking blindfolded on smooth ground.

If a slope is available, gaiting the horse in a straight line and in circles on the slope may augment subtle signs of neurologic deficit. It is not unusual for the gait to appear more normal when the horse is trotted in a straight line on a flat surface. However, if a horse is turned loose in a paddock and observed as it changes speeds and makes sudden turns, the signs may be observed more readily.

It is common for the clinical signs to be more obvious in the pelvic limbs than the thoracic limbs (Fig. 11–1). Some consider the pelvic limb signs to be one grade worse than the thoracic limbs. Even in mild cases there

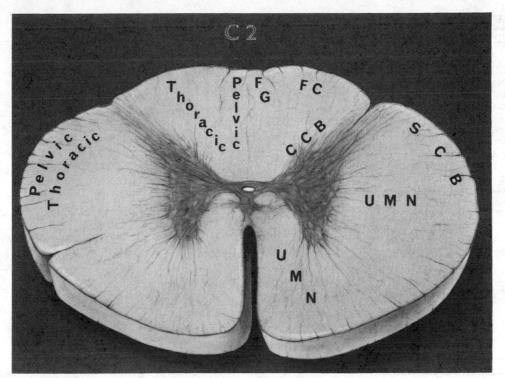

Figure 11–1. Transverse section of cervical spinal cord. The more superficial location of pelvic limb spinocerebellar tracts may explain the more profound signs of ataxia in these limbs. *FG:* Fasciculus gracilis; *FC:* fasciculus cuneatus; *CCB:* cuneocerebellar tract; *SCB:* spinocerebellar tracts; *UMN:* upper motor neuron.

should be some evidence of subtle thoracic limb abnormality. The disparity in signs between the pelvic and thoracic limbs may reflect the more superficial position of the pelvic limb spinocerebellar tracts in the lateral funiculus, where they are contused readily, the greater distance of the pelvic limbs from the center of gravity of the horse, or possibly the greater percentage of upper motor neuron synapses in the grey matter of the cervical intumescence.

As a rule, the clinical signs are fairly symmetric, reflecting disturbance of the ascending general proprioception pathways (ataxia) and descending upper motor neuron pathways (paresis). Rarely are there unequivocal signs of disturbance of the ascending general somatic afferent pathway (pain). See Table 11–1 for differential analysis.

Occasionally an affected horse may show abnormal resistance to flexion of the neck to one or both sides. This occurs only with more severe malarticulation and those with significant degenerative osteoarthropathy of the synovial articulations. Many horses with CSM will not show this increase in neck resistance to movement.

Horses that develop degenerative osteoar-

thropathy of their cervical vertebral articular processes have exostoses that may compress the adjacent spinal cord. The clinical signs will be similar to those described here. These horses may show pain or resistance on flexion of the neck away from the side of the bone lesion. More often these lesions occur in older horses, and the age of onset of clinical signs is later than is usual for CSM. How these lesions relate to the overall pathogenesis of the vertebral abnormalities of CSM is unknown.

Radiography. Careful evaluation of cervical radiographs will usually show the site of the stenosis of the cervical vertebral canal.[10, 81, 101] These should include a normally extended neck, flexed neck, and occasionally a neck extended as much as possible. All seven cervical vertebrae should be evaluated. With severe lesions the stenosis may be obvious on visual examination. Measurement of the vertebral foramina and the amount of flexion between vertebrae will more reliably indicate the site of the stenosis, and myelography should confirm this in most patients. Always evaluate the articular processes as well as the vertebral foramina and bodies. If a degenerative osteoarthropathy of the synovial articula-

TABLE 11–1. DIFFERENTIAL DIAGNOSIS OF THREE COMMON EQUINE SPINAL CORD DISEASES

Disease	Breed Predilection	Age of Onset	Rate of Onset	Progression of Signs
Cervical stenotic myelopathy	Thoroughbred (male)	<6–24 mo.	Often sudden	Static to variable
Equine degenerative myelopathy	None	<1–12 mo.	Always slow	Slow with static periods
Equine protozoal myelitis	Standardbred	1–3 yr. Any adult	Slow to fast	Usually rapid

Degree of Deficit	Limbs Involved	Symmetry of Signs	Muscle Atrophy	CSF
Mild to moderate	Pelvic more than thoracic	Usually symmetric	None	Usually normal
Mild to moderate	Pelvic more than thoracic Pelvic = Thoracic	Always symmetric	None	Normal
Often severe	Any combination	Asymmetric or symmetric	Sometimes	Normal or abnormal

tions has occurred to the extent that it encroaches on the vertebral canal to compress the spinal cord, the osteoarthropathy should be evident on the radiographs.

A normal range of measurements of cervical vertebrae has been established for two different sizes of horses. Two measurements are made and compared with these normal standards. The first is the minimum sagittal diameter. This is the narrowest dorsoventral measurement of the vertebral foramen of each cervical vertebra. The vertebral foramen is the entire passageway through each vertebra for the spinal cord. This measurement is made between the line that represents the roof of the vertebral foramen (the curve in the vertebral arch) and the line representing the floor of the vertebral foramen (the dorsal surface of the body). This is measured for each vertebra at the narrowest part of its foramen.

The minimum flexion diameter is measured on radiographs of the neck held in as much flexion as can be physically made in the anesthetized horse. It measures the size of the vertebral canal at its narrowest point between each pair of cervical vertebrae. This measurement is made between the most craniodorsal point on the body of the caudal vertebra of the pair to the closest portion of the dorsal aspect of the foramen (the arch) of the cranial vertebra of the pair. It is important to appre-

ciate that there is a considerable amount of movement between cervical vertebrae in normal horses. On flexion each vertebra appears to be displaced dorsally into the canal, but this is normal.

Cisternal myelography can be performed using Metrizamide.[10] If a stenosis is apparent on both normally extended and flexed views, the myelogram will confirm the site of stenosis on both views. This is a static stenosis. If the stenosis is only apparent on flexion of the neck, then the myelogram will be normal on the normally extended view and will reveal compression on the flexed view. This is a dynamic stenosis. It is important to recognize that normally on views of the flexed neck, the ventral dye line will become significantly narrow but the dorsal dye line will persist unaltered across each articulation. If the dorsal dye line is also narrowed, this indicates a site of compression.

In horses with degenerative osteoarthropathy involved with the spinal cord compression, this may be more apparent on a myelogram with the neck extended. Ventrodorsal radiographs may be required to diagnose a unilateral compression by the medial encroachment of an enlarged articular process from degenerative osteoarthropathy.

CSF is seldom altered by this condition.

Pathology.   The focal spinal cord lesion

may be only 1 to 2 cm long, and have a remarkable loss of myelin in almost all funiculi, with some evidence of axonal degeneration. In some the dorsal funiculi are spared. In the severe lesion some cavitation may occur in the white matter, and neurons may be depleted from the grey matter and replaced by hypertrophied astrocytes. Secondary Wallerian-type degeneration occurs in the ascending pathways cranial to this focal lesion and in the descending pathways caudal to the focal lesion (Fig. 10–1).

Pathogenesis. The specific cause of the various cervical vertebral abnormalities is unknown. They may result from a number of factors. Although inheritance has often been incriminated, a study of Thoroughbreds with this pathologic diagnosis did not support a genetic basis.[61] Nevertheless, the high incidence of this disease in male Thoroughbreds makes a hereditary predisposition still a consideration. This may be a predisposition for a rapid growth rate that would result in a cervical vertebral defect. A rapid rate of growth causing imbalance between muscle and skeletal structures has been implicated. The syndrome often is seen in young, large, rapidly growing horses with long necks in whom a disparity in growth of the vertebral column and spinal cord may account for the focal stretching of the latter. In addition, nutritional factors may be implicated, as in the canine syndrome.

Prognosis and Therapy. The course of this disease is variable. In most horses the signs remain static or slowly progress. Occasionally they improve but reports of complete recovery are rare.

There is no safe, practical therapy for this condition. Medical therapy to reduce any spinal cord edema associated with acute lesions at best is only temporary. Surgical procedures have been developed and the specific procedure advocated depends on the nature of the stenosis.[129-131] Careful radiography is necessary to define these. A dynamic stenosis is apparent only when the neck is flexed and results from excessive movement of a caudal vertebra at one of the cervical vertebral articulations. It is more common to find this at the C3–C4 or C4–C5 articulation. The surgery that is advocated is arthrodesis of the affected articulation with the neck in extension. This procedure utilizes a ventral approach to the cervical vertebrae, and the intervertebral disk and a portion of the adjacent vertebrae are replaced by a core of bone to fuse the vertebral bodies. This will prevent further dynamic stenosis at

that site and allow the injured spinal cord to recover by remyelination of those intact axons that have lost their myelin from the compression and by allowing the horse to compensate for the lesions that persist. In many of the horses that have been operated on, improvement in clinical signs has occurred and a few have returned to their original function. Response has been best in the more acutely affected horses.

There is always danger to the riders and drivers of these horses that their residual proprioceptive deficit may cause them to stumble and fall. This danger will always exist with these operated horses and must be clearly understood by all concerned with the postoperative use of one of these horses. The long-term effect of this operative procedure also remains to be determined. Although claims have been made that this disease is not inherited, its prevalence in the Thoroughbred breed makes a genetic predisposition highly likely. Attempts to statistically prove a genetic basis have not yet been successful. Based on the information available, I cannot recommend breeding clinically affected animals with or without surgery.

Horses with a static stenosis, one that is present in all positions of the neck, are not candidates for this surgery. Only a decompressive procedure would prevent further stenosis. Dorsal decompressive laminectomies have been performed on horses with a static stenosis. Those that have survived the immediate postoperative difficulties have shown improvement in their clinical signs. The dangers associated with the use of horses following vertebral arthrodesis are the same for these horses.

ATLANTO-OCCIPITAL MALFORMATION OF ARABIAN HORSES (OAAM). Arabian horses of either sex may be born with an atlanto-occipital malformation that may seriously compromise the spinal cord at birth or shortly after.[69, 83, 136] In most there is no discernible atlanto-occipital joint, with complete symmetric fusion of the atlas with the occipital bone. If the joint is present it is malformed and not functional, and the vertebral foramen of the atlas may be extremely narrow cranially. The axis may be displaced ventrally, with the dens articulating ventral to the malformed body of the atlas. In some, the dens may be hypoplastic. Despite this deformity in the vertebral canal between the atlas and the axis, the spinal cord compression in the older Arabian horse has usually occurred within the foramen of the atlas, which is reduced markedly in size. In newborn foals the compression may occur at the atlantoaxial luxation.

The signs of cranial cervical spinal cord compression may be present at birth and cause inability to stand or severe symmetric ataxia and paresis if the foal can stand. Extending the neck to nurse may be difficult and cause the foal to fall. Occasionally there may be an audible click at the site of the malformation when the head is moved. This is probably due to movement at the atlantoaxial luxation. Some foals are born with no clinical neurologic signs and develop them in the first few weeks or months. This suggests that at birth the vertebral foramen of the atlas was large enough for the size of the spinal cord, and the spinal cord escaped compression by the luxation. As the foal grew the foramen failed to remodel and enlarge simultaneous with the growing spinal cord, which became progressively more compressed at this site. Once the neurologic signs are apparent, they progress at a moderate rate. In most of the animals examined the gait has a remarkable spastic quality, especially in the thoracic limbs. They may stumble and fall to either side or backward. Their signs usually are more pronounced than those of most horses with the CSM syndrome.

An important diagnostic feature is the posture of the neck. It is more extended than normal and appears stiff owing to the lack of mobility at the atlanto-occipital joint. Palpation reveals the abnormality of the joint. The transverse process (wing) of the atlas usually is reduced in size, and if the paracondylar process of the occipital bone is palpable, the normal space between the paracondylar process and wing of the atlas may not be felt. They either will be immovable, or there will be limited motion between them.

Radiographs will confirm this diagnosis and reveal the degree of deformity. A myelogram will show the specific site of spinal cord compression.

There is sufficient evidence to support a familial autosomal recessive inheritance as the basis for this disease. Breeding studies are necessary to confirm this and to understand the nature of the inheritance. All known cases have been observed in Arabian horses.[69] This malformation represents a disturbance in the normal development of the caudal occipital and cranial cervical sclerotomes with occipitalization of the atlas and atlantalization of the axis.

Other sporadic cervical vertebral malformations have been observed in the horse with and without spinal cord compression.[48, 55, 83] Most are palpable or can be diagnosed by radiography.

THORACOLUMBAR VERTEBRAL MALFORMATIONS. Thoracolumbar vertebral malformations have been reported sporadically in horses and other farm animals with and without spinal cord compression.[72, 92] No cause for the malformation has been defined.

BOVINE VERTEBRAL MALFORMATION. An atlantoaxial subluxation has been reported in Holstein cattle and one crossbreed with onset of signs of cervical compressive myelopathy from birth to 1 year.[71, 132] The dens was small or absent and the axis was displaced ventral to the atlas. The atlas was fused to the occipital bones in many of these calves.

EQUINE SYNOVIAL CYST. A synovial cyst related to the synovial capsule of the articular processes of cervical vertebrae has been found as the cause of cervical spinal cord compression in horses of many breeds, from 1 to 6 years old.[49] Most have been at the C5–C6 or C6–C7 articulation. They cause a progressive course of clinical signs referable to a cervical spinal cord lesion. These have all been diagnosed at necropsy. Careful myelography and ventrodorsal radiographs are needed to diagnose this lesion. The cause is unknown.

NEOPLASIA

Lymphosarcoma. In cattle lymphosarcoma often may develop in the epidural space at any level of the spinal cord and produce clinical signs referable to the area of the spinal cord that is compressed. This usually affects adult cattle (3 years or older) but can occur in animals that are under 1 year of age. The signs may be slow or rapid in onset and are usually progressive.[45]

Finding evidence of this lesion in other sites in the body and in the blood helps confirm the suspicion, but it can occur at this site without involvement of any other organ and no evidence of leukemia on the hemogram. A significantly elevated lymphosarcoma antibody titer may help implicate this disease. Lack of an antibody titer on the agar gel immunodiffusion test does not preclude this disease.[45]

In one instance of a cow with this lesion in the vertebral foramen of C4, before persistent signs of ataxia and paresis occurred the animal occasionally would collapse when it lowered its head to eat from the floor. Although the majority of lymphosarcomatous neoplasms are confined to the epidural space, they have rarely been found on the inner surface of the dura and in the bones of the vertebral column.

Neurofibroma.[58] Neurofibromas are found most often in cattle of all ages. I have observed a neurofibroma in a 2-month-old calf with signs of a thoracolumbar focal spinal cord lesion. These frequently are seen in various peripheral nerves in cattle at slaughter houses, with no evidence of having produced neurologic signs.

Extramedullary neoplasms are rare in horses.[128] I have observed an intradural extramedullary lymphoreticular neoplasm compressing and infiltrating the C8 and T1 segments of a 1½-year-old quarter horse. The signs appeared quite suddenly, and the horse was unable to get up 24 hours later. The signs suggested a caudal cervical spinal cord lesion. The thoracic limbs were more paretic than the pelvic limbs. The pelvic limbs were severely hypertonic, had normal flexor and plus 3 patellar reflexes, and pain was perceived readily. The thoracic limbs were hypotonic, hyporeflexic, and hypalgesic. The neck could readily be flexed laterally.

Extravertebral neoplasms may invade the vertebral canal and compress the spinal cord. I have observed a fibrosarcoma invade the vertebral canal at the T16–T17 articulation in a 6-year-old male Appaloosa. A 6-month-old male Standardbred was examined for a 3-day course of a right pelvic limb deficit that progressed to paraparesis and inability to rise in the pelvic limbs. A pheochromocytoma was diagnosed with a metastasis in the azygos vein, its spinal branch at T10–T11, and the associated internal ventral vertebral venous plexus. The latter compressed the spinal cord.

EPIDURAL ABSCESS. Abscesses frequently occur in the extradural space of cattle, sheep, and pigs.[39] They may involve the adjacent bone or be restricted to the epidural space. The adjacent spinal cord becomes compressed. The temperature, pulse, and respiration may be normal, but chronic abscesses often are associated with an elevated plasma protein level because of the increased globulin fraction. *Corynebacterium pyogenes, Streptococcus* species, or *Staphylococcus* species are isolated most frequently. *Corynebacterium ovis* (pseudotuberculosis) may occur in sheep. Only in exceptional cases does the abscess invade the dura and break into the leptomeninges. Since the abscess is usually restricted to the epidural space, there are usually no inflammatory cells in the CSF. This is a rare lesion in adult horses. I have observed an abscess of the lumbosacral canal in a young foal with invasion of the meninges of the cauda equina and conus medullaris.

Other compressive lesions have been reported.[17, 51, 109]

INFLAMMATION

Protozoal Myelitis. Horses are susceptible to a protozoal myelitis and encephalitis.[11, 12, 14, 32, 41, 81, 102, 108] (See Case No. 8, Chapter 24.) The identity and life cycle of the protozoan remain unknown.

Electron microscopic studies show that the organism is in the phylum Protozoa, suborder Apicomplexa.[115] The best evidence to date identifies the organism as a *Sarcocystis* species. It has many similarities to *Toxoplasma gondii* but significant differences. There is no evidence that toxoplasmosis of the nervous system occurs in horses. Most publications that have implied this are probably examples of this protozoan that is presumed to be a *Sarcocystis* species.[32, 41] There were no toxoplasma antibody titers in any of our horses with this protozoal disease that were studied. Some of these horses did have antibody titers to *Sarcocystis bovicanis*–like antigens. A similar sporozoan encephalomyelitis has been reported in sheep.[57]

Schizonts and free merozoites have been found in cell cytoplasm in the spinal cord but more commonly free in extracellular spaces.[115] Most commonly, free merozoites parasitized pericytes of capillaries, but they also were found in cytoplasm of macrophages, neurons, axons, and neutrophils in the spinal cord lesion as well as intravascularly. Study of the different developmental stages of schizonts and the recognition of endopolygeny in the late stage of schizogony have permitted tentative diagnosis of the protozoan as a *Sarcocystis* species. The presence of merozoites in neutrophils within blood vessels is suggestive that one route of CNS infection is hematogenous.

This disease occurs most commonly in young adult horses but there is no age limitation. It has not yet been observed in foals. There is a higher incidence of this disease in Standardbreds but all breeds are susceptible. This breed predilection may reflect the form of management of these horses and the peculiarities of the protozoan's life cycle, which remain to be defined.

This organism can produce focal, multifocal, or diffuse lesions in the spinal cord or brain. Most commonly it affects the spinal cord, and the clinical signs reflect a focal lesion.

The onset of clinical signs is variable. Most

have a mild onset but a fairly rapidly progressive course. A few are very slow initially and are often confused with a musculoskeletal lameness. In these horses there may be a number of unsuccessful treatments for the presumed musculoskeletal disease before the signs are recognized as neurologic in origin. A few patients have a peracute onset. Most of these lesions progress, but in some the progress of the disease stops and clinical signs remain static for weeks to months.

The clinical signs will reflect the portion of the spinal cord that is affected. Because the lesion is inflammatory, the neurologic signs are often asymmetric, with one limb much more affected than the other. The lesion affects grey matter as readily as white matter, and if this involves the intumescence, there may be clinical signs of grey matter disease. These include neurogenic atrophy, hypotonia and hyporeflexia for the ventral grey column, and hypalgesia for the dorsal grey column.[104] A caudal cervical spinal cord lesion first may produce an ipsilateral thoracic limb deficit, followed by an ipsilateral hemiparesis, followed by tetraparesis and ataxia. A thoracolumbar lesion may cause an inability to back up, and the horse may collapse on its pelvic limbs and sit like a dog.

This is a common disease in our hospital. In a study of equine neurologic diseases at the New York State College of Veterinary Medicine, approximately one fourth of the diagnoses were equine protozoal encephalomyelitis.[50, 81] Although the hospital population of Standardbreds is approximately 30 per cent, this breed makes up 70 per cent of the horses diagnosed as having equine protozoal encephalomyelitis. This would reflect a genetic predisposition or an environmental factor in the management of these horses. From the survey of the other North American veterinary colleges, all diagnoses of this disease have been made at institutions east of the Rocky Mountains or in horses that originated east of the Rockies. This may be related either to the intensity of the diagnostic search for this disease or to the nature of the life cycle of the infectious agent.

This is the most presumptive diagnosis when adult horses present with evidence of a progressive focal thoracolumbar lesion or progressive hemiparesis, or progressive symmetric tetraparesis that is severe with more serious thoracic limb deficit, or asymmetric deficit with neurogenic atrophy.

Rarely this organism has been related to focal destruction of LMN cell bodies in the spinal cord ventral grey column or brain stem motor nuclei with loss of cell bodies and replacement by reactive astrocytes. This may occur without involvement of the adjacent parenchyma or may precede that involvement. Such a focal selective lesion is provocative for one form of invasion of the CNS being over the motor nerves to muscles which are the only direct access to these motor nuclei. This is further support for the protozoan being a *Sarcocystis* species. I have observed this lesion in the ventral grey column of the L6 and S1 segments of the spinal cord with profound neurogenic atrophy of the muscles innervated by the cranial gluteal nerve (middle and deep gluteal and tensor fasciae latae) and moderate atrophy of the caudal thigh and leg muscles innervated by the sciatic nerve. This clinical deficit occurred two months before ataxia and paresis occurred in both pelvic limbs and was associated with a necrotizing inflammatory lesion in the white matter bilaterally.

The lesion is a necrotizing nonsuppurative encephalomyelitis. It consists of a proliferative inflammation of grey matter and white matter, with a variable degree of necrosis of myelin, and axonal degeneration. Hemorrhage occurs occasionally. The inflammatory cells are mostly mononuclear and include lymphocytes, plasma cells, and macrophages, usually in a perivascular arrangement. The macrophages also may be free in the tissues. A few eosinophils usually are present, as well as multinucleated giant cells. Frequently, a similar nonsuppurative meningitis accompanies this parenchymal lesion. Glial cells proliferate. Neuronal degeneration occurs on the edge of necrotic lesions. In a few patients protozoal organisms are abundant. They mostly are contained in macrophage cytoplasm. A few form rosettes in neuronal cytoplasm or free in the tissues. In many patients these are difficult to find.

CSF will often be abnormal in these patients. This includes mild to moderate elevations of protein and pleocytosis. Lymphocytes and mononuclear cells predominate. Occasionally xanthochromia is present. CSF with these abnormalities may also have variable elevation of the enzymes CK, AST, and LDH. Rarely will one or more of these be elevated without other changes in the CSF. Lumbar CSF is more likely to show an abnormality with a myelitis. It is important to recognize that normal CSF does not preclude this diagnosis. I have been amazed at how severe a myelitis can be without altering the CSF.

Indications for this diagnosis include signs of a moderately progressive lesion in a mature horse, asymmetry of signs, signs of grey matter disease, signs of severe ataxia and paresis, and involvement of only a single animal on a farm (see Table 11–1).

This same disease can occur in the brain stem, cerebellum or cerebrum, or both, and produce clinical signs referable to that area. These are considered with the appropriate neuroanatomic system.

Because of the nature of the organism and the recognized value of antifolic acid drugs for treating toxoplasmosis, it is rational to consider such therapy for this disease. The objectives should be clear that the primary purpose is to stop the progress of the disease. It must be recognized that no recovery can occur where the disease has destroyed cell bodies and axons. Any improvement must depend on resolution of edema and hemorrhage, remyelination of intact axons, and compensation by unaltered components of the nervous system.

We have used the following therapy on a number of horses. The disease has progressed in most despite therapy. A few have remained static and a few have improved. The latter observations have warranted further use and study of this treatment with owners who realize the objectives of the therapy and are cooperative.

For a 1000-lb horse the therapy consists of three days of intravenous administration of sulfonamides such as Sulfa-Plex (Butler) at 250 cc per dose twice a day, and one month of daily oral administration of pyrimethamine (Daraprim, Burroughs Wellcome) at 5 tablets (125 mg) per dose twice a day, and a sulfatrimethoprim combination (Septra, Burroughs Wellcome) at 10 tablets per dose twice a day. Tribrissen may be used for the sulfonamide-trimethoprim combination therapy.

Corticosteroids should be avoided. There is indication that they may enhance the progress of the disease.

It is hoped that future investigations will further define the identity of the causative agent, its life cycle, and a serologic assay to help diagnose the condition. If this is a *Sarcocystis* agent as proposed, then most likely the horse is the intermediate host. It may be an aberrant intermediate host, or the invasion of the nervous system may be an abnormal site for the intermediate stages of the organism

in the horse. The definitive host that harbors the digestive tract stage of development of the organism may be a carnivore or rodent.[40]

This disease is not highly contagious on a farm. There is no indication that it passes between horses that have contact directly or indirectly. Its sporadic occurrence in a few horses each year on farms with a large population of horses would support a life cycle as proposed for a Sarcocystis organism. Identity of the definitive host would make it possible to prevent the disease by eliminating this host from the property.

Equine Herpesvirus 1—Myeloencephalopathy and Vasculitis. Equine herpesvirus type I rhinopneumonitis may produce a diffuse multifocal ischemic or hemorrhagic myelopathy and encephalopathy with leptomeningeal vasculitis.[13, 16, 36, 43, 44, 53, 60, 61, 73, 76, 77, 81, 87, 96, 100, 110, 119, 127] The equine rhinopneumonitis virus causes mild upper respiratory disease in horses of all ages and abortion in pregnant mares. Occasionally, neurologic signs have accompanied outbreaks of abortion and respiratory disease caused by this virus. The neurologic syndrome also may occur as the only illness on a farm. Although adults are most commonly affected, the disease also occurs in young foals. Occasionally the onset is associated with stress.[53]

The neurologic signs usually are sudden in onset but vary in severity from mild ataxia to severe paralysis. After a few days the signs generally do not progress significantly. Mild ataxia may be transient and be followed by complete recovery, or rapidly progress to tetraparesis and lateral recumbency in a 2- to 3-day period. Some horses become recumbent in 24 hours. These horses rarely recover and a few may die rapidly. Some cases with mild ataxia may improve, but retain some permanent gait abnormality. Despite the severity of the signs, bladder paralysis commonly occurs in early stages, and the animal may dribble urine constantly from an enlarged bladder and the tail may be hypotonic. This is unique to this disease and has no clear explanation. Most often the signs are symmetric in the pelvic limbs. Occasionally, the signs are asymmetric. Even a severe hemiparesis may result. Sometimes the onset of neurologic signs is preceded or accompanied by a fever and/or mild respiratory signs.

In a few instances the signs that are sudden in onset are referable to a diffuse cerebral or brain stem lesion. I have observed an extensive hemorrhagic infarction of the brain stem cause recumbency and severe tendency to roll from the disturbance to the vestibular nuclei. Many horses with spinal cord lesions are also quite depressed.

CSF may be xanthochromic and contain a significant elevation of protein, with the normal number of leukocytes or only a slight pleocytosis. The organism may be isolated from the respiratory system or buffy coat of the serum.

The spinal cord lesion usually is a diffuse myelopathy consisting of foci of myelin degeneration and axonal swelling in the white matter of one or more funiculi that are often linear and oriented along the route of a penetrating blood vessel. Sometimes a portion of the grey matter is involved. Occasionally, a few lipid-filled macrophages are present in the lesion, but the general lack of inflammatory cells in the necrotic lesion is remarkable. Sometimes there is hemorrhage associated with this degenerative lesion. Careful study of the leptomeningeal blood vessels often reveals a vasculitis, especially of small arteries. Thrombosis may be observed in autopsies performed shortly after signs began.

Similar lesions may be found in the brain without necessarily producing clinical signs. Ischemic or hemorrhagic infarcts may occur in the brain stem or cerebrum, along with a vasculitis of leptomeningeal or cerebrocortical blood vessels.

It is assumed that the parenchymal lesions are caused by interruption of the blood supply related to the vasculitis and thrombosis that are present. This produces the disseminated focal areas of degeneration or necrosis. The vasculitis is thought to result from the direct effect of the virus on the endothelium and adventitia of the vessel.[61] Inclusion bodies have not been found.

The virus has been isolated from the diseased nervous tissue of horses.[16, 76, 110, 127] The same disease and lesions have been reproduced by inoculating experimental horses with the recovered virus.[127]

This diagnosis should be suspected when a neurologic disease is sudden in onset with little change after 2 to 3 days, involves more than one horse on a farm, is associated with recent abortions or upper respiratory disease on the farm, causes disturbance of bladder function, and is reflected in abnormal CSF determinations. Demonstration of a rising serum neutralization titer to the equine herpesvirus will help confirm the diagnosis.

Because of the nature of the lesion, prompt therapy with high levels of corticosteroids may be beneficial, but they should be used for only a short period at the acute phase of the disease. Prolonged high level dosage may cause viral recrudescence and more extensive upper respiratory disease. Spontaneous recovery often occurs in mildly ataxic and paretic animals. Most recover in a 1- to 4-week period. A few require months. Recumbent animals have been reported to get up after 4 to 21 days,[16, 76] but this is rare.

Although most clinical signs are referable to the spinal cord, occasionally the brain stem and cerebral lesions also produce clinical signs referable to the area of destruction.

Although this disease more commonly occurs in unprotected animals, it has occurred on farms that have regularly vaccinated their horses for the upper respiratory disease. These vaccines have not protected consistently against the neurologic form. A newer, killed vaccine claims to protect horses against the neurologic form as well, and this remains to be determined.

Experimentally horses with circulating serum-neutralizing antibodies can be viremic with the equine herpes virus 1 agent circulating in leukocytes. The virus can spread from infected leukocytes to adjacent endothelial cells of cerebrospinal vasculature without an extracellular phase. Vasculitis is initiated in the endothelial cells of arteries and veins, and parenchymal lesions are the result of these vascular lesions.

A few years ago a number of outbreaks of this disease occurred a few days following the use of a new rhinopneumonitis vaccine. This is no longer on the market.

This neurologic disease occasionally occurs as an outbreak involving large numbers of animals. For this reason it is important to isolate all sick animals as soon as possible from further contact with healthy animals. The efficacy of vaccination at the onset of the outbreak is unknown.

Equine Nonsuppurative Myelitis. Occasionally, a mature horse is presented with moderately progressive signs of a fairly symmetric ataxia and paresis, and a mild diffuse nonsuppurative myelitis is found at necropsy. No obvious microbial agents have been found. Whether this condition is related to the protozoal disease or is a separate entity is not known at this time.

Viral Leukoencephalomyelitis of Goats. A leukoencephalomyelitis occurs in goats and is caused by a C-type retrovirus (CAEV, caprine arthritis-encephalitis virus).[21-25, 28, 29, 91, 121, 123]

Gross Path

This is a persistent virus that has a very high rate of infection in goats. The incidence of subclinical infection is high. Clinical signs of this disease are most common in young kids less than 5 months of age, but they are occasionally observed in adults of any age. Most commonly the signs reflect a major focus of the lesion in the spinal cord or caudal brain stem and cerebellum. Rarely the signs reflect a major cerebral lesion.

The clinical signs of myelitis will vary with the location of the lesion. The onset may be a paraparesis and pelvic limb ataxia that progresses to tetraparesis and ataxia of all four limbs. Occasionally the signs do not progress beyond the paraparesis. In others the signs begin as a tetraparesis and ataxia of all four limbs. In a few the signs are predominantly hemiparesis or hemiplegia from a major lesion on one side of the cervical spinal cord. Kids with brain stem encephalitis usually have all their clinical signs related to the disturbance of this segment of the brain. If the signs begin as a myelitis, they rarely progress to an encephalitis.

Although the lesion is thought to begin initially as a demyelinating lesion and predominate in white matter, the proliferative inflammatory stage may involve grey as well as white matter; if the lesions are in the cervical or lumbosacral intumescence, there will be a loss of muscle tone and reflexes that reflect this grey matter lesion.

Once clinical signs begin in some component of the nervous system, they usually progress fairly rapidly in that focal area. Usually within 7 to 14 days the clinical signs reach their full development. Experimentally these lesions may persist for months. Because of the poor prognosis, most goats are euthanatized at this stage of the disease.

Cerebrospinal fluid is usually abnormal with a mononuclear pleocytosis and protein elevation. Occasionally neutrophils are present but not eosinophils. These CSF changes may be severe. One study of 25 patients with viral leukoencephalomyelitis (CAE) showed the following CSF determinations: leukocytes, 0 to 710 (median, 23) per cu mm; protein, 24 to 3500 (median, 80) mg per dl; cells-to-protein ratio, < 0.10 to 3.72 (median, 0.24). Another report on 10 goats with this disease gave a range of 5 to 1800 leukocytes per cu mm, with a median of 475 and a predominance of mononuclear cells. Other CSF evaluations reported are included in these ranges.

The lesion is often visible on examination of transverse sections of the gross specimen. The affected area will be enlarged, firm, and a yellow to brown color. This granulomatous lesion consists of a massive accumulation of mononuclear inflammatory cells, lipid-filled macrophages, and astrocytes in regions of extensive necrosis of axons and myelin. In some areas of these lesions, axons may be observed surrounded by macrophages and no myelin. This is an indication of the demyelinating stage of this disease. The lesion is widely disseminated, and collections of inflammatory cells are often observed widely distributed in other areas of the spinal cord and brain. In some goats the lesion is widely disseminated with multiple areas of destruction in the spinal cord and not one major focal granulomatous lesion.

There is evidence that the inflammatory response in this lesion may be an immunopathologic reaction to viral antigen on cell surfaces of infected tissue. In immunosuppressed animals these significant lesions do not develop.[26]

This virus also affects the lungs, producing a mild nonsuppurative interstitial pneumonitis, and joints, producing an arthritis. Usually the clinical signs of pneumonitis are mild or not observed, but lesions may be evident in goats with the neurologic disease. The arthritic form of the disease is most often observed in goats 1 year or older.[1, 29, 30] Occasionally older goats that are autopsied because of their chronic joint disease will be found to have a leukoencephalitis that was not apparent clinically.

Because of the primary involvement of the nervous system and synovial membranes by this agent, it has been referred to as the caprine arthritis-encephalitis virus (CAEV). Infected goats can be identified by the presence of serum antibodies against this virus.

There is evidence that the virus persists in blood leukocytes despite circulating antibody and is shed only in the colostrum and milk from infected does. If a doe is known to have had a kid with this disease or has an antibody titer to this virus, subsequent kids should not be allowed to nurse that doe as a means of preventing their infection. They can be raised on cow's colostrum and milk or on milk from uninfected does.

Parasitic Myelitis—Cerebrospinal Nematodiasis

Parelaphostrongylus tenuis—GOATS AND SHEEP. In goats and sheep the migration of the adult nematode, *Parelaphostrongylus tenuis,* through the spinal cord and brain can produce a variety of clinical signs, depending on where the greatest damage occurs.[2, 5, 6, 65, 80, 134] This parasite is the meningeal worm of white-tailed deer, and has a neurotrophic life cycle in that species without producing clinical signs.[3, 4] The organism has an intermediate stage of development in a mollusk. In goats and sheep, most of the clinical signs are referable to the spinal cord lesion and consist of lameness, paresis, and ataxia of one or both pelvic limbs, paraplegia, hemiparesis, tetraparesis and ataxia of all four limbs, and tetraplegia. The presence of profound deficits in the pelvic limbs and mild thoracic limb abnormality suggests multifocal lesions that are consistent with an infectious disease such as this. Mild vestibular signs and blindness also have been caused by the migration of the parasite in the brain. Death may occur. The signs are often progressive, and change as the migratory route changes; they may remain static or even improve spontaneously. A few patients have a focal skin lesion caused by continual rubbing or scratching by the animal. These lesions are usually on the trunk and are oriented dorsoventrally in the pattern of a dermatome. These may relate to the parasitic involvement of selected dorsal roots or dorsal grey column.

One study of 14 patients with the pathologic diagnosis of meningoencephalomyelitis due to *Parelaphostrongylus tenuis* infection showed the following CSF determinations: leukocytes, 6 to 1000 (median, 67.5) cells per cu mm; 70 per cent of the samples contained eosinophils; protein, 34 to 360 (median, 78) mg per dl; cells-to-protein ratio, 0.19 to 9.15 (median, 0.59). Occasionally hemorrhage occurs in the CSF from the organism and xanthochromia may be evident. The presence of eosinophils is highly indicative of this disease. These rarely occur in CSF without parasitism.

This diagnosis should especially be considered whenever more than one animal in a flock is affected with a neurologic syndrome, and yet they do not all show the same clinical signs, suggesting the multifocal nature of the lesion.[7, 89] This clinical disease is seen most commonly in the fall and winter after sheep and goats have been on pasture, where they can ingest the larval infected mollusks that are obligatory in the life cycle of this parasite.

A number of anthelmintics have been tried for the treatment and prophylaxis of this disease.[114] These include diethylcarbamazine (Caricide) with dexamethasone (Azium), levamisol (Ripercol), and thiabendazole. None has been tested adequately for its efficacy. For the patient with neurologic disease, diethyl-

carbamazine with dexamethasone is recommended. For the prophylactic treatment of a flock, levamisol is recommended.

Strongylus vulgaris—HORSES. In horses, migration of the larval form of *Strongylus vulgaris* may produce signs of spinal cord disease.[74, 75, 98, 120, 124] This is an abnormal route for this species of equine parasite. More often the migration is in the brain, but spinal cord lesions do occur. The clinical signs depend on the location of the lesion. They are usually sudden in onset. In theory, this is a progressive disease, and the signs progress and change as the larva migrates. However, this is dependent on the continual migration of the larva. CSF studies should reflect the destruction produced and the reaction to the parasite, as was noted in the goats with cerebrospinal nematodiasis.

The larvae of *Setaria* species have been found in the CNS of horses with progressive neurologic signs.[47] In this country equine cerebrospinal nematodiasis appears to be a rare disease.

Hypoderma bovis—CATTLE. The development of paraparesis and pelvic limb ataxia in cattle that occurs within 24 hours of treatment with systemic insecticides has been blamed on the death of the first instar larva of *Hypoderma bovis* located extradurally in the vertebral canal. Experimental studies do not indicate any relationship of these signs to the parasite. Although the larva may produce some lesions in the epidural tissues, there are no lesions in the adjacent spinal cord or spinal nerves. It is concluded that those cattle that develop these signs are particularly susceptible to the neurotoxicity of the drug that is used.[66]

DEGENERATION

Degenerative Myeloencephalopathy in Horses. A slowly progressive symmetric ataxia, spasticity, and paresis have been observed in young horses and zebras that have a diffuse degenerative myeloencephalopathy.[81, 82, 86] The age at onset may vary from birth to 2 years, but it appears most often in the first few months of life. The signs are slowly progressive and may begin in the pelvic limbs, but soon involve the thoracic limbs. In many patients the thoracic limb deficit is as pronounced as the pelvic limb deficit. In a few the pelvic limb signs are much worse.

The neurologic signs usually suggest an anatomic diagnosis of a focal cervical spinal cord lesion or diffuse spinal cord lesion affecting white matter. In most horses it is not possible to distinguish the clinical signs of this disease from those of a horse with cervical stenotic myelopathy. When the forelimb signs are as pronounced as those in the pelvic limbs, this diagnosis should be suspected.

Laboratory studies on blood and CSF are all normal. Plain and contrast radiographs as well as myelograms are normal.

There are no gross lesions in the central nervous system. On examination with the microscope, a diffuse degeneration of neurons in the white matter of all spinal cord funiculi is seen. It is most pronounced in the dorsolateral aspect of the lateral funiculus (spinocerebellar tract) and in the ventral funiculus adjacent to the ventral median fissure (sulcomarginal tracts). This is a bilaterally symmetric lesion that is most developed in the thoracic spinal cord segments and usually decreases in the lumbar and cervical segments. In severely affected patients the lesion spreads throughout the lateral and ventral funiculi. The dorsal funiculi are usually spared. The most obvious lesion in these areas is the lack of myelin followed by a significant proliferation of astrocytes and their processes in the degenerate area. Careful study will show axonal loss from these areas as well. Swollen eosinophilic (dystrophic) axons are present mostly in the grey matter, and are especially prominent in the nucleus of the dorsospinocerebellar tract in the thoracic segments, and in the gracilic and cuneate nuclei of the medulla. Neuroaxonal dystrophy also occurs variably in the lateral cervical, olivary, vestibular, oculomotor, pretectal, and thalamic nuclei. Therefore this is a multisystem degenerative disease of the nervous system.

This disease should be suspected in young horses with slowly progressive pelvic and thoracic limb ataxia, spasticity, and paresis, especially if the signs begin in the first few months (see Table 11–1). Because the clinical signs resemble those of cervical stenotic myelopathy and the lesions are often not recognized at autopsy, this disease can easily be overlooked. In the hospital population at the New York State College of Veterinary Medicine, this disease is more common than cervical stenotic myelopathy.

The cause of the disease is unknown. The lesions are similar to some of the heredodegenerative diseases of humans,[27, 52] sheep,[20] and cats.[139] The disease has been recognized in a family of zebras, suggesting an inheritance factor.[53] I have observed it in an unrelated zebra. However, in horses it has been recognized in several breeds. Because of the involvement of almost all of the common breeds of horses, an exogenous cause is suspected. As further support for an environmental cause, I recently diagnosed this disease in twins that were from an Arabian-Appaloosa mating. I have observed this to occur on the same farm in the offspring of mares in successive years and in related offspring, which could suggest a familial or environmental basis. I suspect the latter. It is possible that with careful study, more than one form and cause of this disease may be discovered. Some similar clinical signs and lesions have been observed in nutritional deficiency diseases in sheep[15] and rats,[38, 95] and in an ataxic condition of unknown cause in the red deer,[9, 126, 138] and in a plant poisoning in cattle. Deficiencies of copper and vitamin E have been implicated in these reports. To date there is no evidence of these deficiencies in horses with this disease, but further investigation is necessary. Recent studies have defined the copper requirement in ponies and the role of molybdenum in this requirement.[33, 34] Some plant poisonings will produce somewhat similar lesions in cattle, sheep, and horses. Organophosphates may also produce somewhat similar lesions in domestic and laboratory animals. Careful study of the environment of these horses, their diet, and the various anthelmintics to which they are exposed is necessary to attempt to understand the pathogenesis of this disease.

Haloxon Neurotoxicity in Sheep. Sheep exposed to the organophosphate anthelmintic haloxon may develop a neurotoxic response.[8, 78, 137] Acute intoxications are rare, but occasionally a delayed response occurs about 3 to 5 weeks after treatment with this compound. Experimental studies suggest that older sheep are more susceptible. Clinical experience has not supported this.

The clinical signs are fairly rapid in onset, and usually remain static. Over a period of 3 to 4 months of observation the signs neither progress nor improve. Signs are all in the pelvic limbs, and consist of a symmetric spastic paraparesis and ataxia. The sheep are alert, responsive, and strong in the thoracic limbs. They run around with their pelvic limbs in a partially flexed, crouched position, and often with the dorsal surface of the hoof on the ground. There is still voluntary function in the limbs, but the strength and coordination are reduced. The limbs are hypertonic, and reflexes are normal to hyperactive. There is no atrophy and no obvious loss of pain sensation.

The lesions are unremarkable. Swollen axons have been found in the sciatic nerve and lumbar spinal cord.

Resistance of some sheep to this intoxication was found to be related to the amount of an esterase present in their plasma.[8] This enzyme was gene-determined, and when present in sufficient amounts protected the sheep against haloxon. Cholinesterase levels are not depressed significantly when the first neurologic signs appear. A similar organophosphate-induced paraparesis occurs in cattle.[88]

Swayback—Sheep, Goats. An ataxic condition associated with a copper deficiency has been described in sheep and goats and is sometimes referred to as enzootic ataxia.[15, 18, 19, 62, 117, 123] Myelin deficiency is found in specific spinal cord tracts, and neuronal degeneration occurs in brain stem and spinal cord neurons. Subcortical cavitation may occur in the cerebrum. The spinal cord tracts most severely affected are in the dorsolateral aspect of each lateral funiculus and the tracts adjacent to the ventral median fissure on each ventral funiculus. They are bilaterally symmetrical lesions.

Clinical signs may be present at birth and reflect lesions of the spinal cord, or brain, or both. In some the clinical signs do not occur until around 2 to 4 months of age, and initially they consist of a paraparesis and pelvic limb ataxia that usually progresses to affect all four limbs. This is a slowly progressive degenerative disorder of specific populations of neurons that is related to copper deficiency in the dam and offspring.

Nutritional Myelopathy—Pigs. A rapidly progressive spinal cord disorder has been reported in young pigs 3½ to 6 months old.[84] Most of these pigs develop a pelvic limb ataxia and paresis that progresses to paraplegia. Bilaterally symmetric spinal cord demyelination and copper deficiency were found in these pigs.

We have observed a syndrome in young pigs about 4 months old that consists of a symmetric paresis and ataxia of the pelvic limbs. The signs progress for a few weeks until the pigs may have difficulty rising on the pelvic limbs, then the signs remain static. Only pelvic limb signs have been observed. Extensive degeneration of myelin and axons has been observed in the thoracolumbar spinal cords of these pigs and in peripheral nerves. A nutritional basis is suspected. Serum copper levels have been below normal, but the lesion is more extensive than what has been reported in swayback. Studies on the pathogenesis of this disease are in progress.

Some clinicians have observed a rapidly progressive paraparesis and pelvic limb ataxia in 3-month-old pigs fed solely on milk.[133] Treatment with vitamin A was followed by recovery in about a 2-week period. This relationship, if any, remains to be proved.

Arsanilic Acid Poisoning in Pigs. Organic arsenicals are added to the rations of pigs as growth promoters and to prevent swine dysentery. Arsanilic acid is most commonly used. Accidental overdosage results in intoxication.[56, 64, 68] Ataxia is an early sign and may predominate in the pelvic limbs and resemble a thoracolumbar spinal cord lesion. However, the clinical signs are diffuse in their anatomic origin. A drunken ataxic gait with stumbling to either side is an early sign. The signs are often worse in the pelvic limbs but all four limbs are affected. Paresis follows ataxia, and pigs become severely paraparetic and "dog-sit," then become tetraparetic and are unable to rise. When severely affected they may lie in recumbency, with the forelimbs extended caudally and the hindlimbs cranially. They remain alert and responsive. Other signs that have been observed, usually transiently, include head tremor, head tilts, circling, and blindness. One report describes seizures, especially upon forced activity.[103]

The onset and severity of signs is directly related to the toxic level of arsenical in the ration. Early withdrawal of the arsenical may result in complete spontaneous recovery. Lesions develop after a few days of signs and include degeneration of myelin and axons in optic nerves, optic tracts, and peripheral nerves.

Embolic Myelopathy. Spinal cord infarction associated with fibrocartilaginous emboli in spinal vasculature has been reported in horses and a pig.[94, 125, 135] In the horse, the infarct and emboli were in the C6 and C7 segments. Intervertebral disk extrusion was assumed by the presence of fibrocartilage on the outside of the dura. A pony was autopsied 6 months after a sudden neurologic disorder referable to the cervical intumescence. Infarction was found in the C6 and C7 segments, and an intervertebral disk degeneration occurred at the C6–C7 articulation. In the sow, the emboli and infarcts occurred in the lumbosacral spinal cord, associated with degeneration of the L5–L6 intervertebral disk and a fracture of the growth plate on the caudal aspect of L5.

Myelin Disorder of Charolais Cattle. In Charolais cattle a progressive symmetric gait disorder begins at about 1 year of age.[93] The gait is stiff and stumbling, and worse in the pelvic limbs. The animals may become recumbent and have extreme difficulty getting up. Except for an occasional head bob, there are no other signs of intracranial disease. Multiple plaques of abnormal myelin are present in the brain and spinal cord white matter. The pathogenesis is unknown, but this disease may have a familial basis.

NEOPLASIA—INTRAMEDULLARY

Intramedullary neoplasms are rare in large animals. They present clinically similar to extramedullary neoplasms and are difficult to differentiate. Myelography is needed for the differential diagnosis.

MALFORMATION

Myelodysplasia in Calves. Calves born with a moderate to severe pelvic limb ataxia and spastic paresis that is not progressive usually have a focal or diffuse thoracolumbar myelodysplasia. Severe ataxia often predominates over milder loss of voluntary motor function. Sometimes the pelvic limb movements are simultaneous, moving together in a hopping fashion. The same simultaneous bilateral response occurs on stimulation of the flexor reflex but not the patellar reflex. Occasionally a vertebral column malformation accompanies the myelodysplasia and is palpable or visible on radiographs.

A number of different malformations have been observed, but the incidence of any one kind has been insufficient to establish any familial tendencies. These are considered to be sporadic developmental disorders of unknown cause.

The various malformations include meningomyelocele, segmental hypoplasia, diplomyelia within a single vertebral canal, diastematomyelia with two spinal cords in separate vertebral canals, and a variety of forms of disorganized parenchyma and hydromyelia and syringomyelia usually over a number of segments.

Arthrogryposis and cleft palate have been reported along with cervical spinal cord dysraphism in Charolais cattle.[70]

Hamartomas in Foals. A newborn female Thoroughbred foal was observed from birth with episodes of muscle spasms in the pelvic limbs, caudal abdominal muscles, and other lumbar hypaxial muscles, and sweating caudal to the midlumbar area. These episodes lasted from less than a minute to up to one hour and occurred irregularly many times a day. Between these episodes the foal was normal on neurologic evaluation. It ran, played, and kicked like any other normal foal. There was a mild skeletal deformity in the cranial thoracic region. The dorsal aspect of the ribs was depressed on the right just caudal to the scapula, and the ribs bulged on the opposite side. Radiographs confirmed a scoliosis that was most severe at the T7 to T8 region with convexity to the left.

At necropsy the scoliosis was confirmed but there was no stenosis of the vertebral canal. The spinal cord was markedly enlarged from the sixth through the eighth thoracic segments. A portion of the enlargement was a large syrinx in the dorsal columns. The main enlargement was a mass of disorganized grey and white matter that involved the entire transverse section. This was diagnosed as a hamartoma.

The relationship of the clinical signs to this is unknown as is the explanation for why the animal could function normally with its pelvic limbs.

A 9-month-old female Standardbred was normal until 7 months of age when pelvic limb ataxia and paresis related to a mid-thoracic scoliosis and kyphosis were first noticed. At necropsy the vertebral canal was widened at the site of the most significant vertebral malformation at T7 and T8. The spinal cord was enlarged from an intradural mass located predominantly in the dorsal funiculi that was diagnosed as a hamartoma. The delay in onset of neurologic signs is unexplained.

REFERENCES

1. Adams, D. S., Crawford, T. B., and Klevfer Anderson, P.: A pathogenetic study of the early connective tissue lesions of caprine arthritis-encephalitis. Am. J. Pathol., 99:257, 1980.
2. Alden, C., Woodson, F., Mohan, R., and Miller, S.: Cerebrospinal nematodiasis in sheep. J. Am. Vet. Med. Assoc., 166:784, 1975.
3. Anderson, R. C.: The development of *Pneumostrongylus tenuis* in the central nervous system of white-tailed deer. Pathol. Vet., 2:360, 1965.
4. Anderson, R. C., Lankester, M. W., and Strelive, U. R.: Further experimental studies of *Pneumostrongylus tenuis* in cervids. Can. J. Zool., 44:851, 1966.
5. Anderson, R. C., and Strelive, U. R.: The effect of *Pneumostrongylus •tenuis* (Nematoda: Metastrongyloidea) in kids. Can. J. Comp. Med., 33:280, 1969.
6. Anderson, R. C., and Strelive, U. R.: Experimental

cerebrospinal nematodiasis *(Pneumostrongylus tenuis)* in sheep. Can. J. Zool., *44*:889, 1966.

7. Baharsefat, M., Amjadi, A. R., Yamin, B., and Ahoura, P.: The first report of lumbar paralysis in sheep due to nematode larvae infestation in Iran. Cornell Vet., *63*:81, 1972.

8. Baker, N. F., Tucker, E. M., Stormont, C., and Fisk, R. A.: Neurotoxicity of haloxon and its relationship to blood esterases of sheep. Am. J. Vet. Res., *31*:865, 1970.

9. Barlow, R. M., Butler, E. J., and Purves, D.: An ataxic condition in red deer *(Cervus elaphus).* J. Comp. Pathol., *74*:519, 1964.

10. Beech, J.: Metrizamide myelography in the horse. J. Am. Vet. Radiol. Soc., *20*:22, 1979.

11. Beech, J.: Equine protozoan encephalomyelitis. Vet. Med. Small Anim. Clin., *69*:1562, 1974.

12. Beech, J., and Dodd, D. C.: Toxoplasma-like encephalomyelitis in the horse. Vet. Pathol., *11*:87, 1974.

13. Bitsch, V, and Dam, A.: Nervous disturbances in horses in relation to infection with equine rhinopneumonitis virus. Acta Vet. Scand., *12*:134, 1971.

14. Brown, T. T., Jr., and Patton, C. S.: Protozoal encephalomyelitis in horses. J. Am. Vet. Med. Assoc., *171*:492, 1977.

15. Chalmers, G. A.: Swayback (Enzootic ataxia) in Alberta lambs. Can. J. Comp. Med., *38*:111, 1974.

16. Charlton, K. M,. Mitchell, D., Girard, A., and Corner, A. H.: Meningoencephalomyelitis in horses associated with equine herpesvirus infection. Vet. Pathol., *13*:59, 1976.

17. Cho, C. Y., Cook, J. E., and Leipold, H. W.: Angiomatous vascular malformation in the spinal cord of a Hereford calf. Vet. Pathol., *16*:613, 1979.

18. Cordy, D. R.: Enzootic ataxia in California lambs. J. Am. Vet. Med. Assoc., *158*:1940, 1971.

19. Cordy, D. R., and Knight, H. D.: California goats with a disease resembling enzootic ataxia or swayback. Vet. Pathol., *15*:179, 1978.

20. Cordy, D. R., Richards, W. P. C., and Bradford, G. E.: Systemic neuraxonal dystrophy in Suffolk sheep. Acta Neuropathol., *8*:133, 1967.

21. Cork, L. C.: Differential diagnosis of viral leukoencephalomyelitis of goats. J. Am. Vet. Med. Assoc., *169*:1303, 1976.

22. Cork, L. C., and Davis, W. C.: Ultrastructural features of viral leukoencephalomyelitis of goats. Lab. Invest., *32*:359, 1975.

23. Cork, L. C., Hadlow, W. J., Crawford, T. B., Gorham, J. R., and Piper, R. C.: Infectious leukoencephalomyelitis of young goats. J. Infect. Dis., *129*:134, 1974.

24. Cork, L. C., Hadlow, W. J., Gorham, J. R., Piper, R. C., and Crawford, T. B.: Pathology of viral leukoencephalomyelitis of goats. Acta Neuropathol., *29*:281, 1974.

25. Cork, L. C., and Narayan, O.: The pathogenesis of viral leukoencephalomyelitis-arthritis of goats. I. Persistent viral infection with progressive pathologic changes. Lab. Invest., *42*:596, 1980.

26. Cork, L. C., and Narayan, O.: Pathogenesis of goat viral leukoencephalomyelitis-arthritis. *In* Abstracts of the American College of Veterinary Pathologists, 1981.

27. Cowen, D., and Olmstead, E. V.: Infantile neuraxonal dystrophy. J. Neuropathol. Exp. Neurol., *22*:175, 1963.

28. Crawford, T. B., and Adams, D. S.: Caprine arthri-

tis-encephalitis: Clinical features and presence of antibody in selected goat populations. J. Am. Vet. Med. Assoc., *178*:713, 1981.

29. Crawford, T. B., Adams, D. S., Cheevers, U. P., and Cork, L. C.: Chronic arthritis in goats caused by a retrovirus. Science, *207*:997, 1980.

30. Crawford, T. B., Adams, D. S., Sande, R. D., Gorham, J. R., and Henson, J. B.: The connective tissue component of the caprine arthritis-encephalitis syndrome. Am. J. Pathol., *100*:443, 1980.

31. Crowhurst, F. A., Dickinson, G., and Burrows, R.: An outbreak of paresis in mares and geldings associated with equid herpesvirus. Vet. Rec., *109*:527, 1981.

32. Cusick, P. K., Sell, D. M., Hamilton, D. P., and Hardenbrok, H. J.: Toxoplasmosis in two horses. J. Am. Vet. Med. Assoc., *164*:77, 1974.

33. Cymbaluk, N. F., Schryver, H. F., and Hintz, H. F.: Copper metabolism and requirement in mature ponies. J. Nutr., *111*:87, 1981.

34. Cymbaluk, N. F., Schryver, H. F., Hintz, H. F., Smith, D. F., and Lowe, J. E.: Influence of dietary molybdenum copper metabolism in ponies. J. Nutr., *111*:96, 1981.

35. Dahme, E., and Schebitz, H.: Zur Pathogenese der spinalen Ataxie des Pferdes unter Zugrundelegung neurer Befunde. Zbl. Veterinaermed., *17*:120, 1970.

36. Dalsgaard, H.: Enzootic paresis in horses as a consequence of outbreaks of rhinopneumonitis (virus abortion). Medlemsbl. Danske Dyrlaegeforen, *3*:71, 1970.

37. Dimock, W. W., and Errington, B. J.: Incoordination of equidae: Wobblers. J. Am. Vet. Med. Assoc., *95*:261, 1939.

38. Dipaolo, R. V., Kanfer, J. N., and Newberne, P. M.: Copper deficiency and the central nervous system. Myelination in the rat: Morphological and biochemical studies. J. Neuropathol. Exp. Neurol., *33*:226, 1974.

39. Doige, C. E.: Pathologic changes in the lumbar spine of boars. Can. J. Comp. Med., *44*:382, 1980.

40. Dubey, J. P.: Coyote as a final host for Sarcocystis species of goats, sheep, cattle, elk, bison, and moose in Montana. Am. J. Vet. Res., *41*:1227, 1980.

41. Dubey, J. P., Davis, G. W., Koestner, A., and Kiryu, K.: Equine encephalomyelitis due to a protozoan parasite resembling *Toxoplasma gondii.* J. Am. Vet. Med. Assoc., *165*:249, 1974.

42. Falco, M. J., Whitwell, K., and Palmer, A. C.: An investigation into the genetics of "wobbler disease" in Thoroughbred horses in Britain. Equine Vet. J., *8*:165, 1976.

43. Fankhauser, R.: Entzündliche Gefässveränderungen als Grundlage von Rückenmarksläsionen beim Pferd. Schweiz. Arch. Tierheilk., *110*:171, 1968.

44. Fankhauser, R., and Gerber, H.: Zerebrale Vaskulitis beim Pferd. Arch. Exp. Vet. Med., *24*:61, 1970.

45. Ferrer, J. F.: Bovine lymphosarcoma. Compend. Contin. Ed., *2*:S235, 1980.

46. Fraser, H., and Palmer, A. C.: Equine incoordination and wobbler disease of young horses. Vet. Rec., *80*:338, 1967.

47. Frauenfelder, H. C., Kazacos, K. R., and Lichtenfels, J. R.: Cerebrospinal nematodiasis caused by a Filarid in a horse. J. Am. Vet. Med. Assoc., *177*:359, 1980.

48. Funk, K. A., and Erickson, E. D.: A case of atlantoaxial subluxation in a horse. Can. Vet. J., 9:120, 1968.
49. Gerbert, H., Fankhauser, R., Straub, R., and Veltschi, G.: Spinale Ataxie beim Pferd, verursacht durch synoviale Cysten in der Halswirbelsäule. Schweiz. Arch. Tier., 122:95, 1980.
50. Gerstman, B. B.: Equine protozoal myeloencephalitis. Senior Seminar, N.Y. State College of Veterinary Medicine, April 1980.
51. Gilmour, J. S., and Fraser, J. A.: Ataxia in a Welsh Cob Filly due to a venous malformation in the thoracic spinal cord. Equine Vet. J., 9:40, 1977.
52. Greenfield, J. G.: The Spino-Cerebellar Degenerations. Oxford, England, Blackwell Scientific Publications, 1954.
53. Greenwood, R. E. S., and Simpson, A. R. B.: Clinical report of a paralytic syndrome affecting stallions, mares and foals on a Thoroughbred stud farm. Equine Vet. J., 12:113, 1980.
54. Greet, T. R. C., Jeffcott, L. B., Whitwell, K. E., and Cook, W. R.: The slap test for laryngeal adductory function in horses with suspected cervical spinal cord damage. Equine Vet. J., 12:127, 1980.
55. Guffy, M. M., Coffman, J. R., and Strafuss, A. C.: Atlantoaxial luxation in a foal. J. Am. Vet. Med. Assoc., 15:754, 1969.
56. Harding, J. D. J., Lewis, G., and Done, J. T.: Experimental arsanilic acid poisoning in pigs. Vet. Rec., 83:560, 1968.
57. Hartley W. J., and Blakemore, W. F.: An unidentified sporozoan encephalomyelitis in sheep. Vet. Pathol., 11:1, 1974.
58. Helfer, D. H., and Stevens, D. R.: Spinal neurofibroma in a sheep. Vet. Pathol., 15:784, 1978.
59. Hooper, P. T., Best, S. M., and Campbell, A.: Axonal dystrophy in the spinal cords of cattle consuming the Cycad palm, Cycas media. Aust. Vet. J., 50:146, 1974.
60. Jackson, T., and Kendrick, J. W.: Paralysis of horses associated with equine herpesvirus I infection. J. Am. Vet. Med. Assoc., 158:1351, 1971.
61. Jackson, T. A., Osburn, B. I., Cordy, D. R., and Kendrick, J. W.: Equine herpesvirus 1 infection of horses: Studies on the experimentally induced neurologic disease. Am. J. Vet. Res., 38:709, 1977.
62. Jensen, R., Maag, D. D., and Flint, J. C.: Enzootic ataxia from copper deficiency in sheep in Colorado. J. Am. Vet. Med. Assoc., 133:336, 1958.
63. Jones, T. C., Doll, E. R., and Brown, R. G.: The pathology of equine incoordination (ataxia or "wobblers" of foals). Proc. Am. Vet. Med. Assoc., 91st Annual Meeting, 1954, 139–149.
64. Keenan, D. M.: Acute arsanilic acid intoxication in pigs. Aust. Vet. J., 49:229, 1973.
65. Kennedy, P. C., Whitlock, J. H., and Roberts, S. J.: Neurofilariosis, a paralytic disease of sheep. I. Introduction, symptomatology and pathology. Cornell Vet., 42:118, 1952.
66. Khan, M. A.: Significance of "spinal-stage" Hypoderma larvae in systemic insecticide toxicity. Res. Vet. Sci., 10:355, 1969.
67. Krunajcvic, T., and Bergsten, G.: Luxation of the cervical spinal column as a cause of wobbles in a foal. Acta Vet. Scand., 9:112, 1968.
68. Ledet, A. E., Duncan, J. R., Buck, W. B., and Ramsey, F. K.: Clinical, toxicological and pathological aspects of arsanilic acid poisoning in swine. Clin. Toxicol., 6:439, 1973.
69. Leipold, H. W., Brandt, G. W., Guffy, M., and Blauch, B.: Congenital atlanto-occipital fusion in a foal. Vet. Med. Sm. Anim. Clin., 69:1312, 1974.
70. Leipold, H. W., Cates, W. F., Radostits, O. M., and Howell, W. E.: Spinal dysraphism, arthrogryposis and cleft palate in newborn Charolais calves. Can. Vet. J., 10:268, 1969.
71. Leipold, H. W., Strafuss, A. C., Blauch, B., Olson, J. R., and Guffy, M.: Congenital defect of the atlanto-occipital joint in a Holstein-Friesian calf. Cornell Vet., 62:646, 1972.
72. Lerner, D. J., and Riley, G.: Congenital kyphoscoliosis in a foal. J. Am. Vet. Med. Assoc., 172:274, 1978.
73. Little, P. B.: Viral involvement in equine paresis. Vet. Rec., 95:575, 1974.
74. Little, P. B.: Cerebrospinal nematodiasis of equidae. J. Am. Vet. Med. Assoc., 160:1407, 1972.
75. Little, P. B., Lewin, U. S., and Fretz, P.: Verminous encephalitis of horses: Experimental induction with Strongylus vulgaris larvae. Am. J. Vet. Res., 35:1501, 1974.
76. Little, P. B., and Thorsen, J.: Disseminated necrotizing myeloencephalitis: A herpes associated neurological disease of horses. Vet. Pathol., 13:161, 1976.
77. Liu, I. K. M., and Castleman, W.: Equine posterior paresis associated with equine herpesvirus 1 vaccine in California. Equine Med. Surg., 1:397, 1977.
78. Malone, J. D.: Toxicity of haloxon. Res. Vet. Sci., 5:17, 1964.
79. Matthias, D., Dietz, O., and Reckenberg, R.: Zur Klinik und Pathologie der spinalen Ataxie der Fohlen. Arch. Exp. Veterinaermed., 19:43, 1965.
80. Mayhew, I. G., de Lahunta, A., Georgi, J. R., and Aspros, D. G.: Naturally occurring cerebrospinal Parelaphostrongylosis. Cornell Vet., 65:56, 1976.
81. Mayhew, I. G., de Lahunta, A., Whitlock, R. H., Krook, L., and Tasker, J. B.: Spinal cord disease in the horse. Cornell Vet., 68[Suppl.]:6, 1978.
82. Mayhew, I. G., de Lahunta, A., Whitlock, R. H., and Geary, J. C.: Equine degenerative myeloencephalopathy. J. Am. Vet. Med. Assoc., 170:195, 1977.
83. Mayhew, I. G., Watson, A. G., and Heissan, J. A.: Congenital occipitoatlantoaxial malformations in the horse. Equine Vet. J., 10:103, 1978.
84. McGavin, M. D., Ranby, P. D., and Tammemagi, L.: Demyelination associated with low liver copper levels in pigs. Aust. Vet. J., 38:8, 1962.
85. Milne, D., Gabel, A., Chrisman, C., and Fetter, A.: Diagnosis and pathology of the wobbler syndrome (spondylolisthesis): A preliminary study. Proc. Am. Assoc. Eq. Pract., 19:303, 1973.
86. Montali, R. J., Bush, M., Sauer, R. M., Gray, C. M., and Xanten, W. A., Jr.: Spinal ataxia in zebras. Vet. Pathol., 11:68, 1974.
87. Moyer, W., and Rooney, J. R.: An epidemic central nervous system disease in horses. Proc. Am. Assoc. Equine Pract., 19:307, 1973.
88. Nicholson, S. S.: Bovine posterior paresis due to organophosphate poisoning. J. Am. Vet. Med. Assoc., 165:280, 1974.
89. Nobel, T. A., and Olafson, P.: Spinal nematodiasis in sheep. Refuah Vet., 13:51, 1956.
90. Olafson, P.: "Wobblers" compared with ataxic ("swingback") lambs. Cornell Vet., 32:301, 1942.

91. O'Sullivan, B. M., Eaves, F. W., Baxendell, S. A., and Rowan, K. J.: Leucoencephalomyelitis of goat kids. Aust. Vet. J., *54*:479, 1978.

92. Palmer, A. C.: Stenosis of the cervical vertebral canal in a yearling ram. Vet. Rec., *109*:53, 1981.

93. Palmer, A. C., Blakemore, W. F., Barlow, R. M., Frazer, J. A., and Ogden, A. L.: Progressive ataxia of Charolais cattle associated with a myelin disorder. Vet. Rec., *91*:592, 1972.

94. Pass, D. A.: Posterior paralysis in a sow due to cartilaginous emboli in the spinal cord. Aust. Vet. J., *54*:100, 1978.

95. Pentschew, A., and Schwarz, K.: Systemic axonal dystrophy in vitamin E deficient rats. Acta Neuropathol., *1*:373, 1962.

96. Platt, H., Singh, H., and Whitwell, K. E.: Pathological observations on an outbreak of paralysis in broodmares. Equine Vet. J., *12*:118, 1980.

97. Pohlenz, J., and Schulz, L. C.: Rückenmarksveränderungen bei der spinalen Ataxie des Pferdes in iher Abhängigkeit von Ort und Grad der Veränderungen am Halswirbelskelett. Deutsch. Tieraerztl. Wschr., *73*:533, 1966.

98. Pohlenz, J., Schulze, D., and Eckert, J.: Spinale Nematodosis beim Pferd, verursacht durch *Strongylus vulgaris*. Deutsch. Tieraerztl. Wschr., *72*:510, 1965.

99. Prickett, M. E.: Equine spinal ataxia. Proc. Am. Assoc. Equine Pract., *14*:147, 1968.

100. Pursell, A. R., Sangster, L. T., Byars, T. D., Divers, T. J., and Cole, J. R., Jr.: Neurologic disease induced by equine herpesvirus 1. J. Am. Vet. Med. Assoc., *175*:473, 1979.

101. Rantanen, N. W., Gavin, P. R., Barbee, D. D., and Sonde, R. D.: Ataxia and paresis in horses. Part II. Radiographic and myelographic examination of the cervical vertebral column. Compend. Contin. Ed., *3*:S161, 1981.

102. Reed, S. M., Bayly, W. M., Traub, J. L., Gallina, A., and Miller, L. M.: Ataxia and paresis in horses. Part 1. Differential diagnosis. Compend. Contin. Ed., *3*:S88, 1981.

103. Rice, D. A., McMurray, C. H., McCracken, R. M., Bryson, D. G., and Maybin, R.: A field case of poisoning caused by 3-nitro-4-hydroxyphenyl arsenic acid in pigs. Vet. Rec., *106*:312, 1980.

104. Rooney, J. R.: Two cervical reflexes in the horse. J. Am. Vet. Med. Assoc., *162*:117, 1973.

105. Rooney, J. R.: Biomechanics of Lameness. Baltimore, Williams & Wilkins, 1969.

106. Rooney, J. R.: Clinical Neurology of the Horse. Kennett Square, Pa., KNA Press, 1971.

107. Rooney, J. R.: Equine incoordination. I. Gross morphology. Cornell Vet., *53*:411, 1963.

108. Rooney, J. R., Prickett, M. E., Delaney, F. M., and Crowe, M. W.: Focal myelitis and encephalitis in horses. Cornell Vet., *60*:494, 1970.

109. Rowe, C. L.: Hemivertebra in a goat. Vet. Med. Sm. Anim. Clin., *74*:211, 1979.

110. Saxegaard, F.: Isolation and identification of equine rhinopneumonitis virus (equine abortion virus) from cases of abortion and paralysis. Nord. Vet.-Med., *18*:504, 1966.

111. Schebitz, H., and Schulz, L. C.: Zur Pathogenese der spinalen Ataxie beim Pferd—Spondylarthrosis, klinische Befunde. Deutsch. Tieraerztl. Wschr., *72*:496, 1965.

112. Schebitz, H., and Dahme, E.: Spinal ataxia in the horse. Proc. Am. Assoc. Equine Pract., *14*:133, 1968.

113. Schulz, L. C., Schebitz, H., Pohlenz, J., and Mechlenburg, G.: Zur Pathogenese der spinalen Ataxie des Pferdes—Spondylarthrosis pathologisch-anatomische Untersuchungen. Deutsch. Tieraerztl. Wschr., *72*:502, 1965.

114. Shoho, C.: Prophylaxis and therapy in epizootic cerebrospinal nematodiasis of animals by 1-diethylcarbamyl-4-methyl-piperazine dihydrogen citrate: Report of second field trial. Vet. Med., *49*:459, 1954.

115. Simpson, C. F., and Mayhew, I. G.: Evidence for Sarcocystis as the etiologic agent of equine protozoal myeloencephalitis. J. Protozool., *27*:288, 1980.

116. Smith, M. C.: The diagnostic value of caprine cerebrospinal fluid analysis. Int. Goat Sheep Res. J., in press.

117. Smith, R. M., Fraser, F. J., Russell, G. R., and Robertson, J. S.: Enzootic ataxia in lambs: Appearance of lesions in the spinal cord during foetal development. J. Comp. Pathol., *87*:119, 1977.

118. Spaull, G., Palmer, A. C., Allsopp, J. D., and Hughes-Parry, E. M. R.: Wobbler syndrome (cervical stenosis) in a Percheron colt. Vet. Rec., *107*:362, 1980.

119. Sprinkle, T.: Diagnosis-equine rhino. Norden News, *50*:16, 1975.

120. Stavrou, D.: Zur zerebrospinalen Nematodosis der Equiden. Berl. Münch. Tierärztl. Wochenschr., *24*:471, 1967.

121. Stavrou, D., Deutschländer, N., and Dahme, E.: Granulomatous encephalomyelitis in goats. J. Comp. Pathol., *79*:393, 1969.

122. Steel, J. D., Whittem, J. H., and Hutchins, D. R.: Equine sensory ataxia (wobblers). Aust. Vet. J., *35*:442, 1959.

123. Summers, B. A., Appel, M. J. G., Greisen, H. A., Ebel, J. G., Jr., and de Lahunta, A.: Studies on viral leukoencephalomyelitis and swayback in goats. Cornell Vet., *70*:372, 1980.

124. Swanstrom, O. G., Rising, J. L., and Carlton, W. W.: Spinal nematodiasis in a horse. J. Am. Vet. Med. Assoc., *155*:748, 1969.

125. Taylor, H. W., Vandevelde, M., and Firth, E. C.: Ischemic myelopathy caused by fibrocartilaginous emboli in a horse. Vet. Pathol., *14*:479, 1977.

126. Terlecki, S., Done, J. T., and Clegg, F. G.: Enzootic ataxia of red deer. Br. Vet. J., *120*:311, 1964.

127. Thorsen, J., and Little, P. B.: Isolation of equine herpesvirus type I from a horse with an acute paralytic disease. Can. J. Comp. Med., *39*:358, 1975.

128. Traver, D. S., Moore, J. N., Thornburg, L. P., Johnson, J. H., and Coffman, J. R.: Epidural melanoma causing posterior paresis in a horse. J. Am. Vet. Med. Assoc., *170*:1400, 1977.

129. Wagner, P. C., Bagby, G. W., Grant, B. D., Gallina, A., Ratzlaff, M., and Sande, R.: Surgical stabilization of the equine cervical spine. Vet. Surg., *8*:7, 1979.

130. Wagner, P. C., Grant, B. D., Bagby, G. W., Gallina, A. M., Sande, R. D., and Ratzlaff, M.: Evaluation of cervical spinal fusion as a treatment in the equine wobbler syndrome. Vet. Surg., *8*:84, 1979.

131. Wagner, P. C., Grant, B. D., Gallina, A., and Bagby, G. W.: Ataxia and paresis in horses. Part III. Surgical treatment of spinal cord compression. Compend. Contin. Ed., 3:S192, 1981.

132. White, M. E., Pennock, P W., and Seiler, R. J.: Atlanto-axial subluxation in five young cattle. Can. Vet. J., 19:79, 1978.

133. White, P.: Personal communication, 1982.

134. Whitlock, J. H.; Neurofilariosis, a paralytic disease of sheep. II. *Neurophilaria cornellensis* n.g.n. sp. *(Nematoda filaroidia),* a new nematode parasite from the spinal cord of sheep. Cornell Vet., 42:125, 1952.

135. Whitwell, K. E.: Causes of ataxia in horses. Practice, 2:17, 1980.

136. Whitwell, K. E.: Craniovertebral malformations in an Arab foal. Equine Vet. J., 10:125, 1978.

137. Williams, J. F., Dade, A. W., and Benne, R.: Posterior paralysis associated with anthelmintic treatment of sheep. J. Am. Vet. Med. Assoc., 169:1307, 1976.

138. Wilson, P. R., Orr, M. B., and Key, E. L.: Enzootic ataxia in red deer. N. Z. Vet. J., 27:252, 1979.

139. Woodard, J. C., Collins, G. H., and Hessler, J. R.: Feline hereditary neuraxonal dystrophy. Am. J. Pathol., 74:551, 1974.

12

VESTIBULAR SYSTEM—SPECIAL PROPRIOCEPTION

The vestibular system is the primary sensory system that maintains the animal's balance or its normal orientation relative to the gravitational field of the earth. This orientation is maintained in the face of linear or rotatory acceleration and tilting of the animal. The vestibular system is responsible for maintaining the position of the eyes, trunk, and limbs in reference to the position or movement of the head at any time.

ANATOMY AND PHYSIOLOGY

RECEPTOR

The receptor for special proprioception, the vestibular system, develops in conjunction with the receptor for the auditory system (SSA). They are derived from ectoderm but are contained in a mesodermally derived structure. Together these are the components of the inner ear. The ectodermal component arises as a proliferation of ectodermal epithelial cells on the surface of the embryo adjacent to the developing rhombencephalon. This is the otic placode, which subsequently invaginates to form an otic pit and otic vesicle (otocyst), breaking away from its attachment to the surface ectoderm. This saccular structure undergoes extensive modification of its shape, but always retains its fluid-filled lumen and surrounding thin epithelial wall as it becomes the membranous labyrinth of the inner ear. Special modification of its epithelial surface at predetermined sites forms the receptor organ for the vestibular and auditory systems.

Corresponding developmental modifications occur in the surrounding paraxial mesoderm to provide a supporting capsule for the membranous labyrinth. This fluid-filled ossified structure is the bony labyrinth, contained within the developing petrose portion of the temporal bone.

The membranous and bony labyrinths are formed adjacent to the first and second branchial arches and their corresponding first pharyngeal pouch and first branchial groove. The first branchial groove gives rise to the external ear canal; the first pharyngeal pouch forms the auditory tube and the mucosa of the middle ear cavity. The intervening tissue forms the tympanum. The ear ossicles are derived from the neural crest of branchial arches 1 (malleus and incus) and 2 (stapes). These become components of the middle ear associated laterally with the tympanum (malleus), and medially with the vestibular window of the bony labyrinth of the inner ear (stapes).

Anatomically, the bony labyrinth in the petrosal bone consists of three communicating fluid-filled portions. These are the large vestibule, and three semicircular canals and the cochlea which arise from the vestibule. These contain perilymph, a fluid similar to CSF, from which it probably is derived. There are two openings in the bony labyrinth, the vestibular and cochlear windows, which are named according to the component of the bony labyrinth in which they are located. Each is covered by a membrane, and the stapes is inserted in the membrane covering the vestibular window.

The ectodermally derived membranous labyrinth consists of four fluid-filled compartments, all of which communicate. These are contained within the components of the bony

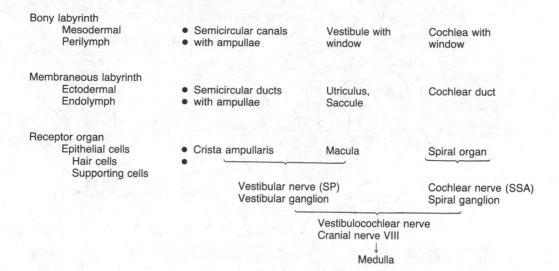

Bony labyrinth Mesodermal Perilymph	● Semicircular canals ● with ampullae	Vestibule with window	Cochlea with window
Membraneous labyrinth Ectodermal Endolymph	● Semicircular ducts ● with ampullae	Utriculus, Saccule	Cochlear duct
Receptor organ Epithelial cells Hair cells Supporting cells	● Crista ampullaris ●	Macula	Spiral organ
	Vestibular nerve (SP) Vestibular ganglion		Cochlear nerve (SSA) Spiral ganglion

Vestibulocochlear nerve
Cranial nerve VIII
↓
Medulla

labyrinth and include the saccule and utriculus within the bony vestibule, three semicircular ducts within the bony semicircular canals, and a cochlear duct within the bony cochlea. The three semicircular ducts are the anterior (vertical), posterior (vertical), and lateral (horizontal). Each semicircular duct is oriented at right angles to the others; thus rotation of the head around any plane causes endolymph to flow within one or more of the ducts. Each semicircular duct connects at both ends with the utriculus, which in turn connects to the saccule by way of the intervening endolymphatic duct and sac. The saccule communicates with the cochlear duct by the small ductus reuniens. The endolymph contained within the membranous system is thought to be derived from the blood along one wall of the cochlear duct, and is absorbed back into the blood through vessels surrounding the endolymphatic sac.

Crista Ampullaris. At one end of each membranous semicircular duct there is a dilation called the ampulla. On one side of the membranous ampulla, a proliferation of connective tissue forms a transverse ridge called the crista (Fig. 12–1). This is lined on its internal surface by columnar epithelial cells, the neuroepithelium. On the surface of the crest is a gelatinous structure that is composed of a protein-polysaccharide material called the cupula, which extends across the lumen of the ampulla. The neuroepithelium is composed of two basic cell types, hair cells and supporting cells.[2, 14-16, 22, 45, 49] The neurons of the vestibulocochlear nerve are derived from placode ectoderm. The dendritic zone of the neurons of the vestibular portion of the vestibulocochlear nerve is in synaptic relationship to the hair cells. The hair cells have on their luminal surface 40 to 80 "hairs" or modified microvilli (stereocilia) and a single modified cilium (kinocilium). They project into the overlying cupula. Movement of fluid in the semicircular duct causes deflection of the cupula, which is oriented transversely to the direction of flow of endolymph. This bends the stereocilia and is the source of stimulus by way of the hair cell to the dendritic zone of the vestibular neuron that is in synaptic relationship with the plasmalemma of the hair cell.

There is one membranous ampulla with its crista ampullaris in one end of each semicircular duct. Because the three semicircular ducts are all at right angles to each other, movement of the head in any plane or angular rotation stimulates a crista ampullaris and the vestibular neurons. They function in dynamic equilibrium.

The vestibular neurons are tonically active, and their activity is excited or inhibited by deflection of the cupula in different directions.[49] Each semicircular duct on one side can be paired to a semicircular duct on the opposite side by their common position in a parallel plane. These synergic pairs are the left and right lateral ducts, the left anterior and right posterior ducts, and the left posterior and right anterior ducts. While movement in the direction of one of these three planes stimulates the vestibular neurons of the crista of one duct, they are inhibited in the opposite duct of the synergic pair. For example, rotation of the head to the right causes the endolymph to flow in the right lateral duct so that the cupula is

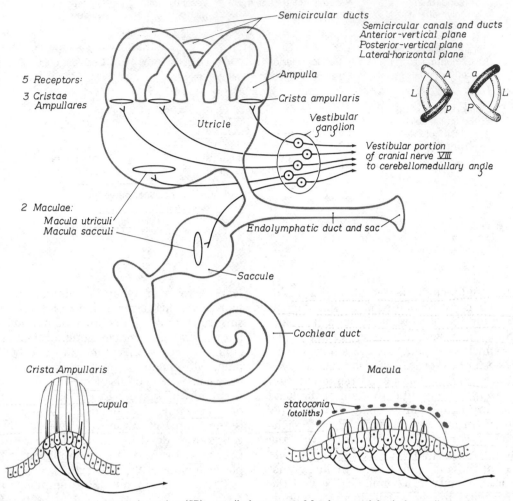

MEMBRANOUS LABYRINTH-VESTIBULAR RECEPTORS

Figure 12–1. Special proprioception (SP)—vestibular system. Membranous labyrinth–vestibular receptors.

deflected toward the utriculus, and the cupula of the left lateral duct is deflected away from the utriculus. This causes increased activity of vestibular neurons on the right side and decreased activity on the left, and results in a jerk nystagmus to the right side. The anatomic orientation of stereocilia relative to the kinocilium on the surface of the crista is responsible for the difference in activity relative to the direction of the cupula deflection. Deviation of the stereocilia toward the kinocilium increases vestibular neuronal activity. These receptors are not affected by a constant velocity of movement but respond to acceleration or deceleration, especially when there is rotation of the head.

Macula. A similar receptor is present in the utriculus and saccule located in the bony vestibule, on one surface of each of these sac-like structures (see Fig. 12–1). At this point the labyrinth is thickened in the shape of an oval plaque called the macula. The surface of the thickened connective tissue is covered by columnar epithelial cells. This neuroepithelium is composed of hair cells and supporting cells. Covering the neuroepithelium is a gelatinous material, the otolithic membrane. On the surface of this membrane there are calcareous crystalline bodies known as statoconia (otoliths). Similar to the hair cells of the cristae, the macular hair cells have projections of their luminal cell membrane—stereocilia and kinocilia—in the overlying otolithic membrane. Movement of the otoliths away from these cell processes is the initiating factor in stimulating an impulse in the dendritic zone of the vestibular neurons that are in synaptic relationship with the base of the hair cells. The macula in the saccule is oriented in a vertical direction (sagittal plane), while that of the utriculus is in a horizontal direction (dorsal plane); thus, gravitational forces continually affect the position of the otoliths in relationship to the hair cells. These are responsible for the sensation of the static position of the head and linear acceleration or deceleration. They function in static equilibrium. The macula of the utriculus may be more important as a receptor for sensing changes in posture of the head, while the macula of the saccule may be more sensitive to vibrational stimuli and loud sounds.

VESTIBULOCOCHLEAR NERVE— CRANIAL NERVE VIII—VESTIBULAR DIVISION

The dendritic zone is in synaptic relationship with the hair cells of the crista ampullaris and macula utriculi and macula sacculi. The axons course through the internal acoustic meatus with those of the cochlear division. The cell bodies of these bipolar-type neurons are inserted along the course of the axons within the petrosal bone, and form the vestibular ganglion. After leaving the petrosal bone through the internal acoustic meatus with the cochlear division of the vestibulocochlear nerve, the axons pass to the lateral surface of the rostral medulla, at the cerebellomedullary angle. This is at the level of the trapezoid body and attachment of the caudal cerebellar peduncle to the cerebellum. The vestibular neurons penetrate the medulla between the caudal cerebellar peduncle and the spinal tract of the trigeminal nerve, and terminate in telodendria at one of two sites. The majority terminate in the vestibular nuclei. A few directly enter the cerebellum by way of the caudal peduncle, and have terminations in the fastigial nucleus and flocculonodular lobe. These form the direct vestibulocerebellar tract.

VESTIBULAR NUCLEI

There are four vestibular nuclei on either side of the dorsal part of the medulla adjacent to the lateral wall of the fourth ventricle (Fig. 12–2).[7] From the level of the rostral and middle cerebellar peduncles, they extend caudally to the level of the lateral cuneate nucleus in the lateral wall of the caudal portion of the fourth ventricle. The four nuclei are grouped into rostral, medial, lateral, and caudal vestibular

nuclei. The rostral vestibular nucleus is located ventromedial to the middle and rostral cerebellar peduncles, dorsal to the motor nucleus of the trigeminal nerve (Plate 7). The medial and lateral vestibular nuclei are located ventromedial to the confluence of the three cerebellar peduncles with the cerebellum (Plate 6). They are dorsal to the descending facial neurons. The medial nucleus continues caudally adjacent to the caudal nucleus in the dorsal medulla to the level of the lateral cuneate nucleus (Plate 5). The caudal cerebellar peduncle is dorsolateral to the caudal vestibular nucleus. The spinal tract of the trigeminal nerve and its nucleus are ventrolateral to the caudal vestibular nucleus in the medulla. The lateral vestibular nucleus is located only at the level of the confluent cerebellar peduncles (Plate 6). The caudal vestibular nucleus is caudal to the lateral vestibular nucleus and continues caudally to the level of the lateral cuneate nucleus. These vestibular nuclei receive afferents primarily from the vestibular division of the vestibulocochlear nerve. In addition, some afferents enter from the fastigial nucleus of the cerebellum.

There are numerous projections from the vestibular nuclei (see Fig. 12–2).[28, 29, 36] These can be grouped into the following pathways:

Spinal Cord. The vestibulospinal tract descends in the ipsilateral ventral funiculus through the entire spinal cord, terminating in all segments on interneurons in the ventral grey column (Plate 1). These interneurons are facilitatory to ipsilateral alpha and gamma motor neurons to extensor muscles, inhibitory to the ipsilateral alpha motor neurons to flexor muscles, and some interneurons cross to the opposite ventral grey column and are inhibitory to the contralateral alpha and gamma motor neurons to extensor muscles (Fig. 12–3). Thus the effect of stimulation of the vestibulospinal tract is an ipsilateral extensor tonus, ipsilateral facilitation of the stretch reflex mechanism, and contralateral inhibition of this mechanism. In the cat the cell bodies of the axons in the vestibulospinal tract are in the lateral vestibular nucleus.

The medial vestibular nucleus projects axons into the medial longitudinal fasciculus, which descends in the dorsal portion of the ventral funiculus through the cervical and cranial thoracic segments, influencing the alpha and gamma motor neurons by way of interneuronal activation.

Through these spinal cord pathways, the position and activity of the limbs and trunk

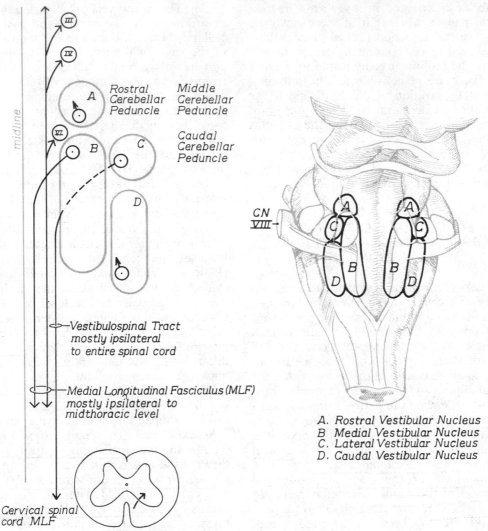

A. Rostral Vestibular Nucleus
B. Medial Vestibular Nucleus
C. Lateral Vestibular Nucleus
D. Caudal Vestibular Nucleus

Figure 12–2.   Vestibular nuclei and tracts.

can be coordinated with movements of the head.

Brain Stem

1. Axons course rostrally in the medial longitudinal fasciculus and reticular formation to influence the nuclei of the cranial nerves VI, IV, and III. This provides coordinated conjugate eyeball movements associated with changes in position of the head. When the brain stem is severely contused by a head injury, these pathways are interfered with and eyeball movement cannot be elicited by changing the position of the head. This is a sign that usually indicates a poor prognosis because of the severity of the associated lesion.

2. Axons project into the reticular formation. Some of these provide afferents to the

vomiting center located there, which is the pathway underlying motion sickness.

3. The pathway for conscious projection of the vestibular system is not well defined. It usually is considered to be similar to the auditory system, and is mediated by way of axons that project rostrally through the midbrain to the contralateral medial geniculate nucleus of the thalamus. Synapse occurs here, and the axons of the medial geniculate neurons project by way of the internal capsule to the gyri of the temporal lobe, primarily the rostral suprasylvian gyrus.

Cerebellum.   Axons of vestibular nuclear neurons project to the cerebellum through the caudal cerebellar peduncle, and terminate mostly in the flocculus of the hemisphere and

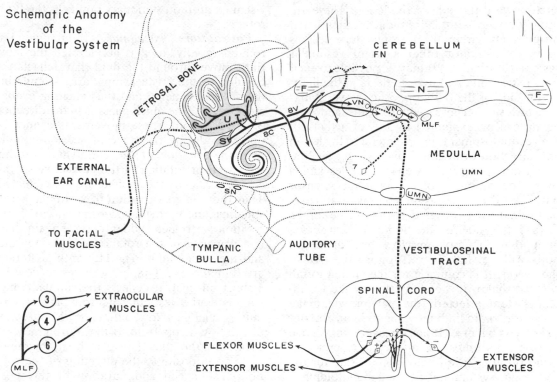

Figure 12–3. Schematic anatomy of the vestibular system. *N*: nodulus; *F*: flocculus; *FN*: fastigial nucleus; *UMN*: upper motor neuron; *MLF*: medial longitudinal fasciculus; *VN*: vestibular nucleus; *8V*: cranial nerve VIII, vestibular portion; *8C*: cranial nerve VIII, cochlear portion; *U*: utricle; *S*: saccule; *SN*: sympathetic neurons; *3*: oculomotor nucleus; *4*: trochlear nucleus; *6*: abducent nucleus; *7*: facial nucleus.

the nodulus of the caudal vermis (the flocculonodular lobe), and the fastigial nucleus. The fastigial nucleus is the most medial of the cerebellar nuclei (Plate 5).

Through these pathways the vestibular system functions to coordinate the eyeballs, trunk, and limbs with movements of the head. It maintains equilibrium during active and passive movement and when the head is at rest.

SIGNS OF VESTIBULAR DISEASE

Vestibular disease produces varying degrees of loss of equilibrium causing imbalance and ataxia. Strength is not interfered with, and therefore no paresis is observed. As a rule the disturbance is unilateral or asymmetric, and the signs are those of an asymmetric ataxia with preservation of strength.

UNILATERAL DISEASE

Unilateral disease of the peripheral receptor is characterized by asymmetric ataxia—loss of

balance with preservation of strength. The same asymmetric ataxia occurs with disease of the vestibular nuclei, but usually the lesion also involves the adjacent descending upper motor neuron pathways and paresis is observed and/or the ascending spinocerebellar pathways and general proprioceptive ataxia is observed. Thus, the observation of paresis and/or general proprioceptive ataxia in an animal with an asymmetric vestibular ataxia is evidence that the lesion is in the medulla of the brain stem. The vestibular signs can be grouped into those that reflect disturbed tonus in axial and appendicular muscles, and those that reflect disturbance of eyeball coordination.

Abnormal Posture and Ataxia

Loss of coordination between head, trunk, and limbs causes imbalance and is reflected in a head tilt with the more ventral ear directed toward the side of the vestibular disturbance. The trunk will tip, fall, or even roll toward the side of the lesion. The trunk may be flexed laterally, with the concavity directed toward the side of the lesion. The animal may tend to circle toward the side of the lesion. These are usually circles with short radii. (Animals that propulsively circle from frontal lobe lesions have no ataxia or other signs of vestibular system disturbance.) It may be possible to elicit mild hypertonia and hyperreflexia in the limbs on the side of the body opposite the vestibular system lesion. These signs of trunk and limb ataxia can be explained by loss of activity of the vestibulospinal tract ipsilateral to the lesion and direction of ataxia. This removes facilitation from ipsilateral extensor muscles and a source of inhibition of contralateral extensor muscles. The unopposed contralateral vestibulospinal tract causes the trunk to be forced toward the side of the lesion by excessive, unopposed extensor muscle tonus. The entire body will tip, fall, or roll toward the side of the lesion. It is common for the animal to fall when it shakes its head. With only the vestibular system affected, the patient will make very short rapid limb movements in an attempt to keep its balance. It has no loss of knowledge of where its limbs are in space (general proprioception). Vision helps compensate for the vestibular system deficit, and blindfolding a patient with a vestibular system lesion may accentuate the clinical signs. Be cautious when you do this with large animals so that they do not fall and injure themselves or observers.

Nystagmus

Normal Vestibular Nystagmus. The sign of disturbed vestibular input to the neurons that innervate extraocular muscles is abnormal nystagmus. Nystagmus is an involuntary rhythmic eyeball oscillation either with equal movements (pendular) or a quick and slow phase (jerk) that can occur in any plane. The direction of the jerk nystagmus is ascribed to that of the quick phase. Both eyeballs usually are affected simultaneously and in the same direction. These oscillations normally are induced by any rapid head movement. Rapid dorsoventral flexion and extension of the animal's head and neck elicits a vertical nystagmus. Similar side to side movements of the head elicit a horizontal nystagmus. The quick phase of the nystagmus is in the direction of the rotation. This can be elicited readily in most normal animals and is called vestibular nystagmus or physiologic nystagmus. It is a normal reflex in which the slow component is initiated by way of the labyrinth, and the fast component results from function of a brain stem center. This reflex helps to maintain

visual fixation on stationary points as the body rotates.

Postrotatory Nystagmus. If an animal is rotated rapidly, as it is accelerated the labyrinth moves around the fluid that deflects the cupulae of the cristae ampullaris, stimulating the vestibular nerve and thus eliciting eyeball movements. The quick phase is in the direction of the rotation. These movements cannot be observed during the stage of acceleration. In time the rotation of the endolymph reaches the speed of rotation of the labyrinth. At this constant velocity the cupulae are not deflected. Thus there is no alteration of vestibular nerve stimulus, and nystagmus does not occur. If the rotation is stopped suddenly, once again there is a disparity in the rotation of the labyrinth and the endolymph. The labyrinth is stationary, but the endolymph continues to flow for a short interval; it deflects the cupulae which stimulates the vestibular neurons, and nystagmus is elicited. Now, however, the direction of the flow is opposite to that during acceleration, and the quick phase of the nystagmus is directed opposite to the direction of the rotation. The speed and duration of this postrotatory vestibular nystagmus are variable, but should be about equal when the response to spinning is compared for both directions.

Vestibular disease is suspected when there is a different response to spinning in one direction as compared with the other. As a rule, when the patient is rotated in a direction opposite to the side of a peripheral receptor lesion, postrotatory nystagmus is depressed. This postrotatory test stimulates both labyrinths. However, the labyrinth on the side opposite the direction of rotation is stimulated more because it is farther away from the axis of rotation. This may explain the abnormal postrotatory nystagmus that is observed with unilateral vestibular disease. On spinning away from the side of the lesion, the diseased labyrinth is farthest from the axis of rotation. It cannot be stimulated properly because of the lesion and a depressed postrotatory response is observed.

This test can readily be performed in patients small enough to be picked up and held with your arms extended. The holder points the head of the animal away from the body and spins in a circle as fast as possible for 6 or 7 revolutions and stops suddenly. The patient's eyes are observed by the examiner. This is repeated in the opposite direction. For some large dogs it is possible to secure them in a rotating desk chair and spin them with the chair. Rarely is this response difficult to elicit in a normal animal.

Caloric Nystagmus. The individual labyrinths can be tested separately by the caloric test. Irrigation of the external ear canal with ice cold water for 3 to 5 minutes causes the endolymph to flow in the semicircular ducts.[32] This normally induces a jerk nystagmus directed to the side opposite the one being stimulated. If the peripheral receptor on the side being tested is nonfunctional because of a disease process, no nystagmus will be observed from the caloric test. Covering the patient's eyeballs may prevent voluntary repression of the response by fixation on an object in the environment. Despite this, sometimes the animal resists this procedure and makes the test unreliable. In some normal dogs, even prolonged irrigation with cold water has failed to elicit nystagmus. Asymmetric responses suggest a deficit on the side being tested. Warm water irrigation has been even less reliable. Because of the difficulty in performing this procedure and its unreliability, I do not use it in evaluating the vestibular system.

Abnormal Nystagmus. When the head is held in its normally extended position or if held flexed laterally to either side or held extended fully. no nystagmus is found. In vestibular system disease a nystagmus may be observed. If it is seen when the head is in its normal extended position, it is called a spontaneous, or resting, nystagmus. If it is induced by holding the head fixed in lateral flexion or full extension, it is called a positional nystagmus. These are forms of abnormal nystagmus.

In peripheral receptor disease the nystagmus is either horizontal or rotatory, and *always* in a direction (quick phase) away from the side of the lesion. The direction of rotatory nystagmus is defined by the change in the 12 o'clock position of the limbus during the quick phase. This direction does not change when the position of the head is changed. With disease of the vestibular nuclei or vestibular pathways in the cerebellum, the nystagmus may be horizontal, rotatory, or vertical, and may change in direction with changes in position of the head. Thus vertical nystagmus, or nystagmus that changes in direction on changing position of the head, is suggestive of central involvement of the vestibular system. However, many patients with central vestibular system lesions will have abnormal nystagmus directed to the opposite side and other features of the examination must be used to localize the lesion.

In some patients with severe vestibular system disturbance there is a slight head oscillation that corresponds to the rate of the spontaneous nystagmus. In addition, occasionally there is an eyelid contraction concomitant with the nystagmus. This is probably elicited reflexly.

Postural Reactions—Strabismus

Most postural reactions are normal except for the righting response. Usually the patient experiences difficulty righting itself, with an exaggerated response toward the side of the lesion. In patients with severe imbalance, it may be difficult to hold them securely in order to perform these postural reactions. It is essential that the ground surface be not slippery and provide good traction for the patient. When the head is extended in the tonic neck reaction, the eyeballs should remain in the center of the palpebral fissure in the dog and cat. This often fails to occur on the side of the vestibular disturbance, and results in a dropped or ventrally deviated eyeball.

In ruminants, it is normal for the eyeballs to deviate ventrally on neck extension. In horses there is normally a slight ventral deviation. In both species it is more pronounced in the eyeball ipsilateral to a vestibular system lesion.

Occasionally, in vestibular disease an eyeball is noticed deviated ventrally or ventrolaterally without extension of the head and neck. This appears as a lower motor neuron strabismus, but can be corrected by moving the head into a different position or by inducing the patient to move its eyeballs to gaze in different directions. This is referred to as a vestibular strabismus. There is no paralysis of the cranial nerves that innervate the extraocular muscles. Moving the head horizontally from one side to the other will elicit a normal degree of adduction and abduction of each eyeball. The ventrally deviated eyeball is on the side of the lesion in the vestibular system. Sometimes the opposite eyeball may appear to be deviated dorsally.

Signs of vestibular disturbance are only occasionally accompanied by vomiting.

Paradoxical Central Vestibular Disease

With unilateral peripheral vestibular system lesions, the head and body tilt are always toward the side of the lesion. With few exceptions, the same occurs with lesions of the central components of the vestibular system.

These exceptions are, therefore, referred to as paradoxical signs.

Some unilateral lesions in the central vestibular pathways, especially with unilateral involvement of the cerebellar medulla and peduncles, produce a head tilt and ataxia directed toward the side opposite the lesion.[33] These are usually destructive space-occupying lesions such as gliomas, granulomatous meningoencephalitis (reticulosis), or other neoplasms.

Experimental ablation of the caudal cerebellar peduncle dorsal to the medulla on one side will produce a head tilt toward the opposite side and nystagmus toward the lesion.[45] If the vestibular nuclei are included in this lesion, the head will tilt toward the side of the lesion and the nystagmus will be directed toward the opposite side. Similarly, ablation of one flocculus and the nodulus will produce a paradoxical syndrome with the head and body tilted away from the side of the floccular lesion.

Usually these natural lesions interfere with the general proprioceptive system afferent to the cerebellum. This produces a mild GP ataxia and postural reaction deficit, always on the same side as the lesion. This observation is the most reliable for locating the side of the lesion.

BILATERAL DISEASE

Bilateral peripheral vestibular disease with complete loss of function is characterized by symmetric ataxia—loss of balance of either side, with strength preserved. There is no postural asymmetry. The patient often stays crouched on the ground with its limbs spread apart. It may crawl along in this posture, occasionally staggering or falling to either side. Some will walk without much loss of balance.

A characteristic jerky side to side head movement often accompanies these signs. Wide excursions of the head to either side accompany the bilateral disturbance of head orientation.

Nystagmus is not observed, and with bilateral destruction of the receptor organs no normal vestibular nystagmus can be elicited by head movement or caloric testing.

DISEASES OF THE VESTIBULAR SYSTEM

PERIPHERAL

Congenital Peripheral Vestibular Disorder. I have observed varying degrees of peripheral vestibular disturbance in litters of German shepherd puppies and Siamese kittens.[48] The onset of signs is usually around 3 to 4 weeks of age. The signs often regress or are compensated for by 2 to 4 months of age. A return to normal function may occur, but recurrences have been noted in the few months following recovery. Head tilt is the most salient sign. Ataxia is often mild. There is usually no abnormal nystagmus. In fact, normal vestibular nystagmus usually cannot be elicited by moving the head. In at least one Siamese cat the peripheral vestibular disorder was accompanied by deafness. Some animals remain permanently affected. Pathologic studies have revealed no inflammatory lesion, but have not been adequate to substantiate or obviate a degenerative disease or malformation. The close relationship of affected litters suggests an hereditary basis, but this remains to be proved.

A congenital, presumably vestibular system abnormality has been recognized in related litters of Burmese cats. The signs are present at or shortly after birth, when rolling is constant in the severely affected kittens. Others show a head tilt and asymmetric ataxia. The signs appear to be nonprogressive. No lesions have been seen in the brains or in inner ears that were preserved with formalin, decalcified, and serial sectioned. Viral isolation studies have been unrewarding. A familial basis is suspected for this congenital disease.

An acute head tilt, circling, and mild ataxia have been observed in one or more puppies in litters of Doberman pinschers.[9] The onset of signs was between 3 and 12 weeks of age. Occasionally deafness occurred and forelimb hypermetria was observed in a few puppies. For some dogs, the signs of vestibular system abnormality resolved spontaneously or were compensated for in a few months. In others these signs persisted unchanged. Those dogs that were deaf did not recover their hearing.

A congenital peripheral vestibular system disturbance was reported in one litter of English cocker spaniels at their birth.[3] They recovered or compensated with no recurrence of signs. One recovered after ten weeks but the signs recurred 2 weeks later and still persisted at 50 weeks of age.

Clinical signs of bilateral peripheral vestibular system disturbance and deafness have been observed in beagles raised in a breeding colony. These signs are present from the time the puppies could first walk or normally respond to environmental noise. A genetic basis is suspected but not proved. A similar syndrome has been observed sporadically in the Akita breed.

Feline Idiopathic Vestibular Disease: Idiopathic-Vestibular Neuropathy.[13] This acquired syndrome is seen in cats of all ages. In the northeast it occurs in the summer and early fall. It occurs suddenly as severe unilateral ataxia characterized by a head tilt and tendency to fall or roll toward the side of the head tilt. It may appear initially to the owner that the cat is unable to get up and walk. However, there is no loss of strength or ability to initiate voluntary movement. The cat is so disoriented as to its position in space that it is reluctant to move. If suddenly picked up, the cat grasps violently for a supporting surface and usually turns rapidly toward the side of the head tilt. If the cat can be supported without struggling or rolling, normal postural reactions will be elicited. These cats have no cerebral disturbance and are extremely alert and responsive. They often stay crouched against a wall and cry distressfully. Initially these signs may appear to be bilateral, with the cat stumbling and showing wide head excursions, but one side will usually predominate.

For the first 72 hours a spontaneous nystagmus occurs in a direction opposite the head tilt. This is usually horizontal, but occasionally it is rotatory. At the onset, a head oscillation may occur simultaneous with the nystagmus. After 3 to 4 days the spontaneous nystagmus disappears, but an abnormal positional nystagmus may be elicted on altering the position of the head. The direction always remains opposite to the side of the head tilt.

As the animal becomes more willing to ambulate, it walks with a broad base and tilts to one side, with the tail often extended straight up. If it turns its head suddenly, it often staggers to the side to which it is tilted. Occasionally, it staggers to the opposite side. Sometimes the trunk sways from side to side. This is called truncal ataxia.

By 7 days the animal moves around more freely, but still with a head tilt and tendency to lean and stagger in that direction. Over the next 2 to 3 weeks the gait continues to improve. The head tilt may be the only persisting residual sign, and that may disappear.

In a cat that has recovered from or compensated for this lesion the signs may be completely absent except when the animal suddenly is stressed, and then a mild degree of disturbance of balance may be apparent.

Experimental labyrinthectomy in the cat produces a syndrome identical to that observed in many of the cases of feline vestibular disease.[8] The ability of these experimental cats to compensate has been determined to be dependent on functional vestibular components of the brain stem and cerebellum, particularly the fastigial nucleus of the cerebellum. The role of the cerebellum in this compensation has been disputed.[41]

The pathogenesis of the feline disease is unknown. Although occasionally associated with a previous or concurrent upper respiratory disease, such a history is lacking in most cases. Microscopic study shows no evidence of an inflammatory lesion in the inner ear. In one cat hemorrhage was evident in the membranous labyrinth. Necropsy studies have been inadequate to determine cytologic changes in the hair cells of the receptor organs. No consistent evidence of an intoxication has been forthcoming. The absence of obvious lesions in most necropsies supports an intoxication of the eighth cranial nerve or its vestibular receptors or abnormal dynamics of the endolymphatic fluid.

The prognosis for recovery is good. Until the pathogenesis is understood, no therapy is recommended. Many drugs have been used, including antibiotics, corticosteroids, antimotion drugs, calcium, and vitamins, but there is no concrete evidence that these increase the rate of recovery.

It is important to distinguish this idiopathic disease from otitis media-interna because only the otitis requires therapy. The peracute onset of solely peripheral vestibular signs and the absence of disease of the external and middle ears on otoscopic examination and normal radiographs of the temporal bones warrant the diagnosis of idiopathic vestibular disease.

Canine Idiopathic Vestibular Disease. A neurologic disturbance occurs most commonly in older dogs that, on careful neurologic evaluation, appears to be similar to that described for the feline vestibular disease.[5, 43] Unfortunately, many of these patients appear to be so incapacitated at the onset of the disease that the signs are attributed mistakenly to a brain stem lesion, and the syndrome is diagnosed as "stroke." This term refers to a cerebrovascular accident that occurs in humans associated with chronic vascular disease and the acute blockage of a cerebral blood vessel or its rupture and subsequent hemorrhage. Similar vascular disease in domestic animals is uncommon; however, signs indicative of cerebrovascular dysfunction occasionally do occur and should be referable to brain stem or cerebral involvement, or both. This is not the case with these older dogs, and it is important to distinguish this fact for prognostic reasons.

The signs of the canine patient with acute vestibular disturbance all are referable to the vestibular system. They are similar to those described for the feline vestibular disease, but occur at any time during the year and may be less pronounced and resolve more quickly. Vomiting may occur during the first few days of the disease. If the dog is severely affected and incapacitated by the disease, the examiner may not recognize that the signs represent a peripheral vestibular disorder until a complete neurologic examination has been performed. Normal strength and postural reactions may be masked by the ataxia and spatial disorientation. Spontaneous recovery is usually complete with no persistent signs.

It is important to distinguish this idiopathic benign disorder, which resolves spontaneously without therapy, from otitis media-interna, which requires vigorous antibiotic therapy and may have recurrent or persistent signs. The idiopathic disease is characterized by a peracute onset of a head tilt, asymmetric ataxia, and rotatory nystagmus without facial paresis, Horner's syndrome, or signs of central nervous system involvement. The absence of otitis externa, abnormal tympanums, and abnormal radiographs of the temporal bones further supports this diagnosis. In both the cat and dog idiopathic disorders, facial paresis, and Horner's syndrome do not occur. The presence of these clinical signs with signs of a peripheral vestibular disorder suggest otitis media-interna or a space-occupying lesion or injury of the temporal bone.

The cause of the idiopathic disorder is unknown. It could result from abnormal dynamics of the endolymphatic fluid with a mild disturbance to its production, circulation, or absorption. An intoxication of the vestibular system receptors may be involved. A neuritis of the vestibular component of the eighth cranial nerve or a mild otitis media-interna seems unlikely, based on the few necropsies that have been performed and revealed no lesions.

These dogs with the idiopathic disorder should be handled in a manner similar to the cats. There is no specific therapy. Confinement over the period of most severe disorientation will help the patient and provide the veterinarian with the opportunity to reevaluate the patient to be sure of the diagnosis. Recurrent episodes have been observed in these dogs on

the same or the opposite side but it is not common.

Otitis Media and Otitis Interna. Vestibular signs occur in animals when the middle ear inflammation indirectly or directly affects the function of the membranous labyrinth.[43, 46, 47] Varying degrees of unilateral vestibular disturbance appear which consist of asymmetric ataxia with strength preservation. Sometimes only a head tilt and positional nystagmus are evident. The onset is acute or chronic, and the signs are often less severe than in the idiopathic vestibular disease. Frequently, these signs are accompanied by an ipsilateral facial paresis to palsy, or in small animals a Horner's syndrome, or both. These occur if the otitis media disturbs the function of the facial and sympathetic nerves, respectively. The latter course through the middle ear in the dog and cat.[4] Unilateral deafness may occur in all species but is difficult to determine clinically.

Otoscopic examination of the external acoustic meatus and tympanum may reveal lesions of the tympanum and exudate in the middle ear. Likewise, radiographic examination may reveal the middle ear inflammation if it is extensive, filling the bulla with thick exudate, or if it affects the bone of the bulla, producing an osteitis and changing its appearance on the radiograph. The normal detail of the bony labyrinth may be obliterated. Although otitis media is most commonly associated with otitis externa, it is not dependent on it. The nasopharnx is also a source of infection by way of the auditory tube. Extension of the infection from the middle and inner ear locations to the meninges takes place more often in cats and pigs. Brain stem signs then accompany the peripheral vestibular signs.

The middle and inner ear inflammation may be bilateral, but if the disturbance to vestibular function is not the same the signs are asymmetric and predominate in one direction.

Occasionally, the inflammatory lesion severely affects both labyrinths, and there is complete loss of peripheral vestibular function. Signs of bilateral peripheral vestibular disease with complete loss of function prevail. Deafness often accompanies these vestibular signs, and bilateral facial palsy has been observed.

When otitis media is suspected, the external ear canal or middle ear cavity should be cultured. Most animals will respond to prolonged oral and topical antibiotics. Occasionally surgery is necessary. Sometimes neurologic signs persist or recur.

This condition is common in calves[24] and

pigs.[30] In calves, where it is recognized early, it usually responds well to antibiotic therapy. Rarely are surgical procedures required. In pigs, streptococcal organisms have most commonly been isolated.

In horses peripheral vestibular disturbance and facial paresis have occurred with otitis media-interna. Response to antibiotic therapy may be complete or residual signs may persist. In a few horses with these signs, excessive enlargement of the proximal portion of the stylohyoid bone has been observed with ossification around the tympanic bulla in the absence of guttural pouch disease. Guttural pouch mycosis often causes inflammation and abnormal bone proliferation of the stylohyoid and tympanohyoid at the articulation with the temporal bone lateral to the bulla. However, signs of peripheral vestibular system disturbance are rarely associated with guttural pouch mycosis. A tympanosclerosis has been observed radiographically in horses associated with signs of peripheral vestibular system disease and facial paresis to paralysis.[18] In most of these patients external injury was thought to be related to the clinical signs and osseous lesions.

Polyneuropathy–Neuritis. Unilateral or bilateral signs of peripheral vestibular disease have been observed with facial paresis or paralysis in mature dogs without evidence of otitis media. In some instances, there has been an associated hypothyroidism and pituitary chromophobe adenoma. Response to thyroid therapy has been unsatisfactory in most patients.

A few patients have been observed with no associated endocrine disease and have resolved spontaneously.

Horses with polyneuritis–neuritis of the cauda equina may have mild signs of peripheral vestibular disturbance from involvement of the eighth cranial nerve. The signs of the cauda equina neuritis will predominate.

Injury. Head injuries may fracture the petrosal bone and cause bleeding from the external ear canal through a ruptured tympanum. The vestibular signs may be masked by the signs referable to an accompanying brain stem contusion. If the signs are primarily limited to disturbance of the peripheral receptor the prognosis is better, since compensation may occur if the cerebellum and brain stem are intact. Facial paralysis may accompany the petrosal bone injury.

Degeneration. Prolonged therapy with high doses of aminoglycoside antibiotics has been found to cause degeneration of the labyrinthine receptors of the vestibular or auditory systems or both.[23, 26, 51-54] These include streptomycin, dihydrostreptomycin, kanamycin, gentamicin, neomycin, and vancomycin. Streptomycin most often affects the vestibular system receptors in cats, whereas the other drugs more commonly affect the auditory receptor, but both receptors are susceptible to damage by all of these drugs. The clinical signs of peripheral vestibular system disturbance are usually unilateral but occasionally are bilateral. If the clinical signs of vestibular system disturbance are recognized early, recovery may occur on withdrawal of the drug. Hearing does not usually return. The peripheral receptor degeneration is documented. More recent investigations do not support any primary degeneration of neurons in brain stem nuclei.[23]

In the southeastern part of the United States, where the blue tail lizard is common, many veterinarians believe that acute peripheral vestibular system disturbance occurs in cats shortly after they eat the tail of this lizard.[1] Additional signs include vomiting, trembling, salivation, and hyperirritability from more diffuse nervous system involvement. Most cats respond spontaneously. A few deaths have occurred.

Neoplasia. Neurofibroma of the vestibulocochlear nerve usually produces signs of unilateral peripheral vestibular disturbance prior to its compression of the brain stem and the additional signs that accompany such compression.

Neoplasms that involve the temporal bone may produce peripheral vestibular system disturbance, often with a facial paresis or paralysis. Fibrosarcoma, osteosarcoma, chondrosarcoma and squamous cell carcinoma have been reported.[40] These are often evident on radiographs.

CENTRAL

Signs of vestibular system disturbance referable to disease of the vestibular nuclei or their neuronal pathways are similar to those seen in peripheral vestibular system disease.[31] Vestibular signs usually only seen with disease of the central pathways include consistently vertical nystagmus, nystagmus that changes direction with different positions of the head, and a persistent tendency to roll in one direction. The latter may occur to a limited degree with peripheral disease.

The lesion is localized to the central pathways mostly by the presence of signs that accompany the brain stem involvement of other functional systems. Evidence of upper motor neuron paresis and general proprioceptive ataxia is the most useful sign. Cerebellar signs, cranial nerve deficits (other than facial), and disturbances to the sensorium from lesions that involve the ascending reticular activating system also localize the vestibular disturbance to the brain stem pathways (Fig. 12–4). Beware of the paradoxical vestibular syndrome. Cerebellar lesions that affect the vestibular system in the caudal cerebellar peduncle or flocculonodular lobules may cause a vestibular head tilt, strabismus, and ataxia on the side opposite that of the lesion. The lesion is localized by observing the side that shows the deficient postural reactions from the lesion in the general proprioceptive or upper motor neuron systems, or both.

Inflammation—Meningoencephalitis. Canine distemper, toxoplasmosis, cryptococcosis, and the diffuse form of granulomatous encephalitis (inflammatory reticulosis)[6] are lesions that are disseminated widely through the central nervous system, and often include the central vestibular pathways. In the focal form of granulomatous encephalitis, a focal space-occupying lesion often occurs on one side of the cerebellar medulla.[42] This sometimes produces the paradoxical central vestibular syndrome.

In cats, the viral agent that produces feline infectious peritonitis also affects the meninges and ependymal surfaces and the adjacent parenchyma of the CNS.[27, 44] In some patients the nervous system lesion predominates and may be accompanied by a chronic uveitis of the eyeball. Chronic illness characterized by partial anorexia and persistent fever that are unresponsive to antibiotic therapy, accompanied by uveitis and mild signs of neurologic disturbance somtimes referable to the cerebellar vestibular systems, are typical of this disease. In one study, pelvic limb weakness, abnormal nystagmus and seizures were the most common signs observed in this disease.[21] CSF may be remarkably altered, with a large pleocytosis of

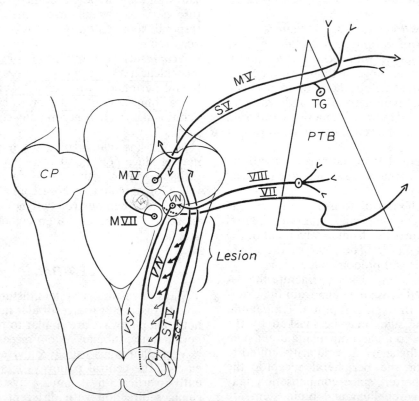

Figure 12–4.   Diagram of cranial neuronal anatomy related to a granuloma that produced right-sided vestibular signs of ataxia and head tilt, complete right facial analgesia without denervation of muscles of mastication, and mild right hemiparesis and general proprioceptive ataxia in a 5-year-old pony. (From Cornell Vet., *40*:622, 1970.) *CP*: cerebellar peduncles; *MV*: motor neurons of trigeminal nerve; *MVII*: motor facial neurons; *SV*: sensory neurons of trigeminal nerve; *TG*: trigeminal ganglion; *STV*: spinal tract of trigeminal nerve; *VIII*: cranial nerve VIII, vestibular portion; *VN*: vestibular nucleus; *VST*: vestibulospinal tract; *SCT*: spinocerebellar tracts; *PTB*: petrous temporal bone.

mostly mononuclear cells and a few neutrophils, and a protein content of 200 to 400 mg per dl. The gamma globulin fraction of serum protein often is increased markedly.

An aberrant parasite wandering through the central vestibular system may produce severe signs of vestibular disturbance. *Cuterebra* larvae have been found in cats. Adult *Parelaphostrongylus tenuis* may affect this area in sheep and goats. Larval forms of *Hypoderma bovis* and *Hypoderma lineatum* have been observed in the cerebellomedullary area of horses.

In ruminants, the bacterium *Listeria monocytogenes* causes inflammation of the brain stem with signs referable to this location, including vestibular disturbance. Varying degrees of upper motor neuron paresis, head tilt, abnormal nystagmus, facial paresis, and depression are typical of this disease. These cattle are usually older than 12 months.

Young goats with signs of cerebello-pontine-medullary disease are most commonly affected with listeriosis or CAE viral encephalitis. The CSF evaluations may be similar. If there is a predominance of leukocytes, listeriosis should be suspected. CAEV encephalitis is more common in goats less than six months old. Occasionally *Parelaphostrongylus tenuis* infection produces lesions in this area with clinical signs. The presence of eosinophils in the CSF would strongly indicate this diagnosis.

In horses the most common brain lesion of protozoal encephalitis is in the caudal brain stem. The signs associated with this lesion often include disturbance of the central components of the vestibular system. Occasionally this disease occurs acutely and causes a horse to be unable to get up from UMN paresis and severe vestibular disorientation.

Although the equine herpesvirus 1 often produces brain lesions, most clinical signs are referable to the lesions in the spinal cord. I observed one adult horse with a severe hemorrhagic infarction of one side of the medulla due to the effect of this virus on the vessels of the medulla. This horse went down acutely with severe disorientation and loss of balance. It constantly tried to roll itself towards the side of the lesion.

Neoplasia. Neoplasms at the cerebello-medullary angle affect the vestibular system.[31, 33, 35] Signs of neurologic disturbance are progressive. Neoplasms at this location often are not accompanied by an increased CSF pressure at the cerebellomedullary cistern. The contents of the CSF vary. It may be normal or similar to that seen with viral inflammations, or show markedly elevated protein levels without a commensurate increase in white blood cells. Cranial nerve deficits such as facial paresis or hypalgesia are more common in small animals with neoplastic disease than with inflammatory disease at this site.

The neoplasm may be at the surface of the parenchyma, compressing it—e.g., a meningioma, neurofibroma, medulloblastoma, choroid plexus papilloma, or lymphosarcoma—or it may be located within the parenchyma, infiltrating and compressing the adjacent tissue—e.g., a glioma, granulomatous encephalitis, or a metastatic neoplasm.

Although neoplasms are more common in older animals, they occasionally occur in young animals.[34] Occasionally extramedullary intracranial neoplasms, including those in the caudal fossa, may be present and produce clinical signs for 1 to 2 years before the patient becomes incapacitated. A choroid plexus papilloma at the fourth ventricle first produced signs in an 18-month-old dog. Clinical signs were evident for 27 months before euthanasia was requested.[20] I have observed a slow-growing pontine meningioma that extended caudally into the cerebellomedullary area produce neurologic signs for over 18 months and the dog was still able to stand and walk. Lymphosarcoma commonly occurs in young cats. Although it is more often epidural in the vertebral canal, it occasionally occurs intracranially and may be located at the cerebellomedullary angle.

Degeneration. Thiamine (vitamin B_1) deficiency occurs most commonly in cats and mink fed all-fish diets that contain thiaminase.[17] Occasionally, it follows chronic anorexia without vitamin therapy. Terminally, there is a hemorrhagic necrosis bilaterally symmetric in the brain stem periventricular grey matter, which includes lateral geniculate nuclei, oculomotor nuclei, caudal colliculi, and vestibular nuclei. The earliest signs of the disease are usually a mild vestibular ataxia, followed by seizures with marked head ventroflexion. Pupils may be dilated and poorly responsive to light. Terminally, there is semicoma, continual crying, opisthotonus, and persistent extensor tonus. Prompt therapy with 1 to 2 mg of thiamine intramuscularly in the early stages of the disease results in complete remission of signs. Sometimes signs of acute vestibular disturbance accompany a prolonged period of inappetence, and complete remission of signs follows thiamine therapy.

Dogs may develop the same disease if their food is cooked before feeding.[37, 38] This destroys the available thiamine. There is usually a spastic paraparesis initially, followed by recumbency, seizures, coma, and death.

Injury. Intracranial injury may affect the central vestibular pathways in addition to other functional systems in the brain stem. The degree of vestibular disturbance manifested depends on the degree of disturbance of the other functional system (UMN, ARAS) which would mask the vestibular disturbance. Abnormal nystagmus may be the only sign of vestibular disturbance evident in the tetraplegic, semicomatose patient.

CONGENITAL NYSTAGMUS

Congenital spontaneous nystagmus occurs in humans as an inherited functional abnormality, or secondary to congenital lesions in the visual system of the infant, including albinism. The nystagmus is usually pendular.

A congenital, rapid, pendular nystagmus occasionally occurs in one or more in a litter of puppies. It usually resolves spontaneously in a few weeks. The cause is unknown.

In cattle, a congenital rapid pendular nystagmus, usually horizontal, is observed in many breeds and usually persists for the life of these animals.[25, 39] It does not appear to interfere with vision. It is most apparent on ophthalmoscopic examination of the fundus of the eye. There is no obvious abnormality of the visual system or other clinical sign of extraocular neuromuscular or vestibular system abnormality. Pigmentation is normal. It is usually observed sporadically, but a high percentage of Guernsey cows in one herd were affected. The heritability of this congenital nystagmus is unknown.

In cats, congenital nystagmus is most often observed with varying degrees of ocular albinism where a larger portion of optic nerve axons cross in the chiasm than normal. The Siamese breed is most often affected, and the condition persists for the life of the cat. It also occurs in some cats with the Chédiak-Higashi syndrome, in which pigmentation and melanin granules are abnormal.[12]

I observed congenital nystagmus in a female Belgian sheepdog and three of her six offspring from one litter. The nystagmus was usually pendular with a variable frequency, but it was often very rapid. There was no obvious visual deficiency. Occasionally, the head was held tipped to one side. No ataxia was evident. Necropsy of the three littermates revealed a lack of development of an optic chiasm. The optic nerve fibers continued into the ipsilateral optic tract without decussation. Two of these dogs were 4 years old at the time of necropsy and their nystagmus had not changed.

Congenital nystagmus may be a result of abnormal sensory input to the system that controls eye movements.[11] In the albino cat there is excessive contralateral projection of optic nerve axons and in the Belgian sheepdog there is almost a complete lack of any contralateral projection.

REFERENCES

1. Adair, H. S., Jr.: Blue-tail lizard. Auburn Vet., *9*:117, 1953.
2. Ades, H. W., and Engström, H.: Form and innervation of the vestibular epithelia. First Symposium on the Role of Vestibular Organs in Space Exploration, NASA. Scientific and Technical Information Division, Office of Technological Utilization, Washington, D.C., U.S. Government Printing Office, 1965, 23–42.
3. Bedford, P. G. C.: Congenital vestibular disease in the English cocker spaniel. Vet. Rec., *105*:530, 1970.
4. Blauch, B., and Strafuss, A. C.: Histologic relationships of the facial (7th) and vestibulocochlear (8th) cranial nerves within the petrous temporal bone in the dog. Am. J. Vet. Res., *35*:481, 1974.
5. Blauch, B., and Martin, C. L.: A vestibular syndrome in aged dogs. J. Am. Anim. Hosp. Assoc., *10*:37, 1974.
6. Braund, K. G., Vandevelde, M., Walker, T. L., and Redding, R. W.: Granulomatous meningoencephalitis in six dogs. J. Am. Vet. Med. Assoc., *172*:1195, 1978.
7. Brodal, A.: Anatomical aspects on functional organization of the vestibular nuclei. Second Symposium on the Role of Vestibular Organs in Space Exploration, NASA—SP115. Scientific and Technical Information Division, Office of Technological Utilization, Washington, D.C., U.S. Government Printing Office, 1966, 119–142.
8. Carpenter, M. B., Fabrega, H., and Glinsmann, W.: Physiological deficits occurring with lesions of labyrinth and fastigial nucleus. J. Neurophysiol., *22*:222, 1959.
9. Chrisman, C. L.: Vestibular disease. Vet. Clin. North Am., *10*:103, 1980.
10. Coats, A. C.: Vestibular neuronitis. Trans. Am. Acad. Ophthalmol. Otolaryngol., *73*:395, 1969.
11. Collewijn, H., Winterson, B. J., and Dubois, M. F. W.: Optokinetic eye movements in albino rabbits: Inversion in anterior visual field. Science, *199*:1353, 1978.
12. Collier, L., Bryan, G. M., and Prieur, D. J.: Ocular manifestations of the Chediak-Higashi syndrome in four species of animals. J. Am. Vet. Med. Assoc., *175*:587, 1979.
13. de Lahunta, A.: Feline vestibular disease. *In* Kirk, R. W. (ed.): Current Veterinary Therapy III. Philadelphia, W. B. Saunders, 1968.

14. Engström, H.: The first-order vestibular neuron. Fourth Symposium on the Role of the Vestibular Organs in Space Exploration, NASA—SP187. Scientific and Technical Information Division, Office of Technological Utilization, Washington, D.C., U.S. Government Printing Office, 1968, 123–135.

15. Engström, H.: Form and organization of the vestibular sensory cells. In Stahle, J. (ed.): Vestibular Function on Earth and in Space. New York, Pergamon, 1970, 87–96.

16. Engström, H., Lindeman, H. H., and Ades, H. W.: Anatomical features of the auricular sensory organs. Second Symposium on the Role of Vestibular Organs in Space Exploration, NASA—SP115. Scientific and Technical Information Division, Office of Technological Utilization, Washington, D.C., U.S. Government Printing Office, 1966, 33–46.

17. Everett, G. M.: Observations on the behavior and neurophysiology of acute thiamine deficiency in cats. Am. J. Physiol., 141:439, 1944.

18. Firth, E. C.: Vestibular disease and its relationship to facial paralysis in the horse: A clinical study of 7 cases. Aust. Vet. J., 53:560, 1977.

19. Holliday, T. A.: Clinical signs of acute and chronic experimental lesions of the cerebellum. Vet. Sci. Commun., 3:259, 1979–1980.

20. Indrieri, R. J., Holliday, T. A., Selcer, R. R., Ackerman, N., and Taylor, J. L.: Choroid plexus papilloma associated with prolonged signs of vestibular dysfunction in a young dog. J. Am. Anim. Hosp. Assoc., 16:263, 1980.

21. Kornegay, J. N.: Feline infectious peritonitis: The central nervous system form. J. Am. Anim. Hosp. Assoc., 14:580, 1978.

22. Lowenstein, O.: The functional significance of the ultrastructure of the vestibular end organs. Second Symposium on the Role of Vestibular Organs in Space Exploration, NASA-SP115. Scientific and Technical Information Division, Office of Technological Utilization, Washington, D.C., U.S. Government Printing Office, 1966, 73–90.

23. Lundquist, Per-G., and Wersäll, J.: Sites of action of ototoxic antibiotics after local and general administration. In Stahle, J. (ed.): Vestibular Function on Earth and in Space. New York, Pergamon, 1970, 267–274.

24. Mahin, L.: Symptoms and treatment of unilateral labyrinthitis in a calf. Vet. Rec., 107:448, 1980.

25. McConnon, J. M., White, M. E., Smith, M. C., Stem, E. S., and Hickey, G.: Congenital pendular nystagmus in dairy cattle. J. Am. Vet. Med. Assoc., in press.

26. McGee, T. M., and Olszewski, J.: Streptomycin sulfate and dihydrostreptomycin toxicity, behavioral and histopathological studies. Arch. Otolaryngol., 75:295, 1962.

27. Montali, R. J., and Strandberg, J. D.: Extraperitoneal lesions in feline infectious peritonitis. Vet. Pathol., 9:109, 1972.

28. Nyberg-Hansen, R.: Origin and termination of fibers from the vestibular nuclei descending in the medial longitudinal fasciculus. An experimental study with silver impregnation methods in the cat. J. Comp. Neurol., 122:355, 1964.

29. Nyberg-Hansen, R., and Mascitti, T. A.: Sites and mode of termination of fibers of the vestibulospinal tract in the cat. J. Comp. Neurol., 122:369, 1964.

30. Olson, L. D.: Gross and microscopic lesions of middle and inner ear infections in swine. Am. J. Vet. Res., 42:1433, 1981.

31. Palmer, A. C.: Pathogenesis and pathology of the cerebellovestibular syndrome. J. Small Anim. Pract., 11:167, 1970.

32. Palmer, A. C.: A test for vestibular function in sheep. Br. Vet. J., 114:307, 1958.

33. Palmer, A. C., Malinowski, W., and Barnett, K. C.: Clinical signs including papilloedema associated with brain tumours in twenty-one dogs. J. Small Anim. Pract., 15:359, 1974.

34. Patnaik, A. K., Erlandson, R. A., Lieberman, P. H., Fenner, W. R., and Prata, R. G.: Choroid plexus carcinoma with meningeal carcinomatosis in a dog. Vet. Pathol., 17:381, 1980.

35. Pedersen, N. C., Holliday, T. A., and Cello, R. M.: Feline infectious peritonitis. In Proceedings of the American Animal Hospital Association, 1974.

36. Petras, J. M.: Afferent fibers to the spinal cord. The terminal distribution of dorsal root and encephalospinal axons. Med. Serv. J. Can., 22:668, 1966.

37. Read, D. H., and Harrington, D. D.: Experimentally induced thiamine deficiency in Beagle dogs: Clinical observations. Am. J. Vet. Res., 42:984, 1981.

38. Read, D. H., Jolly, R. D., and Alley, M. R.: Polioencephalomalacia of dogs with thiamine deficiency. Vet. Pathol., 14:103, 1977.

39. Rebhun, W.: Diseases of the bovine orbit and globe. J. Am. Vet. Med. Assoc., 175:171, 1979.

40. Rendano, V. T., de Lahunta, A., and King, J. M.: Extracranial neoplasia with facial nerve paralysis in two cats. J. Am. Anim. Hosp. Assoc., 16:921, 1980.

41. Robles, S. S., and Anderson, J. H.: Compensation of vestibular deficits in the cat. Brain Res., 147:183, 1978.

42. Russo, M. E.: Primary reticuloses of the central nervous system in dogs. J. Am. Vet. Med. Assoc., 174:492, 1979.

43. Schunk, K. L., and Averill, D. R. Jr.: Peripheral vestibular syndrome in the dog: A review of 83 cases. J. Am. Vet. Med. Assoc., in press.

44. Slausson, D. O., and Finn, J. P.: Meningoencephalitis and panophthalmitis in feline infectious peritonitis. J. Am. Vet. Med. Assoc., 160:729, 1972.

45. Spoendlin, H.: Some morphological and pathological aspects of the vestibular sensory epithelia. Second Symposium on the Role of Vestibular Organs in Space Exploration, NASA-SP115. Scientific and Technical Information Division, Office of Technological Utilization, Washington, D.C., U.S. Government Printing Office, 1966, 99–116.

46. Spreull, J. S. A.: Otitis media of the dog. In Kirk, R. W. (ed.): Current Veterinary Therapy V. Philadelphia, W. B. Saunders Co., 1975.

47. Spreull, J. S. A.: Treatment of otitis media in the dog. J. Small Anim. Pract., 5:107, 1964.

48. Stirling, J., and Clarke, M.: Congenital peripheral vestibular disorder in two German Shepherd Dogs. Aust. Vet. J., 57:200, 1981.

49. Wersäll, J., and Lundquist, Per-G.: Morphological polarization of the mechanoreceptors of the vestibular and acoustic systems. Second Symposium, Role of Vestibular Organs in Space Exploration, NASA. Scientific and Technical Information Division, Office of Technological Utilization, Washington, D.C., U.S. Government Printing Office, 1966, 57–72.

50. Wilson, V. J., Wylis, R. M., and Marco, L. A.: Projection to the spinal cord from the medial and descending vestibular nuclei of the cat. Nature, 215:429, 1967.

51. Winston, J.: Clinical problems pertaining to neurotox-

icity of streptomycin group of drugs. Arch. Otolaryngol., *58*:255, 1953.

52. Winston, J., Lewey, F. H., Parenteau, A., Marden, P. A., and Cramer, F. B.: An experimental study of the toxic effects of streptomycin on the vestibular apparatus of the cat. I. Central nervous system. Ann. Otol. Rhinol. Laryngol., *57*:738, 1948.

53. Winston, J., Lewey, F. H., Parenteau, A., Marden,

P. A., and Cramer, F. B.: Further experimental studies of the toxic effects of streptomycin on the central vestibular apparatus of the cat. Ann. Otol. Rhinl. Laryngol., *58*:988, 1949.

54. Winston, J., Lewey, F. H., Parenteau, A., Spitz, E., and Marden, P. A.: Toxic effects of dihydrostreptomycin upon the central vestibular mechanism of the cat. Ann. Otol. Rhinol. Laryngol., *62*:121, 1953.

CEREBELLUM

DEVELOPMENT

An understanding of the development of the cerebellum is pertinent to the determination of its normal microscopic characteristics and the pathogenesis of diseases that affect it.[2-6, 18, 57, 109, 124, 161, 162]

The cerebellum is the dorsal portion of the metencephalon; the ventral portion is the pons. The cerebellum develops from the alar plate region of the metencephalon (Fig. 13–1). Its first appearance is a dorsal bulge of the alar plate which extends the alar plate tissue dorsally and medially in the roof plate, in which the growths from each side eventually meet. This first growth is called the rhombic lip, arising from the side of the rhomboid fossa of the fourth ventricle. This rhombic lip consists of proliferating cells from the germinal zone adjacent to the fourth ventricle.

Two routes of migration issue from these germinal cells. One involves the migration of differentiating mantle layer cells into the substance of the rhombic lip. These immature neurons no longer divide but continue to grow and mature, and give rise to the layer of Purkinje neurons found throughout the cerebellar cortex and the neurons of the cerebellar nuclei located in the medulla of the cerebellum. The second migration involves actively dividing germinal cells that migrate to the surface of the rhombic lip, where they continue to be located as the folia develop in the cerebellum. This superficial layer of cells, the external germinal layer, continues mitosis, producing a zone of germinal cells composed of up to 10 to 12 layers of cells. Differentiation occurs along the inner aspect of these cells, and those cells that have stopped dividing migrate into the substance of the cerebellum to form the granule neuron layer between the Purkinje neurons and the white matter of the folium. The external germinal layer also contributes the few neurons (stellate cells) found in the most superficial of the three layers of the cerebellar cortex, the molecular layer. The three layers of the definitive cerebellar cortex are from external to internal, the molecular layer, the Purkinje neuron layer, and the granule layer. The folds produced on the surface of the cerebellum are called folia.

Purkinje neurons are formed and begin differentiation early in the development of the embryo.[123, 125] The internal germinal layer adjacent to the fourth ventricle completes its activity prior to birth, leaving only a layer of ependyma to line the fourth ventricle. The external germinal layer is active late in gestation and after birth in some species. The granule cell neurons are formed from the external germinal layer later in gestation than the Purkinje neurons, and their formation is not complete until the postnatal period. The degree of cerebellar development at birth correlates with the amount of motor function and coordination seen in the newborn animal.[66, 127] The foal and calf that walk at birth have a more completely developed cerebellum than the kitten, the puppy, or the human baby, who are helpless at birth. As the brain, including the cerebellum, of these latter species develops, their motor function and coordination for ambulation improve. A direct correlation has been shown between the development of the cerebellar cortex and mobility in the kitten.

In the calf, the formation of Purkinje neurons is completed at about 100 days of gestation. After that no more Purkinje neurons are formed. Those that are present continue to grow and mature (differentiate) in conjunction

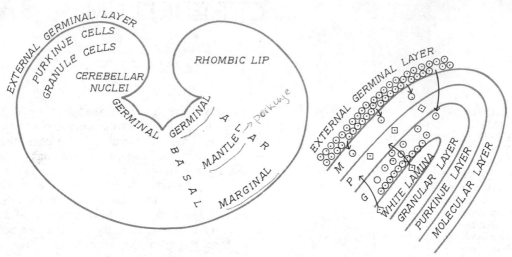

METENCEPHALON   CEREBELLAR FOLIUM – CORTEX

Figure 13-1. Development of the cerebellum.

with the continued development of the cerebellum. In the horse, ox, sheep, and pig, the external germinal layer is more active late in gestation and has mostly exhausted its germinal role prior to birth. In the calf the cerebellar primordium appears at 37 days. The external germinal layer appears at 57 days of gestation and is maximal in thickness by 183 days, when it is composed of six cell layers. Following that it slowly decreases in thickness, reaching a layer two cells thick by 2 months postnatally, and completely disappearing by 6 months postnatally. In the kitten and puppy the external germinal layer reaches maximum thickness in the first postnatal week and starts to decrease in size after the second postnatal week.[174] The granule neuron layer is present at birth but poorly populated and continues to grow in size for up to 10 weeks postnatally.[161] External germinal layer cells will persist for up to 60 to 84 days in the kitten, 75 days in the puppy. When the cells have all migrated into the molecular and granule neuron layers only the leptomeninges remain on the surface of the molecular layer.

ANATOMY

The cerebellum consists of a central median region, the vermis, named for the worm-like contortions it presents caudally, and a lateral hemisphere on each side of the vermis (Figs. 13–3, 13–4).[15, 16] The cerebellum is divided into two disproportionate regions: the large body of the cerebellum, and the small flocculono-

dular lobe. These two regions are separated by the uvulonodular fissure (Fig. 13–4). The flocculonodular lobe, also known as the archicerebellum or vestibular cerebellum, is confined to the ventral aspect of the cerebellum near its center. The nodulus is the most rostral part of the caudal vermis that is adjacent to the fourth ventricle. It connects laterally by a

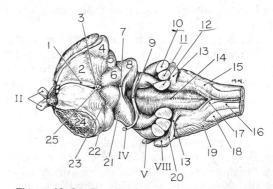

Figure 13–2. Dorsolateral view of the brain stem. *1*: stria habenularis thalami; *2*: dorsal aspect of thalamus; *3*: habenular commissure; *4*: lateral geniculate body; *5*: medial geniculate body; *6*: rostral colliculus; *7*: commissure of caudal colliculi; *8*: caudal colliculus; *9*: decussation of trochlear nerves in rostral medullary velum; *10*: middle cerebellar peduncle; *11*: caudal cerebellar peduncle; *12*: rostral cerebellar peduncle; *13*: dorsal cochlear nucleus; *14*: median sulcus in fourth ventricle; *15*: nucleus cuneatus lateralis; *16*: fasciculus cuneatus; *17*: fasciculus gracilis; *18*: spinal tract of trigeminal nerve; *19*: superficial arcuate fibers; *20*: ventral cochlear nucleus; *21*: brachium of caudal colliculus; *22*: optic tract; *23*: brachium of rostral colliculus; *24*: cut surface between cerebrum and brain stem, internal capsule; *25*: pineal body; *II*: optic nerve; *IV*: trochlear nerve; *V*: trigeminal nerve; *VIII*: vestibulocochlear nerve.

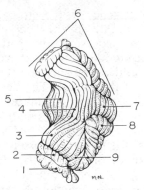

Figure 13–3. Dorsolateral view of the cerebellum. *1*: ventral paraflocculus; *2*: dorsal paraflocculus; *3*: dorsal surface of cerebellum; *4*: fissura prima; *5*: vermis portion of rostral lobe; *6*: right cerebellar hemisphere; *7*: vermis portion of caudal lobe; *8*: paramedian lobule; *9*: ansiform lobule.

peduncle on each side to the flocculus, a small lobule on the ventral lateral aspect of the cerebellar hemisphere. The much larger body of the cerebellum, consisting of vermis and hemispheres, is divided into rostral and caudal lobes by the primary fissure. Within each lobe the folia are grouped into named lobules that reside in different portions of the vermis and hemispheres.

The cerebellum is attached to the brain stem by three groups of neuronal processes on each side, the cerebellar peduncles (Fig. 13–2,

Plates 4 to 9). Although arranged in a medial to lateral plane in which they attach to the cerebellum, they are named from rostral to caudal based on their connections with the brain stem. The caudal cerebellar peduncle connects the spinal cord and medulla with the cerebellum. It contains primarily afferent processes. The middle cerebellar peduncle connects the transverse fibers of the pons with the cerebellum, and is solely afferent to the cerebellum. The rostral cerebellar peduncle connects the cerebellum with the mesencephalon, and contains mainly efferent processes passing out of the cerebellum.

When the cerebellum is sectioned transversely or longitudinally, an extensive area of white matter in the center is seen. This is the cerebellar medulla that sends branches of white matter out into the overlying folia. As a group, these branches are called the arbor vitae because of their resemblance to the branches of a tree. Individually, each is the white lamina of a folium. The arbor vitae is covered by the three layers of the cerebellar cortex. In the cerebellar medulla there are situated collections of neurons that comprise the cerebellar nuclei (Plate 5). In domestic animals these are organized into three nuclei, from medial to lateral on each side of the median plane. They are called the fastigial, interpositional, and lateral (dentate) nuclei, respectively.

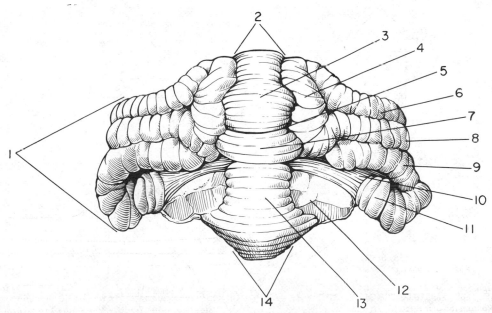

Figure 13–4. Cerebellum, ventral surface. *1*: left cerebellar hemisphere; *2*: caudal vermis; *3*: uvula; *4*: paramedian lobule; *5*: uvulonodular fissure; *6*: ansiform lobule; *7*: nodulus; *8*: dorsal paraflocculus; *9*: ventral paraflocculus; *10*: flocculonodular peduncle; *11*: flocculus; *12*: cerebellar peduncles (cut surface); *13*: lingula; *14*: rostral vermis.

The cerebellar cortex, which is composed of three layers, forms the outer portion of each folium and is similar throughout the cerebellum.[126] The folial surface is covered by leptomeninges. Adjacent to this is the outer relatively cell-free molecular layer. It is composed mostly of the axons and telodendria of granule neurons and the dendritic zones of Purkinje neurons. This bounds the middle layer, which is a single layer of large flask-shaped neurons, the Purkinje neuron layer, which in turn bounds the inner layer of granule neurons. The granule neuron layer is thick and consists of numerous granule cell neurons, the cell bodies of which are small and dark-staining, giving it a characteristic cellular appearance. This layer varies in thickness from 5 to 6 cells at the bottom of a folium to 15 to 20 cells at the top of a folium.

The cerebellar cortex is uniquely organized for the distribution of afferent information (Fig. 13–5). There are two major types of afferents to the cerebellum: mossy and climbing fibers.[69] The more abundant mossy fibers have a widespread origin in the brain stem and spinal cord. As they pass into the cerebellum, collaterals of these processes synapse in the cerebellar nuclei on neuronal cell bodies. The main process enters a folium by way of its white matter, passes into the granule layer, and terminates in synaptic relationship with the dendritic zone of the granule neurons within the granule layer. The axon of the granule neuron courses through the Purkinje neuron layer into the molecular layer, in which it branches and courses parallel to the longitudinal axis of the folium. The dendritic zone of the Purkinje neuron is a maze of branched axons that is arranged in one plane in the molecular layer. This flat plane of neuronal processes is oriented transversely to the longitudinal axis of the folium. By this arrangement, the axon of the granule neuron traverses the dendritic zone of numerous Purkinje neurons. Synapse occurs between these processes. This network can be likened to telephone wires (granule neuron axons) coursing from one telephone pole (dendritic zone of a Purkinje neuron) to another.

Climbing fibers are the axons of olivary neurons that enter the cerebellum through the caudal cerebellar peduncle.[41] Collaterals synapse on neurons in the cerebellar nuclei. The main axon continues into a cerebellar folium by way of its white matter, passes through the granule neuron and Purkinje neuron layers into the molecular layer, and arborizes in synaptic relationship with a Purkinje neuron dendritic zone.

These mossy and climbing fibers are facilitatory at their synapse with neurons of the cerebellar nuclei and the granule neurons and

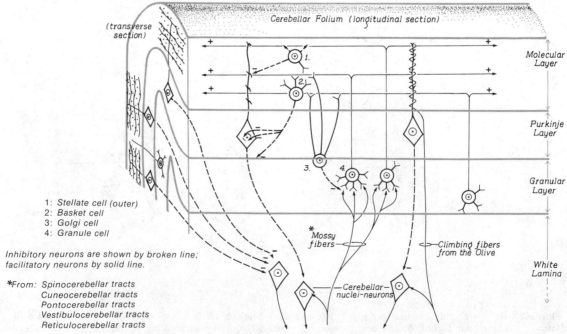

1: Stellate cell (outer)
2: Basket cell
3: Golgi cell
4: Granule cell

Inhibitory neurons are shown by broken line; facilitatory neurons by solid line.

*From: Spinocerebellar tracts
Cuneocerebellar tracts
Pontocerebellar tracts
Vestibulocerebellar tracts
Reticulocerebellar tracts

Figure 13–5. Microscopic anatomy of the cerebellum.

Purkinje neurons, respectively. The granule neurons are facilitatory to the Purkinje neurons. The stellate neurons of the molecular layer (outer and basket) are inhibitory interneurons to the Purkinje neurons. The Golgi neurons of the granule layer are inhibitory interneurons to the granule neurons.[67] The only axon that projects from the cerebellar cortex (an efferent axon) is that of the Purkinje neurons.[65] These axons pass through the granule layer into the folial white matter and then to the cerebellar nuclei. A few Purkinje neuron axons leave the cerebellum through the caudal peduncle and terminate in the vestibular nuclei. The Purkinje neuronal telodendria are inhibitory to the neurons on which they terminate. This inhibition is mediated by the neurotransmitter gamma-aminobutyric acid.[36] The efferent axons that project from the cerebellum to the brain stem are all from the neurons of the cerebellar nuclei, except for the few direct cerebellovestibular processes from Purkinje neurons. It would seem that the major role of the cerebellar cortex is to modulate the continual facilitation of neurons of cerebellar nuclei by way of Purkinje neuron inhibition.

In order for the cerebellum to function as a coordinator of muscular activity and regulator of muscle tone, it must receive afferent information to provide it with knowledge of where the limbs, trunk, and head are in space. Thus afferents of the general and special proprioceptive systems must project to the cerebellum. In addition, it must be apprised of the voluntary activity being induced. Thus it receives afferents from the upper motor neuron system.

CEREBELLAR AFFERENTS

General Proprioception. Spinocerebellar tracts enter mostly through the caudal cerebellar peduncle, with a few via the rostral cerebellar peduncle.

Cuneocerebellar tracts enter via the caudal cerebellar peduncle.

Special Proprioception. Vestibulocerebellar tracts enter directly and indirectly from the vestibular nuclei, via the caudal cerebellar peduncle.

Most of the proprioceptive neurons project to the folia of the cerebellar vermis or the adjacent paravermal folia.

Special Somatic Afferent—Visual and Auditory. Tectocerebellar processes enter directly by way of the rostral cerebellar peduncle and project mostly to the head area of the vermis. Others enter via the pons and middle cerebellar peduncle.

Upper Motor Neuron

OLIVARY NUCLEI. Extrapyramidal nuclei of the telencephalon and brain stem project information to the cerebellum mostly through the olivary nuclei. These nuclei are located in the ventrolateral portion of the caudal medulla (Plates 3, 4). They extend rostrally to just caudal to the facial nucleus, and caudally to a level just caudal to the obex. They consist of three components on each side, which vary in size throughout the length of the nuclei. Where they are most developed, they have the appearance of three fingers oriented obliquely from dorsomedial to ventrolateral just dorsal and lateral to the pyramid and medial lemniscus. The hypoglossal axons course along their lateral border. The axons of the neurons in the olivary nuclei cross the midline and join the contralateral caudal cerebellar peduncle. These are the source of the climbing fibers to the cerebellum. These olivary neurons are activated by neurons of the upper motor neuron system and by spinal cord afferents.

PONTINE NUCLEUS. Axons from the cerebral cortex in all areas of the hemisphere project information to the cerebellum by way of the pontine nucleus. This is the corticopontocerebellar pathway. These cerebral neurons reach this nucleus via the internal capsule, the crus cerebri, and the longitudinal fibers of the pons. Axons leave the longitudinal fibers and synapse on ipsilateral pontine neurons. The neuronal cell bodies of the pontine nucleus surround the longitudinal fibers of the pons (Plates 8, 9). The axons of the cell bodies of the pontine nucleus cross the midline, forming the transverse fibers of the pons and the contralateral middle cerebellar peduncle. This peduncle projects for the most part to the cerebellar hemisphere. There is a direct relationship in the evolution of skilled motor function and the development of the motor cortex, pons, and cerebellar hemispheres. In humans the transverse fibers of the pons extend caudally over the trapezoid body, and the vermis of the cerebellum is buried by the development of the hemispheres.

RED NUCLEUS. Rubrocerebellar processes enter the cerebellum through the rostral cerebellar peduncle.

RETICULAR FORMATION. Reticulocerebellar processes enter by way of the caudal cerebellar peduncle.

CEREBELLAR EFFERENTS[65]

Cerebellar Cortex. Purkinje cell axons, derived mostly from the flocculonodular lobe, project directly to the vestibular nuclei via the caudal cerebellar peduncle.

Cerebellar Nuclei

1. Fastigial nucleus neurons project to vestibular nuclei and the reticular formation by way of the caudal cerebellar peduncle.

2. Interposital nucleus neurons project to the red nucleus and the reticular formation by way of the rostral cerebellar peduncle.

3. Lateral nucleus neurons project to the red nucleus, the reticular formation, the pallidum, and the ventral lateral nucleus of the thalamus through the rostral cerebellar peduncle.

When the rostral cerebellar peduncle enters the mesencephalon, most of its efferent axons decussate in the tegmentum in the ventral tegmental decussation (Plate 10). This is at the level of the caudal colliculus caudal to the rubrospinal decussation. These axons cross to the opposite side to terminate in the contralateral red nucleus, the ventral lateral nucleus of the thalamus, or the pallidum.

A feedback circuit to the cerebral cortex exists by way of the direct projection of the cerebellar lateral nucleus to the contralateral ventral lateral nucleus of the thalamus, which in turn projects to the cerebrum passing through the internal capsule (Fig. 13–6). An indirect route from the cerebellum to the cerebrum exists in its projection to the contralateral red nucleus and pallidum, both of which have projections to the ventral rostral nucleus of the thalamus; this in turn projects to the cerebrum.

There are very few efferent cerebellar axons that project in the spinal cord to directly influence the lower motor neuron.[134] The cerebellum functions through influence over the upper motor neuron tracts that descend the spinal cord to affect lower motor neuron activity.

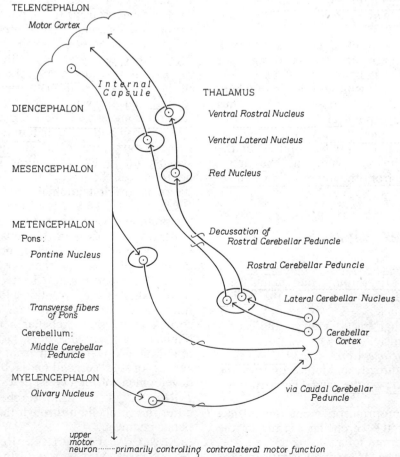

Figure 13–6. Role of the cerebellum in control of motor function: feedback circuit to cerebral cortex from the cerebellum.

FUNCTION

The cerebellum functions as a regulator, not as the primary initiator of motor activity.[63] It functions to coordinate and "smooth" movements induced by the upper motor neuron in relation to the posture of the animal to provide synergy of muscular activity. The cerebellum also functions in the maintenance of equilibrium and in the regulation of tone to preserve the normal position of the body while at rest or during motion.

In summary, the cerebellar nuclei that continually facilitate brain stem neurons in turn are regulated by the inhibitory function of the Purkinje neurons of the cerebellar cortex. The degree of activity of these Purkinje neurons depends on the afferent information reaching them directly by way of the climbing fiber afferents and indirectly via the mossy fiber afferents.

The rostral and vermal portions of the cerebellum are concerned primarily with the inhibition of lower motor neurons to extensor muscles of the neck and thoracic limbs.[34, 35] It thus participates in the overall function of the upper motor neuron to maintain support of the body against gravity.[177]

In an attempt to correlate structure and function, the cerebellum has been divided topographically in different ways.[93, 100] On a phylogenetic basis the cerebellum can be divided into three regions. The archicerebellum primarily includes the flocculonodular lobe, which is concerned with vestibular system activity. The paleocerebellum includes primarily the vermis of the rostral lobe and adjacent hemisphere and is mostly concerned with spinal cord function and postural tonus. The neocerebellum includes part of the vermis of the caudal lobe and most of the cerebellar hemisphere and is more concerned with regulation of skilled movements.

The cerebellum can also be divided into three bilateral longitudinal zones of cortex and related nuclei. The medial zone includes the vermis and fastigial nuclei and is concerned with regulation of tone for posture and locomotion and equilibrium of the entire body. The intermediate zone includes the paravermal cortex and interpositial nuclei and is more concerned with adjusting tone and posture to regulate more skilled movements. The lateral zone includes the lateral portion of each hemisphere and the lateral nuclei. This zone functions in regulating skilled movements of the limbs. This portion is more highly developed in primates, in which skilled limb and hand movements are more common.

SIGNS OF CEREBELLAR DISEASE[51, 52, 93]

Cerebellar disease does not cause the loss of any single function, but a general inadequacy of motor response. As a rule the cerebellum is affected diffusely by disease processes, and the patient typically presents with a bilaterally symmetric ataxia (motor ataxia) with strength preserved. With unilateral lesions, the signs of ataxia are usually ipsilateral to the lesion. Be aware of the paradoxical vestibular syndrome that occurs with unilateral cerebellar medullary and peduncle lesions that affect vestibular components of the cerebellum. With these lesions, the signs of ataxia may be contralateral to the lesion.

Cerebellar disease does not cause paresis. In severe disease the patient may be incapacitated by its ataxic condition and be unable to stand, but voluntary movements are elicited easily with normal strength. Spasticity and ataxia are most commonly observed in the gait. When severely affected, the animal may disorient and fall to either side, forward, or backward. The ataxic gait is characterized by an inability to regulate the rate, range, and force of a movement, which is called dysmetria. The dysmetria usually presents as a hypermetria, an overmeasurement in the gait response observed as greater movements of the limbs than normal in all ranges of motion. Observation of the gait or postural reactions reveals a raised threshold to response. The onset of the voluntary movement is delayed, and the response, once initiated, is exaggerated. After the delay, the limb is raised too high on protraction, and then forcefully returned to the bearing surface. Inadequate Purkinje neuron inhibition of the cerebellar nuclei results in the delay in cessation of a voluntary movement, and thus a hypermetric response occurs.

Involvement of the flocculonodular lobe or fastigial nuclear area of the cerebellum may cause vestibular system disturbance, with loss of equilibrium, abnormal nystagmus, bizarre postures, and a broad-based staggering gait with jerky movements and a tendency to fall to the side or backward, especially if the thoracic limbs are elevated.

Unilateral cerebellar lesions produce ipsilateral signs of spasticity, dysmetria, hypermetria, and abnormal postural reactions. Vestibular disturbances with unilateral cerebellar lesions may cause a disturbance in balance and head tilt toward or away from the side of the lesion. The latter may occur with the lesions above the medulla in the cerebellar peduncles on one side. (See discussion of paradoxical vestibular syndrome in Chapter 12.) The abnormal nystagmus may be present only on holding the head flexed to one side, with the quick phase directed toward the side to which the head is directed. In others the direction of the horizontal or rotatory nystagmus may be consistently toward or away from the side of the suspected lesion; occasionally it is vertical.

Occasionally with unilateral lesions of the cerebellar medulla affecting the fastigial or interposital nuclei, pupillary dilation occurs that is slowly responsive to light.[93] The third eyelid may protrude and the palpebral fissure may be enlarged. The pupillary changes occur in the eye ipsilateral to an interposital nuclear lesion and contralateral to a fastigial nuclear lesion.

The resting posture may show a broad-based stance with the thoracic limbs, and a truncal ataxia which is a swaying of the body from side to side, forward and backward, or occasionally dorsoventrally. These may appear as gross jerky movements of the entire body. A fine head tremor is characteristic of cerebellar cortical disease, and usually is augmented by the initiation of voluntary movements such as are observed as the head reaches for food. This is an intention tremor, a form of dysmetria involving the head. In severe cerebellar abnormality the patient may be in lateral recumbency, unable to right itself to stand, with its head and neck extended in a position of opisthotonos.

The rostral lobe of the cerebellum is especially inhibitory to the stretch reflex mechanism of antigravity muscles (extensor muscle tone). Lesions in this area may result in opisthotonos with rigidly extended thoracic limbs. In some instances the pelvic limbs will be flexed forward under the body by hypertonia of the hypaxial muscles that flex the hips. If the rostral lobe lesion involves the ventral lobules, the pelvic limbs may be rigidly extended away from the body, similar to the thoracic limbs.[93, 168]

Muscle tone usually is increased in domestic animals with cerebellar disease. Reflexes are normal to hyperactive. Postural reactions generally are intact, but the response is usually delayed in its onset and then exaggerated.

Spasticity is evident in these reactions. This is most apparent in the hopping responses. Proprioceptive positioning is usually normal. Abnormal nystagmus is observed only occasionally. If the head is extended and support is withdrawn suddenly, instead of returning to its normal position the head may descend ventrally further than normal. This excessive excursion is referred to as a rebound phenomenon and is a sign of lack of cerebellar control.

It has been found that animals with significant cerebellar cortical disease fail to respond to the menace maneuver normally used to test the visual system. In the presence of normal vision and facial muscle strength, these animals fail to close their eyelids when threatened by a menacing gesture. Varying degrees of this deficit have been observed in horses, cattle, pigs, dogs, and cats with cerebellar cortical lesions. It is known that the entire central visual pathway to the visual cortex as well as the facial neurons of cranial nerve VII must be intact for this normal response to take place. Therefore, it may be assumed that the pathway between the visual cortex and the facial nucleus must pass through the cerebellum; alternatively this deficit reflects a loss of cerebellar facilitation of cortical activity in the motor area. The latter inhibitory effect could prevent the ability of cortical neurons to activate facial neurons for this response.

If an anatomic pathway exists between the cerebrum and facial nucleus that traverses the cerebellum, it may involve a corticopontocerebellar or a corticotectopontocerebellar pathway. I have observed unilateral cerebellar lesions in the dog and horse that produce a lack of this menace response on the same side as the lesion. This would agree with the predominance of optic nerve fibers crossing through the optic chiasm to reach the contralateral visual cortex and the crossing back of corticopontocerebellar pathways at the pontine nucleus and transverse fibers of the pons (see Fig. 14–7).

A number of correlations of clinical signs to loss of function of specific areas of the cerebellum have been determined for experimental and natural lesions (see p. 263).

CEREBELLAR SYNDROMES[51, 52]

CONGENITAL CEREBELLAR DISEASES

In this text the congenital cerebellar diseases includes neonatal syndromes, in which the

Clinical Signs	Cerebellar Area
Opisthotonos, forelimb hyperextension, hindlimb hip flexion—hindlimb extension if the lesion reaches ventral aspect.	Rostral lobe
Hypotonia, hypermetria, intention tremor.	Caudal lobe
Dysequilibrium—drunken, broad-based staggering gait, loss of balance, abnormal nystagmus.	Flocculonodular lobe
Paradoxical vestibular signs—head tilt opposite to side of lesion, nystagmus toward lesion	Cerebellar peduncles: mostly caudal, dorsal to the medulla.
Dilated pupil, partial third eyelid protrusion, enlarged palpebral fissure.	Cerebellar nuclei: fastigial, interposital

clinical signs are present at birth, and postnatal syndromes, in which the onset of signs is some time after birth but reflects a proven or presumed inherited deficit in cell metabolism. They will be discussed in two groups based on the time of onset of clinical signs (Table 13–1).

Neonatal Syndromes

Animals whose signs are present at birth or by the time they are able to ambulate usually do not have progressive signs. Those diseases that have occurred during fetal development and are no longer active at the time of ambulation have no reason to produce progressive signs. A few abiotrophies that have been recognized that occur prenatally or that commence prenatally and continue postnatally usually produce no obvious indication of progression of clinical signs.

In this group are included the prenatal or neonatal viral infections, malformations due to hereditary or unknown cause, and the prenatal or neonatal cerebellar cortical abiotrophies.

Viral infection[187]

CATS: FELINE PANLEUKOPENIA VIRUS.[32, 43-47, 103, 111, 112, 114, 128, 130-132] A congenital, nonprogressive cerebellar ataxia was recognized in cats at least as early as 1888.[91] A genetic basis could not be established for this disease, and in 1965 Kilham and Margolis reported on the possible relationship of this cerebellar disease to a viral-induced malformation.[112] Their studies on viral-induced cerebellar hypoplasia in the rat, hamster, and cat are outstanding research contributions. In 1967 Johnson, Margolis, and Kilham reported the identification of the viral agent as the feline panleukopenia virus.[103] Subsequent studies by Csiza further confirmed this agent as the cause of cerebellar lesions in kittens.[43] A number of reported cases

on feline cerebellar malformations may in fact be the result of this infection.[32, 77, 128]

In utero or perinatal inflammation of the brain with the feline panleukopenia virus produces a profound effect on the developing cerebellum. The major destruction is usually in the cells of the external germinal layer, which is actively proliferating and differentiating granule neurons at the time of birth and for the first few weeks of life. Destruction of this layer produces hypoplasia of the granule cell layer, or granuloprival hypoplasia. Preformed growing Purkinje neurons may also be destroyed by the infection. In some cases, the destruction is so severe that only a few rudimentary folia remain over the medulla of the cerebellum. Although lesions occasionally occur elsewhere in the brain and spinal cord, usually they are minimal and do not cause clinical signs. Postnatal infections with this agent, even though it may cause systemic disease, rarely cause inflammation of the central nervous system resulting in clinical signs.

The diagnostic feature of this disease is exemplified by fairly symmetric, nonprogressive cerebellar signs of all portions of the body that are present in a kitten at the onset of ambulation, around 3 to 4 weeks of age. Spasticity with markedly incoordinated dysmetric limb movements, truncal swaying, and loss of balance are usually observed. A fine head tremor is occasionally observed, but abnormal nystagmus is unusual.

As the kitten grows and becomes more active, the signs become more obvious. However, the lesion is not progressive. The destruction occurred in the perinatal period and no longer continues. Compensation for the cerebellar deficit is usually minimal, and the signs persist for the duration of the animal's life.

As in many of the cerebellar disorders, there is no obvious correlation between the degree of cerebellar lesion and severity of the clinical

TABLE 13–1. CONGENITAL CEREBELLAR DISEASES

1. Neonatal Syndromes: Signs present at birth or at onset of ambulation
   A. Viral infection
      Cats—Feline panleukopenia virus
      Cattle—Bovine virus diarrhea virus
         Akabane virus
         Bluetongue virus
      Sheep—Akabane virus
         Bluetongue virus
      Swine—Hog cholera virus
      Dogs—Canine herpesvirus
   B. Malformation
      Cerebellar hypoplasia-dysplasia with lissencephaly
       Wire-haired fox terrier
       Irish setter
      Cerebellar hypoplasia-dysplasia with polymicrogyria
       Hereford cattle—autosomal recessive
      Cerebellar hypoplasia
       Chow chow dog
       Shorthorn cattle—autosomal recessive
      Miscellaneous malformations
       Dogs, cattle
   C. Congenital hypomyelongenesis-dysmyelinogenesis
   D. Abiotrophy
      Beagles—possible inheritance
      Samoyeds—possible inheritance
      Irish setter—autosomal recessive
      Hereford cattle—suspected inheritance
      Welsh mountain and Corriedale sheep (daft lambs)—autosomal recessive
      Cats—olivopontocerebellar atrophy
2. Postnatal Syndromes: Signs begin a few weeks to months postnatally—Abiotrophies
   A. Dogs
      Kerry blue terrier—autosomal recessive
      Gordon setter—autosomal recessive
      Rough-coated collie—autosomal recessive
      Airedale terrier—possible inheritance
      Finnish harrier—possible inheritance
      Bernese mountain dog—possible inheritance
   B. Horses
      Arabian—presumed recessive inheritance
      Gotland pony—autosomal recessive
   C. Cattle
      Holstein Friesian—presumed recessive inheritance
   D. Swine
      Yorkshire—presumed recessive inheritance

disorder. Rarely, kittens with characteristic clinical signs of cerebellar disease show no obvious lesion in the cerebellum or elsewhere in the brain or spinal cord.

CATTLE: BOVINE VIRUS DIARRHEA VIRUS.[28, 30, 60, 106, 135, 172] In 1968 Kahrs first noticed the possible relationship of calves born with cerebellar ataxia and infections of pregnant dams with the bovine virus diarrhea (BVD) agent.[104] Further clinicopathologic and epidemiologic studies supported this relationship.[105-108] Affected newborn calves that have not consumed colostrum have a detectable serum antibody titer to the BVD agent. Experimental exposure of susceptible pregnant cattle to the BVD agent resulted in the birth of ataxic calves with cerebellar lesions similar to those of the spontaneous disease.[28-30, 172, 185, 186] Final confirmation of the relationship was obtained by sequential study of calf fetuses obtained surgically from cattle infected with the BVD agent at 150 days of gestation.[30] Acute cerebellar lesions with leptomeningeal inflammation, necrosis of external germinal cells, focal parenchymal hemorrhages, and folial edema occurred at 17 and 21 days after inoculation. By 42 days, the cerebellar lesion was complete and the inflammation was subsiding. The residual lesions seen at term consisted of varying degrees of folial degeneration with cavitation. Most calves with this lesion were infected between 100 and 200 days of gestation.

This lesion cannot be summarily referred to as hypoplasia. Only the failure to produce granule neurons from the external germinal cells that were destroyed by the virus can be referred to as hypoplasia. The massive destruction of the preformed Purkinje neurons and folial white matter is a direct degeneration of differentiated growing tissue due to the virus and inflammatory response. The terminal lesion is a cerebellar degeneration or atrophy, only one component of which can be referred to as hypoplasia.

In a few calves with severe cerebellar lesions, cavitated areas can be found scattered through the cerebrum, especially in the occipital lobes. These prosencephalic lesions are the result of the inflammation that occurred in that part of the brain. Clinical signs due to these lesions have not been observed. Ocular lesions have also been observed in spontaneous and experimental examples of the disease.[19, 27] These consist of retinal atrophy, optic neuritis, cataract, and micro-ophthalmia with retinal dysplasia. The acute ocular inflammation also has been found to occur 17 to 21 days after exposure of susceptible cattle to the BVD agent.

The degree of cerebellar lesion observed at term varies considerably from slight gross deformity to almost complete absence of any cerebellar tissue. In the latter, only a small bar of smooth parenchyma may remain over the fourth ventricle where the cerebellum is normally located.

Clinical signs of cerebellar ataxia are usually

symmetric and vary from recumbency with opisthotonos and extensor rigidity of the limbs to a mildly spastic hypermetric gait and slight head tremor. Abnormal nystagmus may occur in animals with severe lesions.

The degree of clinical deficit does not necessarily correlate with the severity of cerebellar lesions. The signs present at birth do not worsen with age. Usually they remain the same for as long as the calf is observed. In a few instances, calves with this disease that could not stand to walk for several days subsequently stood and seemed to compensate and improve in their ability to ambulate. No change was observed over a maximum of 2 weeks.

CATTLE: AKABANE VIRUS.[42, 58, 88, 90, 96, 140, 142, 153, 191] In Australia, Japan, and Israel, a syndrome of arthrogryposis and hydranencephaly has been observed in cattle and sheep with these lesions occurring singly or in combination. Epidemiologic, clinical, and pathologic study of the spontaneous disease and subsequent experimental studies have confirmed this syndrome to be due to the *in utero* infection of the embryo-fetus with the Akabane virus. The disease is limited to those geographic areas where the appropriate vector that carries the virus and infects susceptible ruminants is indigenous. The hydranencephaly results from the viral destruction of germinal cells that give rise to neocortical neurons and the destruction of preformed cerebral cortex predominantly in the neopallium. Clinical signs are referable to the cerebral lesion: dullness, propulsive activity, and blindness. In a few instances with severe cerebral lesions, cerebellar lesions occur and contribute to the clinical signs.

A congenital hydranencephaly and cerebellar hypoplasia has been reported in a herd of Holstein-Friesian cattle in British Columbia, Canada. Cerebellar and cerebral signs were observed.[83] The etiology remains undetermined, though a viral pathogenesis is suspected.

CATTLE: BLUETONGUE VIRUS.[136, 166] The bluetongue virus that produces disease in adult sheep may also produce hydranencephaly in fetal calves exposed to the virus. Similarly, in a few severely affected calves, cerebellar lesions may also occur. Signs of the cerebral lesion predominate.

SHEEP.[38, 145, 146] There is no viral inflammation that selectively destroys only the cerebellum of fetal lambs. Both the Akabane and bluetongue viruses can destroy fetal cerebellar tissue to varying degrees but always in association with severe cerebral lesions that result in hydranencephaly.

Pathogenetic studies on the bluetongue virus show that the most severe cerebral and cerebellar lesions occur when the fetus is infected at 50 to 58 days of gestation.[145, 146] The immature neural cells appear to be especially susceptible at this time to necrosis by this agent.

SWINE.[70, 192] Hog cholera vaccine virus administered to susceptible pregnant sows has been found to produce numerous lesions in fetal pigs, including lesions of the cerebellum. Clinical signs are usually most referable to the diffuse failure of myelination of the spinal cord, brain stem, and cerebellum, which results in a severe whole-body constant tremor associated with voluntary muscular effort. (See discussion of congenital hypomyelinogenesis in Chapter 7.)

DOGS: CANINE HERPESVIRUS INFECTION.[159] There is no viral disease yet recognized in the dog that selectively affects the cerebellum of the fetus or newborn puppy. Occasionally, when a litter of puppies is infected with the canine herpesvirus during the first week of life, a puppy will survive the systemic effects of the agent and be left with a residual cerebellar ataxia due to the destructive effect of the virus on varying components of the cerebellum.

The recently recognized canine parvovirus that has antigenic similarity to the feline panleukopenia virus produces some similar clinical signs in young and adult dogs. However, no nervous system lesions have been observed in the experimental or natural disease in newborn puppies, growing puppies, or adults.[7, 8]

Malformation. A number of malformations have been observed that are either of unknown cause or related to an inherited trait. Microscopic studies of the malformations have not been suggestive of an *in utero* viral inflammation.

I have observed a marked cerebellar dysplasia and cerebral lissencephaly in 2 out of 3 wire-haired fox terriers in a litter and in 3 out of 10 Irish setters in a litter. In both instances, the cerebellum was symmetrically small, less than one-third the normal size; the reduced size was due primarily to failure of formation of the cortex. The rudimentary folia in the wire-haired fox terrier had no normal cortical organization of neurons. Purkinje neurons were haphazardly distributed through masses of granule cells. From the time they could ambulate, these puppies had a severe cerebellar ataxia with difficulty standing and an inability to walk more than a few feet without falling to either side, forward or backwards. One wire-haired fox terrier was raised to 4 years of age. The cerebellar ataxia did not change, but sporadic generalized seizures began shortly after 1 year of age. The latter has been reported in other dogs with lissencephaly.

Lissencephaly has not been reported to result from inflammation associated with an infectious agent. It has been observed without cerebellar lesions in Lhasa apso dogs.[84] A genetic cause is suspected but has not been proved. Viral isolation studies in Irish setters at 4 months of age did not reveal any agent present at the time and the lesion did not indicate an inflammation.

A hereditary encephalopathy due to an autosomal recessive trait has been reported in Hereford calves.[10, 143] The multiple malformations observed included widely dilated lateral ventricles, polymicrogyria of the cerebral hemispheres, malformed mesencephalon with stenosis of the aqueduct, and a cerebellar malformation with severe cerebellar cortical dysplasia. Additionally, cataracts and retinal dysplasia with detachment were observed. These calves are usually unable to get up from birth.

Complete absence of the cerebellar vermis or its caudal portion has been observed as the only lesion in dogs and cattle.[62, 77, 141] In some of these patients, hydrocephalus has been observed. The etiology of these malformations is unknown. Similar hypoplasia-aplasia of the cerebellar vermis, medulla and corpus callosum has been observed in a goat.[184] An autosomal recessive micrognathia and cerebellar hypoplasia was reported in an Aberdeen Angus herd.[68] The cerebellum was one-third the normal size.

Recently, a predominantly microscopic cerebellar hypoplasia was reported in chow-chow dogs that exhibited a persistent cerebellar ataxia from birth.[116] The lack of any Purkinje neurons and depleted granule cell population have been attributed to a genetic defect thought to be transmitted as an autosomal recessive trait. Other reports describe gross and microscopic lesions of cerebellar hypoplasia in unrelated dogs.[110, 167]

A similar autosomal, recessive, cerebellar, cortical hypoplasia has been reported in Shorthorn cattle.[74, 148]

Congenital Hypomyelinogenesis-Dysmyelinogenesis. This disease is described in Chapter 7 under congenital tremor that affects the entire body and is the primary clinical sign.

Other signs of cerebellar disturbance may accompany this diffuse myelin deficiency. Viral and genetic causes have been defined for some examples of this disease. Others have been observed sporadically and the cause has not been determined.

Abiotrophy. Microscopic examination of the cerebellar cortex of some animals with cerebellar ataxia at birth has revealed degenerative changes usually most evident in the Purkinje neurons. This has been called an abiotrophy, which indicates a degeneration due to an intrinsic abnormality in the Purkinje neuron's metabolic structure that does not permit its survival. Abiotrophy refers to the lack (*a-*) of a vital (*bios-*) substance necessary for the nutritional (*-trophy*) life of that cell.[81, 82] This is more frequently observed as a postnatal clinical syndrome due to an inherited defect. It is recognized that the Purkinje neuron is susceptible to many intrinsic and extrinsic insults and its degenerative changes are not specific.[31] Because of the absence of any recognized extrinsic and intrinsic causes in the congenital cerebellar ataxias that follow, an abiotrophy is assumed and in some there is evidence for a genetic cause.

DOGS. I have observed a cerebellar cortical degeneration in two beagles from a litter of six and in three litters of Samoyeds. In all instances, the signs were present at the onset of ambulation. Progression of signs was not obvious but may have occurred insidiously over months in the Samoyeds. The beagles showed severe cerebellar ataxia of all portions of the body with remarkable hypermetria of all limbs, truncal ataxia, and a head tremor. The Samoyeds were distinctly different, as the ataxia was most profound in the pelvic limbs. The pelvic limbs were carried forward under the body and were spastic and obviously hypermetric. The thoracic limbs were only mildly spastic and slightly hypermetric on postural reaction testing.

In the cerebellar cortex of the beagles, there was a diffuse absence of Purkinje neurons and some decrease in granule neurons. In scattered folia, these cells were still present but swollen axons were abundant in the granule layer. These are usually considered to be axons of Purkinje neurons, and in some areas in these dogs, they could be found to arise from axon hillocks of the Purkinje neuron. In the Samoyeds, the swollen axons of Purkinje neurons in the granule layer were the most profound lesion. There was no obvious loss of Purkinje or granule neurons. In both breeds, occasional myelin and axonal necrosis were present in the laminae of folia. This was assumed to be Wallerian degeneration of Purkinje neurons.

Swollen Purkinje neuron axons in the granule layer are a nonspecific indication of an abnormality in the Purkinje neuron. It is seen after injury or in documented cases of Purkinje neuronal degeneration. It should not be a consequence of a failure to develop normally. Therefore, these cases have been described as degenerative lesions that are static by the time the animals are ambulatory.

Although this clinical and pathologic syndrome in the Samoyed has been observed in one litter in Massachusetts and in two in Oklahoma, pedigrees have not been available to implicate a genetic pathogenesis for the lesion.

An autosomal recessive disease has been documented in Irish setters that are presumed to be blind and unable to ambulate owing to their cerebellar lesion.[151] The lesion consists of severe loss of Purkinje neurons, proliferation of astrocytes in the Purkinje cell layer, and degenerative changes in Purkinje neurons that were present, including vacuolization and swollen Purkinje cell axons.

CATTLE. A suspected inherited cerebellar hypoplasia and abiotrophy have been reported in Hereford cattle with nonprogressive signs of cerebellar ataxia present at birth.[97] The paucity of granule neurons and Purkinje neurons suggested a developmental arrest resulting in hypoplasia. The cortical gliosis and evidence of degeneration in surviving Purkinje neurons suggested an abiotrophy. Limited pedigree data suggested inheritance as causative. A syndrome of cerebellar ataxia and seizures was reported in one Ayrshire calf with lesions of cerebellar cortical abiotrophy.[101]

Cerebellar cortical abiotrophy occurs in Angus calves accompanied by a spastic, hypermetric, ataxic gait.[11, 12, 14] The ataxia is preceded by generalized seizures that begin at birth or up to 3 months of age. These seizures are single or multiple and may last for a number of hours. After several episodes of seizures a spasticity and ataxia are evident in the gait. In time both the seizures and spastic ataxia slowly resolve. By 2 years of age some of these calves may be normal. A hereditary basis is proposed for this syndrome. A similar cerebellar cortical abiotrophy was described in a 9-month-old Charolais calf that developed seizures and spastic ataxia at 6 months of age.[37]

SHEEP. Daft lambs are lambs with a severe cerebellar disorder with signs present at birth that are not obviously progressive. The clinical disease was first described in 1945 and the pathology in 1949 when cerebellar cortical degeneration was observed.[99, 190] Although the clinical signs remained static, sequential autopsies indicated that the degenerative lesion in the cerebellar cortex was progressive. Some of the reported signs (blindness, deafness) in a few of the lambs cannot be related to a cerebellar disorder. The disease has been observed in Welsh Mountain sheep in Scotland and Corriedale sheep in Canada.[98, 181] All evidence to date suggests that the disease is inherited as a recessive trait.

CATS. Olivopontocerebellar atrophy has been reported in the cat.[26, 171] Whether this represents a hypoplasia, abiotrophy, or a variant of the many pathologic effects produced by the feline panleukopenia virus remains to be determined. In the latter, severe cerebellar lesions are often accompanied by marked atrophy of the pontine nuclei and transverse fibers. Olivary neuronal cell counts have not been performed.

Postnatal Syndromes

Abiotrophy. Animals with postnatal cerebellar syndromes are normal at birth or at the time they first begin to ambulate. Some time after a period of normal neurologic activity, a cerebellar ataxia commences. The onset and progression of signs varies from slow (weeks to months) to rapid (few days) with a static course or slow progression.

All of these animals have microscopic evidence of cerebellar degeneration. Usually the lesion predominates in the Purkinje neurons with variable degeneration of granule neurons and occasionally medullary nuclear neuronal degeneration. In some instances, brain stem nuclei show evidence of neuronal degeneration.

Where enough data have been available, a genetic basis has been proposed for these abiotrophies. Most of these appear to be non–sex-linked autosomal recessive inherited diseases. Despite the lack of inflammation and the inability to isolate viral agents with tissue culture techniques, a viral pathogenesis cannot be excluded from the continued investigation of these diseases. Neuronal degeneration without evidence of inflammation has been reported in wild mice with type-C RNA virus present in affected neurons.[79] Also, an environmental noxious substance with a predilection for the metabolic apparatus of cerebellar cortical neurons cannot be overlooked in the attempt to understand the pathogenesis of these diseases.

DOGS

Hereditary Cerebellar Cortical and Extrapyramidal Nuclear Abiotrophy in Kerry Blue Terriers.[49, 53, 54, 137] From 1967 to 1970, ten Kerry blue terriers that developed a progressive cerebellar disorder were studied in a kennel in New York State. The onset was between 9 and 12 weeks of age, and both sexes were affected.

Pelvic limb stiffness and mild head tremor were the earliest signs. The gait abnormality progressed to an obvious dysmetric spastic gait and included the thoracic limbs. All movements were jerky, exaggerated, and forceful. The head tremor was exaggerated during intended movements. Strength was normal, and no involuntary adventitious movements occurred. By 8 to 10 weeks of development of the signs, the truncal ataxia became so pronounced that the side to side and to and fro oscillations of the body made linear mobility difficult. Head, trunk, and limb movements became so disorganized that leaping movements and falling backward occurred frequently. There was a poor response to menacing gestures, even though there was no other evidence of facial paresis or a visual deficit. After 20 weeks of progressive signs, the dogs often were unable to coordinate to stand without support.

Sequential autopsies demonstrated a progressive cerebellar cortical degeneration with ultimate loss of Purkinje neurons. As the disease progressed, a bilaterally symmetric degeneration of the olivary nuclei was observed at 3 months of clinical illness. This was followed at 5 to 6 months of illness by a similar symmetric bilateral degeneration of the substantia nigra and then the caudate nuclei. The lesion was considered an abiotrophy. There was no evidence of inflammation. Viral isolation studies and intracerebral inoculation of diseased tissue into puppies and ferrets were unrewarding.

Between 1973 and 1975, three similarly affected Kerry blue terriers were recognized in California, each from a different litter. The clinical illness was first recognized in two dogs at 3 months of age and in one at 4 months. In all, the signs progressed in a fashion similar to those in the New York dogs. Necropsy of one confirmed the similar development of abiotrophy in the cerebellar cortex and extrapyramidal nuclei. Pedigree analysis showed a direct relationship between the affected litters in New York and California.

In the New York kennel alone there were ten affected puppies from 23 offspring in five litters. Six affected puppies could be predicted from 24 offspring of the mating of carrier parents. The large number of observed affected animals in this study is influenced by the small total number of animals studied, and the lack of any litters without affected animals which would be expected in a larger number of matings.

In 1946 Mettler and Goss described an identical abiotrophy in a Kerry blue terrier that was about 1 year old.[137] They called it a striocerebellar degeneration. Study of a film of this dog and the microscopic slides of affected tissue confirmed that this was the same disease.

Since 1975 similarly affected Kerry blue terriers have been recognized in Texas, Washington, Illinois, Ontario, and England. Common ancestors are present in the pedigrees of all these affected dogs. From pedigree analysis and the matings of known carrier animals, a non–sex-linked autosomal recessive inheritance was established for this disease. One confirmed dog in New York and the dog studied in 1946 have no direct relationship to all the other affected dogs, which may indicate a wider dispersion of the recessive gene than originally suspected.

Because of a concerted effort by the breed association to recognize this disease, publish the affected lines, and not breed identified or potential carrier animals, there appears to have been a significant decrease in the incidence in the last few years.

Numerous heredodegenerative diseases in humans involving the cerebellum have been described and usually classified by the anatomic distribution of the lesions.[50, 94, 152] These include cerebello-olivary degeneration and olivopontocerebellar degeneration, some of which have been determined to be hereditary. More recently, patients with olivopontocerebellar degeneration have been found with degeneration of the substantia nigra and basal nuclei.[115, 118, 170]

The temporal sequence of abiotrophy in these dogs suggests a functional or anatomic relationship between these nuclear groups. In olivopontocerebellar degeneration the neuronal degeneration of the olive and pons has been described as a transsynaptic retrograde chain degeneration of neurons which synapse on neurons (Purkinje neuron and granule neuron) that have already degenerated. In these Kerry blue terriers the pontine nucleus did not degenerate, and the neurons of the substantia nigra and caudate nuclei that did degenerate do not synapse in the cerebellum.

The substantia nigra and caudate nuclei are anatomically and functionally connected via the dopaminergic nigrostriatal pathway.[17, 33, 72, 73] With pharmacologic or anatomic destruction of this system, neuronal argyrophilia and depletion occur, but not the severe necrosis and "ballooning" degeneration observed in these dogs.

An alternative pathogenesis to this multisystem degeneration may be that these cellular groups have a similar biochemical characteristic or metabolic requirement that is deficient or becomes abnormal, and accounts for the pattern of degeneration observed.[160] Although dopamine is a neurotransmitter between the substania nigra and caudate nucleus, it does not function in the cerebellar cortex, in which gamma aminobutyrate is the inhibitory neurotransmitter.

It has been proposed that an excitotoxic mechanism involving glutamic acid neurotransmitter systems may account for the cerebellar cortical and caudate nuclear lesions in these dogs.[138]

Gordon Setters.[40, 55, 178] A cerebellar cortical abiotrophy occurs in Gordon setters with clinical onset between 6 and 36 months of age. Most are recognized by 18 months of age. The onset is later than that recognized in most other breeds, and the initial clinical signs are mild and progress at a slow rate. This often makes the exact time of onset difficult to establish accurately. Under experimental conditions the onset was observed between 6 and 10 months of age.

The earliest signs are a slight spasticity and hypermetria of the thoracic limbs. Owners describe these as a clumsy or prancing gait. The signs are usually more obvious in the thoracic limbs. As the dysmetria worsens, a truncal ataxia occurs with lurching of the trunk in any direction. Neck extension causes the dog to lose its balance and fall backwards. Head tremor and abnormal nystagmus are evident only after many months of progress of the disease.

Even after 6 to 7 years of slowly progressive signs, these dogs can usually still stand to walk but often show severe disorientation in addition to their spastic dysmetric gait. They may stumble in any direction. One patient had a few episodes of sudden recumbency with an opisthotonic posture. This lasted a few minutes before resolving to the previous signs of cerebellar disease. These episodes were considered as cerebellar seizures.

Lesions consist of active degeneration and loss of Purkinje neurons and a reduction of granule neurons. Although this lesion occurs throughout the cerebellum, one study showed a predominance in the dorsal vermis and paravermal (pars intermedia) regions.[40] Pedigree analysis and breeding studies have implicated an autosomal recessive inherited basis for this disease.

Because the clinical signs have been mild enough not to be recognized and not to interfere with breeding, many affected dogs in addition to carriers have been bred, which accounts for the widespread occurrence of this disease. By 1982 over 50 dogs from numerous states in the United States had been diagnosed with this disease. The disease was diagnosed in a Gordon setter in Europe.[182]

The breed association has recognized this as an inherited disease and is in the process of adopting measures to control its spread through genetic control.

Rough-Coated Collie. A similar clinical syndrome has been documented in rough-coated collies in Australia.[87] The onset occurs from 4 to 12 weeks, but the signs in the majority of dogs begin around 6 weeks of age and usually progress fairly rapidly over 1 to 4 weeks. Signs first occur in the pelvic limbs but rapidly spread to all muscles of the body. Although the signs reflect the cerebellar cortical degeneration that is apparent, there is a loss of neurons from the cerebellar nuclei and nuclei in the brain stem and a Wallerian degeneration in the lateral and ventral funiculi of the spinal cord. An autosomal recessive inheritance has been substantiated for this disease in collies.

Others. Cerebellar degenerations have been documented in families of Airedale terriers,[39] Finnish harriers,[180] and Bernese mountain dogs[80] in which a genetic basis was suggested. I have observed similar isolated examples of this disease in one or more of a single litter of the following breeds: Labrador retriever, golden retriever, cocker spaniel, Cairn terrier, and Great Dane.

An autosomal recessive inherited ataxia has been described in smooth-haired fox terriers[20, 21] and Jack Russell terriers.[89] These dogs are normal until 10 to 16 weeks of age, when the abnormal gait is first observed. The clinical signs slowly progress over the ensuing weeks. The description of the clinical signs emphasizes a cerebellar ataxia and/or general proprioceptive tract ataxia. To date, all pathologic descriptions have described only symmetric lesions in the spinal cord white matter with significant involvement of the spinocerebellar tracts. No cerebellar lesions have been reported.

HORSES[117]

Arabian. Similar descriptions of cerebellar ataxia have been reported in Arabian horses or part-Arabian horses in Australia, the United States, and England.[64, 76, 150, 175, 176, 188] The onset of signs is usually from birth to a few months of age. Signs may progress rapidly at first, then remain stabilized or slowly progress. In all cases, a symmetric spasticity of all four limbs is prominent. The degree of dysmetria-hypermetria of the limbs varies from mild to severe. If the horse is startled or the head is suddenly elevated, it may back up, raise its forelimbs off the ground with both rigidly extended, and frequently fall over backwards. The trunk, including the head, often sways side to side as the animal runs. An intentional head tremor is a consistent finding but abnormal nystagmus is not observed. Most affected Arabians have normal vision but fail to respond to menacing gestures by closing their eyelids. A few older Arabians have shown a similar clinical and pathologic syndrome of rapid onset of cerebellar ataxia and head tremor with Purkinje neuronal lesions. The onset of signs in these animals was between 9 and 24 months of age.[165]

There is no significant gross cerebellar abnormality, but microscopic study reveals a widespread loss of Purkinje neurons and frequently a paucity of granule neurons. The lesion varies from folium to folium with relative sparing of some. Evidence of active degeneration is infrequent. Viral isolation studies have been unrewarding and a hereditary basis is presumed.

Gotland Pony. A similar clinical and pathologic syndrome has been described in Gotland ponies with the onset of signs from birth to 6 months.[21, 22] Clinical signs are slowly progressive, and an automosal recessive inheritance has been documented for this disease.

CATTLE

Holstein Friesian. An acute onset of a cerebellar ataxia has been described in Holstein cattle beginning at 3 to 9 months of age.[189] The signs progress rapidly over the first few days, then remain static or very slowly progressive. Most calves ultimately become unable to get up but a few have remained ambulatory.

The gait is characterized by a wide-based posture and marked spasticity of the limbs with varying degrees of hypermetria. There is a characteristic posture of an extended neck with ears retracted, palpebral fissures widened, and a dorsomedial strabismus (the medial angle of the pupil is directed dorsally). Abnormal nystagmus may be observed. These calves have normal vision but often lack a menace response. Their ataxia and stumbling into objects has been misinterpreted as blindness by the owner. Despite the presence of marked limb rigidity and occasionally opisthotonos, these calves remain alert and responsive and have remarkably preserved strength.

The alert sensorium, intact vision, and preserved strength clearly differentiate this disease from polioencephalomalacia (cerebrocortical necrosis), which produces an acute onset of signs in similarly aged calves. Hematologic and CSF studies are normal.

The cerebellar lesion consists of focal areas of loss of Purkinje neurons, evidence of Purkinje neuron degeneration, and gliosis in the Purkinje layer. Occasionally neurons in the cerebellar nuclei have been affected. Pedigree studies have implicated a single bull in the pedigrees of all patients studied to date. A form of recessive inheritance is presumed for this disease.

Another form of hereditary cerebellar cortical abiotrophy with evidence of more extensive degeneration throughout the brain has been reported in Holstein calves.[102] The onset was reported to be from 6 weeks to 5 months of age, with progression of signs until the calves were unable to stand.

SWINE. I have observed cerebellar cortical abiotrophy in Yorkshire pigs. Two different lesions have been observed in two separate clinical syndromes.

Sixteen pigs were studied from seven litters with related parents on four different farms.[78] These pigs were normal until 3 to 5 weeks of age, when a sudden onset of pelvic limb stiffness occurred, followed rapidly by ataxia. The ataxia progressed to the thoracic limbs and recumbency occurred in a few days. Despite being recumbent, these pigs were extremely alert, struggled vigorously with all limbs but, when held up to test postural reactions, rarely would initiate a voluntary movement. Abnormal nystagmus was occasionally observed. No head tremor was seen. Pigs were observed for as long as 4 months. They remained recumbent and unable to rise to a sternal posture, yet they were able to eat and grew well.

The most significant lesion consisted of multiple enlargements of Purkinje neuronal axons (torpedoes) as they coursed through the granule neuron layer. There was minimal loss of

Purkinje neuronal cell bodies, and the granule neuron population was normal. A mild increase in the number of axonal swellings was observed in the pigs with the clinical syndrome that were kept for 4 months.

In a second group of Yorkshire pigs, 14 were affected from five litters with related parents. The sudden onset of stiffness and ataxia that rapidly progressed to recumbency occurred between 1 and 4 weeks of age. The lesion predominated in the vermal and paravermal folia and consisted of complete absence of the external germinal layer and marked loss of Purkinje and granule neurons in the associated cortex. There was little evidence of active neuronal degeneration.

Viral isolation studies on representatives of both groups of Yorkshire pigs were unrewarding. At present, a genetic pathogenesis is suspected.

LABORATORY ANIMALS AND HUMANS. Both viral-induced cerebellar lesions and hereditary cerebellar cortical abiotrophies have been described in laboratory animals. It was the study of a viral-induced cerebellar hypoplasia in rats and hamsters that first led to the discovery of a similar spontaneous disease in domestic animals caused by the feline panleukopenia virus.[56, 112, 147, 187]

Many inherited cerebellar cortical diseases have been described in the laboratory-raised house mouse (Mus musculus).[173] The genetic basis for these diseases has been thoroughly described, and colonies of these mice are maintained for research purposes. Some examples include a line of mice referred to as Lurchers, which have an autosomal dominant mutation that is responsible for a cerebellar cortical abiotrophy with loss of neurons from both the Purkinje and granule neuron layers.[179] The Nervous mouse is a line in which an autosomal recessive trait is related to a Purkinje neuron abiotrophy.[120, 121] Purkinje cell degeneration is another disease in mice in which an autosomal recessive mutation is responsible for severe Purkinje neuron abiotrophy and less severe granule neuron abiotrophy.[122, 139] Weaver mutant mice have a recessively inherited defect in Bergman glial cells, which results in a failure of granule neurons to migrate and populate the granule layer of the cerebellum.[163, 164] In each of these examples, the degree of neuronal population susceptibility to the genetic defect varies as well as the anatomic portion of the cerebellum that is affected.

As continued research on mice with abiotrophy attempts to unravel the biochemical basis for the neuronal defect, the findings may be applicable to the numerous abiotrophies recognized in domestic animals.

In utero viral inflammations are well described in humans, with the effect of the rubella virus infection most closely resembling the bovine virus diarrhea disease that results in ocular lesions.[25, 196]

Numerous heredodegenerative diseases involving the cerebellum have been described and are usually classified by the anatomic distribution of the lesions.[1, 24] These include cerebello-olivary degeneration and olivopontocerebellar degeneration, some of which have been determined to be hereditary. Some cases of olivopontocerebellar degeneration have been associated with degeneration of the substantia nigra and basal nuclei, similar to that recognized in the Kerry blue terrier.[115, 118, 170]

If ultrastructural, pharmacologic, and biochemical studies can elucidate the pathogenesis of these abiotrophies in laboratory or domestic animals, a significant contribution may be made to the understanding of the possible therapy for similar diseases in humans.

Storage Disease. Cerebellar signs may accompany the signs of storage disease in the CNS in cats and dogs—the leukodystrophies and lipodystrophies. These are most common in the Cairn and West Highland white terriers with globoid cell leukodystrophy, whose signs begin either as a mild paraparesis and pelvic limb ataxia, or as a hypermetric ataxia from cerebellar involvement.

One 4-year-old wire-haired dachshund had progressive signs of cerebellar ataxia for over 1 year. There was no clinical evidence of involvement of any other system. At necropsy there was extensive loss of Purkinje cell bodies, but the few that remained had a swollen cytoplasm containing a lipid material. Similar swollen neurons were present in numerous brain stem nuclei and the spinal cord grey matter. Cerebral cortical involvement was less. This was an unusual presentation of a lipodystrophy that has been classified as an adult case of neuronal ceroid-lipofuscinosis, based on the histochemical and ultrastructural characteristics of the cytoplasmic material.[48, 119] This lesion has been observed in other older dachshunds without clinical signs of cerebellar disease.[183]

I studied a 6-month-old Portuguese water dog with 1 month of progressive clinical signs of predominantly a cerebellar ataxia. At autopsy almost all central nervous system neurons were swollen with an accumulation of material in their cytoplasm. This stored substrate has not been identified.

Cats with gangliosidosis often have a significant component of their clinical signs related to the cerebellar disturbance. These include a head tremor, spasticity, hypermetria, and loss of balance. (See table of storage diseases—Chap. 14.)

ACQUIRED CEREBELLAR DISEASES

The cerebellum is subject to involvement by the same kind of lesions that affect the adjacent brain stem and other portions of the central nervous system. These include inflammations, neoplasia, diffuse degenerations, and injuries.

Inflammations. The cerebellar white matter and cortex are affected commonly in dogs by the canine distemper virus, which causes inflammation and necrosis. *Toxoplasma gondii* and *Cryptococcus neoformans* also can affect the cerebellum in dogs and cats. The white matter of the cerebellar peduncles and medulla is a common site for the lesion of granulomatous encephalitis (inflammatory form of reticulosis). This may be part of a diffuse lesion or a focal space-occupying granulomatous lesion with clinical signs limited to this site. The severe meningitis of the caudal fossa in cats with feline infectious peritonitis may cause cerebellar signs. The same may occur in any animal, but more commonly in calves with bacterial meningitis.

Protozoal encephalitis has been observed in the cerebellum of horses, causing asymmetric signs.

Parasitic migration may occur through the cerebellum and produce signs of a cerebellar or vestibular disturbance, or both. A *Cuterebra* larva has been observed in cats, and a *Hypoderma bovis* larva in the horse. *Parelaphostrongylus tenuis* may produce these signs in sheep and goats.

In all of these patients the cerebellar signs usually are accompanied by other neurologic signs suggestive of a multifocal or diffuse disease process. CSF is also usually abnormal.

Neoplasms. Primary and metastatic neoplasms may involve the cerebellum.[194, 195] These often are unilateral at the cerebellomedullary or cerebellopontine angle, and usually produce ipsilateral signs of cerebellovestibular disturbance. They are diagnosed by the signs of adjacent brain stem involvement, including upper motor neuron paresis, general proprioceptive ataxia, ascending reticular activating system depression, and ipsilateral cranial nerve paralysis (trigeminal, facial, vestibulocochlear, glossopharyngeal, and vagal). The most common neoplasm observed at this site is the choroid plexus papilloma or carcinoma. Others include meningioma, neurofibroma, medulloblastoma, astrocytoma, and reticulosis.

Diffuse Degenerations. A number of plants and fungi have been identified as sources of toxins that produce a diffuse central nervous system disorder with tremors, hyperexcitability, and ataxia. These may include some signs of cerebellar dysfunction. (See discussion of Tetany-Tremors in Chapter 7.)

A storage disease can be induced by toxic inhibition of a specific lysosomal enzyme in livestock that graze specific species of plants. In Australia, species of *Swainsona* can produce alpha-mannosidosis.[197] In Brazil, ingestion of *Solanum fastigiatum* by cattle produces a storage disease that profoundly affects the Purkinje neurons in the cerebellum.[198] These cattle have episodes of cerebellar seizures and ataxia.

Injury. Cerebellar signs may predominate following intracranial injury if this structure has received the main impact of the injury. The domestic animal is capable of remarkable compensation following extensive traumatic lesions of the cerebellar cortex. Lesions that involve the cerebellar nuclei produce more severe deficits and the degree of compensation is less.

REFERENCES

1. Adams, R. D., and Sidman, R. L.: Introduction to Neuropathology. New York, McGraw-Hill Book Company, 1968.
2. Altman, J.: Postnatal development of the cerebellar cortex in the rat. I. The external germinal layer and the transitional molecular layer. J. Comp. Neurol., 145:353, 1972.
3. Altman, J.: Postnatal development of the cerebellar cortex in the rat. II. Phases in the maturation of Purkinje cells and of the molecular layer. J. Comp. Neurol., 145:399, 1972.
4. Altman, J.: Postnatal development of the cerebellar cortex in the rat. III. Maturation of the components of the granular layer. J. Comp. Neurol., 145:465, 1972.
5. Altman, J., and Anderson, W.: Experimental reorganization of the cerebellar cortex. I. Morphological effects of elimination of all microneurons with prolonged x-irradiation started at birth. J. Comp. Neurol., 146:355, 1972.
6. Altman, J., and Anderson, W.: Experimental reorganization of the cerebellar cortex. II. Effects of

elimination of most microneurons with prolonged x-irradiation started at 4 days. J, Comp. Neurol., *149*:123, 1973.

7. Appel, M. J. G.: Canine parvovirus infection—An emerging disease. Laboratory Report: James A. Baker Institute for Animal Health, Cornell University, Ithaca, New York, *3*(1), 1979.

8. Appel, M. J. G., Cooper, B. J., Greisen, H., and Carmichael, L. E.: Status report: Canine viral enteritis. J. Am. Vet. Med. Assoc., *173*:1516, 1978.

9. Baird, J. D., and Mackenzie, C. D.: Cerebellar hypoplasia and degeneration in part Arab horses. Aust. Vet. J., *50*:25, 1974.

10. Baker, M. L., Payne, L. C., and Baker, G. N.: The inheritance of hydrocephalus in cattle. J. Hered., *52*:135, 1961.

11. Barlow, R. M.: Further observations on bovine familial convulsions and ataxia. Vet. Rec., *105*:91, 1979.

12. Barlow, R. M.: Morphogenesis of cerebellar lesions in bovine familial convulsions and ataxia. Vet. Pathol., *18*:151, 1981.

13. Barlow, R. M., and Dickinson, A. G.: On the pathology and histochemistry of the central nervous system in border disease of sheep. Res. Vet. Sci., *6*:230, 1965.

14. Barlow, R. M., Linklater, K. A., and Young, G. B.: Familial convulsions and ataxia in Angus calves. Vet. Rec., *83*:60, 1968.

15. Barone, R., and Belkhayat, A.: La conformation et la nomenclature du cervelet des équids. Rev. Med. Vet., *121*:1013, 1970.

16. Barone, R., and Berujon, J.-B.: La morphologie du cervelet chez le Boeuf. Bull. Soc. Sci. Vet. Med. Comp., *72*:3, 1970.

17. Bedard, P.: The nigrostriatal pathway. A correlative study based on neuroanatomical and neurochemical criteria in the cat and monkey. Exp. Neurol., *25*:365, 1969.

18. Beery, F.: Untersuchungen über die Entwicklung der Motilität und die histologische Differenzierung des Kleinhirns bei der Katze in den eroten Lebenswochen. Schweiz. Arch. Tierheilk., *104*:701, 1962.

19. Bistner, S. I., Rubin, L. F., and Saunders, L. Z.: The ocular lesions of bovine viral diarrhea-mucosal disease. Vet. Pathol., *7*:275, 1970.

20. Bjorck, G., Dyrendahl, S., and Olsson, S. E.: Hereditary ataxia in smooth-haired fox terriers. Vet. Rec., *69*:871, 1957.

21. Bjorck, G., Everz, K.-E., Hansen, H.-J., and Henricson, B.: Cerebellar hypoplasia in the Gotland pony breed. Proceedings 18th World Veterinary Congress, Paris, 1967, 818.

22. Bjorck, G., Everz, K. E., Hansen, H.-J., and Henricson, B.: Congenital cerebellar ataxia in the Gotland pony breed. Zentralbl. Veterinaermed., *20*:341, 1973.

23. Bjorck, G., Mair, W., Olsson, S.-E., and Sourander, P.: Hereditary ataxia in fox terriers. Arch. Neuropathol. [Suppl.], *1*:45, 1962.

24. Blackwood, W., McMenemey, W. H., Meyer, A., Norma, R. M., and Russell, D. S.: Greenfield's Neuropathology. Baltimore, Williams and Wilkins Company, 1963.

25. Boniuk, V., and Boniuk, M.: The congenital rubella syndrome. Int. Ophthalmol. Clin., *8*:487, 1968.

26. Brouwer, B.: Familial olivopontocerebellar hypoplasia in cats. Psychiatry Neurol. Bl. (Amsterdam), *38*:352, 1934.

27. Brown, T. T., Bistner, S. I., de Lahunta, A., Scott, F. W., and McEntee, K.: Pathogenetic studies of infection of the bovine fetus with bovine viral diarrhea virus. II. Ocular lesions. Vet. Pathol., *12*:394, 1975.

28. Brown, T. T.: Pathogenetic Studies of Bovine Viral Diarrhea Infection in the Bovine Fetus. Ph.D. thesis, Ithaca, N.Y., Cornell University, 1973.

29. Brown, T. T., de Lahunta, A., Bistner, S. I., Scott, F. W., and McEntee, K.: Pathogenetic studies of infection of the bovine fetus with bovine viral diarrhea virus. I. Cerebellar atrophy. Vet. Pathol., *11*:486, 1974.

30. Brown, T. T., de Lahunta, A., Scott, F. W., Kahrs, R. F., McEntee, K., and Gillespie, J. H.: Virus-induced congenital anomalies of the bovine fetus. II. Histopathology of cerebellar degeneration (hypoplasia) induced by the virus of bovine viral diarrhea-mucosal disease. Cornell Vet., *63*:561, 1973.

31. Cajal, S., and Ramon, Y.: Degeneration and Regeneration of the Nervous System. New York, Hafner Company, 1959.

32. Carpenter, M. B., and Donald, H.: A study of congenital feline cerebellar malformations. J. Comp. Neurol., *105*:51, 1956.

33. Carpenter, M. B., and Peter, P.: Nigrostriatal and nigrothalamic fibers in the Rhesus monkey. J. Comp. Neurol., *144*:93, 1972.

34. Chambers, W. W., and Spraque, J. M.: Functional localization in the cerebellum. I. Organization in longitudinal corticonuclear zones and their contribution to the control of posture both extrapyramidal and pyramidal. J. Comp. Neurol., *103*:105, 1955.

35. Chambers, W. W., and Spraque, J. M.: Functional localization in the cerebellum. II. Somatotopic organization in cortex and nuclei. Arch. Neurol. Psychiatry, *74*:653, 1955.

36. Chan-Palay, V., Palay, S. L., and Wu, J. Y.: Gamma aminobutyric acid pathways in the cerebellum studied by retrograde and anterograde transport of glutamic acid decarboxylase antibody after in vivo injections. Anat. Embryol., *157*:1, 1979.

37. Cho, D. Y., and Leipold, H. W.: Cerebellar cortical atrophy in a Charolais calf. Vet. Pathol., *15*:264, 1978.

38. Cordy, D. R., and Schultz, G.: Congenital subcortical encephalopathies in lambs. J. Neuropathol. Exp. Neurol., *20*:554, 1961.

39. Cordy, D. R., and Snelbaker, H. A.: Cerebellar hypoplasia and degeneration in a family of Airedale dogs. J. Neuropathol. Exp. Neurol., *11*:324, 1952.

40. Cork, L. C., Troncoso, J. C., and Price, D. L.: Canine inherited ataxia. Ann. Neurol., *9*:492, 1981.

41. Courville, J., and Faraco-Cantin, F.: On the origin of the climbing fibers of the cerebellum: An experimental study in the cat with an autoradiographic tracing method. Neuroscience, *3*:797, 1978.

42. Coverdale, O. R., Cybinski, D. H., and St. George, T. D.: Congenital abnormalities in calves associated with Akabane virus and Aino virus. Aust. Vet. J., *54*:151, 1978.

43. Csiza, C. K.: Feline Panleukopenia Virus as an Etiological Agent of Ataxia: Pathogenesis and Immune Carrier State. Ph.D. thesis, Ithaca, N.Y., Cornell University, 1970.

44. Csiza, C. K., de Lahunta, A., Scott, F. W., and Gillespie, J. H.: Spontaneous feline ataxia. Cornell Vet., 62:300, 1972.

45. Csiza, C. K., Scott, F. W., de Lahunta, A., and Gillespie, J. H.: Pathogenesis of feline panleukopenia virus in susceptible newborn kittens. I. Clinical signs, hematology, serology and virology. Infect. Immun., 3:833, 1971.

46. Csiza, C. K., Scott, F. W., de Lahunta, A., and Gillespie, J. H.: Pathogenesis of feline panleukopenia virus in susceptible newborn kittens. II. Pathology and Immunofluoresence. Infect. Immun., 3:838, 1971.

47. Csiza, C. K., Scott, F. W., de Lahunta, A., and Gillespie, J. H.: Respiratory signs and central nervous system lesions in cats infected with panleukopenia virus: A case report. Cornell Vet., 62:192, 1972.

48. Cummings, J. F., and de Lahunta, A.: An adult case of canine neuronal ceroid-lipofuscinosis. Acta Neuropathol., 39:43, 1977.

49. Deforest, M. E., Eger, C. E., and Basrur, P. K.: Hereditary cerebellar neuronal abiotrophy in a Kerry blue terrier dog. Can. Vet. J., 19:198, 1978.

50. Dejerine, J., and Thomas, A.: L'atrophie olivopontocerebelleuse. Nouv. Iconogr. Salpet., 13:330, 1900.

51. de Lahunta, A.: Comparative cerebellar disease in domestic animals. Compend. Contin. Ed., 2:8, 1980.

52. de Lahunta, A.: Diseases of the cerebellum. Vet. Clin. North Am.: Small Anim. Pract., 10:91, 1980.

53. de Lahunta, A.: Hereditary cerebellar cortical and extrapyramidal nuclear abiotrophy in Kerry blue terriers. Proceedings 20th World Veterinary Congress, Greece, 1975.

54. de Lahunta, A., and Averill, D. R., Jr.: Hereditary cerebellar cortical and extrapyramidal nuclear abiotrophy in Kerry blue terriers. J. Am. Vet. Med. Assoc., 168:1119, 1976.

55. de Lahunta, A., Fenner, W. R., Indrieri, R. J., Mellick, P. W., Gardner, S., and Bell, J. S.: Hereditary cerebellar cortical abiotrophy in the Gordon setter. J. Am. Vet. Med. Assoc., 177:538, 1980.

56. Del Cerro, M., Nathanson, N., and Monjan, A. A.: Pathogenesis of cerebellar hypoplasia produced by lymphocytic choriomeningitis virus infection of neonatal rats. II. An ultrastructural study of the immune-mediated pathology. Lab. Invest., 33:608, 1975.

57. Del Cerro, M. P., and Snider, R. S.: Studies on the developing cerebellum. II. The ultrastructure of the external granule layer. J. Comp. Neurol., 144:131, 1972.

58. Della-Porta, A. J., Murray, M. D., and Cybinski, D. H.: Congenital bovine epizootic arthrogryposis and hydranencephaly in Australia: Distribution of antibodies to Akabane virus in Australian cattle after the 1974 epizootic. Aust. Vet. J., 52:496, 1976.

59. Dickinson, A. G., and Barlow, R. N.: The demonstration of the transmissibility of border disease of sheep. Vet. Rec., 81:114, 1967.

60. Done, J. T., Terlecki, S., Richardson, C., Harkness, J. S., Sands, J. J., Patterson, D. S. P., Sweasey, D., Shaw, I. G., Winkler, C. E., and Duffell, S. J.: Bovine virus diarrhea mucosal disease virus: Pathogenicity for the fetal calf following maternal infection. Vet. Rec., 106:473, 1980.

61. Dow, R. W.: The evolution and anatomy of the cerebellum. Biol. Rev., 17:179, 1942.

62. Dow, R. W.: Partial agenesis of the cerebellum in dogs. J. Comp. Neurol., 72:569, 1940.

63. Dow, R. W., and Moruzzi, G.: The Physiology and Pathology of the Cerebellum. Minneapolis, University of Minnesota Press, 1958.

64. Dungworth, D. L., and Fowler, M. E.: Cerebellar hypoplasia and degeneration in a foal. Cornell Vet., 55:17, 1966.

65. Eager, R. P.: Efferent corticonuclear pathways in the cerebellum of the cat. J. Comp. Neurol., 120:81, 1963.

66. Eccles, J. C.: The development of the cerebellum of vertebrates in relation to the control of movement. Naturwissenschaften, 56:525, 1969.

67. Eccles, J. C., Llinas, R., and Sasaki, K.: Golgi cell inhibition in the cerebellar cortex. Nature, 204:1265, 1964.

68. Edmonds, L., Crenshaw, D., and Selby, L. A.: Micrognathia and cerebellar hypoplasia in an Aberdeen Angus herd. J. Hered., 64:62, 1973.

69. Ekerot, C. F., and Larson, B.: Correlation between sagittal projection zones of climbing and mossy fibre paths in cat cerebellar anterior lobe. Brain Res., 64:446, 1973.

70. Emerson, J. L., and Delez, A. L.: Cerebellar hypoplasia, hypomyelinogenesis, and congenital tremors of pigs associated with prenatal hog cholera vaccination of sows. J. Am. Vet. Med. Assoc., 147:47, 1965.

71. Fankhauser, R.: Cerebelläre Encephalitis beim Rind. Schweiz. Arch. Tierheilk., 103:292, 1961.

72. Fibiger, H. C., McGeer, E. G., and Atmadja, S.: Axoplasmic transport of dopamine in nigrostriatal neurons. J. Neurochem., 21:373, 1973.

73. Fibiger, H. C., Pudritz, R. E., McGeer, P. O., and McGeer, E. G.: Axonal transport in nigrostriatal and nigrothalamic neurons: Effects of medial forebrain bundle lesions and 6-hydroxydopamine. J. Neurochem., 19:1697, 1972.

74. Finnie, E. P., and Leaver, D. D.: Cerebellar hypoplasia in calves. Aust. Vet. J., 41:287, 1965.

75. Fletcher, T. F.: Ablation and histopathologic studies on myoclonia congenita in swine. Am. J. Vet. Res., 29:2255, 1968.

76. Fraser, H.: Two dissimilar types of cerebellar disorder in the horse. Vet. Rec., 78:608, 1966.

77. Frauchiger, E., and Fankhauser, R.: Vergleichende Neuropathologie des Menschen und der Tiere. Berlin, Springer-Verlag, 1957.

78. Gardner, C.: Cerebellar degeneration in three pigs. Senior seminar, Flower Veterinary Library, Ithaca, N.Y., New York State College of Veterinary Medicine, 1972.

79. Gardner, M. B., Henderson, B. E., Officer, J. E., Rongey, R. W., Parker, J. C., Oliver, C., Estes, J. D., and Huebner, R. J.: A spontaneous lower motor neuron disease apparently caused by indigenous type-C RNA virus in wild mice. J. Natl. Cancer Inst., 51:1243, 1973.

80. Good, R.: Untersuchungen uber eine Kleinhirn rindenatrophie beim Hund. Dissertation, University of Bern, Switzerland, 1962.

81. Gowers, W. R.: A lecture on abiotrophy. Lancet, 1:1003, 1902.

82. Gowers, W. R.: The pathology of tabes dorsalis and general paralysis of the insane. Lancet, 2:1591, 1899.

83. Green, H. J.: Congenital hydranencephaly and cerebellar hypoplasia in calves. J. Am. Vet. Med. Assoc., 173:1008, 1978.

84. Greene, C. E., Vandevelde, M., and Braund, K.: Lissencephaly in two Lhasa apso dogs. J. Am. Vet. Med. Assoc., 169:405, 1976.

85. Hamilton, A. F., and Timoney, P. J.: Bovine virus diarrhea-mucosal disease virus and border disease. Res. Vet. Sci., 15:265, 1973.

86. Harding, J. D. J., Done, J. T., Harbourne, J. F., Randall, C. J., and Gilbert, F. R.: Congenital tremor type A III in pigs, and hereditary sex-linked cerebrospinal hypomyelinogenesis. Vet. Rec., 92:527, 1973.

87. Hartley, W. J., Barker, J. S. F., Wanner, R. A., and Farrow, B. R. H.: Inherited cerebellar degeneration in the rough coated Collie. Aust. Vet. Pract., 8:1–7, 1978.

88. Hartley, W. J., De Saram, W. G., Della-Porta, A. J., Snowdon, W. A., and Shepherd, N. C.: Pathology of congenital bovine epizootic arthrogryposis and hydranencephaly and its relationship to Akabane virus. Aust. Vet. J., 53:319, 1977.

89. Hartley, W. J., and Palmer, A. C.: Ataxia in Jack Russell terriers. Acta Neuropathol., 26:71, 1973.

90. Hartley, W. J., Wanner, R. A., Della-Porta, A. J., and Snowdon, W. A.: Serological evidence for the association of Akabane virus with epizootic bovine congenital arthrogryposis and hydranencephaly syndromes in New South Wales. Aust. Vet. J., 51:103, 1975.

91. Herringham, W. P., and Andrews, F. W.: Two cases of cerebellar disease in cats with staggering. Saint Bartholomew's Hospital Report (London), 24:241, 1888.

92. Holden, M.: Unusual ataxia in three Samoyeds. Senior seminar, Flower Veterinary Library, Ithaca, N.Y., New York State College of Veterinary Medicine, 1974.

93. Holliday, T. A.: Clinical signs of acute and chronic experimental lesions of the cerebellum. Vet. Sci. Comm., 3:259, 1979/1980.

94. Holmes, G.: A form of familial degeneration of the cerebellum. Brain, 30:466, 1907.

95. Hulland, T. J.: Cerebellar ataxia in calves. Can. J. Comp. Med. Vet. Sci., 21:72, 1957.

96. Inaba, Y., Kurogi, H., and Omori, T.: Akabane disease, epizootic abortion, premature birth, stillbirth and congenital arthrogryposis-hydranencephaly in cattle, sheep and goats caused by Akabane virus. Aust. Vet. J., 51:584, 1975.

97. Innes, I. M. R., Russell, D. S., and Wilsdon, A. J.: Familial cerebellar hypoplasia and degeneration in Hereford calves. J. Pathol. Bacteriol., 50:455, 1940.

98. Innes, J. R. M., and MacNaughton, W. M.: Inherited cortical cerebellar atrophy in Corriedale lambs in Canada identical with "daft lamb" disease in Britain. Cornell Vet., 40:127, 1950.

99. Innes, J. R. M., Rowlands, W. T., and Parry, H. B.: An inherited form of cortical cerebellar atrophy in (daft) lambs in Great Britain. Vet. Rec., 61:225, 1949.

100. Ito, M.: Recent advances in cerebellar physiology and pathology. Adv. Neurol., 21:59, 1978.

101. Jennings, A. R., and Summer, G. R.: Cortical cerebellar disease in an Ayrshire. Vet. Rec., 63:60, 1951.

102. Johnson, K. R., Fourt, D. L., and Ross, R. H.: Hereditary congenital ataxia in Holstein-Friesian calves. J. Dairy Sci., 41:1371, 1958.

103. Johnson, R. H., Margolis, G., and Kilham, L.: Identity of feline ataxia virus with the feline panleukopenia virus. Nature, 214:175, 1967.

104. Kahrs, R. E.: The relationship of bovine viral diarrhea-mucosal disease to abortion in cattle. J. Am. Vet. Med. Assoc., 153:1652, 1968.

105. Kahrs, R. F., Lein, D. F., Fullen, H. K., de Lahunta, A., Braun, R. K., Brown, T. A., Duncan, R., Kenny, R. M., McKenzie, B., Parsonson, I. M., Scott, F. W., Wilkie, B. D., and DeRock, O.: An epizootiological investigation into bovine viral diarrhea-mucosal disease as the suspected etiological agent of a series of abortions, stillbirths, early neonatal deaths, and congenital cerebellar disease in a New York dairy herd. Paper No. 1. Epizootiology Series from Dept. of Large Animal Medicine, Obstetrics and Surgery, New York State Veterinary College, Cornell University, Ithaca, N.Y., 1969.

106. Kahrs, R. F., Scott, F. W., and de Lahunta, A.: Congenital cerebellar hypoplasia and ocular defects in calves following bovine viral diarrhea-mucosal disease infection in pregnant cattle. J. Am. Vet. Med. Assoc., 156:1443, 1970.

107. Kahrs, R. F., Scott, F. W., and de Lahunta, A.: Bovine viral diarrhea-mucosal disease abortion, and congenital cerebellar hypoplasia in a dairy herd. J. Am. Vet. Med. Assoc., 156:851, 1970.

108. Kahrs, R. F., Scott, F. W., and de Lahunta, A.: Epidemiological observations on bovine viral diarrhea-mucosal disease, virus-induced congenital cerebellar hypoplasia and ocular defects in calves. Teratology, 3:181, 1970.

109. Kaufmann, J.: Untersuchungen über die Frühentwicklung des Kleinhirns beim Rind. Schweiz. Arch. Tierheilk., 101:49, 1959.

110. Kay, W. J., and Budzelovich, G. N.: Cerebellar hypoplasia and agenesis in the dog. J. Neuropathol. Exp. Neurol., 29:156, 1970.

111. Kilham, L., and Margolis, G.: Viral etiology of spontaneous ataxia of cats. Am. J. Pathol., 48:991, 1966.

112. Kilham, L., and Margolis, G.: Cerebellar disease in cats induced by inoculation of rat virus. Science, 148:244, 1965.

113. Kilham, L., Margolis, G., and Colby, E. D.: Cerebellar ataxia and its congenital transmission in cats by feline panleukopenia virus. J. Am. Vet. Med. Assoc., 158:888, 1971.

114. Kilham, L., Margolis, G., and Colby, E. D.: Congenital infections of cats and ferrets by feline panleukopenia virus manifested by cerebellar hypoplasia. Lab. Invest., 17:465, 1967.

115. Klawans, H. O., and Zeitlin, Z.: L-Dopa in parkinsonism associated with cerebellar dysfunction (probable olivopontocerebellar degeneration). J. Neurol. Neurosurg. Psychiatry, 34:14, 1971.

116. Knecht, C. D., Lamar, C. H., Schaible, R., and Pflum, K.: Cerebellar hypoplasia in Chow Chows. J. Am. Anim. Hosp. Assoc., 15:51, 1979.

117. Koch, P., and Fischer, H.: Die Oldenburger Fohlenataxie als Erbkrankheit. Tierärzt Umschau., 5:317, 1950.

118. Konigsmark, B. W., and Lipton, H. O.: Dominant

olivopontocerebellar atrophy with dementia and extrapyramidal signs: A report of a family through 3 generations. J. Neuropathol. Exp. Neurol., 30:133, 1971.

119. Koppang, N.: Canine ceroid-lipofuscinosis—A model for human neuronal ceroid-lipofuscinosis and aging. Mech. Ageing Dev., 2:421, 1973.

120. Landis, S. C.: Granule cell heterotopia in normal and nervous mutant mice of the BALA/c strain. Brain Res., 61:175, 1973.

121. Landis, S. C.: Ultrastructural changes in the mitochondria of cerebellar Purkinje cells of nervous mice. J. Cell Biol., 57:782, 1973.

122. Landis, S. C., and Mullen, R. J.: The development and degeneration of Purkinje cells in pcd mutant mice. J. Comp. Neurol., 177:125, 1978.

123. Lapham, L. W., Lentz, R. D., Woodward, D. J., Hoffer, B. J., and Herman, B. J.: Postnatal development of tetraploid DNA content in the Purkinje neuron of the rat: An aspect of cellular differentiation. In Pease, D. ed., Cellular Aspects of Neural Growth and Regulation—UCLA Forum in Medical Sciences, 14:61, 1971.

124. Larsell, O.: The Comparative Anatomy and Histology of the Cerebellum from Monotremes Through Apes. Minneapolis, University of Minnesota Press, 1970.

125. Lentz, R. D., and Lapham, L. W.: Postnatal development of tetraploid DNA content in rat Purkinje cells: A quantitative cytochemical study. J. Neuropathol. Exp. Neurol., 29:43, 1970.

126. Llinas, R. R.: The cortex of the cerebellum. Sci. Am., 232:56, 1975.

127. Llinas, R. R.: Neurobiology of cerebellar evolution and development. Proceedings First International Symposium of the Institute for Biomedical Research, 1969.

128. Lockhard, I., and Gillian, L. A.: Neurologic dysfunctions and their relation to congenital abnormalities of the central nervous system of cats. J. Comp. Neurol., 104:403, 1965.

129. Mare, C. J., and Kluge, J. P.: Pseudorabies virus and myoclonia congenita in pigs. J. Am. Vet. Med. Assoc., 164:309, 1974.

130. Margolis, G., and Kilham, L,: In pursuit of an ataxic hamster or virus-induced cerebellar hypoplasia. In Bailey, O. D., and Smith, D. E. (eds.): The Central Nervous System. Baltimore, Williams & Wilkins, 1968, 157–183.

131. Margolis, G., and Kilham, L.: Virus-induced cerebellar hypoplasia. In Infections of the Nervous System. Res. Publ. A.R.N.M.D., 44:113, 1968.

132. Margolis, G., Kilham, L., and Johnson, R. H.: The parvoviruses and replicating cells: Insight into the pathogenesis of cerebellar hypoplasia. Progr. Neuropathol., 1:168, 1971.

133. Markson, L. M., Terlecki, S., Shand, A., Sellers, K. C., and Woods, A. J.: Hypomyelinogenesis congenita in sheep. Vet. Rec., 71:269, 1959.

134. Matsushita, M., and Hosoya, Y.: The location of spinal projection neurons in the cerebellar nuclei (cerebellospinal tract neurons) of the cat: A study with horseradish peroxidase technique. Brain Res., 142:237, 1978.

135. McC. Howell, J., and Ritchie, H. E.: Cerebellar malformations in two Ayrshire calves. Pathol. Vet., 3:159, 1966.

136. McKercher, D. G., Saito, J. K., and Singh, K. V.: Serologic evidence of an etiologic role for Blue-

tongue virus in hydranencephaly of calves. J. Am. Vet. Med. Assoc., 156:1044, 1970.

137. Mettler, F. A., and Goss, L. J.: Canine chorea due to striocerebellar degeneration of unknown etiology. J. Am. Vet. Med. Assoc., 108:377, 1946.

138. Montgomery, D. L., and Storts, R. W.: Hereditary striatonigral and cerebello-olivary degeneration in the Kerry blue terrier. Proc. Am. Coll. Vet. Pathol., 31:119, 1980.

139. Mullen, R. J., Eicher, E. M., and Sidman, R. L.: Purkinje cell degeneration, a new neurological mutation in the mouse. Proc. Natl. Acad. Sci. U.S.A., 73:208, 1976.

140. Nobel, T. A., Klopfer, V., and Newmann, F.: Pathology of an arthrogryposis-hydranencephaly syndrome in domestic ruminants in Israel, 1969–1970. Refuah Vet., 28:144, 1971.

141. Oliver, J. E., and Geary, J. C.: Cerebellar anomalies—two cases. Vet. Med. Small Anim. Clin., 60:697, 1965.

142. Omori, T., Inaba, Y., Kurogi, H., Miura, Y., Nobuto, K., Ohashi, Y., and Matsumoto, M.: Viral abortion, arthrogryposis-hydranencephaly syndrome in cattle in Japan, 1972–1974. Bull. Off. Int. Epiz., 81:447, 1974.

143. Orman, H. K., and Grace, O. D.: Hereditary encephalopathy, a hydrocephalus syndrome in newborn calves. Cornell Vet., 54:229, 1964.

144. Osburn, B. I., Clarke, G. L., Stewart, W. C., and Sawyer, M.: Border disease-like syndrome in lambs: Antibodies to hog cholera and bovine viral diarrhea viruses. J. Am Vet. Med. Assoc., 163:1165, 1973.

145. Osburn, B. I., Johnson, R. T., Silverstein, A. M., Prendergast, R. A., Jochim, M. M., and Levy, S. E.: Experimental viral-induced congenital encephalopathies. II. The pathogenesis of bluetongue vaccine virus infection in fetal lambs. Lab. Invest., 25:206, 1971.

146. Osburn, B. I., Silverstein, A. M., Prendergast, R. A., Johnson, R. T., and Parshall, C. J., Jr.: Experimental viral-induced congenital encephalopathies. I. Pathology of hydranencephaly and porencephaly caused by Bluetongue vaccine virus. Lab. Invest., 25:197, 1971.

147. Oster-Granite, M. L., and Herndon, R. M.: The pathogenesis of parvovirus-induced cerebellar hypoplasia in the Syrian hamster, Mesocricetus auratus, fluorescent antibody, foliation cytoarchitectonic, Golgi, and electron microscopic studies. J. Comp. Neurol., 169:481, 1976.

148. O'Sullivan, B. M., and McPhee, C. P.: Cerebellar hypoplasia of genetic origin in calves. Aust. Vet. J., 51:468, 1975.

149. Palmer, A. C.: Pathogenesis and pathology of the cerebello-vestibular syndrome. J. Small Anim. Pract., 11:167, 1970.

150. Palmer, A. C., Blakemore, W. F., Cook, W. R., Platt, H., and Whitwell, K. E.: Cerebellar hypoplasia and degeneration in the young Arab horse; clinical and neuropathological features. Vet. Rec., 93:62, 1973.

151. Palmer, A. C., Payne, J. E., and Wallace, M. E.: Hereditary quadriplegia and amblyopia in the Irish setter. J. Small Anim. Pract., 14:343, 1973.

152. Parker, H. L., and Kernohan, J. W.: Parenchymatous cortical cerebellar atrophy (chronic atrophy of Purkinje cells). Brain, 56:191, 1933.

153. Parsonson, I. M., Della-Porta, A. J., and Snowdon,

W. A.: Congenital abnormalities in fetal lambs after inoculation in pregnant ewes with Akabane virus. Aust. Vet. J., *51*:585, 1975.

154. Patterson, D. S. P., and Sweasey, D.: Lipid hexose: phosphorus ratio as an aid to the diagnosis of congenital myelin defects in lambs and piglets. Acta Neuropathol., *15*:318, 1970.

155. Patterson, D. S. P., Sweasey, D., and Harding, J. D. J.: Lipid deficiency in the central nervous system of Landrace piglets affected with congenital tremor A-III, a form of cerebrospinal hypomyelinogenesis. J. Neurochem., *19*:2797, 1972.

156. Patterson, D. S. P., Sweasey, D., and Hebert, C. N.: Changes occurring in the chemical composition of the CNS during fetal and postnatal development of the sheep. J. Neurochem., *18*:2027, 1971.

157. Patterson, D. S. P., Sweasey, D., Brush, P. J., and Harding, J. D. J.: Neurochemistry of the spinal cord in British saddleback piglets affected with congenital tremor type A-IV, a second form of hereditary cerebrospinal hypomyelinogenesis. J. Neurochem., *21*:397, 1973.

158. Patterson, D. S. P., Terlecki, S., Dore, J. T., Sweasey, D., and Hebert, C. N.: Neurochemistry of the spinal cord in experimental border disease (hypomyelinogenesis congenita) of lambs. J. Neurochem., *18*:883, 1971.

159. Percy, D. H., Carmichael, L. E., Albert, D. M., King, J. M., and Jonas, J. M.: Lesions in puppies surviving infection with canine herpesvirus. Vet. Pathol., *8*:37, 1971.

160. Perry, L., Hansen, S., Berry, K., Currier, D., and Schut, L. J.: Amino acid neurotransmitters in dominantly inherited cerebellar disorders. Symposium Bel-Air, *6*:183, 1980.

161. Phemister, R. D., and Young, S.: The postnatal development of the canine cerebellar cortex. J. Comp. Neurol., *134*:243, 1968.

162. Rakic, P.: Neuron-glia relationship during granule cell migration in developing cerebellar cortex. A Golgi and electronmicroscopic study in *Macacus rhesus*. J. Comp. Neurol., *141*:283, 1971.

163. Rakic, P., and Sidman, R. L.: Organization of cerebellar cortex secondary to deficit of granule cells in weaver mutant mice. J. Comp. Neurol., *152*:133, 1973.

164. Rakic, P., and Sidman, R. L.: Sequence of development and abnormalities leading to granule cell deficit in cerebellar cortex of weaver mutant mice. J. Comp. Neurol., *152*:103, 1973.

165. Reed, S.: Personal communication, 1982.

166. Richards, W. P. C., Crenshaw, G. L., and Bushnell, R. B.: Hydranencephaly of calves associated with natural Bluetongue virus infection. Cornell Vet., *61*:336, 1971.

167. Russell, J. S. E.: Defective development of the cerebellum in a puppy. Brain, *18*:523, 1895.

168. Satterthwaite, W. R., Talbott, R. E., and Brookhart, J. M.: Changes in canine postural control after injury to anterior vermal cerebellum. Brain Res., *164*:269, 1979.

169. Saunders, L. Z., Sweet, J. D., Martin, S. M., Fox, F. H., and Fincher, M. G.: Hereditary congenital ataxia in Jersey calves. Cornell Vet., *42*:559, 1952.

170. Scherer, H. J.: Extrapyramidale Störungen bei der olivopontocerebellaren Atrophie: ein Beitrag zum Problem des lokalen vorzeitigen Alterns. Zentralbl. Ges. Neurol. Psychiat., *146*:406, 1933.

171. Schut, J. W.: Olivopontocerebellar atrophy in a cat. J. Neuropathol. Exp. Neurol., *5*:77, 1946.

172. Scott, F. W., Kahrs, R. F., de Lahunta, A., Brown, T. T., McEntee, K., and Gillespie, J. H.: Virus induced congenital anomalies of the bovine fetus. I. Cerebellar degeneration (hypoplasia), ocular lesions and fetal mummification following experimental infection with bovine viral diarrhea-mucosal disease virus. Cornell Vet., *63*:536, 1973.

173. Sidman, R. L., Green, M. C., and Appel, S. H.: Catalog of the Neurological Mutants of the Mouse. Cambridge, Mass. Harvard University Press, 1965.

174. Smith, D. E., and Downs, I.: Postnatal development of the granule cell in the kitten cerebellum. Am. J. Anat., *151*:527, 1978.

175. Sponseller, M. L.: Equine cerebellar hypoplasia and degeneration. J. Am. Vet. Med. Assoc., *152*:313, 1968.

176. Sponseller, M. L.: Equine cerebellar hypoplasia and degeneration. Proc. Am. Assoc. Equine Pract., *13*:123, 1967.

177. Spraque, J. M., and Chambers, W. M.: Regulation of posture in intact and decerebrate cat. I. Cerebellum, reticular formation, vestibular nuclei. J. Neurophysiol., *16*:451, 1953.

178. Steinberg, S., Troncoso, J. C., Cork, L. C., and Price, D. L.: Clinical features of inherited cerebellar degeneration in Gordon setters. J. Am. Vet. Med. Assoc., *179*:886, 1981.

179. Swisher, D. A., and Wilson, D. B.: Cerebellar dysplasia in lurcher (Lc) mutant mice. Anat. Rec., *181*:489, 1975.

180. Tontitila, P., and Lindberg, L. A.: ETT fall av cerebellar ataxi hos finsk stoväre. Svoman Elainlääkarilehti, *77*:135, 1971.

181. Van Bogaert, L., and Innes, J. R. M.: Cerebellar disorders in lambs. Arch. Pathol., *50*:36, 1950.

182. Vandevelde, M.: Personal communication, 1982.

183. Vandevelde, M., and Fatzer, R.: Neuronal ceroid-lipofuscinosis in older Dachshunds. Vet. Pathol., *17*:686, 1980.

184. Verhaart, W. J. C.: Partial agenesis of the cerebellum and medulla and total agenesis of the corpus callosum in a goat. J. Comp. Neurol., *77*:49, 1942.

185. Ward, G. M.: Bovine cerebellar hypoplasia apparently caused by BVD-MD virus: A case report. Cornell Vet., *59*:570, 1969.

186. Ward, G. M., Roberts, S. J., McEntee, K., and Gillespie, J. H.: A study of experimentally induced bovine viral diarrhea-mucosal disease in pregnant cattle and their progeny. Cornell Vet., *59*:525, 1969.

187. Weiner, L. P., Herndon, R. M., and Johnson, R. T.: Animal models of viral-induced ataxia: Implications for human disease. Adv. Neurol., *21*:373, 1978.

188. Wheat, J. D., and Kennedy, P. C.: Cerebellar hypoplasia and its sequela in a horse. J. Am. Vet. Med. Assoc., *131*:291, 1957.

189. White, M. E., Whitlock, R. H., and de Lahunta, A.: A cerebellar abiotrophy of calves. Cornell Vet., *65*:476, 1975.

190. White, R. G., and Rowlands, W. T.: An hereditary defect of newly-born lambs. Vet. Rec., *44*:491, 1945.

191. Whittem, J. H.: Congenital abnormalities in calves: Arthrogryposis and hydranencephaly. J. Pathol. Bacteriol., *73*:375, 1957.

192. Young, G. A., Kitchell, R. A., Luedke, A. J., and Sautter, J. H.: The effect of viral and other infections of the dam on fetal development in swine. I. Modified live hog cholera viruses—immunological, virological, and gross pathological studies. J. Am. Vet. Med. Assoc., *126*:165, 1955.

193. Young, S.: Hypomyelinogenesis congenita (cerebellar ataxia) in Angus-Shorthorn calves. Cornell Vet., *52*:84, 1962.

194. Zaki, F. A., and Kay, W. J.: Carcinoma of the choroid plexus in a dog. J. Am. Vet. Med. Assoc., *164*:1195, 1974.

195. Zaki, F. A., Liu, S. K., and Kay, W. J.: Calcifying aponeurotic fibroma in a dog. J. Am. Vet. Med. Assoc., *106*:384, 1975.

196. Zimmerman, L. E.: Histopathologic basis for ocular manifestation of congenital rubella syndrome. Am. J. Ophthalmol., *65*:837, 1968.

197. Dorling, P. R., Huxtable, C. R., and Vogel, P.: Lysosomal storage in *Swainsona* spp. toxicosis: An induced mannosidosis. Neuropathol. Appl. Neurobiol., *4*:285, 1978.

198. Riet-Correa, F., Mendez, M. D. C., Schild, A. L., Summers, B. A., and Oliveira, J. A.: Intoxication by *Solanum fastigiatum,* var. *fastigiatum* as a cause of cerebellar degeneration in cattle. Cornell Vet., in press.

VISUAL SYSTEM—SPECIAL SOMATIC AFFERENT SYSTEM

EMBRYOLOGY OF THE EYEBALL
HISTOLOGY OF THE PARS OPTICA
 RETINAE
CENTRAL VISUAL PATHWAY
CLINICAL EVALUATION
DISEASES OF THE VISUAL SYSTEM

EMBRYOLOGY OF THE EYEBALL

The eyeball is derived from neuroectoderm (retina), surface ectoderm (lens, cornea), and mesoderm (cornea, sclera, and uvea). In the bird, ectodermal neural crest contributes to the cornea, sclera, and uvea.[151] This remains to be proven in the mammal.

The neuroectodermal contribution to the eyeball is induced in the open neural tube stage at its rostral end. This is in the portion of the neural tube destined to form the prosencephalon, and subsequently the diencephalon. The "optic field" neuroectoderm is induced initially by the underlying archenteron endoderm beneath the rostral ventral midline of the neural plate. This initially single primordial optic area is influenced by the adjacent rapidly infiltrating head mesenchyme. This particular portion of head mesenchyme is rostral to the notochord, and therefore is designated the prechordal mesenchyme. It includes neural crest cells and helps induce the separation of the initially single optic area of neuroectoderm into two areas that first appear as depressions within the neural tube—the optic pits—in each half of the future prosencephalon. These proceed to grow laterally as evaginations from the neural tube. They are the optic vesicles (Fig. 14–1). There is evidence in lower vertebrates that the prosencephalic cells that contribute to each optic vesicle come from both sides of the prosencephalon.[100] This may relate to the subsequent development of optic nerve axon crossing at the chiasm. Improper separation of the optic area into two primordia by the prechordal mesenchyme leads to the development of the cyclopic malformation with a single median plane eyeball. Veratrum alkaloids ingested by the ewe exert their influence on this development to produce the cyclopic malformation in lambs. This occurs specifically at 14 days of development.

The optic vesicles bulge laterally from the prosencephalon and lie adjacent to the surface ectoderm, where they proliferate and induce the surface ectoderm to proliferate to form the lens placode. As the optic vesicle grows away from the prosencephalon, its connection elongates into the optic stalk. This is the precursor of the pathway of the optic nerve. The protruding lateral surface of the optic vesicle adjacent to the lens placode invaginates so that it comes to lie against the medial surface of the vesicle. This infolding forms the shape of a cup, and the structure is referred to as the optic cup. It is incomplete ventrally, where the optic or choroidal fissure develops. The embryonic hyaloid vasculature enters the developing eye through this fissure. In time, fusion of the edges closes this fissure, except for a small notch. The infolding that produces the optic cup also involves the optic stalk, which provides a path for the optic nerve axons to enter the brain. The two layers of the optic cup differentiate into the retina.

As the optic vesicle invaginates to form the optic cup, the lens placode developing in the surface ectoderm invaginates to form the lens vesicle, which ultimately separates from the overlying surface ectoderm and remains situated at the opening to the optic cup. A fine fibrous connection remains between the inner layer of the optic cup and the posterior surface of the lens vesicle. The anterior cells of the lens vesicle remain cuboidal. The posterior cells elongate and form the primary lens fibers that eventually obliterate the cavity of the lens vesicle. These primary lens fibers lose their nuclei and become the embryonic lens nucleus. The anterior cuboidal cells remain as the lens epithelium. Proliferation and elongation of these cells around the equator of the lens gives rise to the secondary lens fibers. These fibers grow anteriorly between the anterior epithelium and the embryonic nucleus and posteriorly over the embryonic nucleus beneath the lens capsule. Secondary lens fibers are continually formed at the equator for the life of the animal. The characteristics of these lens fibers

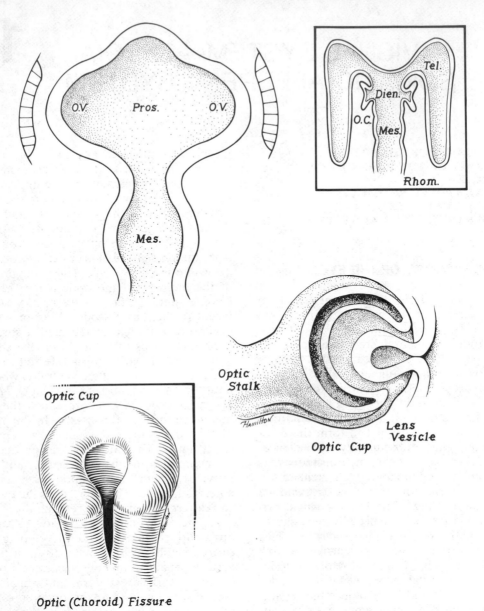

Optic (Choroid) Fissure

Figure 14–1. Development of the eyeball. *O.V.*: optic vesicle; *O.C.*: optic cup; *Tel.*: telencephalon; *Dien.*: diencephalon; *Mes.*: mesencephalon; *Rhom.*: rhombencephalon; *Pros.*: prosencephalon.

impart transparency to the lens. Congenital cataracts develop in the primary lens fibers of the embryonic lens nucleus.[9]

The lens is thought to be partially responsible for the induction of the remaining ectodermal surface cells to form the surface epithelium for the cornea. A rare malformation in cattle is the development of a rudimentary lens within the cornea. This results from the failure of the lens vesicle to separate from the surface ectoderm that ultimately forms the corneal epithelium.

To these primordial ectodermal structures of the eyeball is added the mesodermal-neural crest component. This can be considered as the addition of two layers corresponding to the two basic supporting layers that are formed around the entire central nervous system, the dense protective dura and the thinner vascular pia-arachnoid (Fig. 14–2).

As the loose mesoderm and neural crest surrounding the brain differentiates into the vascular pia-arachnoid (leptomeninges), this process of differentiation continues along the optic stalk and over the optic cup and lens vesicle. The subarachnoid space found between the pia and arachnoid over the brain continues along the optic stalk to the optic

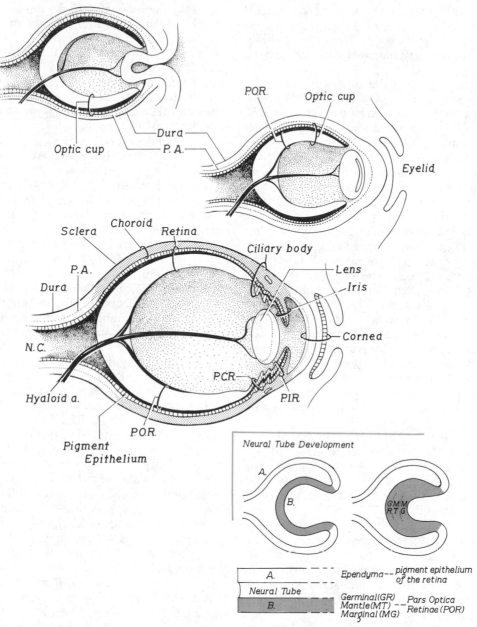

Figure 14–2. Development of the eyeball. *P.A.*: pia arachnoid; *P.O.R.*: pars optica retina; *P.C.R.*: pars ciliaris retina; *P.I.R.*: pars iridica retina; *N.C.*: neural canal.

cup. This is implicated in the spread of disease between the brain and eyeball. At the optic cup the space is obliterated, and the mesoderm-neural crest, homologous with the pia-arachnoid, differentiates into the uveal coat of the eyeball (choroid, ciliary body, and iris) and forms the endothelial layer on the internal surface of the cornea. This initially loose mesoderm-neural crest completely fills the area between the lens vesicle and the corneal endothelium. A space forms in this tissue, leaving the mesoderm-neural crest anteriorly as the corneal endothelium and posteriorly as the body of the iris and pupillary membrane. This space is the anterior chamber, which fills with aqueous. The pupillary membrane is the mesoderm-neural crest situated centrally over the lens. Ultimately, it disintegrates to form the pupil. The space formed in the mesoderm-neural crest between the iris and the lens is the posterior chamber, which also fills with aqueous. The uvea is the vascular tunic of the eyeball that is continuous with the pia-arachnoid, the vascular tunic of the central nervous system, at the optic stalk. The cells of these layers have some similar histologic characteristics.

The space between the fundus of the optic cup and the posterior surface of the lens is the vitreous chamber. The vitreous body that fills it is derived from secretions from the optic cup, the lens, and the enclosed mesenchyme. Hyaloid vessels course in the mesoderm from the base of the brain along the optic stalk in the optic fissure to supply the optic cup, vitreous, and lens. Branches cross through the vitreous to the posterior surface of the lens. These hyaloid vessels normally disappear after birth. Remnants may persist in dogs to around 4 months of age and in cattle to 1 year or more. These are seen emerging from the optic disk that forms at the site of the optic stalk. Abnormal persistence of this hyaloid vasculature to the lens results in cataracts of the posterior lens capsule and accumulation of blood, pigment, and fibrovascular tissue posterior to the lens. This is called persistent hyperplastic tunica vasculosa lentis and persistent hyperplastic primary vitreous.[120, 162, 177] A hereditary basis has been suggested for this in the Doberman pinscher.[211]

As the outer layer of mesoderm-neural crest surrounding the brain differentiates into the dense pachymeninx, the dura, this process of differentiation continues along the optic stalk and optic cup. Over the optic cup this layer forms the fibrous tunic of the eyeball—the sclera. It continues anteriorly deep to the surface ectoderm to form the substance of the cornea, the substantia propria. Thus the fibrous tunic of the brain (dura) and of the eyeball (sclera) have a similar origin which reflects the initial origin of the eyeball from the neural tube.

Differentiation of the optic cup is similar to the differentiation of the neural tube, with two adjacent walls and a space between, the neural canal (Fig. 14–2). The optic vesicle originally consists of proliferating neuroepithelial cells. As the lumen of the vesicle is reduced to a small space by the infolding of the lateral surface, this forms an outer and inner wall to the optic cup. The differentiation of each wall can be compared to that of the neural tube, with the formation of germinal, mantle, and marginal layers. The entire outer layer of the optic cup, which initially proliferated, later regresses to a single layer of cells. Posterior to the ciliary body and adjacent to the choroid,

this is the pigment layer of the retina. Anterior to this it forms the outer layer of the two cell layers that cover the posterior surface of the ciliary body and iris. Thus this differentiated outer layer of the optic cup is homologous to the ependymal layer of the differentiated neural tube that lines the ventricular system and central canal. The inner layer of the optic cup posterior to the ciliary body differentiates into the multilayered sensory portion of the retina, the pars optica retina. Anterior to this, the inner layer differentiates into a single layer of cells to form the inner layer of the two-cell layer that covers the posterior surface of the ciliary body and iris. These two layers of cells, derived from the inner and outer layers of the optic cup, are called the pars ciliaris retinae and pars iridica retinae, respectively, named for the structures they cover. The rostral extent of the pars iridica retinae determines the margin of the iris. Beyond this, the mesoderm of the pupillary membrane degenerates to produce the pupillary space. Improper degeneration of this membrane leaves persistent remnants. This may be a hereditary defect in basenji dogs.[140, 181] The outer nonpigmented layer of cells in the pars iridica retinae proliferates to form the smooth muscle cells of the dilator muscle of the iris. Thus, ectodermal cells are forming muscle in this site.

In the inner layer of the optic cup posterior to the ciliary body, the neuroepithelial cells proliferate as the germinal layer (Fig. 14–3). With development, this layer differentiates into three layers of neurons. The outer layer of cells (toward the sclera) forms the photoreceptor neurons. These line the slit-like lumen, remnant of the neural canal, and are homologous to the ependymal layer. Two other layers of neurons differentiate, and include the layer of bipolar neurons and the ganglion cell neurons. These are homologous to the mantle layer of the neural tube. The nerve fiber layer, a layer of axons from the ganglion cell neurons, is on the inner surface (toward the vitreous) and is homologous to the marginal layer on the surface of the neural tube. The axons of these ganglion cell neurons course to the optic stalk and grow through it back to the brain to form the optic nerve.[205] As these axons penetrate the optic stalk, some optic stalk cells degenerate.[224] Others differentiate into glial cells of the optic nerve. The oligodendroglia of the optic stalk myelinate the axons of ganglion neurons. Myelination occurs in the optic nerve from the brain to the eyeball. This is apparent in the white color of

DEFINITIVE LAYER   *EXTERNAL (SCLERAL) SURFACE*   *EMBRYONIC DERIVATIVE*

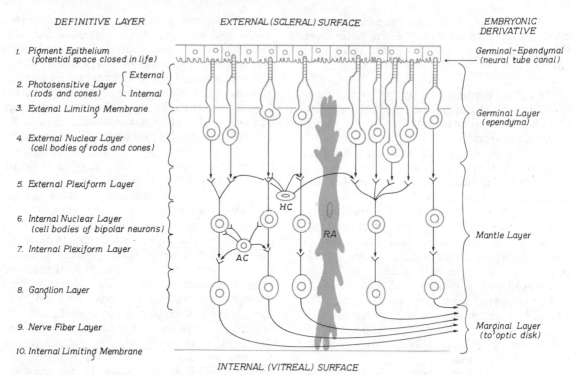

1. *Pigment Epithelium (potential space closed in life)* — *Germinal–Ependymal (neural tube canal)*

2. *Photosensitive Layer (rods and cones)* { *External* / *Internal* }

3. *External Limiting Membrane* — *Germinal Layer (ependyma)*

4. *External Nuclear Layer (cell bodies of rods and cones)*

5. *External Plexiform Layer*

6. *Internal Nuclear Layer (cell bodies of bipolar neurons)*

7. *Internal Plexiform Layer* — *Mantle Layer*

8. *Ganglion Layer*

9. *Nerve Fiber Layer* — *Marginal Layer (to optic disk)*

10. *Internal Limiting Membrane*

INTERNAL (VITREAL) SURFACE

Figure 14–3. Microscopic anatomy of the pars optica retinae. *HC*: horizontal cell (interneuron); *AC*: amacrine cell (interneuron); *RA*: radial astrocyte (Müller's neuroglial cell).

the optic disk, which is seen in the back of the eyeball (fundus) where the optic nerve attaches. No myelination occurs in the nerve fiber layer of the retina. There are more ganglion neurons produced than actually survive in the fully developed retina.[98] Their normal development and survival is dependent on their forming synapses on neurons in the central nervous system—i.e., lateral geniculate nucleus, rostral colliculus, pretectal nucleus. Those ganglion neurons that do not make these synapses degenerate. In the chicken, up to 20 per cent of the ganglion neuron population degenerates in normal retinal development.

In dogs and cats at birth, the single layer of ganglion cell neurons is separated from an outer thick layer of undifferentiated cells which represent the primordia of the photoreceptor neurons and the bipolar cell neurons. These become separated by the external plexiform layer in the first 7 days of life so that the definitive three layers of neurons are established. Radioautographic studies in kittens have established that all of the ganglion neurons are present throughout the retina by 1 day after birth as are all the neurons in the

other two layers in the central part of the retina.[222] Peripherally the germinal cells destined to be neurons in the internal and external nuclear layers continue to proliferate up to 3 weeks after birth. The histologically mature retina is apparent by 6 weeks of age in the dog, which coincides approximately with the development of visual function.[8] The pupillary reflex is demonstrable by 3 weeks. The various media of the eyeball are not transparent until 5 to 6 weeks after birth.[68]

The following sequence of development of the eye has been observed in the dog.[8]

Gestational day:

15—Well-developed optic vesicle and lens placode.

19—Invagination of optic vesicle to form the optic cup.

25—Lens vesicle separated from the surface ectoderm. Multicellular inner layer of optic cup differentiated into outer nuclear (mantle) and inner marginal zones. Outer layer of optic cup is a single-celled, thick layer. Retinal development progress from central to peripheral in the optic cup inner layer as a "wave of maturation."

33—Inner neuroblastic (ganglion neuron) layer separated from outer neuroblastic layer. Formation of optic nerve. Eyelid buds meet and adhere.

Birth:

Retina consists of outer neuroblastic layer, inner plexiform layer, and ganglion neuron and nerve fiber layers.

Postnatal days:

7–13—Formation of inner and outer nuclear layers of retina.

16>35—Distinct inner and outer segments of rods and cones.

14—Eyelids separate (9 days in kittens).

In contrast to the dog with its short gestational period, the bovine newborn eyeball is fully developed. Studies have shown that the bovine eyeball appears well developed by the end of the second trimester of gestation.[27]

The following sequence of development has been observed in the bovine embryo-fetus.

Gestational size (mm), days (approximate):

6 mm, 25–30 days—Well-developed optic vesicle and lens placode.

10 mm, 30 days—Optic cup and lens vesicle separated from surface ectoderm. Multicellular inner layer of optic cup differentiated into outer nuclear (mantle) and inner marginal zones.

14-33 mm, 40–50 days—Separated inner and outer nuclear layers of pars optica retina.

20-40 mm, 40–50 days—Nerve fiber layer formed. Single-celled thick epithelial layer formed from a multilayered outer wall of the optic cup.

24 mm, 40 days—Well-formed optic nerve.

40 mm, 50 days—Eyelid buds meet and adhere.

410 mm, 150–180 days—All layers of the retina present.

Birth:

Eyelids are separated.

HISTOLOGY OF THE PARS OPTICA
RETINAE[54, 167, 203, 234]

Ten layers will be described, progressing from the outer (scleral) surface to the inner (vitreal) surface (Fig. 14–3).

Pigment Epithelium of the Retina.[235] This epithelium comprises a single layer of cuboidal cells, with their base on a basement membrane apposed to the choroid, and their apex facing the photosensitive layer across the potential space of the neural tube (lumen of the optic cup). Numerous processes of the apical cytoplasm and cell membrane interdigitate with the processes of the rods and cones. In cats this is quite elaborate with specialized sheet-like projections from the apical surface of the pigment epithelium ensheathing the external segments of the cones and the rods to a lesser degree.[165] This close arrangement may facilitate the role of the pigment epithelium in the regeneration of rhodopsin, the visual pigment in the rods, and the removal of degenerate rod membranous lamellae by phagocytosis.[2, 73, 135, 240] Many melanin granules occupy the apical cytoplasm of the pigment cells throughout the retina, except over the area occupied by the tapetum lucidum in the choroid. The presence of these pigment granules partly accounts for the dark color of the nontapetal portion of the fundus observed with the ophthalmoscope. The tapetum lucidum in the choroid is rendered more visible by the absence of melanin pigment in this epithelium. These pigment epithelial cells and the photoreceptor neurons are nourished by the vessels in the choriocapillaris layer of the choroid. This layer is adjacent to the scleral side of the pigmented epithelial cells. Exchange of substances between these vessels and the photoreceptor neurons must pass through the pigment epithelial cells.

Photosensitive Layer (Layer of Rods and Cones). This layer, divided into two segments, represents the dendritic zone of the sensory special somatic afferent neuron, the photoreceptor cell.[203, 204, 223, 235] The external and internal segments of the layer are composed of modifications of the cell processes and bodies of the rod and cone cells. The external segment consists of parallel lamellae within the elongate cell processes. These are orderly stacks of flattened, double-membrane sacs in the form of disks. These membranes are oriented transversely to the axis of the cell process. They are formed at the base of the external segment from the modified cilium located there.[212] These membranes migrate distally and are cast off at the outer portion, where they are phagocytized by the pigment epithelial cells. In the rods these membranes contain the visual pigment, rhodopsin, the photoreceptor substance responsible for light absorption and the initiation of the visual stimulus. A similar substance, iodopsin, is in the cone membranous lamellae. The rod cells are sensitive to low levels of illumination (night vision). Cone cells respond to high levels of illumination (day vision) and are responsible for initiating color vision.

The external segment is connected to the internal segment by a slender stalk containing a modified cilium. The internal segment, called the ellipsoid, is elongate in rods and oval in cones, and composed mostly of endoplasmic reticulum and numerous mitochondria. It is a modification of the cell body of these photoreceptor special somatic afferent neurons.

External Limiting Membrane. This "membrane" consists of the junctional complexes between the photoreceptor cells and the supporting radial astrocytes (the cells of Müller). These latter cells surround and support all the neural elements of the retina between the basal lamina of these cells, the internal limiting membrane, and the external limiting membrane on the scleral side of external nuclear layer.

External Nuclear Layer. This layer is composed of the cell bodies with nuclei of the photoreceptor special somatic afferent neurons. The cone nuclei are located adjacent to the external limiting membrane. The rod nuclei are smaller and constitute most of this layer. They extend in several layers toward the inner (vitreal) surface of the retina. In the dog retina, it is estimated that the ratio of the number of rod cells to cone cells is about 18 to 1. The number of cone cells increases toward the central area of the retina. Axons of the rod and cone cells course vitreally into the next layer. Rod cells predominate in the retinas of all the domestic animals that have been studied.

External Plexiform Layer. This is a layer primarily composed of the axons and telodendria of the photoreceptor cells and the axons and dendritic zones of the bipolar neurons and their synaptic arrangements. Intermingled with these are the cell processes of the horizontal cells, an interneuron transmitting between different groups of photoreceptor cells.[124]

Internal Nuclear Layer. This layer primarily consists of the cell bodies (nuclei) of bipolar neurons. These are the second neurons in the visual pathway, and like the photoreceptor cells, they are restricted to the retina. They connect photoreceptor neurons with ganglion cells in the visual pathway. The axon courses from the external plexiform layer, in which the dendritic zone is located, through the internal nuclear layer (cell body), into the internal plexiform layer, in which the telodendria are located. The cell body with its nucleus is situated along the course of this axon, accounting for its bipolar characteristic. On the external, scleral, surface of this internal nuclear layer the cell bodies with nuclei of the horizontal cells are located. On the opposite internal (vitreal) surface, the cell bodies of another interneuron, the amacrine cell, are located. These latter interneurons are in synaptic contact with bipolar cells, ganglion cells, and other amacrine cells. In addition, the nuclei of the radial astrocytes are located in this layer.

Whereas many rod cells are in synaptic contact with one bipolar cell, there may be only one cone cell synapsing on one bipolar cell. Thus there is a convergence of rod cell activity on the bipolar neurons.

Internal Plexiform Layer. This layer primarily is composed of the axons and telodendria of the bipolar cells and the axons and dendritic zones of the ganglion cells and their synaptic arrangements. In addition, the processes of the amacrine cells extend throughout the layer.[123, 125]

Ganglion Layer. This neuronal layer contains the cell bodies with nuclei of the third special somatic afferent neuron in the visual pathway.[215] These are large cell bodies that form an incomplete layer 1 to 2 cells thick between the internal plexiform layer and the nerve fiber layer. It is this neuron that transmits visually induced impulses to the brain by way of its axons in the optic nerve. Nissl substance is evident in the cytoplasm of these cell bodies. These cell bodies vary in size from 6 to 35 microns in diameter.[218] The smallest cell bodies have axons that project predominantly to the rostral colliculus. Medium-sized cell bodies have axons that mostly project to the lateral geniculate nucleus. There may be functional differences between medial and lateral portions of the retina.[220] Mean ganglion neuron size is greater in the lateral (temporal) retina than in the medial (nasal) retina, suggesting a greater projection from the lateral retina (medial visual field of each eye) to the thalamus and occipital cortex. There is an increased number of ganglion cells in the area centralis, and the smaller cell bodies predominate.[213]

Nerve Fiber Layer. This layer consists of the axons of the ganglion neurons coursing on the vitreal surface of the retina to the optic disk. The axons are unmyelinated until they penetrate the sclera at the optic disk. Their myelination at this point accounts for the white color of the optic disk. The nerve fiber layer is thickest in the vicinity of the optic disk. The intermingling of scleral fibers with the axons of ganglion neurons at the point of origin of the optic nerve is called the lamina cribrosa. Stellate astrocytes are located in this nerve fiber layer.

Internal Limiting Membrane. This is formed by the basal cell membrane of the radial astrocyte and a basement membrane; it is the vitreal boundary of the retina.

Area Centralis. In humans there is a round area for most distinct vision located dorsolateral to the optic disk, and called the macula (spot), fovea, or central area. In this area the retina is composed of only cones in the photoreceptor layer, and other modifications occur to facilitate the function for most acute vision. Neuromuscular mechanisms provide that for most acute close-up vision such as reading, the light is focused on this central area in each eyeball. Domestic animals have various modifications of this area.[167] In no species of domestic animal is it readily seen with the ophthalmoscope, except possibly some cats. In the cat, it may be identified as a pale streak or oval part in the area of the tapetum lucidum dorsolateral to the optic disk in which the blood vessels (arterioles) converge (Fig. 14–4).[214] The area itself is devoid of any large blood vessels. In this area centralis in the cat, there is an increase in the number of cone cells relative to rods in the photoreceptor layer, with an overall decrease in the thickness of the external nuclear layer. The length of the outer segments of the photoreceptor cells is increased. The bipolar and ganglion neurons are increased in number. The axons in the nerve fiber layer form an arc as they leave the area centralis and course to the optic disk. If the area centralis is defined as a region of the pars optica retinae in which the ganglion neuron density increases to a peak, then in all ungulates this is evident as a streak of high cell density extending horizontally dorsal to the optic disk.[89] This increase in ganglion neurons is maximal near the lateral end of the visual streak, which corresponds approximately to the location of the area centralis in cats.

The optic disk, the origin of the optic nerve, varies in shape from round to oval to triangular.[1, 21, 142, 147, 236] It is usually slightly ventrolateral to the posterior pole of the eyeball and varies in its relationship to the tapetum lucidum. In toy breeds it may be in the retina entirely below the area of the tapetum lucidum. In medium-sized breeds it is usually half over the inferior border of the tapetum lucidum. In large breeds it may be entirely over the area of the tapetum lucidum.[236] In horses and cattle it is just below the inferior border of the tapetum lucidum. In cats it is always over the area of the tapetum lucidum.

CENTRAL VISUAL PATHWAY[37, 171]

OPTIC NERVE[153]

The growth of the ganglion neuronal axons through the embryonic optic stalk produces the optic nerve, cranial nerve II. The optic nerve is in fact a tract of the central nervous system based on its origin in the optic vesicle and its histologic characteristics. It is surrounded by meninges, including a subarachnoid space. It contains neuroglial cells similar

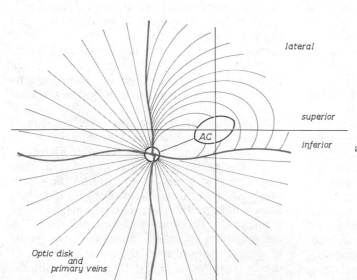

lateral

superior

inferior

AC

Optic disk
 and
primary veins

Figure 14–4.   Relationship of optic disk and area centralis in the retina of the cat.

to those of the brain and has no Schwann cells. The oligodendrocytes are the source of the myelin for the axons in the optic nerve. Leptomeningeal fibers course through the nerve as septa. The optic nerves course caudally in the orbit, surrounded by their meninges and extraocular muscles. They enter the skull through the optic canals of the presphenoid bone and join on the rostroventral aspect of the brain stem, rostral to the hypophysis at the optic chiasm.

OPTIC CHIASM-OPTIC TRACT[217]

At the optic chiasm in domestic animals a majority of the axons in each optic nerve cross, destined to influence the contralateral cerebral hemisphere (Fig. 14–5). This corresponds to the pattern that most modalities that can be localized in space (general proprioception, general somatic afferent) are represented contralaterally in the brain.[44, 91]

In most fish and birds, all the optic nerve axons cross in the optic chiasm. In mammals, partial decussation develops in relationship to the development of a binocular field of vision with frontal positioning of the eyeballs, and the ability to perform coordinated conjugate eyeball movements, including convergence. In primates, in whom this is most developed, the degree of decussation is slightly over 50 per cent. It is estimated that in the cat the degree of decussation is 65 per cent, in dogs 75 per cent, and in the horse, ox, sheep, and pig 80 to 90 per cent. On this basis the cat most closely resembles the primate in degree of decussation, frontal positioning of the eyeballs, and presumably conjugate movement of the eyeballs. As the visual system becomes more complex along with the capability for binocular vision, there is less decussation in the optic chiasm.

The axons that cross in the chiasm come from ganglion neurons on the medial (nasal) aspect of the retina (Fig. 14–5). Axons from ganglion neurons on the lateral (temporal) aspect of the retina remain ipsilateral in their course through the central visual pathway. Neuroanatomic studies in the cat have determined that this division between medial and lateral portions of the retina based on the axons that cross in the chiasm is a vertical line

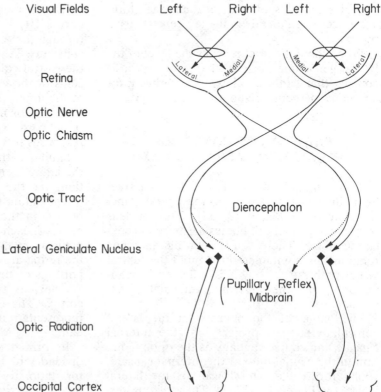

Visual Fields

Retina

Optic Nerve

Optic Chiasm

Figure 14–5. Central visual pathway for conscious perception. (From Vet. Clin. North Am., *3*:491, 1973.)

Optic Tract

Lateral Geniculate Nucleus

Optic Radiation

Occipital Cortex

approximately through the area centralis.[206, 214] This was initially determined by cutting one optic tract and studying the retrograde degeneration that occurred in the ganglion neurons of the retina whose axons were severed (Fig. 14-6). Studies using horseradish peroxidase injected into the lateral geniculate nucleus have further confirmed this nasotemporal division of the retina.[39]

The optic tracts course caudodorsolateral over the side of the diencephalon, progressing from ventral to lateral to caudal to the internal capsule, reaching the lateral geniculate nucleus, which is the caudodorsolateral protrusion of the thalamus (Plates 15, 14, 13, 12).[55, 112] Each tract contains axons mostly from the medial retina of the contralateral eyeball and the lateral retina of the ipsilateral eyeball. The visual field is defined as the area in space observed by each eyeball when fixed at any one moment. Therefore, the lateral half of the visual field of each eyeball will stimulate the medial retina, and the medial half of the visual field will stimulate the lateral retina. Thus each optic tract contains the neurons in which light generates an impulse from the same half of the visual field of each eyeball. That is, the left optic tract contains the neurons stimulated by light from the right half of the visual field of the left and right eyeballs. Objects in the right visual fields of each eyeball, therefore, are represented mainly in the left central visual pathway.

When the optic tract reaches the level of the lateral geniculate nucleus, there are two basic courses that can be followed: a pathway for conscious perception and a reflex pathway.

PATHWAY FOR CONSCIOUS PERCEPTION—VISUAL CORTEX

Approximately 80 per cent of the optic tract fibers in the cat terminate in the lateral geniculate nucleus (Plates 13, 12). This nucleus contains neuronal cell bodies organized in specific laminae. There is a retinotopic anatomic relationship maintained throughout the central visual pathway.[26, 133] This is reflected in laminations of the lateral geniculate nucleus.[44, 72, 75, 76, 79, 87, 88, 96, 115, 116, 145, 194, 216]

The axons of the neurons in the lateral geniculate nucleus project into the internal capsule and course caudally as the optic radiation in the caudal limb of the internal capsule, which forms the lateral wall of the lateral ventricle (Plates 13, 12).[150] These axons ter-

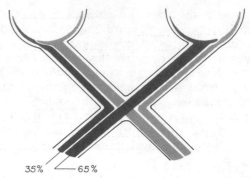

Figure 14–6. Origin in retinal ganglion neuron layer of axons in the optic tract of the cat.

minate in the cerebral (visual) cortex on the lateral, caudal, and medial aspects of the occipital lobe.[72, 95] The gyri that compose this area include the caudal part of the marginal and ectomarginal gyri (laterally), the occipital gyrus (caudally), and the splenial gyrus (medially). This pathway from optic tract, to lateral geniculate nucleus, to optic radiation, to visual cortex, must be intact for normal conscious visual perception to occur.

Various portions of the visual cortex have connections to the visual cortex of the opposite hemisphere, to the motor cortex of both hemispheres, to the cerebellum by way of the pons, to the tegmentum and the nuclei of cranial nerves III, IV, and VI directly or indirectly through the rostal colliculus, and to the rostral colliculus. A tectospinal tract descends from the rostral colliculus through the ventral funiculus of the cervical spinal cord to contribute to the upper motor neuron that influences the lower motor neurons in the grey matter of the spinal cord.[152] Through these pathways, motor responses to visual stimuli can be mediated.

Similar to the arrangement in the optic tract, the lateral geniculate nucleus, the optic radiation, and the visual cortex on one side of the brain contain neurons stimulated by light from objects in the contralateral half of the visual field of each eyeball. This is a retinotopic pathway in that specific anatomic portions of the retina are represented in specific anatomic portions of the optic tract, the lateral geniculate nucleus, the optic radiation, and the visual cortex. These retinal areas have a specific representation in the visual field of each eyeball.

In primates the visual cerebral cortex is divided into the functional areas. Area 17 is for stationary object vision. Areas 18 and 19 function in panoramic vision for movement, spatial relationship, and depth perception. For normal object vision interaction is required between the visual cortex and the rostral colliculus. For normal panoramic vision interaction is required between the visual cortex and the mesencephalic tegmentum. Removal of the rostral colliculus on one side produces hemianopsia in the contralateral visual field for object vision. Bilateral rostral collicular lesions produce complete blindness for still objects. Visual perception of movement and spatial orientation are lost with lesions in the mesencephalic tegmentum. Unilateral lesions of the tegmentum produce a contralateral deficit and cause severe torsion of the head so that it tilts more than 90 degrees to the side opposite the lesion. Blindfolding corrects this postural dystonia, indicating its visual basis.[48, 49]

In cats functional differences between the medial and lateral portions of the retinal ganglion neurons have been found. Those in the lateral retina have a greater projection to the thalamus and visual cortex. More of the medial retinal ganglion neurons project to the rostral colliculus. After bilateral removal of the visual cortex of the occipital lobe, some visual orienting responses persist.[170, 208] These cats can detect objects introduced into the lateral visual field of each eye presumably by using their rostral collicular projection, which is more abundant from the medial (nasal) retina. Total bilateral rostral colliculectomy causes immediate inattention to all visual stimuli and loss of both visual placing and the menace responses. These functions return in a few days to a week. It is obvious that the cerebral cortex and midbrain have extensive interaction in mediating visually guided behavior.

REFLEX PATHWAY[86]

Approximately 20 per cent of the optic tract axons in the cat pass over the lateral geniculate nucleus to terminate in the pretectal area or rostral colliculus (Plates 13, 12, 11).[145] The pretectal area functions in the pupillary reflex pathway. The axons that course into the rostral colliculus follow the brachium of the rostral colliculus, which lies between the rostral colliculus and the lateral geniculate nucleus. The rostral colliculus is also a laminated structure, and in addition to the optic tract axons it receives axons from the cerebral cortex (especially the visual cortex) and the spinal cord (spinotectal tract). Axons of cell bodies in the rostral colliculus project to the tegmentum of the midbrain and medulla to influence nuclei

of cranial nerves III, IV, and VI (tectobulbar fibers), to the spinal cord to influence ventral grey column general somatic efferent neurons (tectospinal tract), to the thalamus for feedback to the cerebral cortex, and to the cerebellum.[152] These pathways function in the coordination of head, neck, and eyeball movements in response to visual stimuli.

CLINICAL EVALUATION

Clinical Tests.[46, 180] Vision can be tested by watching the patient walk in a strange environment or through a maze of obstacles.

The menace test consists of making a menacing gesture with the hand directed at each eyeball while the other eyeball is covered. With a cooperative patient the medial and lateral aspects of each eyeball (retina) can be tested. Care must be taken not to touch any of the facial hairs or to create too much air turbulence. In the stoic patient it may be necessary to tap the eyelids being tested, so that the animal is aware of the test. The entire peripheral and central visual pathway must be intact for a response to occur. This is a learned response and often is absent in young animals. In general it is usually present by 1 to 2 weeks in foals and calves and by 10 to 12 weeks in puppies.

The response observed is closure of the palpebral fissure and sometimes retraction of the eyeball or head away from the gesture. The facial nucleus and nerve must be intact for palpebral closure to occur. Based on the observation of numerous kinds of lesions located in the optic radiation and visual cortex, it can be concluded that these areas are necessary for the perception of vision required in the menace response. Experimental studies have defined a role for the rostral colliculus in the normal menace response, but the rarity of lesions limited to one or both rostral colliculi does not permit any similar clinical conclusion.

In all domestic animals it has been observed that diffuse cerebellar cortical degenerative lesions cause a failure of the menace response bilaterally, with no visual deficit and normal facial nerve function. It is assumed either that the pathway that mediates this response from visual cortex to the facial nucleus passes through the cerebellum (Fig 14–7) or that the cerebellar lesion causes inhibition of the cerebrocortical neurons involved in this response. If there is an anatomic pathway through the cerebellum for this response, it may involve a corticopontocerebellar pathway. Alternatively, it may involve the rostral colliculus via

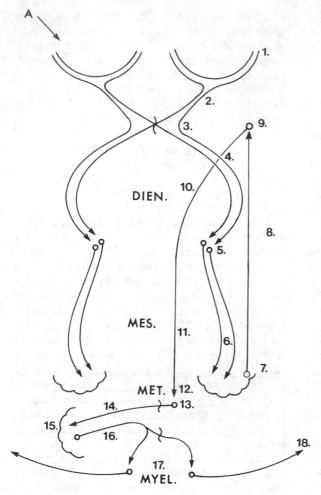

Figure 14–7. An anatomic pathway of the menace response: *1*: retina; *2*: optic nerve; *3*: optic chiasm; *4*: optic tract; *5*: lateral geniculate nucleus; *6*: optic radiation; *7*: visual cortex; *8*: internal capsule, association fiber; *9*: motor cortex; *10*: internal capsule, projection fiber; *11*: crus cerebri; *12*: longitudinal fibers of pons; *13*: pontine nucleus; *14*: transverse fibers of pons and middle cerebellar peduncle; *15*: cerebellar cortex; *16*: efferent cerebellar pathway; *17*: facial nuclei; *18*: facial muscles—orbicularis oculi. ⟨ indicates axons crossing the midline of the brain. A lesion in the left cerebellar hemisphere would prevent a menace response directed at the left eyeball from its lateral visual field (*A*) because 65 to 90 percent of the optic axons cross in the chiasm.

a corticotectopontocerebellar or more direct corticotectocerebellar pathway.[114]

In the horse and dog, a unilateral menace response deficit with normal vision has been observed to accompany large unilateral cerebellar lesions on the same side as the deficit. This may be explained by the crossing that occurs from the cerebrum to the cerebellum at the pontine nucleus.

The pupillary light reflex response was described in Chapter 6. The cones are probably the most receptive to this bright light stimulus. This tests the peripheral visual pathway and central pathway to the level of the thalamus and pretectum only. The oculomotor nucleus and nerve mediate the motor response. Loss of the pupillary response due to lesions in the afferent visual pathway usually occurs only with a severe lesion.

Clinical Signs.[46] (See Tables 14–1, 14–2.) The degree of visual deficit depends on the location and extent of the lesion in the visual pathway.

Lesions that destroy the retina or optic nerve in one eye cause blindness and a normal to partially dilated pupil in that eyeball. This does not usually cause any disorientation of the gait, nor any head tilt or neck curvature in domestic animals. In birds, this may cause a head tilt toward the blind eye. There is no palpebral closure in response to a menacing gesture in the affected eyeball. Light directed into the blind eyeball produces no response in either eyeball. Light directed into the normal eyeball causes both pupils to constrict. In the pupillary reflex pathway, the afferents cross both in the optic chiasm and in the pretectum to influence both oculomotor nuclei. It is through this pathway that the environmental light causes complete to partial constriction of the pupil of the blind eyeball. As you swing the light slowly from one eye to the other, both pupils constrict

TABLE 14–1.   CLINICAL SIGNS OF VISUAL DEFICIT

Test	Right Optic Nerve	Right Cranial Nerve III	Right Postorbital	Right Optic Tract	Right Visual Cortex
			Lesions		
Left eye (OS)					
Pupil	Normal size	Normal size	Normal size	Normal size	Normal size
	Light in OS	Light in OS	Light in OS	Light in OS	Light in OS
	Both constrict	Only OS constricts	Only OS constricts	Both constrict	Both constrict
Menace	Present	Present	Present	Mostly absent	Mostly absent
Right eye (OD)					
Pupil	Normal to partial dilation	Complete dilation	Complete dilation	Normal size	Normal size
	Light in OD	Light in OD	Light in OD	Light in OD	Light in OD
	Neither constrict	Only OS constricts	Neither constricts	Both constrict	Both constrict
Menace	Absent	Present	Absent	Mostly present	Mostly present

when the light is directed into the normal eye, but as the light swings into the affected eye, the pupil is dilating from the previous constriction and cannot respond to the direct stimulus. If the normal eye is covered, the pupil of the affected eye will dilate.

Bilateral retinal or optic nerve disease that is total causes complete blindness, with both pupils widely dilated and unresponsive to light directed into either eyeball. Optic neuritis is the most common cause of this kind of deficit. Ordinarily it takes very severe retinal or optic nerve lesions to prevent the pupils from constricting to a bright source of light. In most instances vision will disappear before the pupillary light reflex. Therefore, an animal may be blind from retinal or optic nerve disease and still have pupils responsive to a bright source of light. Usually there is some abnormality in this response and in the normal room light both pupils are slightly dilated. If blindness occurs slowly and the animal is confined to a small environment, the visual deficit may not be noticed. Blind animals may adjust well to their normal surroundings.

Unilateral lesions in the optic tract, lateral geniculate nucleus, optic radiation, or visual cortex result in a visual deficit in the contralateral visual field of each eyeball. Because of the degree of decussation, the visual deficit can usually be appreciated only in the contralateral eyeball. This is referred to as a hemianopsia because there is a visual deficit in 50 per cent of the total visual field. In the dog, this represents about a 25 per cent retinal dysfunction in the ipsilateral eyeball and a 75

TABLE 14–2.   NEURO-OPHTHALMOLOGY: REVIEW OF CLINICAL SIGNS

Extraocular:
    Size of palpebral fissue—musculus levator palpebrae (III): frontalis (VII) in large animals.
        Narrow: oculomotor nerve paralysis (ptosis) with strabismus and mydriasis; sympathetic paralysis—Horner's syndrome; facial paralysis in large animals; and atrophy of muscles of mastication.
        Wide: Facial paralysis in small animals.
    Protrusion of the third eyelid: sympathetic paralysis—Horner's syndrome; tetanus—when stimulated; facial paralysis—when the eye is menaced; severe depression in cats; and hyperplasia of the gland of the third eyelid.
    Strabismus: Vestibular system disturbance—ventrolateral, inconstant; oculomotor nerve paralysis—ventrolateral, constant; abducent nerve paralysis—medial, constant; and trochlear nerve paralysis—dorsal deviation of medial angle-constant.
    Nystagmus—vestibular system disturbance: peripheral disease—nystagmus to opposite side; congenital blindness—pendular; and congenital nystagmus—pendular.
    Sensory perception—trigeminal nerve: ophthalmic nerve to eyeball (cornea)—neurotrophic keratitis; maxillary nerve to eyelids laterally; and ophthalmic nerve to eyelids medially.

Intraocular:
    Size of pupil:
        Mydriasis: oculomotor nerve paralysis (ptosis) with strabismus; optic nerve paralysis with total blindness; glaucoma; iris atrophy; and retinal disease.
        Miosis: sympathetic paralysis—Horner's syndrome; acute intracerebral disease—released oculomotor nuclear function; ocular pain—oculopupillary reflex; and iritis.
    Examination: menace (vision), and pupillary light reflex.

per cent retinal dysfunction in the contralateral eyeball.

In the dog and cat the visual deficit is most evident by the failure of the menace response. It may be difficult to detect as the animal moves in its surroundings. Occasionally, an object may be bumped on the side opposite the lesion, but often there is no evidence of visual deficit. Unilateral blindfolding and maze testing of the animal may help demonstrate the deficit. In the horse and ruminants with 80 to 90 per cent crossing of optic nerve axons there is a greater tendency to walk into objects on the side of the visual deficit, contralateral to the lesion.

In all domestic animals there is a poor or absent palpebral closure response to menacing gestures to the eyeball contralateral to the lesion. If the examiner is careful, this test can be performed reliably without using a transparent barrier between the hand and the eyeball to prevent air currents and direct contact with the facial hairs.

It is important to cover the eyeball not being tested and to menace the other eyeball from both its medial and lateral sides. The deficit will be more pronounced from the lateral side (visual field) when there are contralateral lesions in the central visual pathway.

In unilateral lesions caudal to the optic chiasm, the pupillary light reflex responses are usually normal, because of the crossing at the chiasm and pretectal area. The light always should be directed toward the lateral retina in which the area centralis is located. This occasionally may turn a slow response into a normal one. If a lesion completely destroys one optic tract, careful evaluation may determine that the pupillary light reflex is decreased when the light is directed into the eye contralateral to the optic tract lesion. This is because of the major crossing of optic nerve axons at the optic chiasm and crossing back of pretectal neurons in the caudal thalamus to the oculomotor neurons on the same side as the eye being tested.[197]

Bilateral lesions in the optic tracts and area of the lateral geniculate nucleus, if complete, produce total blindness and dilated pupils unresponsive to light. More often the lesions are partial and clinical signs are difficult to determine. Canine distemper encephalitis often produces extensive lesions in the optic tracts without obvious clinical deficit of vision or pupillary function.

Bilateral lesions in the optic radiations, or the visual cortex, or both, cause complete blindness with normal pupillary light reflexes.

DISEASES OF THE VISUAL SYSTEM[101, 118, 185]

RETINA—OPTIC NERVE[28, 45, 57, 61, 136, 146, 183, 190, 192, 210]

1. There are many examples in veterinary medicine of hereditary retinal degenerations, called progressive retinal atrophy (PRA), which slowly produce blindness over a period of many months to years. Many have been shown to be hereditary, for example, in Gordon and Irish setters, miniature and toy poodles, Norwegian elkhounds, malamutes, and others.[5-7, 16-20, 38, 156-159, 161, 233] In this disease there is a slowly progressive degeneration of the photoreceptor cells. In some breeds in the early stages this may be restricted to only one type of photoreceptor cell—the rod cells in Norwegian elkhounds (night blindness), and cone cells in Alaskan malamutes (hemeralopia or day blindness).[122, 186-188] Terminally in these diseases pupils are dilated and unresponsive to light. Cats develop a retinal degeneration that predominates in the area centralis. This is due to a dietary deficiency of taurine.[4, 23, 80, 84, 85] Cats have a unique metabolism that requires a dietary source of taurine. In its absence, central retinal degeneration occurs. Only when the peripheral retina becomes affected late in the course of the degeneration will clinical signs be evident.

2. Malformation of parts of the eyeball occurs as an hereditary disease in collie dogs. In its more severe manifestation it may produce blindness because of disruption of the retina, or optic nerve, or both.[52, 53, 192, 229, 238, 239] This is referred to as the collie eye syndrome and may include scleral ectasia, or chorioretinal dysplasia, or both. It is a nonprogressive disease. The primary defect may relate to abnormal closure of the choroidal fissure and abnormal pigment epithelium of the retina, retarding development of the retina and choroid.

Retinal dysplasias are abnormal development of the pars optica retinae of the optic cup.[5] Abnormal differentiation of the inner layer of the optic cup results in rosettes of neuroepithelial cells and retinal folds. Inherited retinal dysplasia occurs in the English springer spaniel,[134] American cocker spaniel,[80, 139] Bedlington terrier,[189] Sealyham terrier,[10] and Labrador retriever.[24] These are often not associated with visual deficit but are detected on ocular examination. In some patients there are abnormalities in other components of the eyball, and in Labrador retrievers skeletal abnormality accompanies the retinal dysplasia.[34]

Retinal dysplasias can also result from in utero or perinatal viral infections. This occurs in cats and is caused by the feline panleukopenia virus.[164]

3. Microphthalmia has been observed in kittens born from mothers treated for a prolonged period during gestation with *griseofulvin,* an oral treatment for fungus infections. Other malformations attributed to this teratogen include hydrocephalus, cleft palate, cranium bifidum and exencephaly, spina bifida, and cyclopian malformation. There is no eyeball evident on peripheral examination of the small eyelids and orbit. On microscopic examination of the orbital tissues, neuroepithelium is present. A similar microphthalmia accompanies the severe craniofacial malformation in Burmese kittens that is inherited.

Hereditary microphthalmia has been reported in collies, schnauzers, Australian shepherds, and white Short Horn cattle.[70] Microphthalmia is a sporadic malformation most commonly observed in calves. It often accompanies other malformations of the brain and cranial cavity. In Guernseys it is sometimes accompanied by cardiac malformation and a wry tail. Although no eyeball may be apparent on physical examination of the orbit, eyelids, and conjunctival sac, a rudimentary hypoplastic-dysplastic eyeball is usually present in the orbit. The presence of neuroepithelium is indicative of optic vesicle development. The only evidence of development of the optic stalk may be a tube of meninges extending through the optic canal to the site of the optic chiasm.

4. Bilateral hypoplasia of the optic nerve has been observed in the cat, dog, and horse.[22, 56, 71, 228] The optic disk is markedly diminished in size as are the optic nerve, chiasm, and tracts. The patients are blind from birth, with dilated, unresponsive pupils. Whether these cases are all hypoplasia or some are perinatal degenerations is not known. In dogs it is most common in miniature poodles.

5. Night blindness has been observed in the Appaloosa breed.[232] They often stumble and fall while being ridden during and after dusk and are reluctant to move in the dark. These patients sometimes show abnormal head and eyeball movements as if there was a visual problem. The eyeballs may rotate in the orbit and occasionally show a dorsal deviation of the medial aspect of the eyeball. Ophthalmoscopic examination is normal. A rod cell photoreceptor deficit is assumed, but this remains to be proved. No lesions are observed on histologic examination of the retina. A recessive inheritance is suspected for this condition.

6. Injury to the optic disk or nerve can occur associated with head trauma. Fundic examination should be performed along with the neurologic evaluation of a blind patient with brain injury before attributing the visual deficit to cerebral contusion and edema. In these latter patients dilated pupils may accompany the brain stem or oculomotor nerve compression or contusion, and be misleading as to the cause of the blindness.

7. Optic neuritis is an inflammatory disease that occurs in dogs as a fairly sudden onset of total blindness, usually bilateral with dilated unresponsive pupils, with or without visible abnormalities associated with the optic disk.[31, 80, 149, 207] It is a nonsuppurative inflammatory lesion with necrosis of myelin and axons and often appears as a granulomatous encephalitis (inflammatory form of reticulosis). Therefore, a few patients will show other signs reflecting a more diffuse distribution of the lesion. In many patients the cisternal cerebrospinal fluid is abnormal. This inflammation is sometimes responsive to vigorous corticosteroid therapy. Any relationship of this disease to the canine distemper virus has yet to be determined.[62]

Although the onset of blindness as recognized by the owner appears to be sudden, unilateral or partial visual deficit produced as the lesion progressed may have been overlooked. Careful examination may reveal mild signs of general proprioceptive ataxia or vestibular system deficits referable to lesions in the spinal cord and cerebellomedullary region. Beware that in a few patients this disease will affect the optic nerves and produce blindness, yet the pupils may still respond to a bright light. However, in room light the pupils are usually enlarged.

Other causes of optic neuritis include canine distemper, toxoplasmosis, and cryptococcosis. These usually produce a chorioretinitis that is visible with the ophthalmoscope and other signs of diffuse or multifocal brain and/or spinal cord involvement. Blindness is uncommon in canine distemper encephalitis with optic nerve or tract involvement.

Blindness with dilated unresponsive pupils

occurred in a 10-month-old colt as a result of an acute bilateral optic neuropathy.[119] The onset was closely associated with administration of a recommended dose of oral anthelmintic considered to be safe. An idiosyncratic reaction was suspected. Bilateral retinal and optic nerve degeneration occurred in adult horses, causing blindness with dilated unresponsive pupils. A relationship to prior extensive hemorrhage was proposed as the cause.[69]

8. Neoplasia of the presphenoid bone or meninges ventral to the brain with infiltration of the optic nerves produces bilateral blindness with dilated unresponsive pupils.

9. Optic nerve compression occurs in young growing cattle from stenosis of the optic canals caused by vitamin A deficiency and failure of bone resorption.[209] This is most common in cattle in western North America that are 18 to 24 months old and have been on dry range with no green feed for 3 to 4 months. The blindness is associated with dilated unresponsive pupils. Disk edema may be observed. Occasionally these cattle are mildly ataxic and tremor. They will not respond to treatment with vitamin A.

OPTIC CHIASM[25]

In domestic animals, unlike humans, most pituitary neoplasms grow into the hypothalamus. The normal canine pituitary gland projects caudally away from the optic chiasm. Therefore, enlargement of this gland often does not affect the chiasm.[47]

In one dog, a meningioma developed between the optic chiasm and pituitary gland, causing compression of both. Bilateral blindness with dilated unresponsive pupils occurred. The clinical signs were improved temporarily with corticosteroid therapy.

Occasionally, the cerebral infarction syndrome in cats (see Chapter 7) causes ischemic necrosis of the optic chiasm, resulting in blindness and dilated unresponsive pupils.

OPTIC TRACTS

Bilateral

1. Incomplete bilateral lesions may produce partial bilateral visual deficit with variable pupillary response. This is typical of the inflammation and necrosis caused by the canine distemper virus, which has a predilection for this system. Often no clinical visual deficit is observed.

2. In humans, pituitary neoplasia commonly causes compression of the optic chiasm and tracts because of the rostral location of the pituitary directly ventral to the chiasm, and the lack of a meningeal barrier. In domestic animals, involvement of the optic chiasm is less common because of the caudal position of the pituitary gland and the restrictive dural diaphragma sellae in the ruminant. Occasionally, canine pituitary neoplasms affect one or both optic tracts as the hypothalamus is invaded or compressed by the neoplasm. In a horse with a large pars intermedia neoplasm, sudden blindness followed ischemic necrosis of the adjacent optic tracts. Pupils were dilated and unresponsive to light.[47]

Unilateral

1. Unilateral neoplasms in the hypothalamus and thalamus often encroach upon one optic tract, resulting in a visual deficit (poor menace response) in the contralateral eyeball with normal pupillary responses to light or a slower pupillary response in the eye contralateral to the optic tract lesion when a light is directed into that eye.

Because of the close approximation of the internal capsule and rostral crus cerebri to the optic tract, space-occupying lesions in the lateral hypothalamus, or thalamus, or both, that affect the optic tract usually also affect the internal capsule and rostral crus cerebri. This usually results in a normal gait but contralateral postural reaction deficits.

2. Traumatic or ischemic lesions that cause necrosis of these tissues on one side of the diencephalon can result in the same residual neurologic signs—contralateral visual deficit and postural reaction deficits.

LATERAL GENICULATE NUCLEUS

Unilateral destruction of this nucleus produces signs of visual disturbance similar to those observed with optic tract lesions, a contralateral menace deficit. Pupillary light responses will be normal if the optic tract axons that pass over the lateral geniculate nucleus to the pretectal nucleus are spared. Bilateral destruction of the lateral geniculate nucleus and associated optic tract axons projecting to the brain stem results in blindness with dilated unresponsive pupils. A neoplastic or granulomatous inflammatory lesion could cause this. An abnormality in the retinogeniculate projections and the neuronal organization in this nucleus has been observed in Siamese cats and white Persian tiger cats.[3, 29, 40, 182, 199, 200, 221] There is evidence that more ganglion neurons in the Siamese cat retina project contralaterally, as compared with normally pigmented feline breeds. In the retina the transition from retinal ganglion neurons that project contralaterally to those that project ipsilaterally is more gradual and is centered farther lateral (temporal) to the area centralis instead of at the area centralis. This directly relates to the abnormality observed in the lamination of the lateral geniculate nucleus. The degree of abnormality of the nasotemporal division of the retina varies between individual Siamese cats. It is suggested that a genetic mutation has caused this abnormal routing of ganglion neuron axons from an ipsilateral to a contralateral projection, and this may be related to the genes responsible for coat color. There is no obvious impairment of vision, but in some cats this visual system anomaly has been associated with a congenital bilateral medial strabismus or a congenital nystagmus.[77, 78, 97, 113, 195]

OPTIC RADIATION—VISUAL CORTEX

Unilateral. Unilateral lesions produce hemianopsia recognized in the contralateral eyeball, as previously discussed. Pupillary size and response to light are normal.

1. Neoplastic lesions produce progressive signs of neurologic deficit. Convulsions or changes in behavior may accompany the visual deficit. Frequently, the cerebrospinal fluid pressure is elevated.[47, 60]

2. Traumatic lesions that cause necrosis of these tissues may leave a residual neurologic deficit limited to a contralateral visual deficit. If the entire hemisphere is involved, a contralateral postural reaction deficiency may be seen on neurologic examination. Immediately following the injury the neurologic signs may be more extensive, suggestive of diffuse cerebral disturbance. As the hemorrhage and edema subside, the residual neurologic deficits relate to the areas of tissue necrosis.

3. Cerebral infarction most commonly seen in cats (see Chapter 7) may destroy the optic radiation, or visual cortex, or both in one hemisphere. When the signs of the acute cerebral disturbance resolve after the first few days, it is usual to find a contralateral menace deficit from the visual pathway lesion and a contralateral postural reaction deficit from the lesion in the cerebral pathway for the upper motor neuron and general proprioceptive systems. Neither disturbance may be reflected in the routine activities of the cat. CSF may contain an increased amount of protein (20 to 100 mg per dl) and normal or slightly higher numbers of leukocytes.

4. Unilateral cerebral abscess in the horse caused by *Streptococcus equi* may directly affect the optic radiation and cause a contralateral visual deficit with normal pupils. Expansion of this lesion with accompanying cerebral edema may increase intracranial pressure and cause the occipital lobes to herniate ventral to the tentorium cerebelli. This further compromises the function of the visual cortex bilaterally and causes total blindness if both sides are affected.[47, 173]

Similar signs may occur in ruminants with a *Corynebacterium pyogenes* abscess.

5. In encephalitis caused by *Toxoplasma gondii,* a space-occupying granuloma may be produced in the vicinity of the optic radiation and cause a contralateral visual deficit. CSF should contain inflammatory cells, often with neutrophils and increased amounts of protein.

6. Occasionally, focal protozoal encephalitis occurs in horses and is severe enough in one hemisphere to cause swelling and necrosis and a contralateral visual deficit. This is assumed to be the same organism that causes protozoal myelitis in horses (see Chapter 11).

Bilateral. Total blindness with normal pupils is characteristic of bilateral visual cortex lesions.

1. The same explanation of tentorial herniation for bilateral signs of visual deficit can be offered for any space-occupying cerebral lesion or when the brain swells following injury. Head injury that causes progressive cerebral edema causes blindness. The pupillary activity varies with the degree of brain stem involvement.

2. A malformation, hypoplasia of the prosencephalon with complete absence of cerebral hemispheres, has been observed in calves. The lack of cerebral tissue caused the visual deficit, despite a functional brain stem.

3. Bilateral hydranencephaly in ruminants is caused by an in utero viral infection of the fetus by the Akabane or Blue Tongue virus. Destruction of the visual cerebral cortex and optic radiation causes blindness with normally responsive pupils.

4. Obstructive hydrocephalus compromises the optic radiation in the internal capsule, in which it forms the lateral wall of the dilated

lateral ventricle. Bilateral visual deficit is a common sign of this lesion.

5. In the recovery phase of diffuse ischemic necrosis of the cerebrum caused by an overdose of anesthetic and a prolonged apnea and cardiac arrest, the only residual deficit may be that of blindness with intact pupils. In this situation the cerebral cortex has been compromised.[81, 154]

6. Polioencephalomalacia in cattle and sheep is characterized by severe cerebral disturbance, including blindness in most cases.[138] The visual deficit is due to the necrosis of cerebral cortical tissue in the visual cortex. The pathogenesis of this disease involves an abnormality in thiamine (vitamin B_1) metabolism. Lead intoxication causes a similar acute necrosis of the cerebral cortex and an associated blindness.[36] Similarly, severe water intoxication with cerebral disturbances may lead to blindness.[92]

7. Intoxication by wheat seed fungicide containing mercury causes a chronic degeneration of neurons in the cerebral cortex and their replacement by astrocytes. Convulsions and blindness may appear in the chronic stage of the disease.[111]

8. Chronic inflammation of the cerebral white matter caused by the canine distemper virus may result in a demyelination and astrocytosis of the centrum semiovale, including the optic radiation. This is a sclerosing encephalitis that may produce a unilateral or bilateral visual deficit with normal pupillary function.

9. Infarction of the cerebral white matter by septic vasculitis and thrombosis occurs in thrombotic meningoencephalitis in cattle caused by *Hemophilus somnus*. Visual deficits may result.

Bilateral disseminated cerebral infarcts occurred in a pony associated with the release of a *Strongylus vulgaris* larva from the wall of the brachiocephalic trunk. Bilateral central visual deficit accompanied other signs of the acute diffuse cerebral lesion.

10. Storage Diseases. Storage diseases in the central nervous system result from a deficiency of a specific degradative lysosomal enzyme causing the accumulation of a substrate that is stored in the cytoplasm of neurons, and occasionally in glial cells, macrophages, and cells in other organs (Table 14-3).[13, 108] The enzyme deficiency is usually inherited as an autosomal recessive gene. Each storage disease is named by the nature of the substrate that accumulates. These metabolic disorders are most common in dogs and cats and many are models of comparable diseases in humans.

TABLE 14–3. STORAGE DISEASE IN DOMESTIC ANIMALS[13, 108]

Neuronal

A. Glycolipid[83]
  1. Gangliosidosis[144, 176]
    a. GM$_1$ gangliosidosis[15, 50, 59, 94, 103, 148, 174, 201, 202]
      Beta-galactosidase deficiency
        Siamese cats*, domestic short-haired cat
        Friesian calves, dog
    b. GM$_2$ gangliosidosis (Tay-Sachs)[41, 42, 128, 129, 166, 178]
      Hexosaminidase deficiency
        German short-haired pointer*
        Yorkshire pig*
        Domestic short-haired cat
  2. Sphingomyelin lipidosis (Niemann-Pick)[32, 230]
    Spingomyelinase deficiency
      Cats—Siamese, domestic short-haired
      Dogs—Portuguese water dog (?)
  3. Ceroid lipofuscinosis[43, 74, 106, 109, 160, 169, 226]
    English setters*
    Siamese cat, Chihuahua, dachshund, cocker spaniel, border collie
    Sheep
  4. Glucocerebrosidosis (Gaucher's disease)[82, 132, 225, 227]
    Beta glucosidase deficiency
    Australian silkie terrier*
    Abyssinian cats

B. Glycoprotein
  1. Glycogenosis (Pompe, Cori)[33, 172, 179]
    Alpha-glucosidase deficiency
      Short-horn beef cattle, cat, dog, sheep
  2. Mannosidosis[14, 107, 137]
    Alpha-mannosidase deficiency
      Angus cattle*
      Plants of genus *Swainsona* → inhibitor of lysosomal alpha-mannosidase[99, 110, 242, 243]
    Beta-mannosidase deficiency
      Nubian goats[245-248]

Myelin

  1. Globoid cell (Krabbe)[30, 63, 64-67, 104, 130, 131, 141, 168, 184, 237, 241]
    Beta-galactocerebrosidase deficiency
      Cairn and West Highland white terriers*, beagle, poodle, mongrel, domestic short-haired cat, polled Dorset sheep
  2. Leukodystrophy
    Charolais cattle[155]
    Labrador retriever[143]
    Dalmation[244]

*Autosomal recessive inheritance.

Most of these diseases are expressed in neurons by the accumulation of a complex of lipid, protein, and/or carbohydrate in the neuronal cytoplasm. One inherited enzymatic deficiency in dogs and cats affects central and peripheral nervous system myelin, which degenerates and accumulates in macrophages.

The clinical signs are usually first observed at a few months of age. Occasionally they start at a few weeks of age, especially in cats, and a few canine diseases may not start until around 2 years of age. They are usually slow in onset and progression and are diffuse in origin. Visual deficit occurs if the function of the neurons in the visual cortex and occasionally the ganglion neuron layer of the retina is compromised by the stored substrate. The signs frequently include cerebellar involvement and often the spinal cord.

Table 14–3 lists the majority of the storage diseases that have been recognized in domestic animals.

Patient Report

Signalment. The patient was a 7½-year-old male boxer.

History. Four months prior to admission, the owner noticed that the right thoracic limb seemed to bother the dog. Occasionally, it would slide out laterally, and when standing the dog seemed to favor it by treading continually on it, as if it could not get the limb into a comfortable position. Each time the paw was placed it immediately would be retracted and replaced. One month later, the owner noticed that the right pelvic limb occasionally slid out laterally, especially on slippery floors. In the month before admission the dog showed some difficulty and caution when climbing stairs. The dog ran well on firm footing, without indicating any abnormality to the owner.

Examination. The patient was in good physical condition, alert and responsive. No muscle atrophy was evident. While standing, the right thoracic limb frequently was treaded on the floor, as if the dog either could not find a comfortable position for it or it would not support its weight well in certain positions, and therefore kept moving it to a more satisfactory position. The right pelvic limb frequently slid out laterally on a slippery floor, and was replaced continually. When the dog walked on firm footing little deficit was seen, but on a slippery floor either or both of the right limbs often would slide out laterally on the floor. The patient ran well on a surface that was not slippery.

All flexor reflexes were normal. The patellar reflex on the right side was hyperactive (plus 3), and on the left side was normal (plus 2). Muscle tone was normal. When the dog relaxed, increased resistance often could be induced by manipulating the right pelvic limb. It was not evident in the left pelvic limb or in either thoracic limb. Pain perception was intact from all limbs.

The hopping response with the left limbs was normal, but with the right limbs the response was exaggerated, almost hypermetric in action. The extensor thrust response with the pelvic limbs was slightly asymmetric. Proprioceptive positioning was slow in the right pelvic limb. Placing was usually normal. On tonic neck and eye testing, the right forepaw occasionally knuckled onto its dorsal surface.

Cranial nerve examination was normal except for the visual pathway. The menace response in the right eye was deficient. When the patient was blindfolded unilaterally and walked through a maze, only a minimal difference between the two sides could be seen. There was only a suggestion that the animal had more difficulty with the left eye blindfolded. Pupillary response to light was normal in both eyes, direct and indirect. No fundic abnormalities were noted.

Anatomic Diagnosis. These signs suggest a lesion in the left cerebrum involving visual and sensorimotor cortex, or in the left internal capsule involving the optic radiation and UMN and GP pathways to and from the sensorimotor cortex, or on the left side of the diencephalon affecting the optic tract and internal capsule.

Differential Diagnoses. The age of the dog, progressive nature of the signs, and the localizing nature of the signs all suggest a neoplastic process. Other considerations include a focal granulomatous encephalitis or focal toxoplasma encephalitis.

Ancillary Study. Radiographs of the skull were normal. Cerebrospinal fluid pressure was 410 mm (normal is <170). It was clear and contained 20 mg of protein per dl and <10 cells per cmm.[7] The increased intracranial pressure suggested an expanding space-occupying lesion.

Outcome. The dog was treated with corticosteroids and lived for about 3 months before neurologic signs worsened and euthanasia was performed. At necropsy, an astrocytoma was found in the left cerebral internal capsule and the optic radiation.

REFERENCES

1. Ammann, K., and Müller, A.: Das Bild des normalen Augenhintergrundes beim Pferd. Berl. Münch. Tierärztl. Wochenschr., *81*:370, 1968.
2. Anderson, D. H., Fisher, S. K., and Steinberg, R. H.: Mammalian cones: disc shedding, phagocytosis and renewal. Invest. Ophthalmol., *17*:117, 1978.
3. Antonini, A., Berlucchi, G., Maazi, C. A., and Sprague, J. M.: Behavioral and electrophysiological effects of unilateral optic tract section on ordinary and Siamese cats. J. Comp. Neurol., *185*:183, 1979.
4. Aquirre, G. D.: Retinal degeneration associated with the feeding of dog foods to cats. J. Am. Vet. Med. Assoc., *172*:791, 1978.
5. Aquirre, G., Farber, R., Lolley, R., Fletcher, R. T., and Chader, G. J.: Rod-cone dysplasia in Irish setters: A defect in cyclic GMP metabolism. Science, *201*:1133, 1978.
6. Aquirre, G. D., and Rubin, L. F.: Progressive retinal atrophy in the miniature poodle: An electrophysiologic study. J. Am. Vet. Med. Assoc., *160*:191, 1972.
7. Aquirre, G. D., and Rubin, L. F.: Rod-cone dysplasia (progressive retinal atrophy) in Irish setters. J. Am. Vet. Med. Assoc., *166*:157, 1975.
8. Aquirre, G. D., Rubin, L. F., and Bistner, S. I.: Development of the canine eye. Am. J. Vet. Res., *33*:2399, 1972.

9. Ashton, H.: Congenital nuclear cataracts in cattle. Vet. Rec., *100*:505, 1977.

10. Ashton, N., Barnett, K. C., and Sachs, D. D.: Retinal dysplasia in the Sealyham terrier. J. Pathol. Bacteriol., *96*:269, 1968.

11. Baker, H. J.: Inherited metabolic disorders of the nervous system in dogs and cats. *In* Kirk, R. W. (ed.): Current Veterinary Therapy V: Small Animal Practice. Philadelphia, W. B. Saunders Co., 1974.

12. Baker, H. J., Jr., Lindsey, J. R., McKhann, G. M. and Farrell, D. F.: Neuronal GM_1 gangliosidosis in a Siamese cat with beta galactosidase deficiency. Science, *174*:838, 1971.

13. Baker, H. J., Mole, J. A., Lindsey, J. R., and Creel, R. M.: Animal models of human ganglioside storage diseases. Anim. Mod. Biomed. Res. VI Metabolic Diseases, *35*:1193, 1976.

14. Barlow, R. M., MacKellar, A., Neurlands, G., Wiseman, A., and Berrett, S.: Mannosidosis in Aberdeen Angus cattle in Britain. Vet. Rec., *109*:441, 1981.

15. Barnes, I. C., Kelly, D. F., Pennock, C. A., and Randell, J. A. J.: Hepatic beta galactosidase and feline GM_1 gangliosidosis. Neuropathol. Appl. Neurobiol., *7*:463, 1981.

16. Barnett, K. C.: Canine retinopathies. I. History and review of literature. J. Small Anim. Pract., *6*:41, 1965.

17. Barnett, K. C.: Canine retinopathies. II. The miniature and toy poodle. J. Small Anim. Pract., *6*:93, 1965.

18. Barnett, K. C.: Canine retinopathies. III. The other breeds. J. Small Anim. Pract., *6*:185, 1965.

19. Barnett, K. C.: Canine retinopathies. IV. Causes of retinal atrophy. J. Small Anim. Pract., *6*:229, 1965.

20. Barnett, K. C.: Primary retinal dystrophies in the dog. J. Am. Vet. Med. Assoc., *154*:804, 1969.

21. Barnett, K. C.: Variations of the normal ocular fundus of the dog. Am. Anim. Hosp. Assoc. Proc., *39*:1, 1972.

22. Barnett, K. C., and Grimes, T. D.: Bilateral aplasia of the optic nerve in a cat. Br. J. Ophthalmol., *58*:663, 1974.

23. Barnett, K. C., and Burger, I. H.: Taurine deficiency retinopathy in the cat. J. Small Anim. Pract., *21*:521, 1980.

24. Barnett, K. C., Bjorck, G. B., and Koch, E.: Hereditary retinal dysplasia in the Labrador retriever in England and Sweden. J. Small Anim. Pract., *10*:755, 1970.

25. Barnett, K. C., Kelly, D. F., and Singleton, W. B.: Retrobulbar and chiasmal meningioma in a dog. J. Small Anim. Pract., *8*:391, 1967.

26. Bishop, G. H., and Clare, M. C.: Organization and distribution of fibers in the optic tract of the cat. J. Comp. Neurol., *103*:269, 1955.

27. Bistner, S. I., Rubin, L. F., and Aquirre, G. D.: Development of the bovine eye. Am. J. Vet. Res., *34*:7, 1973.

28. Bistner, S. I., Rubin, L. F., and Saunders, L. Z.: The ocular lesions of bovine viral diarrhea-mucosal disease. Pathol. Vet., *7*:275, 1970.

29. Blake, R., and Antoinetti, D. N.: Abnormal visual resolution in the Siamese cat. Science, *194*:109, 1976.

30. Blakemore, W. F., Mitten, R. W., Palmer, A. C., and Patterson, R. C.: Value of a nerve biopsy in diagnosis of globoid cell leukodystrophy in the dog. Vet. Rec., *94*:70, 1974.

31. Braund, K. G., Vandevelde, M., Albert, R. A., and Higgins, R. J.: Central (post-retinal) visual impairment in the dog—a clinical-pathologic study. J. Small Anim. Pract., *18*:395, 1977.

32. Bundza, A., Lowden, J. A., and Charlton, K. M.: Niemann-Pick disease in a poodle dog. Vet. Pathol., *16*:530, 1979.

33. Ceh, L., Hauge, J. G., Svenkervd, R., and Strande, A.: Glycogenoses type III in the dog. Acta Vet. Scand., *17*:210, 1976.

34. Carrig, C. B., MacMillan, A., Brundage, S., Pool, R. R., and Morgan, J. P.: Retinal dysplasia associated with skeletal abnormalities in Labrador retrievers. J. Am. Vet. Med. Assoc., *170*:49, 1977.

35. Chrisp, C. E., Ringler, D. H., Abrams, G. D., Radin, N. S., and Brenkert, A.: Lipid storage disease in a Siamese cat. J. Am. Vet. Med. Assoc., *156*:616, 1970.

36. Christian, R. G., and Tryphonas, L.: Lead poisoning in cattle: Brain lesions and hematologic changes. Am. J. Vet Res., *32*:203, 1971.

37. Cogan, D. G.: Neurology of the Visual System. Springfield, Ill., Charles C Thomas, 1966.

38. Cogan, D. G., and Kuwabara, T.: Photoreceptive abiotrophy of the retina in the elkhound. Pathol. Vet., *2*:101, 1965.

39. Cooper, M. L., and Pettigrew, J. D.: The decussation of the retinothalamic pathway in the cat, with a note on the major meridians of the cat's eye. J. Comp. Neurol., *187*:285, 1979.

40. Cooper, M. L., and Pettigrew, J. D.: The retinothalamic pathways in Siamese cats. J. Comp. Neurol., *187*:313, 1979.

41. Cork, L. C., Munnell, J. F., and Lorenz, M. D.: The pathology of feline GM_2 gangliosidosis. Am. J. Pathol., *90*:723, 1978.

42. Cork, L. C., Munnell, J. F., Lorenz, M. D., Murphy, J. V., Baker, H. J., and Rattazzi, M. C.: GM_2 ganglioside lysosomal storage disease in cats with beta-hexosaminidase deficiency. Science, *196*:1014, 1977.

43. Cummings, J. F., and de Lahunta, A.: An adult case of canine neuronal ceroid lipofuscinosis. Acta Neuropathol., *39*:43, 1977.

44. Cummings, J. F., and de Lahunta, A.: An experimental study of the retinal projections in the horse and sheep. Ann. N.Y. Acad. Sci., *167*:293, 1969.

45. Davis, T. E.: Bone Resorption in Hypovitaminosis A. Ph.D. thesis. Ithaca, N.Y., Cornell University, 1968.

46. de Lahunta, A.: Small animal neuro-ophthalmology. Vet. Clin. North Am., *3*:491, 1973.

47. de Lahunta, A., and Cummings, J. F.: Neuro-ophthalmologic lesions as a cause of visual deficit in dogs and horses. J. Am. Vet. Med. Assoc., *150*:994, 1967.

48. Denny-Brown, D., and Chambers, R. A.: Physiological aspects of visual perception. I. Functional aspects of visual cortex. Arch. Neurol., *33*:219, 1976.

49. Denny-Brown, D., and Fischer, E. G.: Physiological aspects of visual perception. II. The subcortical visual direction of behavior. Arch. Neurol., *33*:228, 1976.

50. Donnelly, W. J. C., Kelly, M., and Sheahan, B. J.: Leukocyte beta galactosidase activity in the diagnosis of bovine GM_1 gangliosidosis. Vet. Rec., *100*:318, 1977.

51. Donnelly, W. J. C., Sheahan, B. J., and Rogers, T. A.: GM_1 gangliosidosis in Friesian calves. J. Pathol., *111*:173, 1973.

52. Donovan, E. F., and Wyman, M.: Ocular fundus

anomaly in the collie. J. Am. Vet. Med. Assoc., *147*:1465, 1965.

53. Donovan, R. H., Carpenter, R. L., Schepens, C. L., and Tolentino, F. I.: Histology of the normal collie eye. I. Topography, cornea, sclera, and filtration angle. Ann. Ophthalmol., *6*:257, 1974.

54. Dowling, J. E.: Organization of vertebrate retinas. Invest. Ophthalmol., *9*:650, 1970.

55. Elgeti, H., Elgeti, R., and Fleischhauer, K.: Postnatal growth of the dorsal lateral geniculate nucleus of the cat. Anat. Embryol., *149*:1, 1976.

56. Ernest, J. T.: Bilateral optic nerve hypoplasia in a pup. J. Am. Vet. Med. Assoc., *168*:125, 1976.

57. Evans, H. E., Ingalls, T. N., and Binns, W.: Teratogenesis of craniofacial malformations in animals. III. Natural and experimental cephalic deformities in sheep. Arch. Environ. Health, *13*:706, 1966.

58. Fagan, R. H.: Canine congenital nystagmus. Seminar, Flower Veterinary Library, Ithaca, N.Y., New York State College of Veterinary Medicine, 1974.

59. Farrell, D. F., Baker, H. J., Herndon, R. M., Lindsey, J. R., and McKhann, G. M.: Feline GM₁ gangliosidosis: Biochemical and ultrastructural comparisons with the disease in man. J. Neuropathol. Exp. Neurol., *32*:1, 1973.

60. Finn, J. P., and Tennant, B. C.: A cerebral and ocular tumor of reticular tissue in a horse. Vet. Pathol., *8*:458, 1971.

61. Fischer, C. A.: Intraocular cryptococcosis in two cats. J. Am. Vet. Med. Assoc., *158*:191, 1971.

62. Fischer, C. A., and Jones, G. T.: Optic neuritis in dogs. J. Am. Vet. Med. Assoc., *160*:68, 1972.

63. Fletcher, T. F., Jessen, C. R., and Bender, A. P.: Quantitative evaluation of spinal cord lesions in canine globoid leukodystrophy. J. Neuropathol. Exp. Neurol., *36*:84, 1977.

64. Fletcher, T. F., Kurtz, H. J., and Stallan, E. M.: Experimental Wallerian degeneration in peripheral nerves of dogs with globoid cell leukodystrophy. J. Neuropathol. Exp. Neurol., *30*:593, 1971.

65. Fletcher, T. F., Kurtz, H. J., and Low, D. G.: Globoid cell leukodystrophy (Krabbe type) in the dog. J. Am. Vet. Med. Assoc., *149*:165, 1966.

66. Fletcher, T. F., Lee, D. G., and Hammer, R. F.: Ultrastructural features of globoid-cell leukodystrophy in the dog. Am. J. Vet. Res., *32*:177, 1971.

67. Fletcher, T. F., Suzuki, K., and Martin, F. B.: Galactocerebrosidase activity in canine globoid leukodystrophy. Neurology, *27*:758, 1977.

68. Fox, M. W.: Postnatal ontogeny of the canine eye. J. Am. Vet. Med. Assoc., *143*:968, 1963.

69. Gelatt, K. N.: Neuroretinopathy in horses. J. Equine Med. Surg., *3*:91, 1979.

70. Gelatt, K. N., and McGill, L. D.: Clinical characteristics of microphthalmia with colobomas of the Australian shepherd dog. J. Am. Vet. Med. Assoc., *162*:393, 1973.

71. Gelatt, K. N., Leipold, H. W., and Coffman, J. R.: Bilateral optic nerve hypoplasia in a colt. J. Am. Vet. Med. Assoc., *155*:627, 1969.

72. Glickenstein, M., King, R. A., Miller, J., and Berkley, M.: Cortical projections from the dorsal lateral geniculate nucleus of the cat. J. Comp. Neurol., *130*:55, 1967.

73. Goldman, A. I., and O'Brien, P. J.: Phagocytosis in the retinal pigment epithelium of the RCS rat. Science, *201*:1023, 1978.

74. Green, P. D., and Little, P. B.: Neuronal ceroid-lipofuscin storage in Siamese cats. Can. J. Comp. Med., *38*:207, 1974.

75. Guillery, R. W.: The laminar distribution of retinal fibers in the dorsal lateral geniculate nucleus of the cat: A new interpretation. J. Comp. Neurol., *139*:339, 1970.

76. Guillery, R. W.: The organization of synaptic interconnections in the laminae of the dorsal lateral geniculate nucleus of the cat. Z. Zellforsch. Mikrosk. Anat., *96*:1, 1969.

77. Guillery, R. W., and Kaas, J. H.: Genetic abnormality of the visual pathways in a "white" tiger. Science, *180*:1287, 1973.

78. Guillery, R. W., and Kaas, J. H.: A study of normal and congenitally abnormal retinogeniculate projections in cats. J. Comp. Neurol., *143*:73, 1971.

79. Guillery, R. W., and Stelzner, D. J.: The differential effects of unilateral lid closure upon the monocular and binocular segments of the dorsal lateral geniculate nucleus in the cat. J. Comp. Neurol., *139*:413, 1970.

80. Gwin, R. M.: Diagnosis and treatment of retinopathies in the dog and cat. *In* Proceedings of the Kal Kan Symposium, Sept. 1978, page 9.

81. Hartley, W. J.: Polioencephalomalacia in dogs. Acta Neuropathol., *2*:271, 1963.

82. Hartley, W. J., and Blakemore, W. F.: Neurovisceral glucocerebroside storage (Gaucher's disease) in a dog. Vet. Pathol., *10*:191, 1973.

83. Hartley, W. J., and Blakemore, W. F.: Neurovisceral storage and dysmyelinogenesis in neonatal goats. Acta Neuropathol., *25*:325, 1973.

84. Hayes, K. C.: Taurine Nutrition for Pets. Nutr. Aids. Quaker Oats Co. Fall, 1981.

85. Hayes, K. C., and Carey, R. E.: Retinal degeneration associated with taurine deficiency in the cat. Science, *188*:949, 1975.

86. Hayhow, W. R.: An experimental study of the accessory optic fiber system in the cat. J. Comp. Neurol., *113*:281, 1959.

87. Hayhow, W. R.: Experimental degeneration of optic axons in lateral geniculate body of the cat. Acta Anat., *37*:281, 1958.

88. Hayhow, W. R.: The cytoarchitecture of the lateral geniculate body in the cat in relation to the distribution of crossed and uncrossed optic fibers. J. Comp. Neurol., *110*:1, 1958.

89. Hebel, R.: Distribution of retinal ganglion cells in five mammalian species (pig, sheep, ox, horse, dog). Anat. Embryol., *150*:45, 1976.

90. Hegreberg, G. A., Thuline, H. C., and Francis, B. H.: Morphologic changes in feline leukodystrophy. Fed. Proc., *30*:341, 1971.

91. Herron, M. A., Martin, J. E., and Joyce, J. R.: Quantitative study of the decussating optic axons in the pony, cow, sheep and pig. Am. J. Vet. Res., *39*:1137, 1978.

92. Heslink, P.: Water intoxication in a calf. Senior seminar, Flower Veterinary Library, Ithaca, N.Y., New York State College of Veterinary Medicine, 1975.

93. Hocking, J. D., Jolly, R. D., and Batt, R. D.: Deficiency of alpha mannosidase in Angus cattle. Biochem. J., *128*:69, 1972.

94. Holmes, E. W., and O'Brien, J. S.: Feline GM₁ gangliosidosis: Charactcrization of the residual liver and beta galactosidase. Am. J. Hum. Genet., *30*:505, 1978.

95. Howard, D. R., and Breazile, J. E.: Normal visual cortical-evoked response in the dog. Am. J. Vet. Res., *33*:2155, 1972.

96. Howard, D. R., and Breazile, J. E.: Optic fiber

projections to dorsal lateral geniculate nucleus in the dog. Am. J. Vet. Res., *34*:419, 1973.

97. Hubel, D. H., and Wiesel, T. N.: Aberrant visual projections in the Siamese cat. J. Physiol., *218*:33, 1971.

98. Hughes, W. F., and McLoon, S. C.: Ganglion cell death during normal retinal development in the chick: Comparisons with cell death induced by early target field destruction. Exp. Neurol., *66*:587, 1979.

99. Huxtable, C. R., Dorling, P. R., and Colegate, S. M.: Mannosidosis induced by Swainsonine—a model to study pathogenetic aspects of neuronal lysosomal storage disease. Proc. Am. Coll. Vet. Pathol., *31*:118, 1980.

100. Jacobsen, M., and Hirose, G.: Origin of the retina from both sides of the embryonic brain: A contribution to the problem of crossing at the optic chiasm. Science, *202*:637, 1978.

101. Jensen, H. E.: Stereoscopic Atlas of Clinical Ophthalmology of Domestic Animals. St. Louis, C. V. Mosby, 1971.

102. Johns, P. R., Rusoff, A. C., and Dubin, M. W.: Postnatal neurogenesis in the kitten retina. J. Comp. Neurol., *187*:545, 1979.

103. Johnson, A. H., Donnelly, W. J. C., and Sheahan, B. J.: The glycosaminoglycan content of liver in bovine GM_1 gangliosidosis. Res. Vet. Sci., *22*:265, 1977.

104. Johnson, G. R., Oliver, J. E., and Selcer, R.: Globoid cell leukodystrophy in a Beagle. J. Am. Vet. Med. Assoc., *167*:380, 1975.

105. Johnson, K. H.: Globoid cell leukodystrophy in the cat. J. Am. Vet. Med. Assoc., *157*:2057, 1970.

106. Jolly, R. D., and West, D. M.: Blindness in South Hampshire sheep: A neuronal ceroid lipofuscinosis. N. Z. Vet. J., *24*:123, 1976.

107. Jolly, R. D., and Thompson, K. G.: The pathology of bovine mannosidosis. Vet. Pathol., *15*:141, 1978.

108. Jolly, R. D., and Hartley, W. J.: Storage diseases of domestic animals. Aust. Vet. J., *53*:1, 1977.

109. Jolly, R. D., Janmaat, A., West, D. M., and Morrison, I.: Ovine ceroid-lipofuscinosis: A model of Batten's disease. Neuropathol. Appl. Neurobiol., *6*:195, 1980.

110. Jones, L. F., Van Kampen, K. R., and Hartley, W. J.: Comparative pathology of Astragalus (locoweed) and Swainsona poisoning in sheep. Pathol. Vet., *7*:116, 1970.

111. Kahrs, R. F.: Chronic mercurial poisoning in swine: A case report of an outbreak with some epidemiological characteristics of hog cholera. Cornell Vet., *58*:67, 1968.

112. Kalil, R.: Development of the dorsal lateral geniculate nucleus in the cat. J. Comp. Neurol., *182*:265, 1978.

113. Kalil, R. E., Jhaveri, S. R., and Richards, W.: Anomalous retinal pathways in the Siamese cat: An inadequate substrate for normal binocular vision. Science, *174*:302, 1971.

114. Kanamura, K., and Brodal, A.: Tectopontine projection in the cat: An experimental anatomical study with comments on pathways for receptive impulses to the cerebellum. J. Comp. Neurol., *3*:371, 1973.

115. Karamanlidis, A. N., and Magras, J.: Retinal projections in domestic ungulates. I. The retinal projections in the sheep and the pig. Brain Res., *44*:27, 1972.

116. Karamanlidis, A. N., and Magras, J.: Retinal projections in domestic ungulates. II. The retinal projections in the horse and ox. Brain Res., *6*:209, 1974.

117. Karbe, E., and Schiefer, B.: Familial amaurotic idiocy in male German shorthair pointers. Pathol. Vet., *4*:223, 1967.

118. Kay, W. J.: Veterinary clinical neurophthalmology: The loss of central vision. *In* Proceedings of the Kal Kan Symposium, 1978.

119. Kelly, D. F., and Pinsent, P. J. N.: Optic neuropathy in a horse. Acta Neuropathol., *48*:145, 1979.

120. Kern, T. J.: Persistent hyperplastic primary vitreous and microphthalmia in a dog. J. Am. Vet. Med. Assoc., *178*:1169, 1981.

121. Kern, T. J., and Riis, R. C.: Optic nerve hypoplasia in three miniature poodles. J. Am. Vet. Med. Assoc., *178*:49, 1980.

122. Koch, S. A., and Rubin, L. F.: Distribution of cones in the hemeralopic dog. J. Am. Vet. Med. Assoc., *159*:1257, 1971.

123. Kolb, H.: The inner plexiform layer in the retina of the cat: Electron microscopic observations. J. Neurocytol., *8*:295, 1979.

124. Kolb, H.: The organization of the outer plexiform layer in the retina of the cat: Electron microscopic observations. J. Neurocytol., *6*:131, 1977.

125. Kolb, H., and West, R. W.: Synaptic connections of the interplexiform cell in the retina of the cat. J. Neurocytol., *6*:155, 1977.

126. Koppang, N.: Canine ceroid lipofuscinosis: A model for human neuronal ceroid lipofuscinosis and aging. Mech. Aging Develop., *2*:421, 1973–74.

127. Koppang, N.: Neuronal ceroid lipofuscinosis in English setters: Juvenile amaurotic familial idiocy in English setters. J. Small Anim. Pract., *10*:639, 1970.

128. Kosanke, S. D., Pierce, K. R., and Read, W. K.: Morphogenesis of light and electron microscopic lesions in porcine GM_2-gangliosidosis. Vet. Pathol., *16*:6, 1979.

129. Kosanke, S. D., Pierce, K. R., and Bay, W. W.: Clinical and biochemical abnormalities in porcine GM_2-gangliosidosis. Vet. Pathol., *15*:685, 1978.

130. Kurczynski, T. W., Fletcher, T. F., and Suzuki, K.: Lactosylceramidases in canine globoid cell leukodystrophy. J. Neurochem., *29*:37, 1977.

131. Kurtz, H. J., and Fletcher, T. F.: The peripheral neuropathy of canine globoid-cell leukodystrophy (Krabbe-type). Acta Neuropathol., *16*:226, 1970.

132. Lange, A. L., Van den Berg, P. B., and Baker, M. K.: A suspected lysosomal storage disease in Abyssinian cats. Part II. Histopathological and ultrastructural aspects. J. S. Afr. Vet. Med. Assoc., *48*:201, 1977.

133. Laties, A. M., and Sprague, J. M.: The projection of optic fibers to the visual centers in the cat. J. Comp. Neurol., *127*:35, 1966.

134. Lavach, J. D., Murphy, J. M., and Severin, G. A.: Retinal dysplasia in the English springer spaniel. J. Am. Anim. Hosp. Assoc., *14*:192, 1978.

135. LaVail, M. M.: Rod outer segment disk shedding in rat retina. Relationship to cyclic lighting. Science, *194*:1071, 1976.

136. Leipold, H. W., and Huston, K.: Congenital syndrome of anophthalmia-microphthalmia with associated defects in cattle. Pathol. Vet., *5*:407, 1968.

137. Leipold, H. W., Smith, J. E., Jolly, R. D., and Eldridge, F. E.: Mannosidosis of Angus calves. J. Am. Vet. Med. Assoc., *175*:457, 1979.

138. Little, P. B., and Sorenson, D. K.: Bovine polioencephalomalacia, infectious embolic meningoencephalitis and acute lead poisoning in feedlot cattle. J. Am. Vet. Med. Assoc., 155:1892, 1969.

139. MacMillan, A. D., and Lipton, D. E.: Heritability of multifocal retinal dysplasia in American cocker spaniels. J. Am. Vet. Med. Assoc., 172:568, 1978.

140. Mason, T. A.: Persistent pupillary membrane in the Basenji. Aust. Vet. J., 52:343, 1976.

141. Mc C. Howell, J., and Palmer, A. C.: Globoid cell leucodystrophy in two dogs. J. Small Anim. Pract., 12:633, 1971.

142. McCormack, J. E.: Variations of the ocular fundus of the bovine species. Vet. Scope, 18:21, 1974.

143. McGrath, J. T.: Fibrinoid leukodystrophy (Alexander's disease). In Andrews, E. J., Ward, B. C., and Altman, N. H. (eds.): Spontaneous Animal Models of Human Disease. New York, Academic Press, 1979.

144. McGrath, J. T., Kelly, A. M., and Steinberg, S. A.: Cerebral lipidosis in the dog. J. Neuropathol. Exp. Neurol., 27:141, 1968.

145. Meikle, T. H., Jr., and Sprague, J. M.: The neural organization of the visual pathways in the cat. Int. Rev. Neurobiol., 6:150, 1964.

146. Morris, M. L., Jr.: Feline degenerative retinopathy. Cornell Vet., 55:295, 1965.

147. Müller, A.: Das Bild des normalen Augenhintergrundes beim Rind. Berl. Münch. Tierarztl. Wochenschr., 82:181, 1969.

148. Murray, J. A., Blakemore, W. F., and Barnett, K. C.: Ocular lesions in cats with GM_1 gangliosidosis with visceral involvement. J. Small Anim. Pract., 18:1, 1977.

149. Nafe, L.: Canine optic neuritis. Compend. Contin. Ed., 3:978, 1981.

150. Niimi, K., and Sprague, J. M.: Thalamo-cortical organization of the visual system in the cat. J. Comp. Neurol., 138:219, 1970.

151. Noden, D. M.: Interactions directing the migration and cytodifferentiation of avian neural crest cells. In Garrod, D. R. (ed.): Specificity of Embryological Interactions. London, Chapman and Hill, 1978.

152. Nyberg-Hansen, R.: The location and termination of tectospinal fibers in the cat. Exp. Neurol., 9:212, 1964.

153. Olson, C. R., and Freeman, R. D.: Eye alignment in kittens. J. Neurophysiol., 41:848, 1978.

154. Palmer, A. C.: Cardiac arrest and cerebrocortical necrosis. Vet. Rec., 80:390, 1967.

155. Palmer, A. C., Blakemore, W. F., Barlow, R. M., Fraser, J. A., and Ogden, A. L.: Progressive ataxia of Charolais cattle associated with a myelin disorder. Vet. Rec., 91:592, 1972.

156. Parry, H. B.: Degenerations of the dog retina. I. Structure and development of the retina of the normal dog. Br. J. Ophthalmol., 37:385, 1953.

157. Parry, H. B.: Degenerations of the dog retina. II. Generalized progressive atrophy of hereditary origin. Br. J. Ophthalmol., 37:487, 1953.

158. Parry, H. B.: Degenerations of the dog retina. VII. Central nonprogressive degeneration due to an anomaly of the ganglion cells and their axons. Br. J. Ophthalmol., 39:29, 1955.

159. Parry, H. B., Tansley, K., and Thomson, L. C.: Electroretinogram during development of hereditary retinal degeneration in the dog. Br. J. Ophthalmol., 39:349, 1955.

160. Patel, V., Koppang, N., Patel, B., and Zeman, W.: Alpha-phenylenediamine-mediated peroxidase deficiency in English Setters with neuronal ceroid lipofuscinosis. Lab. Invest., 30:366, 1974.

161. Peiffer, R. L.: Inherited ocular diseases of the dog and cat. Compend. Contin. Ed., 4:152, 1982.

162. Peiffer, R. L., Gelatt, K. N., and Gwin, R. M.: Persistent primary vitreous and a pigmented cataract in a dog. J. Am. Anim. Hosp. Assoc., 13:478, 1977.

163. Percy, D. H., and Jortner, B. S.: Feline lipidosis. Arch. Pathol., 92:136, 1971.

164. Percy, D. H., Scott, F. U., and Albert, D. M.: Retinal dysplasia due to feline panleukopenia virus infection. J. Am. Vet. Med. Assoc., 167:935, 1975.

165. Pfeffer, B. A., and Fisher, S. K.: Development of retinal pigment epithelial surface structures ensheathing cone outer segments in the cat. J. Ultra. Res., 76:158, 1981.

166. Pierce, K. R., Kosanke, S. D., Bay, W. W., and Bridges, C. H.: Porcine cerebrospinal lipodystrophy (GM_2 gangliosidosis). Am. J. Pathol., 83:419, 1976.

167. Prince, J. H., Diesem, C. D., Eglitis, I., and Ruskett, G. L.: Anatomy and Histology of the Eye and Orbit in Domestic Animals. Springfield, Ill., Charles C Thomas, 1960.

168. Pritchard, D. H., Napthine, D. V., and Sinclair, A. J.: Globoid cell leukodystrophy in polled Dorset sheep. Vet. Pathol., 17:399, 1980.

169. Rac, R., and Giesecke, P. R.: Lysosomal storage disease in Chihuahuas. Aust. Vet. J., 51:403, 1975.

170. Rademaker, G. G. J., and Ter Braak, J. W. G.: On the central mechanisms of some optic reactions. Brain, 71:48, 1948.

171. Rademaker, G. G. J., and Ter Braak, J. W. G.: On the central mechanisms of some optic reactions. Brain, 71:48, 1948.

172. Rafiquzzaman, M., Svenkervd, R., Strande, A., and Hauge, J. G.: Glycogenoses in the dog. Acta Vet. Scand., 17:196, 1976.

173. Raphel, C. F.: Brain abscess in three horses. J. Am. Vet. Med. Assoc., 180:874, 1982.

174. Read, D. H., Harrington, D. D., Keenan, T. W., and Hinsman, E. J.: Neuronal-visceral GM_1 gangliosidosis in a dog with beta galactosidase deficiency. Science, 194:442, 1976.

175. Read, W. K., and Bridges, C. H.: Cerebrospinal lipodystrophy in swine. A new disease model in comparative pathology. Pathol. Vet., 5:67, 1968.

176. Read, W. K., and Bridges, C. H.: Neuronal lipodystrophy: Occurrence in inbred strain of cattle. Pathol. Vet., 6:235, 1969.

177. Rebhun, W. C.: Persistent hyperplastic primary vitreous in a dog. J. Am. Vet. Med. Assoc., 169:620, 1976.

178. Ribelin, W. E., and Kintner, L. D.: Lipodystrophy in the central nervous system in a dog: A disease with similarities to Tay Sachs disease in man. Cornell Vet., 46:532, 1956.

179. Richards, R. B., Edwards, J. R., Cork, R. D., and White, R. R.: Bovine generalized glycogenosis. Neuropathol. Appl. Neurobiol., 3:45, 1977.

180. Roberts, S. R.: A system of testing vision in animals. J. Am. Vet. Med. Assoc., 128:544, 1956.

181. Roberts, S. R., and Bistner, S. I.: Persistent pupillary membrane in basenji dogs. J. Am. Vet. Med. Assoc., 153:533, 1968.

182. Robertson, T. W., Hickey, T. L., and Guillery, R.

W.: Development of the dorsal lateral geniculate nucleus in normal and visually deprived Siamese cats. J. Comp. Neurol., 191:573, 1980.

183. Rogers, K. T.: Experimental production of perfect cyclopia by removal of telencephalon and reversal of bilateralization in somite stage chicks. Am. J. Anat., 115:487, 1964.

184. Roszel, J. F., Steinberg, S. A., and McGrath, J. T.: Periodic acid-Schiff-positive cells in cerebrospinal fluid of dogs with globoid cell leukodystrophy. Neurology, 22:738, 1972.

185. Rubin, L. F.: Atlas of Veterinary Ophthalmoscopy. Philadelphia, Lea & Febiger, 1974.

186. Rubin, L. F.: Clinical features of hemeralopia in the adult Alaskan malamute. J. Am. Vet. Med. Assoc., 159:1696, 1971.

187. Rubin, L. F.: Hemeralopia in Alaskan malamute pups. J. Am. Vet. Med. Assoc., 158:1699, 1971.

188. Rubin, L. F.: Heredity of hemeralopia in Alaskan malamutes. Am. J. Vet. Res., 28:355, 1967.

189. Rubin, L. F.: Heredity of retinal dysplasia in Bedlington terriers. J. Am. Vet. Med. Assoc., 152:260, 1968.

190. Rubin, L. F., and Craig, P. H.: Intraocular cryptococcosis in a dog. J. Am. Vet. Med. Assoc., 147:27, 1965.

191. Rubin, L. F., and Lipton, D. E.: Retinal degeneration in kittens. J. Am. Vet. Med. Assoc., 162:467, 1973.

192. Saunders, L. Z.: Congenital optic nerve hypoplasia in collie dogs. Cornell Vet., 42:67, 1952.

193. Sanderson, A. T., and Anderson, L. J.: Histiocytosis in two pigs and a cow. Conditions resembling lipid storage disorders in man. J. Pathol., 100:207, 1970.

194. Sanderson, K. J.: The projections of the visual field to the lateral geniculate and medial interlaminar nuclei in the cat. J. Comp. Neurol., 143:101, 1971.

195. Sanderson, K. J., Guillery, R. W., and Shackelford, R. M.: Congenitally abnormal visual pathways in mink (Mustela vison) with reduced retinal pigment. J. Comp. Neurol., 154:225, 1974.

196. Sandstrom, B.: Glycogenosis of the central nervous system in the cat. Acta Neuropathol., 14:194, 1969.

197. Scagliotti, R. H.: Current concepts in veterinary neuroophthalmology. Vet. Clin. North Am.: Small Anim. Pract., 10:417, 1980.

198. Scott, F. W., de Lahunta, A., Schultz, R. D., Bistner, S. I., and Riis, R. C.: Teratogenesis in cats associated with griseofulvin therapy. Teratology, 11:79, 1974.

199. Shatz, C.: A comparison of visual pathways in eastern and midwestern Siamese cats. J. Comp. Neurol., 171:205, 1977.

200. Shatz, C. J., and Levay, S.: Siamese cat: Altered connections of visual cortex. Science, 204:328, 1979.

201. Sheahan, B. J., Donnelly, W. J. C., and Grimes, T. D.: Ocular pathology of bovine GM_1 gangliosidosis. Acta Neuropathol., 41:91, 1978.

202. Sheahan, B. J., Roche, E., and Donnelly, W. J. C.: Studies on cultured skin fibroblasts from calves with GM_1 gangliosidosis. J. Comp. Pathol., 87:205, 1977.

203. Shively, J., Epling, G., and Jensen, R.: Fine structure of the canine eye: retina. Am. J. Vet. Res., 31:1339, 1970.

204. Shively, J. N., Epling, G. P., and Jensen, R.: Fine structure of the postnatal development of the canine retina. Am. J. Vet. Res., 32:383, 1971.

205. Silver, J., and Sidman, R. L.: A mechanism for the guidance and topographic patterning of retinal

ganglion cell axons. J. Comp. Neurol., 189:101, 1980.

206. Singleton, M. C., and Peele, T. L.: Distribution of optic fibers in the cat. J. Comp. Neurol., 125:303, 1965.

207. Smith, J. S., de Lahunta, A., and Riis, R. C.: Reticulosis of the visual system in a dog. J. Small Anim. Pract., 18:634, 1977.

208. Sprague, J. M.: The superior colliculus and pretectum in visual behavior. Invest. Ophthalmol., 11:473, 1972.

209. Spratling, F. R., Bridge, P. S., Barnett, K. C., Abrams, J. T., Palmer, A. C., and Sharman, I. M.: Experimental hypovitaminosis A in calves: Clinical and gross postmortem findings. Vet. Rec., 77:1532, 1965.

210. Spratling, F. R., Bridge, P. S., Barnett, K. C., Abrams, J. T., Palmer, A. C., and Sharman, I. M.: Experimental hypovitaminosis A in calves. Vet. Rec., 77:532, 1965.

211. Stades, F. C.: Persistent hyperplastic tunica vasculosa lentis and persistent hyperplastic primary vitreous (PHTVL/PHPV) in 90 closely related Doberman pinschers: Clinical aspects. J. Am. Anim. Hosp. Assoc., 16:739, 1980.

212. Steinberg, R. H., Fisher, S. K., and Anderson, D. H.: Disc morphogenesis in vertebrae photoreceptors. J. Comp. Neurol., 190:501, 1980.

213. Stone, J.: A quantitative analysis of the distribution of ganglion cells in the cat's retina. J. Comp. Neurol., 124:337, 1965.

214. Stone, J.: The naso-temporal division of the cat's retina. J. Comp. Neurol., 126:585, 1966.

215. Stone, J.: The number and distribution of ganglion cells in the cat's retina. J. Comp. Neurol., 180:753, 1978.

216. Stone, J., and Hansen, S. M.: The projection of the cat's retina in the lateral geniculate nucleus. J. Comp. Neurol., 126:601, 1966.

217. Stone, J., and Campion, J. E.: Estimate of the number of myelinated axons in the cat's optic nerve. J. Comp. Neurol., 180:799, 1978.

218. Stone, J., and Keens, J.: Distribution of small and median-sized ganglion cells in the cat's retina. J. Comp. Neurol., 192:235, 1980.

219. Stone, J., Campion, J. E., and Leicester, J.: The nasotemporal division of retina in the Siamese cat. J. Comp. Neurol., 180:783, 1978.

220. Stone, J., Leventhal, A., Watson, C. R. R., Keens, J., and Clarke, R.: Gradients between nasal and temporal areas of the cat retina in the properties of retinal ganglion cells. J. Comp. Neurol., 192:219, 1980.

221. Stone, J., Rowe, M., and Campion, J. E.: Retinal abnormalities in the Siamese cat. J. Comp. Neurol., 180:773, 1978.

222. Tucker, G. S.: Light microscopic analysis of the kitten retina: Postnatal development in the area centralis. J. Comp. Neurol., 180:489, 1978.

223. Tucker, G. S., Hamasaki, D. I., Labbie, A., and Muroff, J.: Anatomic and physiologic development of the photoreceptor of the kitten. Exp. Brain Res., 37:459, 1979.

224. Ulshafer, R. J., and Clavert, A.: Cell death and optic fiber penetration in the optic stalk of the chick. J. Morph., 162:67, 1979.

225. Van den Berg, P. B., Baker, M. K., and Lange, A. L.: A suspected lysosomal storage disease in Abyssinian cats. Part I: Genetic, clinical, and clinical pathological aspects. J. S. Afr. Vet. Med. Assoc., 48:195, 1977.

226. Vandevelde, M., and Fatzer, R.: Neuronal ceroid-lipofuscinosis in older dachshunds. Vet. Pathol., *17*:686, 1980.

227. Van de Water, N. S., Jolly, R. D., and Farrow, B. R. H.: Canine Gaucher disease: The enzymic defect. Aust. J. Exp. Biol. Med., *57*:551, 1979.

228. Weisse, I., and Stötzer, H.: Hypoplasie des Nervus opticus und Kolobom der Papille bei einem jungen Beagle. Berl. Münich. Tierarztl. Wochenschr., *86*:1, 1973.

229. Weisse, I., Stötzer, H., and Seitz, R.: Die neuroepitheliale Invagination, eine Form der Netzhaut-Dysplasie beim Beagle-Hund. Zentralbl. Veterinaermed., *20A*:89, 1973.

230. Wenger, D. A., Sattler, M., Kudoh, T., Snyder, S. P., and Kingston, R. S.: Niemann-Pick disease: A genetic model in Siamese cats. Science, *208*:1471, 1980.

231. Whittem, J. H., and Walker, D.: Neuronopathy and pseudolipidosis in Aberdeen-Angus calves. J. Pathol. Bacteriol., *74*:281, 1957.

232. Witzel, D. A., Riis, R. C., Rebhun, W. C., and Hillman, R. B.: Night blindness in the Appaloosa: Sibling occurrence. J. Equine Med. Surg., *1*:383, 1977.

233. Wolf, E. D., Vainisi, S. J., and Santos-Anderson, R.: Rod-cone dysplasia in the collie. J. Am. Vet. Med. Assoc., *173*:1331, 1978.

234. Wolff, E.: Anatomy of the Eye and Orbit. Philadelphia, W. B. Saunders Co., 1968.

235. Wouters, L., and De Moor, A.: Ultrastructure of the pigment epithelium and the photoreceptors in the retina of the horse. Am. J. Vet. Res., *40*:1066, 1979.

236. Wyman, M., and Donovan, E. F.: The ocular fundus of the normal dog. J. Am. Vet. Med. Assoc., *147*:17, 1965.

237. Yajima, K., Fletcher, T. F., and Suzuki, K.: Canine globoid cell leukodystrophy. Part I. Further ultra-structural study of the typical lesion. J. Neurol. Sci., *35*:179, 1977.

238. Yakely, W. L.: Collie eye anomaly: Decreased prevalence through selective breeding. J. Am. Vet. Med. Assoc., *160*:1103, 1972.

239. Yakely, W. L., Wyman, M., Donovan, E. F., and Fechheimer, N. S.: Genetic transmission of an ocular fundus anomaly in collies. J. Am. Vet. Med. Assoc., *152*:457, 1968.

240. Young, R. W., and Bok, D.: Participation of the retinal pigment epithelium in the rod outer segment renewal process. J. Cell. Biol., *42*:392, 1969.

241. Zaki, F., and Kay, W. J.: Globoid cell leukodystrophy in a miniature poodle. J. Am. Vet. Med. Assoc., *163*:248, 1973.

242. Dorling, P. R., Huxtable, C. R., and Vogel, P.: Lysosomal storage in Swainsona spp. toxicosis: An induced mannosidosis. Neuropathol. Appl. Neurobiol., *4*:285, 1978.

243. Huxtable, C. R., Dorling, P. R., and Walkley, S. U.: Onset and regression of neuraxonal lesions in sheep with mannosidosis induced experimentally with Swainsonine. Acta Neuropathol., *58*:27, 1982.

244. Bjerkas, I.: Hereditary "cavitating" leukodystrophy in dalmatian dogs. Acta Neuropathol., *40*:163, 1977.

245. Hartley, W. J., and Blakemore, W. F.: Neurovisceral storage and dysmyelinogenesis in neonatal goats. Acta Neuropathol., *25*:325, 1973.

246. Cavanagh, K., Dunston, R. W., and Jones, M. Z.: Plasma alpha and beta mannosidase activities in caprine beta mannosidosis. Am. J. Vet. Res., *43*:1058, 1982.

247. Jones, M. Z., and Dawson, G.: Caprine beta mannosidosis: Inherited deficiency of beta-D-mannosidase. J. Biol. Chem., *256*:5185, 1981.

248. Healy, P. J., Seaman, J. T., Gardner, I. A., and Sewell, C. A.: Beta mannosidase deficiency in Anglo Nubian goats. Aust. Vet. J., *57*:504, 1981.

AUDITORY SYSTEM—SPECIAL SOMATIC AFFERENT SYSTEM

ANATOMY

RECEPTOR[9, 37]

The development of the receptor for the auditory system was described with the development of the vestibular system. The cochlea, the coiled portion of the bony labyrinth, is a passageway in the petrosal bone that contains perilymph. The degree of coiling varies with the different species of animal. There are 3.25 turns in the dog cochlea compared with 2.5 in humans. The portion of bone that forms the center or axis of the cochlea is the modiolus. At the base of the modiolus, the cochlea communicates with the vestibule. A shelf of bone projects into the cochlea from the modiolus. This is the spiral lamina that partially divides the cochlea into two portions, and is absent at the apex or most distal extent of the cochlea (Fig. 15-1).

The cochlear duct is the coiled portion of the membranous labyrinth derived from the embryonic ectodermal otocyst that is located inside the cochlea and contains endolymph. It is a tubular structure that is situated between the spiral lamina on the medial wall of the cochlea (adjacent to the modiolus) and the opposite lateral wall of the cochlea. This completes the partitioning of the cochlea into two portions, each filled with perilymph: the scala vestibuli and scala tympani. The scala vestibuli is situated dorsal to the cochlear duct and communicates proximally with the vestibule and distally at the apex of the cochlear duct with the scala tympani. Because the cochlear duct does not reach the apex of the cochlea, this communication is possible. The site of

communication is the helicotrema. The scala tympani is located ventral to the cochlear duct. It communicates distally at the helicotrema with the scala vestibuli. Proximally at the base of the coiled cochlea, it terminates at the cochlear window, which is covered by a membrane. On the other side of the cochlear window is the air-filled cavity of the middle ear in the tympanic bulla. Perilymph fills the scala vestibuli and scala tympani. At the level of the origin of the cochlea from the vestibule, the cochlear duct communicates with the saccule by way of the ductus reuniens.

The cochlear duct is triangular in shape with its base, the stria vascularis and spiral prominence, situated along the outer lateral wall of the cochlea. A thin layer of tissue forms the dorsal border of the cochlear duct, the vestibular membrane. This borders the scala vestibuli and extends from the outer wall (dorsolaterally) to the middle of the medial wall, at the position of the spiral lamina. The basilar membrane, a highly organized layer of collagen-like fibers, extends from the spiral lamina (medially) to the middle of the lateral wall of the cochlea. The spiral organ (organ of Corti) is the sensory epithelium that rests on the basilar membrane, and is composed of several types of supporting cells and hair cells.[9] The hair cells have modified microvilli on their luminal surface, "hairs" or stereocilia. The tips of these cell processes (hairs) are embedded in a proteinaceous membrane, the tectorial membrane, which covers the hair cells and is attached medially along the cochlear duct. The dendritic zone of the cochlear portion of the eighth cranial nerve is in synaptic relationship with the base of the hair cells. Sound waves are transmitted from the air medium of the external ear canal to the solid medium of the tympanum and chain of three ear ossicles, which extend to the vestibular window, to the fluid medium of the perilymph in the scala vestibuli. Wave flow through the scala vestibuli is reflected to the basilar membrane by way of the endolymph of the cochlear duct or the scala tympani through its communication at the helicotrema. Movement of the highly organized basilar membrane causes the hair cells

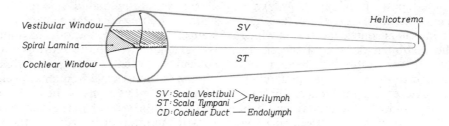

Bony Labyrinth—Cochlea—from Mesoderm

SV: Scala Vestibuli
ST: Scala Tympani ⟩ Perilymph
CD: Cochlear Duct —— Endolymph

Membranous Labyrinth—Cochlear Duct and the Spiral Organ—
from Ectoderm (Otic Placode and Cyst)

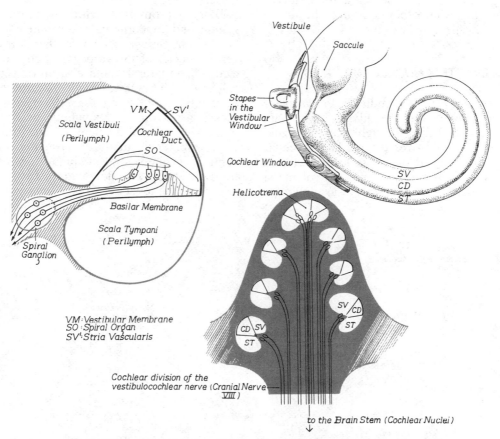

VM: Vestibular Membrane
SO: Spiral Organ
SV': Stria Vascularis

Figure 15–1. Receptor of special somatic afferent system—auditory (SSA).

of the overlying spiral organ to move, and their stereocilia embedded in the tectorial membrane to bend. This action causes an impulse to be generated in the cochlear neurons.[53] The basilar membrane acts like a resonator, and different portions respond maximally to specific frequencies of the sound waves. Low frequencies cause maximal vibration of the basilar membrane at the apex of the cochlear duct. High frequencies affect the proximal portion of the basilar membrane maximally.

CRANIAL NERVE VIII—VESTIBULOCOCHLEAR NERVE—COCHLEAR DIVISION

The neurons of the vestibulocochlear nerve are derived from placode ectoderm associated with the otocyst. The dendritic zone of the cochlear division of the eighth cranial nerve is in synaptic relationship with the base of the hair cells in the spiral organ. The axons course medially into the modiolus. The cell bodies of these bipolar neurons are located in the modiolus at the origin of the spiral lamina, where they form the spiral ganglion. The axons course through the center or axis of the modiolus to the internal acoustic meatus, in which they join the vestibular division of the eighth cranial nerve. In the vestibulocochlear nerve the axons course to the region of the cerebellomedullary angle at the junction of the medulla and pons, caudal to the transverse fibers of the pons. They terminate in telodendria on cell bodies located on the lateral side of the medulla, where the nerve enters. These cell bodies form the cochlear nuclei (dorsal and ventral) which bulge from the lateral side of the medulla, where they appear to be in the vestibulocochlear nerve (Fig. 15–2, Plates 6, 7).

BRAIN STEM NUCLEI AND TRACTS

The axons of the cell bodies in the cochlear nuclei pass into the medulla by two main pathways—ventrally through the trapezoid body and dorsally over the caudal cerebellar peduncle by way of the acoustic stria (Plates 5, 6, 7).[11] Numerous pathways involving a variable number of synapses are available for the auditory system for reflex activity and conscious projection (Fig. 15–2).

Reflexes are mediated by direct influence of neurons of the cochlear nuclei on the brain stem lower motor neuron, or indirectly by transmission through the neurons of the caudal colliculus or other auditory nuclei. Reflex regulation of sound wave frequency occurs by way of the afferent neurons of the cochlear division of the eighth cranial nerve and the cochlear nuclei, the efferent neurons of the motor nucleus of the trigeminal nerve in the pons that innervates the tensor tympani muscle, and the facial neurons that innervate the stapedius muscle.

Other neurons that belong to the auditory system and function in reflex and conscious perception pathways include the dorsal and ventral nuclei of the trapezoid body, the nucleus of the lateral lemniscus, and the caudal colliculus. The neurons of the ventral nucleus of the trapezoid body are scattered without specific arrangement throughout the trapezoid fibers. The dorsal nucleus of the trapezoid body forms a distinctly encapsulated nucleus ventrally in the rostral medulla, dorsal to the trapezoid body and dorsolateral to the pyramid, from the level of the facial nucleus in the

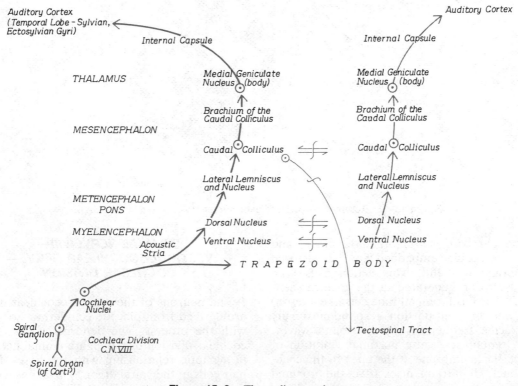

Figure 15–2. The auditory pathway.

medulla to the motor nucleus of the trigeminal nerve in the pons. (Plates 6, 7).[25] The lateral lemniscus is composed mostly of ascending axons in the auditory system, coursing from the rostral medulla through the pons to the caudal mesencephalon on the lateral surface of the brain stem (Plate 8, 9, 10).[17] It contains auditory axons from the cochlear nuclei or the various nuclei of the trapezoid body on the same or opposite sides. The lateral lemniscus is formed medial to the middle cerebellar peduncle and is exposed on the lateral surface of the caudal mesencephalon rostral to the transverse fibers of the pons that form the middle cerebellar peduncle. Embedded along the ventromedial aspect of this lemniscus is the nucleus of the lateral lemniscus (Plate 9). The lateral lemniscus terminates at the caudal colliculus.

The caudal colliculus consists of cell bodies of neurons and axonal processes organized in laminae (Plates 9, 10).[34] It is a reflex center for the auditory system. Efferent axons project to brain stem lower motor neurons by way of the tectobulbar pathways and to the cervical spinal cord through the tectospinal pathway in the ventral funiculus, which arises from the rostral colliculus. Efferent axons project to the thalamus in the brachium of the caudal colliculus located on the lateral side of the mesencephalon ventral to the rostral colliculus (Plates 10, 11). These terminate in the medial geniculate nucleus (Plate 12).

THALAMOCORTICAL PATHWAY

Axons in the conscious projection pathway arise primarily from cell bodies in the caudal colliculus and project in the brachium of the caudal colliculus located on the lateral side of the mesencephalon coursing rostrally to the medial geniculate nucleus of the thalamus.[44] This nucleus extends caudally beside the mesencephalon (Plates 12, 13). It is the specific thalamic projection nucleus for the auditory system and projects axons by way of the internal capsule to the cerebral cortex of the temporal lobe. The auditory sensory cortex is located mostly in the sylvian and ectosylvian gyri. Studies in the dog have localized the auditory conscious projection pathway to the ectosylvian gyrus, in which the various frequencies can be arranged from rostral (high frequency) to caudal (low frequency).[46–48]

The ascending auditory pathway is characterized by diffuseness and a bilateral distribution. Despite this, at the cortical level there is a predominance of contralateral representation of each cochlear duct. Thus impulses stimulated in one cochlear duct are conducted predominantly to the opposite temporal lobe. Crossing occurs at the level of the trapezoid body, between the nuclei of the lateral lemniscus and at the commissure of the caudal colliculus.

DEAFNESS[40, 45]

By recording brain stem auditory evoked potentials, researchers have found that there is evidence of hearing at 10 to 11 days of age in dogs. Audiometry studies first detect hearing perception at 5 days in kittens and 14 days in puppies.[14] These are determined from behavioral responses to pure tones and bands of noise. The frequency range first responded to is located in the outer half of the basal coil and second coil of the cochlea. This may be related to this region of the cochlea having the most advanced blood supply. Normal hearing in dogs usually develops by 4 to 5 weeks of age.

Partial loss of hearing and even unilateral complete loss of hearing are difficult to establish on clinical examination of domestic animals. Complete bilateral deafness usually is caused by direct or indirect interference with the function of the receptor organ. For central lesions to produce deafness, there must be extensive damage to both cerebral hemisphere or to the pathways on both sides of the brain stem. Such lesions most likely would produce severe neurologic deficit referrable to the interference with the other systems adjacent to the auditory pathways. Because of the multitude of brain stem pathways available for the auditory system, there is a large margin of safety for this function. Therefore, when presented with a deaf animal, attention should be directed to those diseases that affect the receptor portion of this system. The best test for total deafness is to confront the sleeping patient with a loud noise. Inability to arouse the patient in this manner is the best evidence of total inability to hear. Less obvious degrees of deafness are difficult to evaluate, and the careful observations of the patient in its own environment by the owner may be the most reliable.

More sophisticated procedures have been developed and include a technique of monitoring changes in respirations in response to hearing sounds, as well as recording electroencephalographic responses to auditory stimuli.[6] Brain stem responses to far field auditory stimuli can be recorded percutaneously from the brains of animals. The various wave forms have been related to specific components of the peripheral and central portions of the auditory system. The procedure of recording brain stem auditory evoked responses (BAER) can be utilized to determine the presence of an auditory defect and the level of the lesion.[7, 49, 50] Impedance auditometry has been developed to evaluate the integrity of the middle ear and conduction components of the auditory system in dogs.[36]

CONDUCTION DEAFNESS AND NERVE DEAFNESS

There are two kinds of peripheral deafness: conduction and nerve deafness. Conduction deafness involves an abnormality in the gaseous or solid media that transmit the sound waves to the perilymph of the cochlea. The receptor is functional and responds to vibrations induced in the petrosal bone by a tuning fork, but does not respond to sound waves that are unable to reach the receptor. Diseases that obliterate the external ear canal, rupture the tympanum, or interfere with the function of the ear ossicles in the middle ear produce conduction deafness.

Nerve deafness involves an abnormality in the receptor organ itself.[2, 26, 27, 41] Congenital deafness has been reported in dogs and cats caused by a lesion—degeneration, hypoplasia, or aplasia—of the cochlear duct and its spiral organ. The signs are permanent. Frequently, the affected animals have a white hair coat.[1, 5, 21, 37, 51] There is a high incidence of congenital deafness in white cats with blue irises in which the white color is dependent on a dominant autosomal gene that has complete penetrance for white fur and incomplete penetrance for the production of a blue iris and deafness.[4, 31, 35, 38]

An epidemiologic survey of congenital deafness in dogs showed a breed predisposition in the Dalmatian, Australian heeler, English setter, Australian shepherd, Boston terrier, Old English sheepdog, and English bulldog.[19] The cocker spaniel has also been implicated, and the condition is seen sporadically in individuals of many other breeds. Congenital deafness has been associated in both dogs with the white coat color and dogs that possess the "merle"

color gene. The bull terrier is white and deafness is reported in that breed. The Australian heeler, Australian shepherd and Old English sheepdog all possess the "merle" color gene and are predisposed to deafness.[28] Pigmentation may be lacking in the iris, retinas, and choroid of these dogs, and the primary defect may involve a neural crest abnormality. Others have observed multiple ocular defects associated with partial albinism and deafness in dogs and suggested a common embryonic developmental defect.[16] A familial trend has been observed in some of these breeds, but the mode of inheritance is not known. The Dalmatian has a high risk for this condition.[3, 32, 52] One study suggested a sex-linked inheritance with varying expression.[3] In most instances, deaf puppies result from the breeding of parents with normal hearing. These cats and dogs with pigmentary disorders and deafness can be compared to children with similar anomalies, referred to as the Waardenburg syndrome.[10]

An inherited deafness is described in the Norwegian Dunkerhound breed.[13] This is a cochlear-saccular degeneration that occurs in the white individuals of this breed, which are homozygous for the merle color gene. About 75 per cent of these white dogs have a hearing loss that varies from complete to partial bilateral or unilateral deafness. In all instances there is evidence of the initial development of hearing before the degeneration begins. The degeneration occurs earlier and faster in those dogs that will become completely deaf. In these dogs the hearing loss is detectable between 2 and 3 weeks of age. Degenerative changes are most pronounced in the basal coil and it decreases apically. Degeneration predominates in the stria vascularis, where the blood supply is markedly reduced, but also involves the hair cells of the spiral organ.

In the deaf Dalmatian, hair cell degeneration occurs in the spiral organ, predominantly in the second coil of the cochlear duct. Ganglion cells and the stria vascularis degenerate in this same region. This is the region of the cochlear duct that is the first to develop and reach full differentiation.

A similar cochlear duct degeneration has been observed in deaf white mink, in which the congenital deafness is an inherited condition associated with the white color gene in the homozygous condition.[12, 15, 20, 42] These deaf mink develop hearing for about 7 days before degeneration begins. The degenerative changes have been related to a regression of the vascular supply to the cochlear duct.

Signs suggestive of a congenital bilateral vestibular disturbance have been observed in beagle puppies that have been born deaf. These include ataxia, abnormal head orientation with occasional continuous bobbing or rotary movements, and a lack of ability to produce nystagmus. Genetic data suggest a recessive inheritance of an abnormality of development of both the vestibular and auditory receptors in the membranous labyrinth.

Ototoxicity occurs following the prolonged use of certain antibiotics.[8, 18, 24, 29, 33] Large amounts of aminoglycoside antibiotics will cause degeneration of the hair cells of the labyrinthine receptors of the vestibular or auditory systems, or both. These antibiotics include streptomycin, dihydrostreptomycin, gentamicin, neomycin, and kanamycin. The specific effect depends on the chemical form of the antibiotic, the dose, and the species receiving it. Once deafness occurs, hearing rarely returns.

Inflammatory disease of the middle ear and inner ear that destroys the receptor of the auditory system produces deafness. This is most obvious in the animal affected bilaterally.[43]

The geriatric patient that is progressively losing its ability to hear probably has a progressive degeneration of the receptor organ or the chain of ossicles in the middle ear.

REFERENCES

1. Adams, E. W.: Hereditary deafness in a family of foxhounds. J. Am. Vet. Med. Assoc., *128*:302, 1956.
2. Altmann, F.: Histologic picture of inherited nerve deafness in man and animals. Arch. Otolaryngol., *51*:852, 1950.
3. Anderson, H., Henrickson, B, Lundquist, P. G., and Wedenberg, E.: Genetic hearing impairment in the Dalmatian dog. Acta Otolaryngol., *232*:1, 1968.
4. Bergsma, D. R., and Brown, K. S.: White fur, blue eyes, and deafness in the domestic cat. J. Hered., *62*:171, 1971.
5. Bosher, S. K., and Hallpike, C. S.: Observations on the histologic features, development, and pathogenesis of the inner ear degeneration of the deaf white cat. Proc. R. Soc. [Biol.] Series B, *162*:147, 1965.
6. Bradford, Z. J., McKinley, J. H., Rousey, C. L., and Klein, D. E.: Measurement of hearing in dogs by respiration audiometry. Am. J. Vet. Res., *34*:1183, 1973.
7. Cazals, Y., Aran, J-M., Erre, J-P, and Guilhaume, A.: Acoustic responses after total destruction of the cochlear receptor: Brainstem and auditory cortex. Science, *210*:83, 1980.
8. Crowell, W. A., Divers, T. J., and Byars, T. D.: Neomycin toxicosis in calves. Am. J. Vet. Res., *42*:29, 1981.
9. Engström, H., and Ades, H. W.: The ultrastructure of the organ of Corti. *In* Friedmann, I. (ed.): The Ultrastructure of Sensory Organs. Amsterdam, North Holland Publishing Co., 1973, 83-151.
10. Faith, R. E., and Woodard, J. C: Animal models of human disease: Waardenburg's syndrome. Comp. Pathol. Bull., *5*:3, 1973.
11. Fernandez, C., and Karapas, F.: The course and termination of the striae of Monakow and Held in the cat. J. Comp. Neurol., *131*:371, 1967.
12. Flottorp, G., and Foss, I.: Development of hearing in hereditarily deaf white mink (Hedlund) and normal mink (Standard) and the subsequent deterioration of the auditory response in Hedlund mink. Acta Otolaryngol., *87*:16, 1979.
13. Foss, I.: Development of hearing and vision, and morphological examination of the inner ear in hereditary deaf white Norwegian Dunkerhound and normal dogs (black and dappled Norwegian Dunkerhounds). M.S. Thesis, Cornell University, 1981.
14. Foss, I., and Flottorp, G.: A comparative study of the development of hearing and vision in various species commonly used in experiments. Acta Otolaryngol., *77*:202, 1974.
15. Foss, I., and Flottorp, G.: Measurements of hearing and morphological examination of the inner ear in deaf white mink (Hedlund) and normal mink (standard). *In* Proceedings of the Seventh International Congress of Electron Microscopy, *3*:761, 1970.
16. Givin, R. M., Wyman, M., Lin, D. J., Ketring, K., and Werling, K.: Multiple ocular defects associated with partial albinism and deafness in the dog. J. Am. Anim. Hosp. Assoc., *17*:401, 1981.
17. Goldberg, J. M., and Moore, R. Y.: Ascending projections of the lateral lemniscus in the cat and monkey. J. Comp. Neurol., *129*:143, 1967.
18. Hawkins, J. R., and Lurie, M. H.: The ototoxicity of dihydrostreptomycin and neomycin in the cat. Ann. Otol. Rhinol. Laryngol., *62*:1128, 1953.
19. Hayes, H. M., Wilson, G. P., Fenner, W. R., and Wyman, M.: Canine congenital deafness: Epidemiologic study of 272 cases. J. Am. Anim. Hosp. Assoc., *17*:473, 1981.
20. Hilding, D. A., Siguira, S., and Nakai, Y.: Deaf white mink: Electron microscopic study of the inner ear. Ann. Otol. Rhinol. Laryngol., *76*:647, 1967.
21. Howe, H. A.: The reaction of the cochlear nerve to destruction of its end organ: A study of deaf albino cats. J. Comp. Neurol., *62*:72, 1935.
22. Hudson, W. R., and Ruben, R. J.: Hereditary deafness in the Dalmatian dog. Arch. Otolaryngol., *75*:213, 1962.
23. Igarashi, M., Alford, B. R., Cohn, A. M., Saito, R., and Watanabe, T.: Inner ear anomalies in dogs. Ann. Otol. Rhinol. Laryngol., *81*:249, 1972.
24. Innes, J. R. M., and Saunders, L. Z.: Comparative Neuropathology. New York, Academic Press, 1962.
25. Irving, R., and Harrison, J. M.: The superior olivary complex and audition: A comparative study. J. Comp. Neurol., *130*:77, 1967.
26. Johnsson, L.-G., and Hawkins, J. E.: Symposium on basic ear research. II. Strial atrophy in clinical and experimental deafness. Laryngoscope, *81*:1105, 1972.
27. Johnsson, L.-G., and Hawkins, J. E.: A direct approach to cochlear anatomy and pathology in man. Arch. Otolaryngol., *85*:43, 1967.
28. Johnston, D. E., and Cox, B.: The incidence in purebred dogs in Australia of abnormalities that may be inherited. Aust. Vet. J., *46*:465, 1970.

29. Kohonen, A.: Effect of some ototoxic drugs upon the pattern and innervation of cochlear sensory cells in the guinea pig. Acta Otolaryngol. (Stockholm) Suppl., 208:1, 1965.

30. Lurie, M. H.: The membranous labyrinth in the congenitally deaf collie and Dalmatian dog. Laryngoscope, 58:279, 1948.

31. Mair, I. W. S.: Hereditary deafness in the white cat. Acta Otolaryngol. (Suppl.) 314:5, 1973.

32. Mair, I. W. S.: Hereditary deafness in the Dalmatian dog. Otorhinolaryngol., 212:1, 1976.

33. McGee, T. M., and Olszewski, J.: Streptomycin sulfate and dihydrostreptomycin toxicity; behavioral and histopathologic studies. Arch. Otolaryngol., 75:295, 1962.

34. Merzenich, M. M., and Reid, M. D.: Representation of the cochlea within the inferior colliculus of the cat. Brain Res., 77:397, 1974.

35. Pcyol, R., Rebillard, M., and Rebillard, G.: Primary neural disorders in the deaf white cat cochlea. Acta Otol., 83:59, 1977.

36. Penrod, J. P., and Coulter, D. B.: The diagnostic uses of impedance audiometry in the dog. J. Am. Anim. Hosp. Assoc., 16:941, 1980.

37. Pujol, R., and Marty, R.: Postnatal maturation in the cochlea of the cat. J. Comp. Neurol., 139:115, 1970.

38. Rebillard, G., Rebillard, M., Carlior. E., and Pcyol, R.: Histophysiological relationships in the deaf white cat auditory systems. Acta Otol., 82:48, 1976.

39. Roberts, S.: Color dilution and hereditary defects in collie dogs. Am. J. Ophthalmol., 63:1762, 1967.

40. Rose, W. R.: Audiology 1: Hearing and deafness. VM/SAC, 72:281, 1977.

41. Saunders, L. Z.: The histopathology of hereditary congenital deafness in white mink. Pathol. Vet., 2:256, 1965.

42. Sigiura, A., and Hilding, D. A.: Cochleo-saccular degeneration in Hedlund white mink. Acta Otol., 69:126, 1970.

43. Spreull, J. S. A.: Treatment of otitis media in the dog. J. Small Anim. Pract., 5:107, 1964.

44. Strominger, N. L., and Oesterreich, R. E.: Localization of sound after section of the brachium of the inferior colliculus. J. Comp. Neurol., 138:1, 1970.

45. Torok, N.: A review of neuro-otology pathogenesis of neuro-otological diseases. Am. J. Med. Sci., 246:154, 1963.

46. Tunturi, A. R.: Audio frequency localization in the acoustic cortex of the dog. Am. J. Physiol., 141:397, 1944.

47. Tunturi, A. R.: Classification of neurons in the ectosylvian auditory cortex of the dog. J. Comp. Neurol., 142:153, 1971.

48. Tunturi, A. R.: The pathway from the medial geniculate body to the ectosylvian auditory cortex in the dog. J. Comp. Neurol., 138:131, 1970.

49. Whidden, S. J., and Redding, R. W.: Evaluation of origins in the brain stem of far field averaged auditory responses in the canine. In Proceedings of the American College of Veterinary Internal Medicine, 1979, page 112.

50. Whidden, S. J., Redding, R. W., and Graves, J.: Evaluation of the normative far field averaged auditory evoked responses in the canine. In Proceedings of the American College of Veterinary Internal Medicine, 1979, page 112.

51. Wolff, D.: Three generations of deaf white cats. J. Hered., 33:39, 1942.

52. Young, G. B.: Inherited defects of dogs. Vet. Rec., 67:15, 1955.

53. Zwislocki, J. J.: Sound analysis in the ear: A history of discoveries. Am. Sci., 69:184, 1981.

VISCERAL AFFERENT SYSTEMS

GENERAL VISCERAL AFFERENT SYSTEM

The visceral afferent system consists of neurons whose dendritic zones are primarily in the viscera of the body, in those tissues that in general are derived from splanchnopleure. The general visceral afferent system consists of neurons with cell bodies located in all of the spinal and many of the cranial ganglia. These are concerned with body temperature, blood pressure, gas concentration and pressure, and movement of viscera. The special visceral afferent system consists of neurons restricted in their location to specific cranial nerves and whose function is limited to taste and smell.

ANATOMY

Receptor—Peripheral Nerves. The receptors of the general visceral afferent system are located throughout the viscera of the body, in which they are stimulated by a number of different modalities.[9, 23] Stretch, distention, or pressure on or in a viscus are the most common modalities. Some receptors are sensitive to chemical changes in the environment. Free endings and a variety of encapsulated ones are found at the dendritic zone of the neurons in this system. The axons course over the peripheral nerves most available to the viscus. In the head these are the facial nerve to the middle ear and blood vessels of the head, the glossopharyngeal nerve to the caudal tongue, pharynx, and carotid body and sinus, and the vagus nerve to the pharynx and larynx. In the tho-

racic and abdominal cavities these are the vagus nerve and the peripheral branches of the sympathetic trunk, the splanchnic nerves. Here in the body cavities the general visceral afferent (GVA) axons course toward the central nervous system in nerves that contain neurons of the parasympathetic and sympathetic portions of the general visceral efferent system (Fig. 16–1). Visceral afferent axons from the peripheral blood vessels course through peripheral nerves to the segmental spinal nerves.

The cell bodies of these GVA neurons are located in the geniculate ganglion of the facial nerve, the distal ganglia of the glossopharyngeal and vagus nerves, and the spinal ganglia of the involved spinal nerves.[5, 22] Recent horseradish peroxidase studies on the esophageal innervation of the dog revealed GVA neurons in both vagal ganglia, the glossopharyngeal ganglion, and the cervical and thoracic spinal ganglia.

Brain Stem Nuclei and Tracts. The axons continue from the various ganglia into the central nervous system. Those axons in the facial, glossopharyngeal, and vagus nerves enter the ventrolateral aspect of the medulla and course to a position near the lateral aspect of the fourth ventricle adjacent to the sulcus limitans. There the axons course rostrally and caudally in a column called the solitary tract (Fig. 16–1; Plates 3, 4). This tract is surrounded by neurons forming the nucleus of the solitary tract, in which the axons in the tract terminate. This solitary tract and its nucleus develop in the alar plate adjacent to the motor column of the general visceral efferent system; therefore, it is found dorsolateral to the parasympathetic nucleus of the facial, glossopharyngeal, and vagal nerves. The solitary tract stands out in myelin-stained sections as a densely stained cylindrical structure surrounded by the unstained cell bodies of its nucleus. It extends from the level of the facial nucleus (special visceral efferent) rostrally to caudal to the obex. Caudally the gracilic and medial cuneate nuclei are dorsal to it. Rostrally the medial vestibular nucleus is dorsal to it.

The nucleus of the solitary tract probably participates mostly in reflex activity and pro-

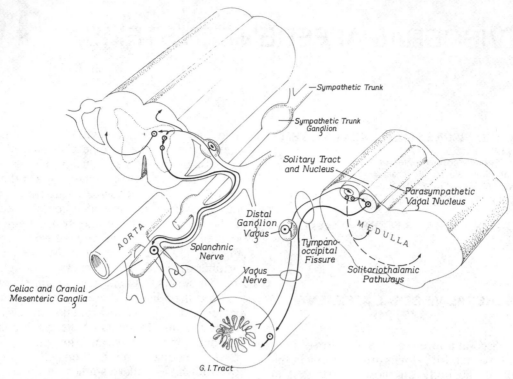

Figure 16–1. General visceral afferent system. Reversal of the GVE sympathetic pathway (conscious perception) and parasympathetic pathway (reflex function).

jects to the cell bodies in the general visceral efferent column directly or indirectly by way of interneurons in the reticular formation that participate in the various metabolic centers regulating visceral function—respiratory, cardiovascular, swallowing, micturition.[15]

Some cell bodies in the nucleus of the solitary tract project axons rostrally in a pathway for conscious projection. These course mostly on the contralateral side of the brain stem in an ill-defined solitariothalamic pathway that closely parallels the medial lemniscus and spinothalamic pathway. These axons terminate at a synapse in the ventral caudal medial nucleus of the thalamus, which in turn projects axons via the internal capsule to the somesthetic cortex.

The axons of the general visceral afferent system receptors in the body cavities that course centrally over the splanchnic nerves follow in a reverse pathway from that taken by the motor neurons of the general visceral efferent system (Fig. 16–1). From the sympathetic trunk the axons course by way of the rami communicantes to the spinal nerve and the dorsal root. The cell body is located in the corresponding spinal ganglion. The axon continues over the dorsal root into the dorsal grey

column of the spinal cord, and terminates on a neuronal cell body located there.

Passing through interneurons in the grey matter, the reflex pathway can be completed by synapse on a preganglionic cell body in the intermediate grey column (T1–L5). The pathway for conscious projection involves synapse of the GVA axon in the dorsal root on a cell body in the dorsal grey column whose axon enters the same or opposite lateral funiculus and courses cranially along with the axons of the spinothalamic system. This is probably a multisynaptic system which follows the same course as that of the spinothalamic system (general somatic afferent), including synapse in the ventral caudal lateral thalamic nucleus for projection to the somesthetic cortex.

There is some evidence that from the body cavities, the GVA neurons in the vagus nerve are concerned mostly with reflex activity, and those entering the spinal cord by way of the sympathetic trunk are concerned mostly with the conscious projection of visceral afferent stimuli—the source of "visceral pain."[20]

In addition to these pathways from the dendritic zone to the central nervous system, there is now evidence that some GVA neurons reside entirely within the wall of the viscus in an enteric plexus in which intrinsic reflex activity can occur.

FUNCTIONAL CONCEPTS

Most smooth muscle regulation is involuntary, and occurs at a reflex level not reaching the level of conscious perception. The enteric plexus within the wall of the bowel may function autonomously, independent of its extrinsic nerve supply and the central nervous system. Pacemaker activity has been recognized in selected areas of the bowel. Visceral surfaces are mostly insensitive to many of the stimuli to which the surface of the body is sensitive. There is no conscious perception of touching, pinching, or cutting normal viscera. This is exemplified by the rumenotomy or cesarian section, which are performed with local anesthesia of the body wall and parietal peritoneum. The wall of the rumen or uterus is incised without anesthesia and without discomfort to the patient.

Conscious perception of visceral sensation—visceral pain—occurs following tension or distention of the wall of the viscus or traction on its mesentery. Diseased, inflamed visceral surfaces are sensitive to touching and cutting. Loss of blood supply (ischemia) to the wall of the viscera is a source of visceral pain.

Visceral pain is poorly localized to its specific source, being reflected as a dull, deep pain in the body cavity. This may reflect the fact that compared with the general somatic afferent system there are fewer general visceral afferent neurons, and they are stimulated only occasionally by modalities that are conducted to the level of conscious perception. Thus the cerebrum has little experience with localizing the source of these modalities, which come from structures that cannot be visualized. This provides part of the basis for the phenomenon of referred pain, in which a specific area of the body surface is hypersensitive and is perceived to be where the pain is coming from.

In referred pain the visceral pain is referred to the surface of the body supplied by sensory neurons whose axons terminate in the same segment of the spinal cord and on the same cells as the visceral afferents (Fig. 16–2). Thus there is a dermatomal distribution to referred visceral pain, and the surface of the body can be mapped to represent the areas of pain

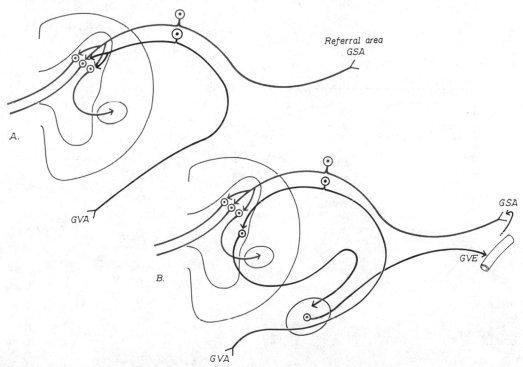

Figure 16–2. Anatomy of the dermatomal rule for referred visceral pain. *A*: Theory of common pool of neurons for GSA and GVA that project to the brain. *B*: Theory of a GVA viscerovisceral reflex arc causing tonic spasm of peripheral blood vessels which alters tissue metabolism with the accumulation of by-products that stimulate the local GSA receptors.

referral for the various visceral organs. For example, the diaphragm is referred to the shoulder and neck region innervated by general somatic afferent neurons in cervical nerves 5, 6, and 7. The stomach is referred to the midthorax region (T6–T9). The ureter is referred to the area of the scrotum (L3, L4). Many theories have been proposed to explain this phenomenon. The common pool theory proposes that both the GSA and GVA neurons synapse in the dorsal grey column on the same cell bodies for the conscious projection pathway by way of the spinothalamic system. The GSA system is stimulated frequently, while the GVA system is stimulated only occasionally. The site of the stimulus from the GSA system is recognized easily on the surface of the body, and the brain has "learned" the source of the stimulus. When the same dorsal grey column neurons are stimulated by excessive activity in the GVA system, the brain misinterprets the source and refers it to the origin of the GSA neurons.

The viscerovisceral reflex arc theory proposes that excessive GVA stimulation causes a reflex spasm of peripheral somatic blood vessels by way of GVE sympathetic motor neurons in the same spinal cord segments (Fig. 16–2). Release or accumulation of abnormal substances at the site of the vasospasm then stimulates the dendritic zone of the GSA neurons in that area of GVE distribution. These impulses are conducted into the segmental dorsal grey column and projected to the somesthetic cortex, which projects the pain to the body surface innervated by the GSA system. In reality, referred pain is rarely recognized and utilized clinically in veterinary medicine. There is anatomic evidence that supports a much more diffuse location of visceral sensory neurons than formerly assumed, which may explain the observation. In the dog, 22 spinal cord segments supply sensory innervation to the stomach.[12]

Bradycardia occurs in some cattle with chronic indigestion and ruminoreticular distention from decreased outflow.[8, 21] This is explained by the stimulation of vagal general

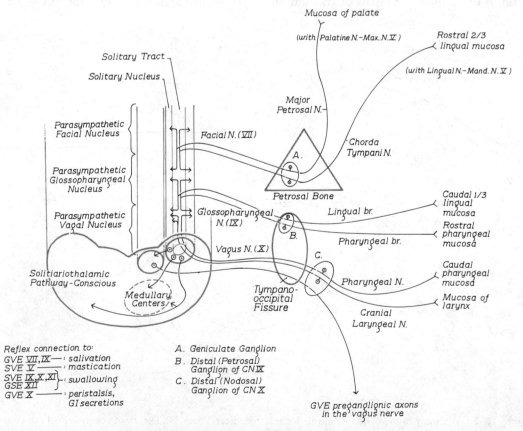

Figure 16–3. Special visceral afferent pathways for taste.

visceral afferent neurons where they are involved in peritoneal lesions associated with the forestomach. Traumatic reticuloperitonitis and the peritonitis associated with abomasal ulcers are the most common causes.

SPECIAL VISCERAL AFFERENT SYSTEM—TASTE

The primary receptors for the sense of taste, the gustatory sense, are responsive to chemical agents taken into the mouth and are organized in the form of small structures, taste buds, associated with the various glossal papillae.[6] Taste buds also occur in the soft palate, pharynx, larynx, lips, and cheeks. The neuroepithelial taste cells surround a pit, the taste pore. Short cytoplasmic processes, taste hairs, protrude into the lumen, in which they are "sensitive" to chemical substances dissolved in the saliva in the pit. There is a rapid turnover of the neuroepithelial receptor cells in the taste bud. Following denervation, the taste bud degenerates and will reform 1 to 2 days after reinnervation of the tongue papilla.[3]

These neuroepithelial receptor cells are in synaptic relationship with the dendritic zone of the special visceral afferent neurons (Fig. 16–3). The cell bodies of these neurons are in the geniculate ganglion of the facial nerve, and the distal ganglia of the glossopharyngeal and vagus nerves. The facial neurons are distributed to the palate and rostral two thirds of the tongue by way of branches of the trigeminal nerve.[4, 22] The glossopharyngeal nerve innervates taste buds in the caudal one third of the tongue and the rostral pharynx. The vagus innervates taste buds in the caudal pharynx and the larynx.

The course and central pathway for reflex activity and conscious perception are the same as those described for the general visceral afferent system neurons in these three cranial nerves. In the cat, taste perception is located primarily in the presylvian gyrus.[7, 16, 17]

The perception of taste is a psychological phenomenon involving the central projection of many afferent systems and the role of higher centers such as the limbic system, which contributes the factors of memory of past experiences.[14] Although the primary afferent is the chemoreceptor in the taste bud, thermoreceptors and mechanoreceptors in the oral cavity and pharynx and olfactory receptors also contribute to the sensation.[13]

SPECIAL VISCERAL AFFERENT SYSTEM—SMELL

The telencephalon can be subdivided on a developmental evolutionary basis into the archipallium, the paleopallium, and the neopallium. The archipallium and paleopallium comprise the rhinencephalon or the "smell brain." On an anatomic and functional basis, the rhinencephalon consists of an olfactory portion (paleopallium) and a nonolfactory portion or limbic system (archipallium). The limbic system has evolved extensively in the higher species of mammals, and in addition to the telencephalon involves nuclei and tracts in the brain stem.

The olfactory (paleopallial) portion of the rhinencephalon is the special visceral afferent system designed for the conscious perception of smell. The nonolfactory portion or limbic system is concerned with the emotional response to afferent stimuli, one of which is the olfactory special visceral afferent system.

The specialized chemoreceptor of the olfactory rhinencephalon is a bipolar neuron located in the olfactory epithelium of the nasal mucosa of the caudal part of the nasal cavity. The cell body and dendritic zone reside in the epithelium. Six to eight long cilia project from the apex of the olfactory cell and lie in the secretion on the surface of the olfactory epithelium, where they are stimulated by chemical substances dissolved in the secretions.[10, 18] The axon courses away from the cell body into the connective tissue of the nasal mucosa, and joins with the other axons to form the olfactory nerves—cranial nerve I. These pass through the foramina in the cribriform plate of the ethmoid bone and into the olfactory bulbs, in which the telodendria synapse with the dendritic zones of the neurons of the olfactory bulb. These are brush (tufted) and mitral cells. Many olfactory neurons converge on a few neurons of the olfactory bulb.

The axons of the mitral cells of the olfactory bulb project through the olfactory tract and lateral olfactory stria to the ipsilateral olfactory cortex over the pyriform lobe (Fig. 16–4, Plates 15, 16). Synapse may occur with neurons in the cortex of the olfactory peduncle (lateral olfactory gyrus), or lateral stria, or in the olfactory tubercle, which is a nucleus located between the lateral and medial olfactory striae. The majority of the central olfactory projections are ipsilateral and project to the pyriform cortex without a relay through a thalamic nucleus.

OLFACTORY RHINENCEPHALON

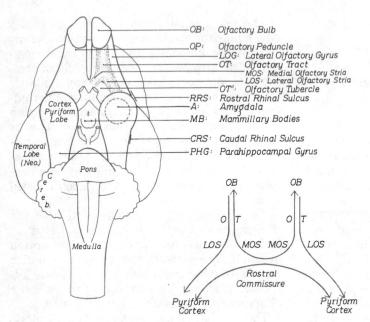

Figure 16–4. Anatomy of the special visceral afferent olfactory system.

The functions of the two olfactory bulbs are correlated by axons of the brush neurons in the olfactory bulb that course through ipsilateral olfactory tract and medial olfactory stria, the rostral commissure, and the contralateral medial olfactory stria and olfactory tract to the contralateral olfactory bulb. The olfactory peduncle includes the olfactory tract and the adjacent cortex of the lateral olfactory gyrus ventral to the rostral lateral rhinal sulcus. Commissural fibers in the rostral commissure also pass between the cortices of the two pyriform lobes.

This is the conscious perception pathway for the olfactory—special visceral afferent—system. The so-called reflex pathway involves projections into the nuclear areas of the limbic system. Axons in the medial olfactory stria enter the septal area (septal nuclei and subcallosal area). Axons in the lateral olfactory stria enter the amygdaloid nucleus and hippocampus. These provide pathways for the olfactory system to enter nuclei of the limbic system.

The development of the olfactory portion of the rhinencephalon (the SVA system) varies extensively among species of mammals. In the dog, the sense of smell is highly developed functionally and anatomically, and this is referred to as a macrosmatic species. Primates are microsmatic, lacking a well-developed olfactory system.

Experimental lesions in one olfactory bulb or peduncle produce unilateral anosmia. Bilateral lesions in the olfactory mucosa,[11] bulbs, peduncles, or pyriform lobes cause complete anosmia. Lesions in any part of the nonolfactory portion of the rhinencephalon, the limbic system, do not interfere with the sense of smell.

Deficiencies in the sense of smell are difficult to verify by clinical testing. The owner's observations of the animal's behavior on sensing the presence of food or game in the field may be more reliable information. Substances such as cloves, cinnamon, perfume, xylol, or benzol can be used, but one must be careful of irritating chemicals that stimulate the general somatic afferent neurons of the trigeminal nerve which are distributed in the nasal mucosa. The most common cause of complete anosmia is severe rhinitis with involvement of the olfactory nasal mucosa. Head injury may cause a shearing off of the olfactory nerves as they pass through the cribriform plate, resulting in anosmia.

REFERENCES

1. Beidler, L. M., and Smallman, R. L.: Renewal of cells within taste buds. J. Cell Biol., 27:263, 1965.
2. Bell, F. R., and Kitchell, R. L.: Taste reception in the goat, sheep, and calf. J. Physiol., 183:145, 1966.
3. Cheal, M., and Oakley, B.: Regeneration of fungi-

form tastebuds: Temporal and spatial characteristics. J. Comp. Neurol., *172*:609, 1977.

4. Chibuzo, G. A., Cummings, J. F., and Evans, H. E.: Surgical procedure for exposure of the chorda tympani in dogs: A ventral approach. Cornell Vet., *69*:295, 1979.

5. Cottle, M. K.: Degeneration studies of primary afferents of the IXth and Xth cranial nerves in the cat. J. Comp. Neurol., *122*:329, 1964.

6. Davies, R. O., Kare, M. R., and Cagan, R. H.: Distribution of tastebuds on fungiform and circumvallate papillae of bovine tongue. Anat. Rec., *195*:443, 1979.

7. Emmers, R.: Localization of thalamic projection of afferents from the tongue in the cat. Anat. Rec., *148*:67, 1964.

8. Ferrante, P., and Whitlock, R. H.: Chronic (vagus) indigestion in cattle. Compend. Contin. Ed., *3*:S231, 1981.

9. Fletcher, T. F., and Bradley, W. E.: Afferent nerve endings in the urinary bladder of the cat. Am. J. Anat., *128*:147, 1970.

10. Graziadei, P. P. C.: The ultrastructure of vertebrate olfactory mucosa. *In* Friedmann, I. (ed.): The Ultrastructure of Sensory Organs. Amsterdam, North Holland Publishing Co., 1973.

11. Houpt, K. A., Shepherd, P., and Hintz, H. F.: Two methods for producing peripheral anosmia in dogs. Lab. Anim. Sci., *28*:173, 1978.

12. Khurana, R. K., and Petras, J. M.: Anatomic demonstration of the afferent innervation of the dog's stomach: A possible implication for visceral pain in humans. Neurology, *32*:A71, 1982.

13. Kitchell, R. L.: Newer knowledge on taste in dogs and cats. Gaines Vet. Symp., *14*:15, 1964.

14. Kitchell, R. L.: Taste perception and discrimination by the dog. Adv. Vet. Sci. Comp. Med., *22*:287, 1978.

15. Morest, D. K.: Experimental study of the projections of the nucleus of the tractus solitarius and the area postrema in the cat. J. Comp. Neurol., *130*:277, 1967.

16. Morrison, A. R., Hand, P. J., and Ruderman, M. I.: Cortical gustatory and facial somesthetic areas of the cat as revealed by an anatomicophysiological technique. Anat. Rec., *172*:462, 1972.

17. Morrison, A. R., and Tarnecki, R.: A new location for the gustatory cortex of the cat. Anat. Rec., *181*:431, 1975.

18. Moulton, D. G., and Beidler, L. M.: Structure and function in the peripheral olfactory system. Physiol. Rev., *47*:1, 1967.

19. Murray, R. G.: The ultrastructure of taste buds. *In* Friedmann, I. (ed.): The Ultrastructure of Sensory Organs, Amsterdam, North Holland Publishing Co., 1973.

20. Paintal, A. S.: Vagal sensory receptors and their reflex effects. Physiol. Rev., *53*:159, 1973.

21. Rebhun, W. C.: Vagus indigestion in cattle. J. Am. Vet. Med. Assoc., *176*:506, 1980.

22. Rhoton, A. L., Jr.: Afferent connections of the facial nerve. J. Comp. Neurol., *133*:89, 1968.

23. Vemura, E., Fletcher, T. F., and Bradley, W. E.: Distribution of lumbar afferent axons in muscle coat of cat urinary bladder. Am. J. Anat., *139*:389, 1974.

NONOLFACTORY RHINENCEPHALON: LIMBIC SYSTEM

ANATOMY
  TELENCEPHALON
  DIENCEPHALON
  MESENCEPHALON
FUNCTION

The prosencephalon consists of two telencephalons and one diencephalon. The diencephalon is composed of the thalamus, hypothalamus, epithalamus, and subthalamus on each side of the third ventricle. Each telencephalon forms a cerebral hemisphere. The cell bodies of the neurons in the cerebrum are located in two general areas. One is on the outside surface of the gyri in the laminations of the cerebral cortex. The other is deep to the surface in basal nuclei. The caudate nucleus, pallidum, and putamen are basal nuclei that function primarily in the extrapyramidal system. The amygdala and septal nuclei function mainly in the limbic system.

The cerebral cortex covers the surface of the cerebrum and can be divided into three general regions based on its evolution. The paleopallium (pall-cloak) consists of the olfactory bulb, olfactory penduncle, and the cortex over the pyriform lobe. The archipallium is the hippocampus, which is an internal gyrus rolled into the lateral ventricle during development. The neopallium is the most recently evolved and comprises the remainder of the cerebrum, which includes all the gyri dorsal to the rhinal sulcus.

Another grouping of brain components is called the rhinencephalon—the "smell" brain. This consists of an olfactory component, the paleopallium (see Chapter 16), and a nonolfactory component, which is referred to as the limbic system. In the telencephalon this includes the archipallium.

The term *limbic system* refers to the anatomic arrangement of the telencephalic neurons and tracts that are components of this system, and are arranged as two incomplete ring-like structures on the medial aspect of the telencephalon at its border with the diencephalon (Fig. 17–1). Limbus refers to border, and these telencephalic structures border the main mass of the cerebral vesicle. The term has been expanded in usage to include the major nuclei and pathways in the rostral brain stem that are connected with these telencephalic structures anatomically and functionally (Table 17–1).

ANATOMY

TELENCEPHALON

The telencephalic components of the limbic system form two "cortical rings" at the border of the diencephalic-telencephalic junction (Fig. 17–1). The inner ring consists of the amygdaloid body, the hippocampus, and the fornix. The outer ring consists of the cingulum, the cingulate gyrus, and the septal area.

The amygdaloid body, one of the basal nuclei of the telencephalon, is a complex of nuclei located in the pyriform lobe deep within the olfactory cortex (Fig. 17–2, Plate 15). A projection pathway, the stria terminalis, passes in the angle between the thalamus and caudate nucleus. It progresses in a caudal, dorsal, rostral, and then in a ventral direction to terminate in the septal area and rostral hypothalamus. A diagonal band courses on the ventral surface of the cerebrum and connects the amygdaloid body with the septal area.

The hippocampus is a unique gyrus of the cerebrum that has been rolled into the lateral ventricle in which it is found, forming part of the medial and ventral wall of the lateral ventricle dorsally, and the medial and dorsal

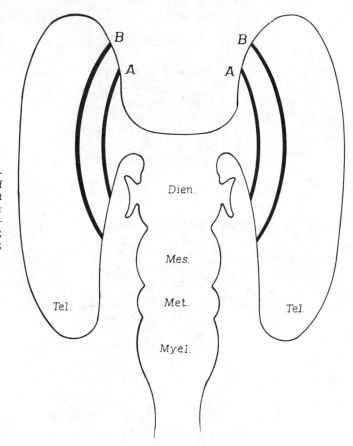

Figure 17–1. Schematic diagram of developing brain vesicles with approximate site of telencephalic components of limbic system at the "border" of the cerebral vesicle. *A*: inner ring—amygdala, hippocampus; *B*: outer ring—cingulate gyrus, septal area; *Tel.*: telencephalon; *Dien.*: diencephalon; *Mes.*: mesencephalon; *Met.*: metencephalon; *Myel.*: myelencephalon.

TABLE 17–1. NONOLFACTORY RHINENCEPHALON: LIMBIC SYSTEM. SUMMARY OF MAJOR STRUCTURES

I. Telencephalon:
  A. Inner cortical ring
      Amygdaloid body
      Hippocampus
         Fimbria-fornix—septal area,
           hypothalamus, mammillary bodies
  B. Outer cortical ring
      Cingulum and gyrus
      Septal area
         Medial forebrain bundle—hypothalamus:
           brain stem LMN—GVE
II. Diencephalon:
  A. Thalamus
      Habenular nucleus
         Stria habenularis thalamus
         Habenular intercrural tract
      Rostral thalamic nucleus
  B. Hypothalamus
      Mammillary bodies
         Mammillothalamic tract
         Mammillotegmental tract—reticular
           formation
III. Mesencephalon:
      Intercrural nucleus—reticular formation

wall of the ventricle ventrally (Plates 12–14). The hippocampus extends from the amygdaloid body in each pyriform lobe in a curve, progressing caudally and then dorsally and rostrally over the diencephalon, from which it is separated by meninges. Dorsal to the caudal thalamus the hippocampi from each side meet at the median plane and a commissure is formed there, the hippocampal commissure. Caudal to the pyriform lobe the hippocampus is covered superficially by the parahippocampal gyrus, which is bounded laterally by the caudal lateral rhinal sulcus and medially where it joins the hippocampus by the hippocampal sulcus (Plate 14). The parahippocampal gyrus is continued dorsally, dorsal to the corpus callosum, by the cingulate gyrus (Plates 12–14).

Axons course to and from the hippocampus along its lateral side, forming the fimbria and crus of the fornix. The two crura meet rostral to the hippocampal commissure and pass rostrally as the bodies of the fornix (Fig. 17–2, Plates 15, 16). After coursing rostrally they

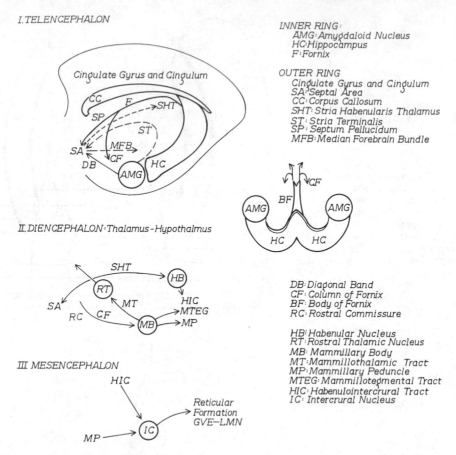

Figure 17–2. Anatomy of the limbic system.

turn ventrally at the level of the rostral commissure; here the two bodies separate and form the distinctly cylindrical columns of the fornix. Each column splits at the rostral commissure and a small bundle courses rostrally into the septal area. The larger portion of the column passes caudal to the rostral commissure (post-commissural column) and ventrally through the hypothalamus on either side of the third ventricle to terminate in the mammillary body on either side (Plates 14, 15). The body and proximal column of the fornix are attached dorsally to the corpus callosum by the septum pellucidum. There are leptomeninges ventral to the body of the fornix rostrally to the level of the interventricular foramen.

The cingulum is the long association tract forming the longitudinal fibers in the white matter of the cingulate gyrus (Fig. 17–2). These fibers course from the parahippocampal gyrus located caudally to the septal area and frontal lobe gyri located rostrally. The cingulate gyrus is the cerebral cortex covering the cingulum that is located dorsal to the corpus callosum and is continuous caudally with the parahippocampal gyrus and rostrally with the septal area (Plates 12–16).

The septal area consists of the subcallosal area, which is the cerebral cortex ventral to the genu of the corpus callosum and the septal nuclei. These septal nuclei are nuclear masses in the ventral septum pellucidum protruding into the lateral ventricle from the medial side. (Plate 16). The septal area connects with the hippocampus by way of the adjacent columns of the fornix, with the amygdaloid body through the diagonal band and stria terminalis, and with the habenular nuclei via the stria habenularis thalamus (Plate 15). The medial forebrain bundle passes caudally from the septal area into the hypothalamus. By way of this pathway, limbic system efferents can influence the hypothalamic centers that control the activity of the general visceral efferent system.

The function of the limbic system involves visceral motor activation. The hypothalamic nuclei serve as the upper motor neuron that regulates the general visceral efferent system.

These hypothalamic nuclei, as well as the brain stem GVE lower motor neuron, receive numerous limbic system efferents.

DIENCEPHALON

In the thalamus the habenular nucleus and the rostral thalamic nucleus function mainly in the limbic system (Fig. 17–2). The habenular nucleus is located adjacent to the third ventricle rostral to the pineal body (Plate 14). It connects with the telencephalic septal area by way of the stria habenularis thalamus located on either side of the dorsal thalamus adjacent to the third ventricle (Plate 15). It connects with the intercrural nucleus of the mesencephalon via the habenulointercrural tract. The rostral thalamic nucleus receives afferents from the mammillary body of the hypothalamus through the mammillothalamic tract (Plates 14, 15). The rostral thalamic nucleus projects predominantly to the cingulate gyrus and adjacent neopallium.

The limbic system component of the hypothalamus is the mammillary body. The paired mammillary bodies are located adjacent to the ventral midline caudal to the infundibulum of the hypophysis in the most caudal portion of the hypothalamus (Plate 14). They connect with the hippocampus by way of the columns of the fornix, and with the rostral thalamic nucleus via the mammillothalamic tract. The paired columns of the fornix and mammillothalamic tracts pass through the hypothalamus adjacent to the third ventricle. In addition to these pathways, the mammillary bodies connect with the mesencephalic tegmentum and the visceral motor column in the medulla through the mammillotegmental tract. The mammillary peduncle courses caudally to the mesencephalic intercrural nucleus.

MESENCEPHALON

The intercrural nucleus is the only limbic system nucleus in the mesencephalon. It is located between the two crus cerebri on the ventral surface of the mesencephalon on the floor of the intercrural fossa (Plates 10, 11). It connects with the habenular nucleus by way of the habenulointercrural tract, the mammillary bodies via the mammillary peduncle, and the reticular formation of the brain stem, which in turn influences the visceral motor column—general visceral efferent lower motor neuron in the medulla.

FUNCTION

The limbic system receives and associates afferent impulses from the olfactory (SVA), optic (SSA), auditory (SSA), exteroceptive (GSA), and interoceptive (GVA) sensory systems. It projects predominantly on the hypothalamus and caudal brain stem primarily influencing the visceral motor column.

The limbic system is involved with mostly emotional or behavioral patterns. Emotion involves visceral reaction, which is controlled largely by the autonomic nervous system. This system is regulated centrally by the hypothalamus, which accounts for the multitude of connections of the limbic system with the hypothalamus.

The limbic system is considered to function in humans as the higher center controlling the psychic and motor aspects of behavior. It is the portion of the brain involved in man's basic drives, sexual activity, emotional experience, memories, and fears and pleasures.[5, 13, 20, 43]

James Papez, professor of neurology at Cornell University, suggested in 1937 that the part of the rhinencephalon now classified as the limbic system was concerned with activity other than the perception of smell.[45] Following his observations of the distribution of the rabies lesions in dogs in these rhinencephalic structures and the bizarre behavior exhibited by the rabid animal, he attributed to these structures a role in the control of normal behavior.

Since then many different experimental procedures and clinical observations have substantiated this role of the limbic system in the control of an animal's behavior. These observations have included the effect of direct stimulation of rhinencephalic structures, the effect of ablation of portions of these structures, and the syndromes produced by diseases causing lesions in these structures.

The specific results have varied even with the use of similar procedures because of the difficulty in the exact placement of stimulating electrodes and the variable spread of electrical excitation to adjacent structures, coupled with the fact that adjacent nuclei may have diametrically opposed functions. Surgical ablations that were repeated often lacked exact specificity. Nevertheless, the general conclusion drawn from all these observations is that the alteration of the animal's behavior suggests either that a basic drive has been satisfied, or that the condition of an unsatisfied basic drive has been created. Some examples of these observations follow.

Self-Stimulation. Self-stimulation experiments were designed in which electrodes were implanted in various specific areas of the limbic system and stimulation occurred when the experimental animal stepped on a lever or bar in the floor of the cage.[12, 44, 55] The response observed was assumed to be pleasurable when it was sought and continually repeated by the animal, even to the exclusion of feeding. A painful experience was assumed when the stimulation was actively avoided. Such self-stimulation of the intercrural nucleus, septal area, and rostral hypothalamus in cats and rats was sought so actively that the animal continually pressed the bar to the exclusion of eating. These areas have been called the pleasure centers. Similar stimulation of the lateral hypothalamus and selected mesencephalic areas resulted in complete avoidance of the source of the stimulus. These were referred to as pain centers.

Direct Stimulation. Direct stimulation of the feline cingulate gyrus, amygdala, or hippocampus results in the production of a psychomotor convulsion, one characterized by a marked abnormal behavior preceding the tonic-clonic somatic motor phase of the convulsion.[17, 21, 37, 39] Expressions of arousal, fear or rage, or both, were observed. Direct stimulation of the temporal lobe in humans under local anesthesia has caused individuals to completely recall a past experience and express the full emotional impact of the event. Upon cessation of the stimulus, the patient does not remember recalling the event.

Experimental Destruction. Ablation experiments have resulted in variable responses, all of which show alteration in the animal's behavior. In cats, amygdalectomy results in unfriendliness and fear or even a rage response—complete sympathetic response with a tendency to attack animate or inanimate objects.[17, 52] Hypersexuality in males and hyperphagia also have been observed. All these behaviors represent unsatisfied basic drives that the animal is attempting to remedy. Amygdalectomy has caused aggressive monkeys to be tame, nonaggressive, sometimes hypersexual, and to show no emotional response when confronted by objects or events that formerly elicited an emotional response. Lesions in the temporal lobe in humans often cause psychomotor convulsions. Removal of the temporal lobe may stop the convulsions, but seriously blunts the emotional response of the individual, and memory of past events is often lost. Bilateral lesions have been pro-

duced in the amygdala in dogs that showed variable degrees of aggressiveness and viciousness. This has seemed to be helpful only in alleviating the aggressive behavior in nervous, fear-biting dogs.

Destruction of the amygdala or hippocampus in cats using aluminum oxide creme directly applied to the area resulted in psychomotor convulsions.

Diseases. Diseases that cause lesions in the temporal lobe in humans often are the source of psychomotor convulsions. Neonatal or childhood trauma, or infectious diseases that cause encephalitis of this area, such as the measles virus, cause damage to the temporal lobe. The temporal lobe is associated closely with the amygdala and hippocampus. Their functions overlap, and the lesions described as in temporal lobe usually involve the hippocampus as well. Psychomotor convulsions in humans are characterized by loss of contact with the external environment and hallucinations of visual events, or often by visceral sensations (smells, tastes) that are pleasing or distasteful. This is accompanied by visceral motor activity such as pupillary dilation, salivation, mastication, fecal and urinary excretions, and a somatic activity consisting of wildly running around as if searching for something, along with a good deal of expression of emotion. It usually culminates in a generalized seizure characterized by falling on one side, opisthotonos, and tonic (rigid extension) and clonic (rapidly alternating contraction and relaxation of a muscle) activity of the limbs, alternating with paddling or running movements of the limbs. Complete recovery follows. The duration may be from 2 to 3 or 10 to 15 minutes.

Psychomotor seizures have been observed in dogs with lesions in the pyriform lobe or hippocampus. When agenized flour is used in dog foods, it causes necrosis in these areas bilaterally and produces this kind of convulsion.[41, 46] Similar necrosis from ischemia of unknown origin produces this behavior, as well as inflammatory lesions caused occasionally by the distemper virus.[47] In dogs psychomotor convulsions have been referred to as "running fits," because before the dog falls on its side and evidences tonic-clonic activity of its extremities along with opisthotonos, it may have a period of running wildly around its environment and barking and growling, completely unaware of anyone or anything. Occasionally, the psychic stage is manifested in what might be called a hallucination. The dog may stand in a corner, barking and growling, with dilated pupils and the hair erect on its back as if it were going to attack an object, although there is nothing there. Extreme fear may be manifested. The dog is usually nonresponsive to the owner during these episodes.

At the present time, the most common cause of convulsions in dogs that are accompanied by a psychic stage with bizarre behavior is lead poisoning. There have not been adequate studies on the distribution of the lesion to determine whether limbic system structures are more affected.

Frontal Lobotomy. Frontal lobe structures are intimately connected with the limbic system and hypothalamus and are involved in the status of an animal's behavior.[15, 18] Frontal lobotomies have been performed in humans and in animals to alleviate violent aggressive behaviors that are destructive in nature. In humans, extensive changes in personality and loss of intellect accompany the loss of aggressive behavior, and therefore the procedure now is seldom used. The results in dogs have been variable.[2, 3, 40, 49]

In one study frontal lobotimies were performed on two groups of aggressive animals.[1] One group consisted of malamutes used as sled dogs that had marked aggression toward one other. The other group of dogs and cats consisted of house pets that had histories of aggressive behavior toward people. The lobotomies performed on the malamutes with interspecies aggression were more successful than those performed on the animals aggressive toward humans. In most instances, the lobotomized malamutes were able to return to the sled dog team and to function without attacking the other dogs. However, this surgical procedure is not without serious sequelae and should be performed only as a last resort.

More recently, electroconvulsive shock therapy has been used alone or together with lobotomies on dogs with aggressive behavior.[30]

Behavioral Abnormalities. Behavioral abnormalities are common in domestic animals.[4, 6–11, 14, 16, 19, 22–29, 31–34, 36, 42, 48, 50, 51, 53, 54, 56] In this textbook these are defined as changes in the animal's normal habits, personality, attitude, reaction to its environment, and its general sensorium. Some of the clinical signs that comprise this abnormal behavior include dullness, lethargy, sleepiness, stupor or semicoma, dementia, failure to recognize owners or familiar environment or objects, inability to learn, destructive behavior, irritability, aggression, vicious behavior, propulsive pacing or circling, hypersexuality, polydipsia, polyphagia, pica, and anorexia.

Normal behavior requires a complex integrated involvement of the entire nervous system but particularly the prosencephalon. Some of these behavioral abnormalities are caused by a lesion in the prosencephalon (cerebrum, thalamus, hypothalamus), and these usually involve some component of the limbic system. Some of these are psychologic disturbances for which there is no recognized structural or metabolic disturbance of brain function and others are inappropriate behavior for the environment in which the animal is expected to live. The latter include aggression or destruction, which are normal animal behaviors but inappropriate in its environment where it is inconvenient or dangerous to the owner or others.

Almost any disturbance of the prosencephalon will cause one or more of these clinical signs of abnormal behavior. A few are more specifically related to individual signs such as polydipsia with pituitary-hypothalamic neoplasia. Encephalitis, neoplasia, intoxications, malformations, injuries, infarcts, and metabolic disorders must all be considered in the differential diagnoses.

A structural or metabolic brain disturbance will be supported as the cause of the behavioral abnormality if there are neurologic deficits other than the abnormal behavior determined on the neurologic examination. Postural reaction deficits, or blindness, or both support the diagnosis of a prosencephalic lesion.

If the neurologic examination is normal, a psychologic disturbance or inappropriate behavior must be considered. Ordinarily all ancillary procedures such as CBC, blood chemistry, cerebrospinal fluid, radiography, electroencephalography, scintigraphy, and computerized axial tomography are normal in dogs with these problems.

The evaluation of animals for the cause of their psychological disturbance or inappropriate behavior requires a detailed analysis of their environment, training, and all their experiences since birth. Frequently, environmental alterations or the lack of or inappropriate training are identified, and with correction the problem can be rectified. Obviously this requires extensive cooperation on the part of the owners. There are numerous publications that deal with recognition, diagnosis and control of these kinds of behavioral abnormalities.

SPRINGER SPANIEL "RAGE" SYNDROME. An episodic behavioral abnormality has been recognized in the English springer spaniel.[35, 38] This disorder occurs in dogs that are normally well-behaved, well-adapted house pets and consists of an episodic change in behavior that lasts a few seconds to a few minutes, with the dog returning to normal again. The first signs may be sudden snapping and a marked bilateral mydriasis with a glazed appearance to the eyes. This often follows a mild provocation such as approaching or petting the dog. A few fine tremors may occur in the pelvic limbs; the dog will often wag its tail, growl, and attack and bite animate or occasionally inanimate objects. This aggression is often directed at just one member of the family with whom it lives. It is completely unresponsive to its normal environment, including the owner. At times the dog may crouch under a table or desk and not allow anyone near it.

The episodes may occur sporadically, weeks apart at first, but often increase in frequency to many times per day. In the majority of dogs the signs begin at around 18 months of age, but the range of onset is three months to about 4 years. It occurs predominantly in male dogs.

High levels of progestins and a vigorous behavioral training program may help control the disease, but neither will completely eliminate all aggressive behavior. All ancillary studies are normal. The electroencephalograph has not been found to produce a consistently abnormal tracing. No light microscopic lesions have been observed in the central nervous system.

This resembles a partial idiopathic seizure involving limbic system structures in that it is an episodic disturbance of brain function that resolves spontaneously and recurs at varying intervals. However, it is completely unresponsive to any anticonvulsant therapy.

It is hoped that neurochemical studies will reveal the basis for this and other behavior disorders in animals.

REFERENCES

1. Allen, B. D., Cummings, J. F., and de Lahunta, A.: The effects of prefrontal lobotomy on aggressive behavior in dogs. Cornell Vet., 64:201, 1974.
2. Andersson, B.: A case of nervous distemper treated with a prefrontal lobectomy. Nord. Vet. Med., 8:17, 1956.
3. Andersson, B., and Olsson, K.: Effects of bilateral amygdaloid lesions in nervous dogs. J. Small Anim. Pract., 6:301, 1965.
4. Antelyes, J.: Objectionable behavior in pet animals. VM SAC, 62:661, 774, 1967.
5. Bandler, R., and Flynn, J. P.: Neural pathways from thalamus associated with regulation of aggressive behavior. Science, 183:96, 1974.
6. Barchas, J. D., Akil, H., Elliott, G. R., Holman, B.

R., and Watson, S. J.: Behavioral neurochemistry: Neuroregulators and behavioral states. Science, 200:964, 1978.
7. Beaver, B. L.: Mental lapse aggression syndrome. J. Am. Anim. Hosp. Assoc., 16:937, 1980.
8. Beaver, B.: Veterinary Aspects of Feline Behavior. St. Louis, C. V. Mosby Co., 1980.
9. Borchelt, P., and Tortora, D. F.: Animal behavior therapy: The diagnosis and treatment of pet behavior problems. In Proceedings of the Animal Meeting of the American Animal Hospital Association, 1979.
10. Borchelt, P. L., and Voith, V. L.: Elimination behavior problems in cats. Compend. Contin. Ed., 3:730, 1981.
11. Brown, C. J., Murphee, O. D., and Newton, J. E. O.: The effect of inbreeding on human aversion in pointer dogs. J. Hered., 69:362, 1978.
12. Bruner, A.: Self-stimulation in the rabbit: An anatomical map of stimulation effects. J. Comp. Neurol., 131:615, 1967.
13. Brutowski, S.: Functions of prefrontal cortex in animals. Physiol. Rev., 45:721, 1965.
14. Caldwell, D. S., and Little P. B.: Aggression in dogs and associated neuropathology. Can. Vet. J., 21:152, 1980.
15. Coffey, F. J.: Ethology and canine practice. J. Small Anim. Pract., 12:123, 1971.
16. Denny, M. R.: Animal Behavior. Chicago, Wiley Interscience Inc., 1979.
17. Egger, M. D., and Flynn, J. P.: Further studies on the effects of amygdaloid stimulations and ablation on hypothalamically elicited attack behavior in cats. In Adey, W. R., and Tokizane, T. (eds.): Progress in Brain Research. Structure and Function of the Limbic System. Amsterdam and New York, Elsevier, 1967.
18. Fox, M. W.: Abnormal Behavior in Animals. Philadelphia, W. B. Saunders Co., 1968.
19. Fox, M. W.: Understanding Your Cat. New York, Coward, McCann, Geoghegan Inc., 1974.
20. Fulton, J. F.: The Frontal Lobes and Human Behavior. Liverpool, Eng., University Press, 1952.
21. Gol, A.: Relief of pain by electrical stimulation of the septal area. J. Neurol. Sci., 5:115, 1967.
22. Hart, B. L.: Medial preoptic-anterior hypothalamic area and sociosexual behavior of male dogs. J. Comp. Physiol. Psychol., 86:328, 1974.
23. Hart, B. L.: Feline Behavior: A Practitioner's Monograph. Santa Barbara, Cal., Veterinary Practice Publishing Co., 1978.
24. Hart, B. L.: Objectionable urine spraying and urine marking in cats: Evaluation of progestin treatment in gonadectomized males and females. J. Am. Vet. Med. Assoc., 177:529, 1980.
25. Hart, B. L.: Olfactory tractotomy for control of objectionable urine spraying and urine marking in cats. J. Am. Vet. Med. Assoc., 179:231, 1981.
26. Hart, B. L.: Progestin therapy for aggressive behavior in male dogs. J. Am. Vet. Med. Assoc., 178:1070, 1981.
27. Hart, B. L., Haugen, C. M., and Peterson, D. M.: Effects of medial preoptic-anterior hypothalamic lesions on mating behavior of male cats. Brain Res., 54:177, 1973.
28. Hart, B. L., and Ladewig, J.: Effects of medial preoptic-anterior hypothalamic lesions on development of sociosexual behavior in dogs. J. Comp. Physiol. Psychol., 93:566, 1979.

29. Henry, J. P.: Mechanisms of psychosomatic disease in animals. Adv. Vet. Sci. Comp. Med., *20*:115, 1976.

30. Hoerlein, B. F.: Advances in canine neurology. Gaines Vet. Symp., *24*:3, 1974.

31. Hopkins, S. G., Schubert, T. A., and Hart, B. L.: Castration of adult male dogs: Effects on roaming, aggression, urine marking and mounting J. Am. Vet. Med. Assoc., *168*:1108, 1976.

32. Houpt, K. A.: Aggression in dogs. Compend. Contin. Ed., *123*:123, 1979.

33. Houpt, K. A.: Clinical behavioral problems: aggression. *In* Kirk, R. W. (ed.): Current Veterinary Therapy: Small Animal Practice VII. Philadelphia, W. B. Saunders Co., 1980.

34. Houpt, K. A.: Equine behavior. Equine Pract., *1*:20, 1979.

35. Houpt, K. A.: Personal communication, 1982.

36. Houpt, K. A., and Wolski, T. R.: Domestic Animal Behavior for Veterinarians and Animal Scientists. Ames, Iowa State University Press, 1982.

37. Hunsberger, R. W., and Bucher, V. M.: Affective behavior produced by electrical stimulation in the forebrain and brain stem of the cat. *In* Adey, W. R., and Tokizane, T. (eds.): Progress in Brain Research. Structure and Function of the Limbic System. Amsterdam and New York, Elsevier, 1967.

38. Jezyk, P. F.: Personal communication, 1982.

39. Kling, A., and Coustan, D.: Electrical stimulation of the amygdala and hypothalamus in the kitten. Exp. Neurol., *10*:81, 1964.

40. Kramer, W., and Beigers, J. D.: Frontale leucotomie bij de hond. Tijdschre. Diergeneesk., *83*:589, 1958.

41. Mellanby, E.: Diet and canine hysteria, experimental production by treated flour. Br. Med. J., *2*:885, 1946 and *2*:288, 1947.

42. Newton, J. E., Dykman, R. A., and Chapin, J. L.: The prediction of abnormal behavior from autonomic indices in dogs. J. Nerv. Ment. Dis., *166*:635, 1978.

43. Olds, J.: The limbic system and behavioral reinforcement. *In* Adey, W. R., and Tokizane, T. (eds.): Progress in Brain Research. Structure and Function of the Limbic System. Amsterdam and New York, Elsevier, 1967.

44. Olds. J.: Pleasure centers in the brain. Sci. Am., *195*:105, 1956.

45. Papez, J.: A proposed mechanism of emotion. Arch. Neurol. Psychiatry, *38*:725, 1937.

46. Parry, H. B.: Canine hysteria in relation to diet. Vet. Rec., *60*:389, 1948.

47. Parry, H. B.: Epileptic states in the dog with special reference to canine hysteria. Vet. Rec., *61*:23, 1949.

48. Pemberton, P. L.: Feline and canine behavior control: Progestin therapy. *In* Kirk, R. W. (ed.): Current Veterinary Therapy: Small Animal Practice VII. Philadelphia, W. B. Saunders Co., 1980.

49. Redding, R. W.: Prefrontal lobotomy of the dog. *In* Proceedings of the Annual Meeting of the American Animal Hospital Association, 1972.

50. Redding, R. W., and Walker, T. L.: Electroconvulsive therapy to control aggression in dogs. Mod. Vet. Pract., *57*:595, 1976.

51. Scott, J. P., and Fuller, J. P.: Dog behavior: The genetic basis. Chicago, University of Chicago Press, 1965.

52. Summers, T. B., and Kaelber, W. W.: Amygdalectomy: Effect in cats and a survey of its present status. Am. J. Physiol., *203*:1117, 1962.

53. Tortora, D. F.: Help! This Animal is Driving Me Crazy. New York, Playboy Press, 1977.

54. Voith, V. L.: Applied animal behavior for the veterinary practitioner. *In* Proceedings of the Annual Meeting of the American Animal Hospital Association, 1980.

55. Wilkinson, H. A., and Peele, T. L.: Intracranial self-stimulation in cats. J. Comp. Neurol., *121*:425, 1963.

56. Wolski, T. R.: Preventing behavior problems in dogs. *In* Kirk, R. W. (ed.): Current Veterinary Therapy: Small Animal Practice VIII. Philadelphia, W. B. Saunders Co., in press.

Chapter
18 SEIZURES—CONVULSIONS

DEFINITION[75, 117]

The terms *seizure, convulsion, epilepsy*, and *fit* are synonyms for a brain disorder expressed as a paroxysmal cerebral dysrhythmia, a paroxysmal transitory disturbance of brain function that has a sudden onset, ceases spontaneously, and has a tendency to recur. The term *epilepsy* is more often used for seizures that are recurrent and of unknown cause, or idiopathic. A seizure is the result of a sudden uncontrolled discharge of neurons. The initial seizure focus may involve only a small number of highly unstable neurons that spontaneously discharge, which induces surrounding neurons to discharge and the seizure spreads or generalizes. The pathogenesis of seizures in veterinary medicine has recently been reviewed.[150] This neuronal hyperexcitability can result from imbalance in excitatory and inhibitory neurotransmitter activity in favor of the former and/or alteration of the cell membrane or the internal cell metabolism, which influences the threshold for depolarization. The period of the seizure is referred to as the ictus, or the attack. The manifestation of these seizure disorders is extremely variable. Any unusual involuntary phenomenon that is episodic and recurrent in nature should be evaluated as a seizure disorder. Such phenomena include loss or derangement of consciousness, excessive or decreased voluntary muscle tone or movement, visceral muscle activity, and altered behavior.

Postictal depression refers to the period of recovery after a seizure when the patient may wander around in confusion, circling or bumping into objects from blindness, or may sleep for a long period. The length and form of postictal depression are variable. There is no correlation between the severity of the seizure and the duration, nature, or severity of the postictal phase. A short, partial seizure may have a longer, more complex postictus than a generalized seizure. As a rule, this postictal phase lasts less than an hour, but much longer periods up to 1 to 2 days can occur that are not necessarily related to a more severe seizure. This probably represents the severe neuronal disturbance "exhaustion" caused by the excessive neuronal activity throughout the nervous system.

CLASSIFICATION

Seizures may be classified as partial or general. Those that begin as partial seizures may generalize subsequently.

Partial Seizures. Partial seizures have an "epileptogenic" or seizure focus that does not spread. The signs seen indicate the location of the seizure focus in the brain. When the seizure focus is in the motor area of the cerebrum there may be contralateral head turning, tonus or clonus of one or more limbs, and flexion of the trunk. In the visual area of the cerebrum there may be light biting and a photogenic seizure, while in the limbic system there may be altered behavior with complex motor activity, including somnolence, confusion, apparent blindness, failure to recognize objects, viciousness, screaming, barking, attacking inanimate objects, voracious or absent appetite, fear behavior, chewing, licking, and jaw snapping.[29] Such activity followed by a generalized seizure is referred to as a psychomotor seizure.

The duration of a partial (focal) seizure is variable. At any time it may spread to become a generalized seizure. The electroencephalogram may localize the seizure focus.[23]

A partial seizure that begins in one group of muscles and slowly spreads to other muscles in the same limb and then to the other ipsilateral limb muscles is called a Jacksonian seizure. It may terminate in a generalized seizure.

It is caused by a structural lesion in the area of the contralateral motor cerebral cortex, and only occasionally occurs in domestic animals.

Dogs that episodically "attack" the base of their tail or episodically run rapidly in circles may have an idiopathic partial seizure disorder and often respond to anticonvulsant therapy.

An almost continual behavior of rapid head movements characterized as "fly catching" has been observed in King Charles spaniels.[48] The onset is usually before 1 year of age. This is assumed to be an idiopathic partial seizure, but no drug has been found effective to control it.

Generalized Seizures. Generalized seizures in veterinary medicine usually are referred to as a grand mal seizure. These have no localizing signs. This is the most common form of seizure in dogs. The severe generalized seizure is characterized by a variable, brief psychic stage or behavioral alteration in which the dog may become restless, seek attention of its owner, or stare into space. This is then followed by a combination of visceral and somatic motor activity as the dog loses contact with its environment and becomes unconscious. Pupillary dilation, excessive salivation, and chewing activity represent the visceral motor activity. The limbs become tonic and are extended rigidly, and the animal falls on its side. A brief period of opisthotonos, marked tonic limb extension, and apnea is followed by or alternated with clonic limb activity and paddling or running movements. This somatic motor activity usually is bilaterally symmetric from the onset and throughout its course. The entire seizure generally only lasts 1 to 2 minutes, but this is variable. Occasionally, there are urinary and fecal excretions during or after the seizure.

In mild generalized seizures the dog may sense an impending disturbance and try to hide or find its owner. This brief period is followed by uncontrollable clonic jerking of the limbs, trunk, and head. The patient may try to walk and stumble and fall or remain in a sternal position. There may be salivation and occasionally vomiting and excretion of urine and feces. These dogs act extremely anxious and confused but remain conscious and try to reach their owners. The seizure may last from a few minutes to 15 to 20 minutes. Occasionally holding and comforting the animal shortens its duration.

Petit mal seizures are mild generalized seizures that consist of an extremely brief (few seconds) loss of consciousness and generalized loss of muscle tone. This seizure has a characteristic electroencephalographic pattern. True petit mal seizures probably do not occur in domestic animals.

Generalized tetanic seizures with rigid tonic extension of the limbs, opisthotonos, and apnea are found in strychnine poisoning and are elicited easily by any form of stimulation to the patient. Such seizures are not accompanied by paddling or running movements, masticatory activity, or salivation, and rarely does the patient lose consciousness.

The degree of partial seizure or the development of a generalized seizure depends on the degree and rate of spread of electrical activity from the initial seizure focus. If the seizure activity remains confined to its initial focus in the motor cortex, the involuntary motor activity is confined to a small muscle group or one limb. If the initial focus is confined to the temporal-pyriform lobe neurons, the seizure manifestation may be limited to episodes of behavior demonstrating fear or hysteria, motor activity such as mastication, or facial muscle twitching.

The seizure generalizes when the electrical activity spreads to the diencephalon, which in turn discharges to both cerebral hemispheres through its diffuse cortical projection nuclei. The ultimate motor activity that is observed results from the upper motor neuron discharge on the entire lower motor neuron of the brain stem and spinal cord.

PATHOGENESIS[137, 150]

Fundamental to all seizures is a small focus of "epileptic" neurons that exhibit some uniquely abnormal characteristics that cause them to intermittently spontaneously depolarize. Only live neurons can participate in a seizure. Neurons normally receive a large number of synapses with inhibitory and facilitatory neurotransmitter activity. The summation of this synaptic activity determines the activity of the neuron. The membrane potential of the neuron which is influenced by these synapses results from the selective movement of sodium and potassium across the cell membrane, and this is dependent on energy generated from aerobic oxidative metabolism in the neuron.

Almost any alteration of the environment of this neuron can result in a spontaneous discharge. If this environmental alteration only involves a small group of neurons and does not spread, it may produce only an abnormal spike on the electroencephalogram. If a larger group of neurons spontaneously discharges, this may result in a focal seizure and a focal dysrhythmia on the electroencephalogram. If the spontaneous discharge spreads, a generalized seizure results with generalized dysrhythmia on the electroencephalogram. The alteration of a neuron's environment to elicit a spontaneous discharge may be structural, biochemical, or unknown. Structural alterations include intracranial organic brain diseases that directly alter brain structure. This may include the neuronal cell body directly or the glial cells in their environment. Extracranial metabolic or toxic disorders may alter the biochemical environment of the neuron in such a way as to result in spontaneous neuronal discharge. Idiopathic seizures occur in individuals who have no definable extra- or intracranial disease. Such individuals have an inherently low seizure threshold and a tendency for neuronal groups to spontaneously depolarize. This may be inherited in some breeds and result from a genetically determined alteration of neurotransmitter synthesis release or degradation. These include the excitatory neurotransmitters acetylcholine, glutamate, and serotonin, and the inhibitory neurotransmitters gamma aminobutyric acid, taurine, and norepinephrine.

SEIZURE THRESHOLD

Each individual has a certain threshold of stimulation for a seizure that is established by the environment of the neuron. If this threshold is exceeded, a seizure will occur. The seizure threshold can be defined as the sum of events that regulate neuronal excitability and include the neuronal cell membrane, the number and location of facilitatory and inhibitory synapses, neurotransmitter synthesis and degradation, and the glial environment. This threshold varies among individuals and may be the underlying cause of most idiopathic epilepsies. Presumably, the metabolic and structural bases for this threshold are established genetically.

The so-called normal individual has a seizure threshold that can be exceeded only by stimuli such as certain convulsant drugs and electric shock treatment. Individuals with the lower seizure threshold can be divided into two groups. In the first group are those in whom seizures can be stimulated by conditions such as fatigue, fever, photic stimulation, hyperventilation, or estrus. In the second are those

individuals with the lowest seizure threshold, who have spontaneous seizures with no detectable stimulus. This is typical of many idiopathic epileptics.

Seizures can be a sign of serious organic brain disease, or of a genetically determined neuronal morphology and physiology that allow spontaneous depolarization. The prognosis obviously is dependent on the underlying cause. It is the responsibility of the examiner to determine this to the best of his or her ability. Educating the client as to the significance of this clinical sign is also an important responsibility of the clinician and may determine the survival of the patient and the success of the therapy.

CAUSES OF SEIZURES[9, 22, 35, 36, 58, 73, 74, 80, 84-86, 118, 120, 125, 140]

Seizures occur when there is an alteration of the environment of the neurons of the prosencephalon. Anything that alters neuronal function in the brain is potentially seizure-producing. The cause of the alteration can be either extracranial or intracranial (Table 18–1).

EXTRACRANIAL

A discussion of extracranial causes that alter neuronal metabolism follows. Usually with these diseases there are no clinical neurologic signs apparent in the interictal period (between seizures).

Hypoglycemia.[88] Functional neoplasms of the beta cells of the pancreatic islets may occur in the dog usually at the age of 5 years or older.[15, 30, 31, 33, 34, 91, 98, 114, 129, 163, 164, 184, 185] Boxers, poodles, and terriers have the highest reported incidence. There is one report in a pony.[146] Typically, the seizures are generalized and occur prior to feeding, when the blood glucose level is at its lowest. Occasionally they occur shortly after eating if the stimulus of eating carbohydrates elicits an outflow of insulin from the neoplastic cells. Seizures are the most common neurologic abnormality, but occasionally evidences of altered behavior, or mild ataxia or paresis, or both, may be presenting signs. A fasting blood glucose level of less than 60 mg per 100 cc is suspicious, and less than 40 mg per 100 cc is diagnostic for hypoglycemia associated with the neurologic

TABLE 18–1. CAUSES OF SEIZURES

EXTRACRANIAL
  Hypoglycemia
    Glycogen storage diseases
    Beta cell neoplasm of pancreas
  Hypoxia
    Cardiorespiratory disease
  Hepatoencephalopathy
  Renal disease
  Hypocalcemia
  Hyperkalemia
  Hyperlipoproteinemia
  Gastrointestinal disease
    Parasitism
    "Garbage" toxicity
INTRACRANIAL
  Inflammations
    Canine distemper encephalitis, toxoplasmosis, cryptococcosis
    Other viral encephalitides: rabies, equine
    Feline infectious peritonitis meningoencephalitis in cats
  Neoplasia
    Primary or metastatic
  Malformations
    Hydrocephalus, lissencephaly-pachygyria
  Injury
  Degenerations
    Polioencephalomalacia in ruminants
    Vitamin A deficiency in calves
    Thiamine deficiency in cats
    Cerebral infarction in cats
    Salt poisoning in pigs
    Intoxications:
      lead, mercury, arsenic, chlorinated hydrocarbons, organic phosphates, hexachlorophene,
        ethylene glycol; radiopaque media for myelography
IDIOPATHIC EPILEPSY

abnormality. Radioimmunoassay of serum insulin may demonstrate excessive levels or, when compared with the plasma glucose in a ratio, the ratio will be higher than that in normal dogs. The clinical signs are most commonly associated with those periods when the blood glucose drops rapidly. Rarely hypoglycemia has been associated with nonpancreatic neoplasms in the dog.[167]

A functional hypoglycemia occasionally is observed in hunting dogs and causes seizures associated with periods of exercise.[88] This is thought to be due to the inability of the dog to mobilize enough liver glycogen into utilizable glucose during periods of heavy use. Feeding the animal before hunting, or providing glucose in the form of candy bars while hunting, may allay the condition. Some young dogs of the toy breeds from 6 to 12 weeks old have a predilection for hypoglycemia. A glucose-6-phosphatase deficiency in puppies, similar to von Gierke's disease in children, results in failure to produce free glucose in the liver. Hypoglycemia may occur during periods of stress. Ketones are often present in the urine in high concentrations. Treatment with 4 cc

per kg of body weight of a 50 per cent glucose solution should alleviate the immediate neurologic signs. Some dogs grow out of the condition in 3 to 4 months. Other metabolic causes of fasting hypoglycemia have been described in puppies.[169] Hypoglycemia may occur transiently in young puppies that are stressed by cold, starvation, gastrointestinal disorders, or other systemic illness.

Pre- and postpartum hypoglycemia have been reported in dogs.[4, 77, 78] Adrenal insufficiency and liver disease may impair gluconeogenesis and glycogen storage and result in hypoglycemia, but this is uncommon.

Liver Disease. Severe liver disease with excess ammonia in the blood can lead to seizures. The most common example of this in the dog is the hepatic encephalopathy associated with portacaval communications.[3, 12, 13, 24, 34, 59, 63, 97, 105, 115, 155, 159, 162, 165, 166, 168, 170, 172, 179, 180, 188]

In the horse the liver necrosis of Theiler's disease may produce seizures along with the other signs of acute hepatic encephalopathy.[72]

Hypocalcemia. Hypocalcemia associated with parturition in the bitch may cause seizures.[87, 142] It also has been reported in hunting dogs following exercise, and in chronic renal disease. Treatment with 4 cc per kg of a 10 per cent solution of calcium gluconate should alleviate the neurologic signs.

Muscle tremors, tonic spasms of limb muscles, tetany, episodic weakness, behavioral alterations, and seizures have been observed in hypocalcemic dogs that have decreased levels of parathormone from parathyroid gland disease.[90, 103, 156] Lymphocytic parathyroiditis has been identified in some of these. They have been successfully managed with oral calcium supplementation with or without vitamin D therapy.[42]

Renal Disease. Occasionally, renal disease associated with prolonged uremia causes seizures in dogs.[20, 139, 175, 176, 186] The acidosis that accompanies this disease near its end stage may be the cause of the neurologic disturbance. Hypoglycemia and hypocalcemia also have been incriminated. This occurs more commonly in young dogs with congenital renal disease.

Hypoxia. Hypoxia from cardiovascular disease or pulmonary disease may cause periodic episodes of collapse or seizures.[18, 21, 27, 40, 43, 50, 64, 93, 96, 101, 102, 143, 144, 147, 148] Repeated seizures may lead to hypoxia of nervous tissue and may be self-perpetuating. Hypoxia is a component of the pathogenesis of neonatal seizures in foals.[66, 121]

Hyperkalemia. Hyperkalemia occurs in adrenocortical insufficiency (Addison's disease) or may follow the sudden withdrawal of steroids after their prolonged use, and seizures may occur.

Hypomagnesemia. This electrolyte disturbance is more often a cause of seizure activity in the bovine species referred to as "grass tetany."

Hyperlipoproteinemia. Seizures have been observed in dogs with defective lipid metabolism causing hyperlipoproteinemia. It has been reported as most common in the miniature schnauzer, with the onset of seizures between 2 and 7 years.[145]

Intestinal Parasitism. Intestinal parasitism in young puppies may be associated with seizures that may be produced by a hypocalcemia, hypoglycemia, or some unknown mechanism. Generalized seizures often occur with winter coccidiosis in young cattle in feedlots in western Canada. The pathogenesis is unknown.

Allergy. There have been some clinical observations of seizures in dogs with food-induced hypersensitivity.[136] The seizures cease following correction of the allergy.

Hyperthermia. Heat stroke occurs when the hypothalamic thermal regulatory centers can no longer maintain normal body temperature when the animal is confined in a poorly ventilated space in a high environmental temperature. Seizures may occur as one of the clinical signs. Be aware that seizures in themselves can elevate the body temperature.

INTRACRANIAL

Intracranial diseases are the more common causes of seizures. Usually, a thorough neurologic examination detects abnormal neurologic signs in the interictal period. The presence of these signs usually indicates structural brain disease.

Inflammation. Encephalitis from any cause that involves prosencephalic structures can be a source of seizures. Canine distemper encephalitis is the most common cause of seizures in the dog associated with encephalitis.[131] The kind of seizure associated with this disease is not specific, but visceral motor activity is often prominent in the form of clonic masticatory activity and salivation, the so-called "chewing gum fits." In addition to the seizures there are usually interictal signs of diffuse neurologic deficit, suggesting multifocal disease. The CSF may be abnormal, with mild elevations of mononuclear cells and protein. Toxoplasmosis or cryptococcal meningoencephalitis also may be causes of seizures in dogs or cats. Feline infectious peritonitis and a nonsuppurative polioencephalomyelitis may cause seizures in cats.[178] Chronic encephalitis of Pug dogs commonly causes seizures.

Neoplasia. Primary or metastatic neoplasms may cause seizures.[16, 119, 122] They are more common in older dogs. Other evidence of focal neurologic disease may be apparent from the interictal neurologic examination. However, if a cerebral neoplasm is slow in growing, does not increase intracranial pressure significantly, and does not affect the sensorimotor cortex or its pathway to and from the brain stem, or the optic radiation and visual cortex, no interictal neurologic deficit may be detected. CSF pressure sometimes is elevated and the protein content may be elevated slightly. The signs, including the frequency of the seizures, are usually progressive.

Malformation. Hydrocephalus is the most common malformation of the prosencephalon, and occasionally causes seizures. Electroencephalography usually indicates this diagnosis, and pneumoventriculography confirms it. Visual deficit and behavioral abnormalities may accompany this malformation, but no one set of signs is diagnostic.

Lissencephaly and pachygyria have been observed in the Lhasa apso. Behavioral abnormalities, with an inability to train properly, and visual deficits appear at an early age, but seizures usually do not occur until near the end of the first year of life. This malformation also was observed in a wire-haired terrier that presented with nonprogressive signs of severe cerebellar abnormality from birth. The cerebellum was reduced markedly in size and dysplastic. There was no evidence of degeneration or previous in utero inflammation. A litter mate with similar ataxia was raised to 4½ years of age. The ataxia persisted unchanged. At 1½ years of age this dog began to have seizures. They occurred at the rate of at least four per month for about 2 years, despite anticonvulsant therapy. In the last year they increased in frequency to one to two weekly.The dog died following a seizure at 4½ years old.

Injury. Trauma to the brain may cause seizures at the time of the initial damage, but more often the seizures do not take place until weeks or months after the injury occurred and the tissue has healed. The cerebral scar is somehow thought to serve as the seizure focus in this condition. These seizures usually only occur in animals that have had signs of a significant intracranial disturbance at the time of injury.

Neuronal Degeneration. Diseases that cause neuronal degeneration often cause seizures.[1, 51]

Polioencephalomalacia in cattle, sheep, and goats usually is related to abnormal metabolism of the thiamine coenzyme. Seizures may accompany the marked neurologic deficit typical of this disease that is destructive to the cerebral cortex. Immediate treatment with thiamine early in the course of the disease may reverse the signs.

Thiamine deficiency occasionally occurs in cats on an all-fish diet that contains a thiaminase, or following a prolonged anorexia.[44] Generalized seizures frequently are elicited by handling the animal. Early treatment with a few milligrams of thiamine alleviates the condition. Cats that are stressed by a systemic infection may be predisposed to thiamine deficiency after a few days of anorexia.

Intoxication with lead in some areas may be a common cause of seizures in dogs and cattle.[189] There are many sources, including paint, linoleum, tarpaper, roofing materials, and batteries. In dogs gastrointestinal and neurologic signs occur together or singly in this disease. The neurologic signs usually involve seizures or abnormal behavior. The seizures are often psychomotor, accompanied by bizarre behavioral abnormalities. The results of blood studies are considered to be nearly pathognomonic for this disease when numerous erythrocytes are observed that are nucleated and have basophilic stippling, in the absence of a severe anemia. Urinary levels of alpha aminolevulinic acid may be elevated. The finding of elevated blood levels of lead is diagnostic. In young growing dogs a radiograph of long bones may show a "lead line" at the metaphysis. Treatment with calcium ethylenediaminetetraacetic acid often results in rapid recovery from the signs.

In calves with lead poisoning the seizures often are associated with propulsive, maniacal activity. Hyperesthesia is pronounced. Odontoprisis and lack of ruminal motility may be noted. Blindness is common.

Intoxication with chlorinated hydrocarbons, hexachlorophene, ethylene glycol,[61] organic phosphates, and mercury may affect neuronal metabolism and cause seizures. Cats are especially susceptible to the chlorinated hydrocarbons used in many flea dip preparations. Strychnine poisoning acts predominantly on the spinal cord inhibitory neurons, but the effects of this toxin may be more widespread in the central nervous system.

Salt poisoning occasionally is observed in pigs fed on garbage high in salt content concomitant with a restriction of their water intake. The toxicity is related to the sodium ion. The seizures are often characterized by a rapid backward movement, with the pig in a sitting position. Signs of diffuse cerebral disease accompany the seizures. The laminar cerebral necrosis often is accompanied by a marked infiltration of eosinophils in this disease.

Water intoxication occurs in calves and possibly pigs when a large volume of water is consumed. Seizures may accompany the other signs of diffuse brain disturbance. In most cases, hemoglobinuria is present. Cardiac arrhythmia is common. Hypo-osmolar serum is diagnostic.

Vitamin A deficiency decreases the CSF absorptive mechanism and may result in a sudden increase in CSF pressure and generalized seizures in cattle. This occurs in 6- to 8-month-old cattle that have been on dry pasture for many weeks without green feed. Most respond to vitamin A therapy.

The water-soluble compounds used for myelography may cause seizures in the first few hours after the procedure.[38] This is due either to the direct effect of the compound on neuronal metabolism or to its osmotic effect on the CSF.

IDIOPATHIC EPILEPSY

Idiopathic epilepsy is a syndrome characterized by repeated episodes of seizures for which there is no known demonstrable clinical or pathologic cause.[2, 6, 17, 41, 67, 68, 76] The diagnosis ultimately is made by examination of the patient and ruling out the extracranial and intracranial diseases that cause seizures. The seizure threshold differs for each individual and is a result of a combination of structural and biochemical features of the neurons and their environment that controls their activity. Genetic factors regulate the developmental mechanisms that establish this seizure threshold. Dogs with idiopathic epilepsy may have a lower threshold as a result of minor alterations of these genetic factors. Pedigree analysis and breeding studies have determined an inherited idiopathic epilepsy in the German shepherd (Alsatian),[47] Belgian Tervuren,[177] keeshond,[182] beagle,[41] and dachshund.[76] It occurs commonly in all breeds of poodle, Saint Bernard, cocker spaniel, Irish setter, Alaskan and Siberian huskies, wire-haired fox terrier, and Labrador and golden retrievers, but has not been proved to be inherited in these breeds. The disease occurs sporadically in almost all breeds and in mongrel dogs.

Seizures usually begin between 1 and 3 years of age, but younger or older onsets occur. They may be preceded by a short aura during which the animal acts as if it knows a seizure is coming. The seizure is usually generalized in type, lasting from one half a minute to 2 minutes. However, a great variety of partial seizures may also be idiopathic.[23] There is no set type of seizure in idiopathic epilepsy for any one animal, but usually the type does not vary within one affected animal. In the large breeds such as German shepherds, Saint Bernards, and Irish setters, the seizures are usually severe and generalized and often occur in multiples. In miniature and toy poodles they are often generalized but mild without loss of consciousness. They develop spasticity and uncontrolled trembling and attempt to crawl to the owner. In the immediate postictal period the patient usually is depressed and occasion-

ally blind. The seizures sometimes recur at fairly regular intervals. The interval varies from one or a few weeks to months between seizures. The frequency of seizures may increase as the dog ages, and occasionally the patient develops status epilepticus, during which death may occur. During the interictal period the patient shows no signs of neurologic disturbance. Some of these patients show abnormalities in their electroencephalograms recorded in the interictal period. Often these seizures can be controlled with proper anticonvulsant therapy.

Idiopathic epilepsy is most common in dogs but occasionally occurs in cats, cattle,[10, 11] and horses. An idiopathic seizure syndrome has been observed in Arabian foals.[99] The onset of generalized seizures is 3 to 9 months of age. After a few weeks these usually cease spontaneously. A familial basis is suspected. A form of idiopathic epilepsy has been observed in horses that seems to be related to the estrus period when estrogen levels are increased. Seizures only occur during these periods in these mares. Occasionally one or more seizures will occur over a few days without identification of a cause and cease spontaneously. This can occur at any age in dogs but more commonly occurs in the young puppy.

EXAMINATION OF THE PATIENT

The following is an example of a dog presented with the chief complaint of seizures. This demonstrates the kind of information the examiner should obtain in attempting to diagnose the cause of seizures.

Chief Complaint. Seizure.

Signalment

AGE. Less than 1 year—canine distemper encephalitis; lead poisoning; hypoglycemia of toy breeds; puppies with severe intestinal parasitism; young dogs with signs of liver disease who may have a portacaval shunt; hydrocephalus; lissencephaly; occasionally idiopathic.

One to 3 years—usual onset of idiopathic epilepsy.

Over 5 years—neoplasia in prosencephalon; hypoglycemia from beta cell neoplasm in pancreas.

BREED. Hypoglycemia of toy breeds; hydrocephalus in toy and brachycephalic breeds; neoplasms in brachycephalic breeds; idiopathic epilepsy in the German shepherd, Belgian Tervuren, keeshond, beagle, dachshund, Saint Bernard, poodle, cocker spaniel, Irish setter,

Alaskan and Siberian huskies, Labrador and golden retrievers; leukodystrophy in Cairn and West Highland white terriers; lipodystrophy in German short-haired pointers and English setters; lissencephaly in the Lhasa apso; portacaval shunts and hyperlipoproteinemia in miniature schnauzers.

SEX. Mammary gland adenocarcinomas metastasize to the brain; seizure threshold may be reduced during estrus.

USE. Hunting dogs may develop hypoglycemia.

History

DESCRIPTION. Obtain a careful description of the seizure. A consistent focal location in partial seizures may indicate the site of a structural lesion. Seizures from intoxicants and in idiopathic epilepsy usually are symmetric, with no lateralizing focal component. Bizarre behavioral abnormalities that precede a generalized seizure may occur in lead poisoning. Seizures in cats with severe flexion of the trunk and neck occur in thiamine deficiency. Idiopathic epileptics usually have short, generalized, seizures.

Transient cerebral ischemia such as from heartworms may produce episodes of transient ataxia and collapse. Episodic collapse may occur in hypoadrenocorticoidism (Addison's disease) and cataplexy. These are not seizure disorders.

ONSET AND COURSE. An explosive onset of continuous seizures, serial or status epilepticus, can occur with neoplasms, intoxicants, or idiopathic epilepsy. A progressive course with more frequent and longer seizures is found with inflammations or neoplasms. Regular intervals are more common in idiopathic epilepsy, but even in that disease they may be progressive. Hypoglycemic seizures often occur just prior to feeding or shortly after feeding. Seizures often follow a high-protein meal in hepatic encephalopathy.

ENVIRONMENT. Investigate the environment of other dogs or litter mates with signs suggestive of canine distemper. A source of intoxicants should be sought, for example: lead—paint, linoleum, wallboard, tarpaper, roofing materials; metaldehyde—snail bait; hexachlorophene—soap; ethylene glycol—antifreeze; chlorinated hydrocarbons, organophosphates—insecticides; fluoroacetate (1080)—rodenticides; mercury—seed treated with fungicide; arsenic—ant poisons, insecticides; phenols—cresol, germicides.

DIET. An all-fish diet may precipitate thiamine deficiency in cats. Engorgement on spoiled garbage may cause seizures in dogs.

PAST MEDICAL HISTORY. Seizures can follow intracranial injuries up to 2 years or longer. Such injuries usually have produced significant signs of cerebral disturbances such as stupor, unconsciousness, blindness, and tetraplegia followed by recovery.

Febrile illness may have been caused by the canine distemper virus. The neurologic form can occur days to weeks later.

Difficult, prolonged birth may produce cerebral lesions from hypoxia or trauma.

Diagnosis of neoplastic disease in other organs may herald a metastasis to the brain.

Previous progressive neurologic deficit that culminated in a seizure suggests organic brain disease.

Evidence of behavior change, polyuria and polydipsia, or a voracious, indiscriminate appetite may suggest hypothalamic involvement by a pituitary neoplasm. Signs of hyperadrenocorticoidism (Cushing's disease) may accompany a pituitary adenoma.

Recent changes in behavior often accompany frontal lobe neoplasia. Episodic behavioral alterations in the young dog may accompany hepatic encephalopathy, or the malformations of lissencephaly and pachygyria.

The primary purpose of the examination of the patient is to establish if the disease producing the seizure is *extracranial* or *intracranial*.

Physical Examination. Other organs that may be diseased and occasionally may produce seizures include the liver, kidney, and cardiorespiratory structures. Diffuse systemic disease may accompany the various encephalitides in the dog.

Neurologic Examination (Fig. 18–1). Abnormalities in the interictal neurologic examination suggest intracranial structural brain disease. Focal signs suggest a neoplasm, infarct, or previous injury. Mild hemiparesis and general proprioceptive deficit only observable on postural reaction testing suggest a contralateral internal capsule or sensory-motor cortex lesion; hemianopsia suggests a contralateral optic tract, optic radiation, or occipital lobe lesion. Circling may occur toward the side of a cerebral lesion. Signs of multifocal central nervous system disease suggest inflammation or multiple neoplastic metastasis. Signs of diffuse neurologic disturbance can occur with inflammatory or degenerative diseases or from metabolic disturbance that is extracranial in origin.

If interictal signs are absent, either extracranial or intracranial disease may be present.

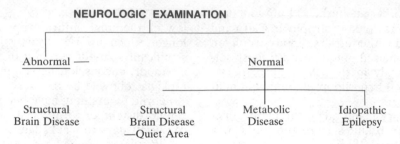

Figure 18–1. The significance of the neurologic examination in seizures.

A small focal area of injury, neoplasia, or inflammation in a "quiet" area of the brain may produce seizures with no definable interictal signs. Most extracranial diseases do not produce interictal signs. The most common extracranial disease is hypoglycemia, followed by hepatoencephalopathy and hypoxia. Dogs with idiopathic epilepsy do not have interictal signs.

Ancillary Examination

LABORATORY FINDINGS. CBC: Lead poisoning—presence of nucleated red blood cells, basophilic stippling, and a low normal packed cell volume; may be normal with viral encephalitis; increased WBC with abnormal differential may accompany suppurative meningoencephalitis; leukocytosis occasionally occurs in portacaval communications; polycythemia—greater than 70 to 75 per cent packed cell volume may produce seizures; hyperviscosity may produce seizures.

BUN: Increased in chronic renal disease; may be decreased in portacaval shunts.

Urinalysis: Signs of renal or liver disease; look for ammonium biurate crystals in hepatic encephalopathy; ketosis occurs in hypoglycemic puppies.

Liver function: BSP—higher than 5 per cent retention of bromsulfalein in 30 minutes suggests diffuse liver dysfunction (or increased indocyanin green retention[32])—most valuable for portacaval communications; serum alanine aminotransferase and alkaline phosphatase may be increased with focal or diffuse liver lesions; ammonia may increase in serum with diffuse liver disease and seizures. The ammonia tolerance test may be abnormal.

Fasting blood glucose: A 24-hour fast is usually sufficient to demonstrate the hypoglycemia from pancreatic neoplasms. Forty-eight hours may be necessary in toy breeds with glycogen storage disease. Less than 60 mg of glucose per dl is suspicious. Less than 40 mg per dl or an increased insulin-glucose ratio is diagnostic.

Calcium: Hypocalcemia may cause tetanic-type seizures in eclampsia, chronic renal disease, especially if congenital, or following parathyroid gland removal or destruction from immune-mediated inflammation.

Acid-base and electrolyte abnormalities (except calcium) rarely cause seizures in dogs.

CSF: Normal in all idiopathic epileptics, most dogs with extracranial metabolic diseases, and some dogs with intracranial organic diseases.

Mild elevation of protein levels with normal cells or mild mononuclear pleocytosis occurs in viral encephalitis or with neoplasia. Pressure may be elevated with neoplasia.

RADIOGRAPHY. In suspected cases of cranial injury or neoplasms that may be adjacent to the bony walls of the cranium, causing erosion, radiographs may help to confirm a diagnosis. Pneumoventriculograms may confirm hydrocephalus. Evidence of metastatic neoplasia on thoracic radiographs may help diagnose similar brain neoplasia.

CEREBRAL ANGIOGRAPHY. Some have found this useful to diagnose space-occupying lesions.

SCINTIGRAPHY. Radioisotope scanning procedures of the brain may help confirm most space-occupying lesions, large infarcts, or granulomas.

ELECTROENCEPHALOGRAPHY. EEG is usually helpful in confirming suspicious cases of hydrocephalus, and may help confirm inflammatory and neoplastic diseases.

COMPUTERIZED AXIAL TOMOGRAPHY. Where available, this has been useful in confirming space-occupying or large inflammatory lesions.

If the signalment and history are appropriate, and all the results of the physical, neurologic, and ancillary examinations are normal, idiopathic epilepsy can be diagnosed.

Examination Summary. The extent of the examination performed on an individual patient with seizures depends on the number of seizures and the age of the patient at the time of the examination. All patients should undergo complete physical and neurologic examinations. In a young dog with only one seizure, this may be sufficient. In the older dog with one seizure, a CBC, BUN, blood calcium and glucose compose the minimum data base. Dogs of any age with recurrent seizures should have a more complete data base with CBC, BUN, blood electrolytes (Ca, Mg, Na, K), glucose, serum alanine aminotransferase, alkaline phosphatase, and cerebrospinal fluid examination. Further study will depend on the differential diagnosis that is under consideration and the facilities available. These may include a BSP retention study, blood ammonia, serum albumin and globulin, serum and CSF antibody titers, radiography, electroencephalography, scintigraphy, and computerized axial tomography.

TREATMENT

Treatment should be directed at the primary disease if it can be recognized.[116, 128] The seizures should be controlled by pharmacologic agents.[25, 106, 124, 127, 135, 138] Primarily three anticonvulsants have been used in veterinary medicine: phenobarbital, primidone, and phenytoin. Based on what are assumed to be effective blood and tissue levels of the drugs, the rapid rate of metabolism of phenytoin in dogs makes it difficult to maintain such levels without high doses and a frequency of administration that may not be practical.[56, 100, 133, 152, 154] In general it is best to initiate therapy with phenobarbital. If that is ineffective it may be slowly replaced by primidone and, if necessary, phenytoin or a combination of drugs.

ANTICONVULSANTS

Phenobarbital.[160] The action of this drug is on the neuronal cell body, preventing initiation of a seizure but not its propagation. It raises the seizure threshold. This drug is effective rapidly, and is especially useful in treatment of status epilepticus. It is the drug of choice for cats. Its disadvantage is the sedation that may follow moderate doses. It is supplied in ⅛ gr (8 mg), ¼ gr (16 mg), and ½ gr (32 mg) tablets for oral use, and in vials of 1 gr (64 mg) and 2 gr (128 mg) for parenteral use. The dose is 1 to 2 mg per kg, bid, or tid.

Some patients will initially be depressed on

this drug but usually recover sensorium in a few days without a decrease in the dose of the drug. Occasonally this drug will make a dog extremely hyperactive or eat and drink excessively.

Primidone (Mylepsin, Mysoline). Primidone is partially metabolized to phenobarbital and phenylethylmalonic acid.[55, 187] All three have anticonvulsant activity. These act directly on the neurons to prevent initiation of a seizure.

Primidone has a rapid anticonvulsant action, but often produces a severe depression and occasionally ataxia. This may be transient as the patient adjusts to the drug. Of all the drugs used for seizures, this may produce the most significant polyphagia, polydipsia, and polyuria; occasionally it produces hyperactivity. Hepatic necrosis is also reported.[79] It is not recommended for cats by the manufacturer.

It is supplied in 50-mg and 250-mg tablets. Therapy should start at 10 to 15 mg per kg per day split into bid or tid doses. This dose can be increased to about 35 mg per kg per day as necessary to control seizures. This gradual increase in dose should avoid the initial fatigue and sedation often experienced at higher doses.[190]

Phenytoin (diphenylhydantoin, Dilantin). This drug does not prevent initiation of a seizure, but stops its spread. It occasionally produces a mild ataxia, and takes about 4 to 7 days to build an effective CNS level.[132, 149, 173] In cats its rate of metabolism is much slower and it may cause an undesirable level of sedation.[14, 174] It is supplied in 30- and 100-mg capsules and 50 mg tablets for oral use. There is no firmly established maximum dosage.[92] The dose used is the amount that will control the seizures. The minimal dose to begin with is 10 mg per kg tid. Usually it will require 20 to 35 mg per kg tid to obtain control or a blood level assumed to be effective (10 μg per ml in humans).[152] Seizure control may require doses as high as 50 to 80 mg per kg tid. The wide dosage range is due to the variable rapid rate of metabolism of this drug in most dogs. Although there have been many claims for its clinical efficacy, this has not been supported by pharmacologic studies. Clinicians feel this drug is more effective in the small breeds of dogs.

Beware of toxicity of phenytoin when chloramphenicol,[153] phenylbutazone, chlorpromazine, diazepam, or halothane is administered simultaneously.

Diazepam (Valium). Diazepam, a benzodiazepine, is used mostly in patients with status epilepticus.[62, 161] It often produces significant sedation, and has received only limited use as a daily therapeutic drug for generalized seizures. Some have thought it useful as a daily anticonvulsant in combination with primidone in large breed dogs at a dose of 5 to 10 mg tid orally. It is supplied as a tablet in 5- and 10-mg quantities.

Alternative Anticonvulsants

Other anticonvulsants used in human medicine have been recommended, but clinical trials in domestic animals are few.

Valproic Acid. Sodium valproate has been recommended when the usual anticonvulsants have been ineffective.[60, 94, 112, 134, 141] This is more often in the larger breed dogs with idiopathic epilepsy. Improved control has been observed in some of these dogs. Dosages ranging from 30 to 180 mg per kg per day split into three administrations have been recommended.

Paramethadione. This is a drug used for petit mal seizures in humans. Preliminary data indicate that it appears to be as effective as the other canine anticonvulsants, but also that it may be especially helpful in those patients found difficult to control with the usual canine anticonvulsants.[126] It was used at a daily dosage of 10 to 60 mg per kg.

Trimethadione and Carbamazepine. Trimethadione and carbamazepine are used in humans for petit mal and generalized seizures, respectively.[57] Their efficacy and side effects in domestic animals are unknown.

Complications

Hepatic complications of varying degree occur with most anticonvulsants. Phenobarbital, primidone, and phenytoin frequently induce microsomal production of alkaline phosphatase, causing an elevation of the serum level.[104, 171] Sometimes serum alanine aminotransferase is increased and occasionally there is a prolonged retention of BSP. Liver necrosis with clinical signs of hepatic dysfunction is infrequent but has been observed with primidone therapy or combinations of primidone and phenytoin.[26, 113, 130] With dogs on long-term therapy, periodic evaluation of liver function is advised. BSP retention, serum gamma-glutamyl transferase, and bile acid determinations are the most valuable for this.[26]

RECOMMENDATIONS

It is important to establish the goals of the therapy with the owner. In most serious idio-pathic epileptics, complete elimination of seizures is unlikely. The goal should be to strive for a decrease in frequency, number, and severity to a level that the owner and patient can endure. Most failures to control seizures are due to inadequate dosage or lack of owner cooperation in administration of the drug.

There are no specific dosage levels or guidelines, except for reliance on experience.[85] It is most important that the drug be given exactly as directed, with no lapses in therapy. A lapse in therapy often produces seizures. If seizures remain uncontrolled, the dosage should be increased progressively until control occurs or drug toxicity is encountered. It is preferable to use a single drug rather than combinations for ease of dosage regulations and to avoid side effects. If necessary, combinations can be used. If a change in drug is considered necessary do not stop the drug in use abruptly, but slowly decrease it as the new drug is initiated.

Clients should be instructed thoroughly that a trial with one or more drugs may be necessary to achieve successful control in their animal. Most seizure patients with progressive organic disease can be controlled at least partially.

Occasionally relapses occur, even in well-controlled patients. The exacerbation of a seizure disorder after successful management does not necessarily indicate the presence of a progressive organic lesion, but just may require more vigorous therapy. Similarly, if the seizures change in pattern, this does not necessarily imply the presence of an organic lesion.

There is often no correlation between the severity and duration of the seizure and the underlying disease. Some idiopathic epileptics have much more serious seizures than dogs with large intracranial neoplasms. The prognosis in serious seizure disorders, including status epilepticus, is not necessarily grave if there is no indication of organic brain disease from the examination. Except in status epilepticus, dogs usually do not die from a seizure.

The decision to treat depends on the nature and frequency of the seizures and the concern of the owner. A single seizure does not require preventive therapy if there is no indication of the cause upon complete examination of the patient. Most dogs that have mild single seizures as often as once every two months need not be treated if the owner can accept this. More frequent seizures and more serious seizures or clusters of seizures should be treated because of the threat of status epilepticus.

Experimentally spontaneous seizures can be

induced by the kindling phenomenon, which involves frequent repeated experimental stimulations of cerebral neurons.[46] There is no evidence to date that there is a greater tendency for more seizures to occur following one clinical seizure because of this kindling phenomenon. This is justification for not instituting anticonvulsant therapy after one single seizure. The kindling phenomenon has been used experimentally to test the efficacy of anticonvulsant drugs in dogs.[183]

THE MANAGEMENT OF STATUS EPILEPTICUS

Status epilepticus is a condition in which seizures are continual, one after the other, with no recovery between them. These can lead to irreversible coma or death, and should be considered a medical emergency. Death is caused by a combination of hyperthermia, circulatory collapse, and acidosis and hypoxia from muscle exertion and impaired respiration.

The seizures must be stopped. The drugs of choice, in the order of their use, are diazepam, phenobarbital, and barbiturate anesthesia.

Diazepam (Valium) is a tranquilizer that enhances presynpatic inhibitory mechanisms.[5] It is particularly useful in stopping the generalized seizures of a status patient, dog or cat. It has a relatively short action, and often needs repeated administration. It is supplied in 2-cc vials with 5 mg per cc, and in 5-mg and 10-mg tablets. In status, it usually is given intravenously in 5- to 10-mg doses every 10 to 15 minutes until the seizures stop. The intramuscular route may be used in a violent patient. If 3 or 4 doses are inadequate, intravenous phenobarbital or pentobarbital should be administered to effect using a dose of 3 to 15 mg per kg. Complete anesthesia with pentobarbital sodium may be required.

The ideal management should include the following steps:

1. Be sure the patient's airway is intact and not obstructed. Administer oxygen if necessary.

2. Place an indwelling intravenous catheter in the patient.

3. Draw blood for complete blood count, glucose, and calcium determinations.

4. Administer 50 per cent dextrose intravenously—2 to 25 cc. (toy poodle to German shepherd). Hypoglycemia may be primary or be secondary to the prolonged generalized seizures.

5. If hypocalcemia is suspected, as in eclampsia, administer slowly 5 to 10 cc of 10 per cent or 20 per cent calcium gluconate.

6. Administer the intravenous anticonvulsant—diazepam, phenobarbital, or pentobarbital anesthesia.

7. Hyperthermia should be treated with icewater baths.

8. As soon as the animal can swallow, oral medication with phenobarbital or primidone should be instituted.

9. Corticosteroids may be administered intravenously (dexamethasone, 1 to 2 mg per kg) to stabilize lysosomes and to prevent catecholamine release.

10. Mannitol, 0.5 to 2.0 gm per kg of 20 per cent solution intravenously, should be considered if there is reason to suspect cerebral cytotoxic edema from prolonged hypoxia.

11. Lactic acidosis may require bicarbonate therapy.

NARCOLEPSY—CATAPLEXY

Narcolepsy is an incurable disorder of the normal sleep mechanism of the central nervous system of unknown cause. In humans the disease consists of four components that vary in severity: excessive daytime sleepiness, cataplexy, hypnagogic hallucinations, and sleep paralysis. In domestic animals cataplexy is the most prominent aspect of the narcoleptic syndrome.[8, 52, 70, 83, 107, 109] Cataplexy is characterized by sudden episodes of collapse with complete inhibition of tone to almost all striated muscles. Muscles of respiration and cardiac muscle are unaffected. Eye muscles may contract, causing eye movement, and occasionally sudden contraction of limb or trunk muscles produces spasmodic motions. The cataplectic event may be either partial, interfering with normal locomotion, or complete, with collapse. Careful study of affected dogs has demonstrated an increased tendency to sleep, but this is not observed as a clinical problem.[95, 108]

During these cataplectic episodes, the EEG records low amplitude, fast activity, typical of paradoxical, fast wave or rapid eye movement (REM) sleep. The EMG shows no recordable muscle tone, which relates to the clinical sign of cataplexy.

Normal sleep consists of 2 major components: slow wave and fast wave sleep. When normal sleep is induced, slow wave sleep occurs first and periods of fast wave sleep are alternated with slow wave sleep throughout the normal sleep period. The anatomic areas concerned with the induction of sleep are in the midline raphe area of the pons for slow wave sleep, with serotonin as a major chemical mediator, and the locus coeruleus of the pons for fast wave sleep, with norepinephrine as the major chemical mediator.[71] These centers act through the ascending and descending activating system of the reticular formation. The EEG recording reflects the activity of the diffuse cortical projection nuclei of the thalamus, which in turn are responding to discharges from the ascending reticular activating system under the direction of the sleep centers in the pons.

During slow wave sleep the EEG is synchronized and shows a regular pattern of high amplitude slow waves. With the EMG a low amplitude activity can be recorded from muscles, reflecting a resting motor tone.

The EEG during fast wave sleep consists of a low amplitude, fast activity, typical of the wake state, yet the individual being recorded is sleeping. Therefore, this is also referred to as paradoxical sleep. During fast wave sleep, the locus ceruleus activates the medullary reticular formation nucleus, whose axons descend the spinal cord and completely inhibit the lower motor neuron somatic efferent neurons.[81, 151] This corresponds to the inactive EMG recording and the atonia demonstrable in the muscles. Because rapid eye movements occur during this phase of sleep it is also referred to as REM sleep. It is during this phase of sleep that dreams occur.

The clinical sign of cataplexy reflects a spontaneous initiation of the fast wave sleep mechanism, with the sudden medullary inhibition of almost all lower motor neurons to muscles resulting in collapse. This is usually reflected in all muscles but may be limited to specific muscle groups. Usually the patient appears to be aware of its environment during these collapse episodes. Occasionally only partial attacks occur resulting in stumbling and partial, but not complete, collapse.

This is an idiopathic disease that may result from neurotransmitter abnormalities. Research studies have documented decreased concentration and/or turnover of serotonin, dopamine, and norepinephrine in these patients.[49] Therapy with drugs such as imipramine and fluoxetine that decrease serotonin uptake may help these patients.[7] Additionally, cholinergic mechanisms may be involved.[39] Anticholinesterases such as physostigmine augment the clinical signs, and atropine sulfate, which blocks acetylcholine, may decrease the signs.

It has been recognized in many breeds of dogs, cats, horses, Shetland ponies, the miniature horse, and the bull.[19, 37, 65, 89, 110, 111, 123, 157] It has been called fainting disease in Shetland ponies and Suffolk draft horses.[158] The disease appears to be inherited as an autosomal recessive disease in Doberman pinschers and Labrador retrievers.[53] The disease may also be inherited in the miniature poodle.

The onset of the disease is usually fairly sudden and by 6 months of age. A pattern of duration and frequency is usually set in the first week or two of the disease and will remain relatively unaltered. Duration may be from a few seconds to 20 minutes. Excitement and feeding may induce the signs. Manual stimulation may terminate the attack. Less commonly, the onset of the disease may not occur until the patient is an adult. A few dogs have been observed with the onset as late as 8 years of age.

In diagnosing this episodic recurrent disturbance of brain function, it is important to differentiate it from a seizure in which there is clinical evidence of uncontrolled paroxysmal neuronal discharge reflected in the animal's sensorium, behavior, and motor activity. In cataplexy there is complete atonia and absence of any discharge to muscles. Myasthenia gravis and hypoadrenocorticism may show progressive weakness and collapse, but will not occur so abruptly or will not spontaneously cease as rapidly as cataplexy. Edrophonium (Tensilon) testing can help confirm myasthenia gravis, and electrolyte studies (showing hyperkalemia) will help confirm hypoadrenocorticism. Similarly, hypoglycemia may produce episodes of ataxia, paresis, and collapse, but these signs will not occur and disappear abruptly and blood glucose levels should confirm or deny this diagnosis. Syncope from cardiac arrhythmias can be ruled out by careful cardiac examination including ECG.

The diagnosis of cataplexy can be substantiated by the clinical response of a severely affected patient to a single intravenous injection of imipramine (Tofranil) at 0.5 mg per kg. In a less frequently affected patient, the clinical signs may be provoked by feeding or by the administration of an anticholinesterase, physostigmine, at 0.05 to 0.1 mg per kg intravenously. These dogs should show a spontaneous attack in 5 to 15 minutes. Some dogs can be controlled with oral imipramine, a tricyclic antidepressant (0.5 to 1.0 mg per kg tid). Other drugs used include the stimulants methylphenidate (Ritalin, at 0.25 mg per kg bid or tid) and dextroamphetamine (Dexedrine, at 5 to 10 mg tid), or phenelzine (Nardil), which is a monoamine oxidase inhibitor. The optimum dose of drug to control cataplexy varies among individuals and must be established by the clinician for each patient. The doses provided here are only guidelines.

A disorder of rapid eye movement sleep, similar to a seizure disorder, was reported in a cat.[69] Violent episodes of motor activity were associated with this phase of the sleep cycle.

REFERENCES

1. Andersson, B., and Olson, S. E.: Epilepsy in a dog with extensive bilateral damage to the hippocampus. Acta Vet. Scand., 1:98, 1959.
2. Atkeson, F. W., Ibensen, A., and Eldrige, E.: Inheritance of an epileptic type character in Brown Swiss cattle. J. Hered., 35:45, 1944.
3. Audell, L., Jönsson, L., and Lannek, B.: Congenital porta-caval shunts in the dog. Zentralbl. Veterinaermed., 21:797, 1974.
4. Austad, R., and Bjerkas, E.: Eclampsia in the bitch. J. Small Anim. Pract., 17:793, 1976.
5. Averill, D. A., Jr.: Treatment of status epilepticus in dogs with diazepam sodium. J. Am. Vet. Med. Assoc., 156:432, 1970.
6. Averill, D. R.: Idiopathic epilepsy. In Andrews, E. J., Ward, B. C., and Altman, H. H. (eds.): Spontaneous Animal Models of Human Disease II. New York, Academic Press, 1979.
7. Babcock, D. A., Narver, E. L., Dement, W. C., and Mitler, M. M.: Effects of imipramine, chlorimipramine, and fluoxetine on cataplexy in dogs. Pharmacol. Biochem. Behav., 5:599, 1976.
8. Baker, T. L., Mitler, M. M. Foutz, A. S., and Dement, W. C.: Diagnosis and treatment of narcolepsy in animals. In Kirk, R. W. (ed.): Current Veterinary Therapy: Small Animal Practice VIII. Philadelphia, W. B. Saunders Co. in press.
9. Barker, J.: Epilepsy in the dog—A Comparative approach. J. Small Anim. Pract., 14:281, 1973.
10. Barlow, R. M., Linklater, K. A., and Young, G. B.: Familial convulsions and ataxia in Angus calves. Vet. Rec., 83:60, 1968.
11. Barlow, R. M.: Further observations on bovine familial convulsions and ataxia. Vet. Rec., 105:91, 1979.
12. Barrett, R. E.: Canine hepatic encephalopathy. In Kirk, R. W. (ed.): Current Veterinary Therapy: Small Animal Practice VII. Philadelphia, W. B. Saunders Co., 1980.
13. Barrett, R. E., de Lahunta, A., Roenigk, W. J., Hoffer, R. E., and Coons, F. H.: Five cases of congenital portacaval shunt in the dog. J. Small Anim. Pract., 17:71, 1976.
14. Barthold, S. W., Kaplan, B. J., and Schwartz, A.: Reversible dermal atrophy in a cat treated with phenytoin. Vet. Pathol., 17:469, 1980.
15. Beck, A. M., and Krook, L.: Canine insuloma. Two surgical cases with relapses. Cornell Vet., 55:330, 1965.
16. Berryman, F. V., and de Lahunta, A.: Astrocytoma in a dog causing convulsions. Cornell Vet., 65:212, 1975.
17. Biefelt, S. W., Redman, H. C., and McClellan, R. O.: Sire and sex-related differences in rates of epileptiform seizures in a purebred beagle dog colony. Am. J. Vet. Res., 32:2039, 1971.
18. Bjork, C. A.: Circulostatic cerebral hypoxic epilepsy. Vet. Med./Small Anim. Clin., 65:33, 1970.
19. Blauch, B. S., and Cash, W. C.: A brief review of narcolepsy with presentation of two cases of narcolepsy in dogs. J. Am. Anim. Hosp. Assoc., 11:467, 1975.
20. Bovee, K.: The uremic syndrome. J. Am. Anim. Hosp. Assoc., 12:189, 1976.
21. Branch, C. E., Beckett, S. D., and Robertson, B. T.: Spontaneous syncopal attacks in dogs: A method of documentation. J. Am. Anim. Hosp. Assoc., 13:673, 1977.
22. Breazile, J. E.: Convulsive disorders in dogs. In Kirk, R. W. (ed.): Current Veterinary Therapy IV. Philadelphia, W. B. Saunders Co., 1971.
23. Breitschweidt, E. B., Braezile, J. B., and Broadhurst, J. J.: Clinical and electroencephalographic findings associated with ten cases of suspected limbic epilepsy in the dog. J. Am. Anim. Hosp. Assoc., 15:37, 1979.
24. Breznock, E. M.: Surgical manipulation of portosystemic shunts in dogs. J. Am. Vet. Med. Assoc., 174:819, 1979.
25. Bunch, S. E.: Anticonvulsant drug therapy in companion animals. In Kirk, R. W. (ed.): Current Veterinary Therapy: Small Animal Practice VIII. Philadelphia, W. B. Saunders Co., in press.
26. Bunch, S. E., Castleman, W. L., Hornbuckle, W. E., and Tennant, B. C.: Hepatic cirrhosis in dogs associated with long-term anticonvulsant drug therapy in dogs. J. Am. Vet. Med. Assoc., 181:357, 1982.
27. Bush, B. M., and Fankhauser, R.: Polycythemia vera in a bitch. J. Small Anim. Pract., 13:75, 1972.
28. Capen, C. C., and Martin, S. L.: Hyperinsulinism in dogs with neoplasia of the pancreatic islets. Pathol. Vet., 6:309, 1969.
29. Cash, W. C., and Blauch, B. S.: Jaw snapping syndrome in eight dogs. J. Am. Vet. Med. Assoc., 175:709, 1979.
30. Caywood, D. D., Wilson, J. W., Hardy, R. M., and Shull, R. M.: Pancreatic islet cell adenocarcinoma: Clinical and diagnostic features of six cases. J. Am. Vet. Med. Assoc., 174:714, 1979.
31. Cello, R. M., and Kennedy, P. C.: Hyperinsulinism in dogs due to pancreatic islet cell carcinoma. Cornell Vet., 47:538, 1957.
32. Center, S. A., Bunch, S. E., Baldwin, B. H., and Hornbuckle, W.: Comparison of BSP and ICG clearance in the cat. Am. J. Vet. Res., in press, 1982.
33. Chrisman, C. L.: Postoperative results and complications of insulinomas in dogs. J. Am. Anim. Hosp. Assoc., 16:677, 1980.
34. Cornelius, L. M., Thrall, D. E., Halliwell, W. H., Frank, G. M., and Kern, A. J.: Anomalous portosystemic anastomoses associated with chronic hepatic insufficiency in six young dogs. J. Am. Vet. Med. Assoc., 167:220, 1975.
35. Croft, P. G.: Fits in dogs: A survey of 260 cases. Vet. Rec., 77:438, 1965.
36. Cunningham, C. G.: Canine seizure disorders. J. Am. Vet. Med. Assoc., 158:589, 1971.
37. Darke, P. G. G.: Narcolepsy in a dog. Vet. Rec., 101:177, 1977.

38. Davis, E. M., Glickman, L, Rendano, V. T. and Short, C. E.: Seizures in dogs following metrizamide myelography. J. Am. Anim. Hosp. Assoc., 17:641, 1981.

39. Delashaw, J. B., Foutz, A. S., Guilleminault, C., and Dement, W. C.: Cholinergic mechanisms and cataplexy in dogs. Exp. Neurol., 66:745, 1979.

40. DiBartola, S. P., and Reynolds, H. A.: Hypoglycemia and polyclonal gammopathy in a dog with plasma cell dyscrasia. J. Am. Vet. Med. Assoc., 180:1345, 1982.

41. Edmonds, H. L., Hegreberg, G. A., VanGelder, N. M., Sylvester, D. M., Clemmons, R. M., and Chatburn, C. G.: Spontaneous convulsions in Beagle dogs. Fed. Proc., 38:2424, 1979.

42. Elissalde, G. S., Woolridge, J. B., Steel, E. G., and Elissalde, M. H.: Treatment of a seizuring hypoparathyroid dog. Canine Pract., 7:14, 1980.

43. Ettinger, S.: Isoproterenol treatment of atrioventricular block in the dog. J. Am. Vet. Med. Assoc., 154:398, 1969.

44. Everett, G. M.: Observations on the behavior and neurophysiology of acute thiamine deficient cats. Am. J. Physiol., 141:439, 1944.

45. Ewing, G. O., Suter, P. F., and Bailey, C. S.: Hepatic insufficiency associated with congenital anomalies of the portal vein in dogs. J. Am. Anim. Hosp. Assoc., 10:463, 1974.

46. Fabisiak, J. P.: The role of cerebral free amino acids and taurine in the kindling models of epilepsy. M.S. Thesis, Cornell University, 1980.

47. Falco, M. J., Barker, J., and Wallace, M. E.: The genetics of epilepsy in the British Alsatian. J. Small Anim. Pract., 15:685, 1974.

48. Farrow, B. R. H.: Personal communication, 1982.

49. Faull, K., Foutz, A. S., Holman, R. B., Anderson, P. J., and Dement, W. C.: Assays of monamine metabolites in CSF samples from control and narcoleptic canines. In Proceedings of the Fourth International Catecholamine Symposium, 1978.

50. Fisher, E. W.: Fainting in boxers—the possibility of vaso-vagal syncope (Adams-Stokes attacks). J. Small Anim. Pract., 12:347, 1971.

51. Fisher, K.: Herdförmig symmetrische Hirngewebsnekrosen bei Hunden mit epileptiformen Krämpfen. Pathol. Vet., 1:133, 1964.

52. Foutz, A. S., Mitler, M. M., and Dement, W. C.: Narcolepsy. Vet. Clin. North Am.: Small Anim. Pract., 10:65, 1980.

53. Foutz, A. S., Mitler, M. M., Cavalli-Sforza, L. L., and Dement, W. C.: Genetic factors in canine narcolepsy. Sleep, 1:413, 1979.

54. Fox, M. W., and Stanton, G.: A developmental study of sleep and wakefulness in the dog. J. Small Anim. Pract., 8:605, 1967.

55. Frey, H. H., Gobel, W. and W. Löscher: Pharmacokinetics of primidone and its active metabolites in the dog. Arch. Int. de Pharmacodyne. 242:14, 1979.

56. Frey, H. H., and Löscher, W.: Clinical pharmacokinetics of phenytoin in the dog: A reevaluation. Am. J. Vet. Res., 41:1635, 1980.

57. Frey, H. H., and Löscher, W.: Pharmacokinetics of carbamazepine in the dog. Arch. Int. Pharmacodyne. Ther., 243:180, 1980.

58. Gastaut, H., Berard-Baider, M., Barraspen, M., and Van Bogaert, L.: Anatomical and clinical study of 19 epileptic dogs. In Baldwin, M., and Bailey, P. (eds.): Temporal Lobe Epilepsy. Springfield, Illinois, Charles C Thomas, 1958.

59. Gofton, H.: Surgical ligation of congenital portosystemic venous shunts in the dog: A report of three cases. J. Am. Anim. Hosp. Assoc., 14:728, 1978.

60. Gram, L., Flachs, H., Wurtz-Jorgensen, A., Painas, J., and Anderson, B.: Sodium valproate, serum level and clinical effect in epilepsy: A controlled study. Epilepsia, 20:303, 1979.

61. Grauer, G. F., and Thrall, M. A.: Ethylene glycol (antifreeze) poisoning in the dog and cat. J. Am. Anim. Hosp. Assoc., 18:492, 1982.

62. Greenblatt, D. J., and Shader, R. I.: Benzodiazepines. N. Engl. J. Med., 291:1011, 1239, 1974.

63. Griffiths, G. L., Lumsden, J. H., and Valli, V. E. O.: Hematologic and biochemical changes in dogs with portosystemic shunts. J. Am. Anim. Hosp. Assoc., 17:705, 1981.

64. Hamlin, R. L., Smetzer, D. L., and Breznock, E. M.: Sinoatrial syncope in miniature schnauzers. J. Am. Vet. Med. Assoc., 161:1022, 1972.

65. Hart, B. L.: Behavioral aspects of canine narcolepsy. Canine Pract., 2:8, 1975.

66. Haughey, K. G., and Jones, R. T.: Meningeal haemorrhage and congestion associated with the perinatal mortality of foals. Vet. Rec., 98:518, 1976.

67. Hegreberg, G. A., and Edmonds, H. L., Jr.: Familial progressive myoclonic epilepsy (Lafora's disease). In Andrews, E. J., Ward, B. C., and Altman, H. H. (eds.): Spontaneous Animal Models of Human Disease II. New York, Academic Press, 1976.

68. Hegreberg, G. A., and Padgett, G. A.: Inherited progressive epilepsy of the dog with comparisons to Lafora's disease of man. Fed. Proc., 35:1202, 1976.

69. Hendricks, J., Morrison, A. R., Farnbach, G. L., Steinberg, S. A., and Mann, G.: A disorder of rapid eye movement sleep in a cat. J. Am. Vet. Med. Assoc., 178:55, 1981.

70. Hendricks, J. C., and Morrison, A. R.: Normal and abnormal sleep in mammals. J. Am. Vet. Med. Assoc., 178:121, 1981.

71. Henley, K., and Morrison, A. R.: A reevaluation of the effects of lesions of the pontine tegmentum and locus coeruleus on phenomena of paradoxical sleep in the cat. Acta Neurobiol. Exp., 34:215, 1974.

72. Hjerpe, C. A.: Serum hepatitis in the horse. J. Am. Vet. Med. Assoc., 144:734, 1964.

73. Holliday, T. A.: Clinical aspects of some encephalopathies of domestic cats. Vet. Clin. North Am., 1:367, 1971.

74. Holliday, T. A.: Epilepsy in cats. Mod. Vet. Pract., 51:14, 1970.

75. Holliday, T. A.: Seizure disorders. Vet. Clin. North Am., 10:3, 1980.

76. Holliday, T. A., Cunningham, J. G., and Gutnich, M. J.: Comparative clinical and electroencephalographic studies on canine epilepsy. Epilepsia, 11:281, 1970.

77. Irvine, C. H. G.: Hypoglycemia in the bitch. N. Z. Vet. J., 12:140, 1964.

78. Jackson, R. F., Bruss, M. L., Growney, P. J., and Seymour, W. G.: Hypoglycemia-ketonemia in a pregnant bitch. J. Am. Vet. Med. Assoc., 177:1123, 1980.

79. Jennings, P. B., Utter, W. F., and Fariss, B. L.: Effects of long-term primidone therapy in a dog. J. Am. Vet. Med. Assoc., 164:1123, 1974.

80. Johnson, J. T.: Tonic seizures in a dog. J. Am. Vet. Med. Assoc., 159:427, 1971.

81. Jones, B. F.: Elimination of paradoxical sleep by

lesions of the pontine gigantocellular tegmental field in the cat. Neurosci. Lett., *13*:385, 1979.

82. Jouvet, M.: The states of sleep. Sci. Am., *216*:62, 1967.

83. Katherman, A. E.: A comparative review of canine and human narcolepsy. Compend. Contin. Ed., *2*:818, 1980.

84. Kay, W.: Epilepsy. In Kirk, R. W. (ed.): Current Veterinary Therapy V. Small Animal Practice. Philadelphia, W. B. Saunders Co., 1974.

85. Kay, W. J.: Epilepsy. Proc. Am. Anim. Hosp. Assoc., *40*:402, 1973.

86. Kay, W. J.: Epilepsy in cats. J. Am. Anim. Hosp. Assoc., *11*:77, 1975.

87. Kirk, G. R., Breazile, J. E., and Kenney, A. D.: Pathogenesis of hypocalcemic tetany in the thyro-parathyroidectomized dog. Am. J. Vet. Res., *35*:407, 1974.

88. Kirk, R. W.: Hypoglycemia. In Kirk, R. W. (ed.): Current Veterinary Therapy III. Philadelphia, W. B. Saunders Co., 1968.

89. Knecht, C. D., Oliver, J., Reading, R., Selcer, R., and Johnson, G.: Narcolepsy in a dog and cat. J. Am. Vet. Med. Assoc., *162*:1052, 1973.

90. Kornegay, J. N., Greene, C. E., Martin, C., Gongacz, E. J., and Melcon, D. K.: Idiopathic hypocalcemia in four dogs. J. Am. Anim. Hosp. Assoc., *16*:723, 1980.

91. Krook, L., and Kenney, R. M.: CNS lesions in dogs with metastasizing islet cell carcinoma. Cornell Vet., *52*:358, 1962.

92. Lefebvre, E. B., Haining, R. G., and Labbe, R. F.: Coarse facies, calvarial thickening, and hyper-phosphatasia associated with long-term anticonvulsant therapy. N. Engl. J. Med., *286*:1301, 1972.

93. Legendre, A. M., Appleford, M. D., Eyster, G. E., and Dade, A. W.: Secondary polycythemia and seizures due to right to left shunting patent ductus arteriosus in a dog. J. Am. Vet. Med. Assoc., *164*:1198, 1974.

94. Löscher, W.: Plasma levels of valproic acid and its metabolites during continued treatment in dogs. J. Vet. Pharmacol. Therap., *4*:111, 1981.

95. Lucas, E. A., Foutz, A. S., Dement, W. C., and Mitler, M. M.: Sleep cycle organization in narcoleptic and normal dogs. Physiol. Behav., *23*:737, 1979.

96. Mahaffey, L. W., and Rossdale, P. D.: Convulsive syndrome in newborn foals. Vet. Rec., *69*:1277, 1957.

97. Marretta, S. M., Pask, A. J., Greene, R. W., and Liu, S.-K.: Urinary calculi associated with porta-systemic shunts in six dogs. J. Am. Vet. Med. Assoc., *178*:133, 1981.

98. Mattheeuws, D., Rottiers, R., De Rijcke, J., De Rick, A., and De Schepper, J.: Hyperinsulinism in the dog due to pancreatic islet cell tumor: A report on three cases. J. Small Anim. Pract., *7*:313, 1976.

99. Mayhew, I. G.: Personal communication, 1982.

100. Maynert, E. W.: The metabolic fate of dyphenylhydantoin in the dog, rat, and man. J. Pharmacol. Exp. Ther., *130*:275, 1960.

101. McGrath, C. J.: Polycythemia vera in dogs. J. Am. Vet. Med. Assoc., *164*:1117, 1974.

102. Meierhenry, E. F., and Liu, S.-K.: Atrioventricular bundle degeneration associated with sudden death in the dog. J. Am. Vet. Med. Assoc., *172*:1418, 1978.

103. Meyer, D. J.: Primary hypoparathyroidism. In Kirk, R. W. (ed.): Current Veterinary Therapy VII.

104. Meyer, D. J., and Noonan, N. E.: Liver tests in dogs receiving anticonvulsant drugs (diphenylhydantoin and primidone). J. Am. Anim. Hosp. Assoc., *17*:261, 1981.

105. Meyer, D. J., Strombeck, D. R., Stone, E. A., Zenoble, R. D., and Buss, D. D.: Ammonia tolerance test in clinically normal dogs and in dogs with portosystemic shunts. J. Am. Vet. Med. Assoc., *173*:377, 1978.

106. Millichap, J. G.: Drug treatment of convulsive disorders. N. Engl. J. Med., *286*:464, 1972.

107. Mitler, M. M., and Foutz, A.: The diagnosis and treatment of narcolepsy in animals. In Kirk, R. W. (ed.): Current Veterinary Therapy VII. Small Animal Practice. Philadelphia, W. B. Saunders Co., 1980.

108. Mitler, M. M., and Dement, W. C.: Sleep studies on canine narcolepsy: Pattern and cycle comparisons between affected and normal dogs. Electroencephalogr. Clin. Neurophysiol., *43*:691, 1977.

109. Mitler, M. M., and Dement, W. C.: Narcolepsy. In Andrews, E., Ward, B., and Altman, N. (eds.): Spontaneous Animal Models of Human Disease. Vol. 2. New York, Academic Press, 1979.

110. Mitler, M. M., Boysen, B. G., Campbell, L., and Dement, W. C.: Narcolepsy—cataplexy in a female dog. Exp. Neurol., *45*:332, 1974.

111. Mitler, M. M., Stowe, O., and Dement, W. C.: Narcolepsy in seven dogs. J. Am. Vet. Med. Assoc., *168*:1036, 1976.

112. Nafe, L. A., Parker, A., and Kay, W. J.: Sodium valproate: A preliminary clinical trial in epileptic dogs. J. Am. Anim. Hosp. Assoc., *17*:131, 1981.

113. Nash, A. S., Thompson, H., and Bogan, J. A.: Phenytoin toxicity: A fatal case in a dog with hepatitis and jaundice. Vet. Rec., *100*:280, 1977.

114. Njoku, C. O., Strafuss, A. C., and Dennis, S. M.: Canine islet cell neoplasia: A review. J. Am. Anim. Hosp. Assoc., *8*:284, 1972.

115. Oliver, J. E.: Hepatic neuropathies—a review. Vet. Med./Sm. Anim. Clin., *60*:498, 1965.

116. Oliver, J. E.: Surgical relief of epileptiform seizures in the dog. Vet. Med./Sm. Anim. Clin., *60*:367, 1965.

117. Oliver, J. E.: Seizure disorders in companion animals. Compend. Contin. Ed., *2*:77, 1980.

118. Oliver, J. E., and Hoerlein, B. F.: Convulsive disorders of dogs. J. Am. Vet. Med. Assoc., *146*:1126, 1965.

119. Palmer, A. C.: Clinical signs associated with intracranial tumors in dogs. Res. Vet. Sci., *2*:326, 1961.

120. Palmer, A. C.: Pathological changes in the brain associated with fits in dogs. Vet. Rec., *90*:167, 1972.

121. Palmer, A. C., and Rossdale, P. D.: Neuropathology of the convulsive foal syndrome. J. Reprod. Fertil. [Suppl.], *23*:691, 1975.

122. Palmer, A. C., Malinowski, W., and Barnett, K. C.: Clinical signs including papilloedema associated with brain tumours in twenty-one dogs. J. Small Anim. Pract., *15*:359, 1975.

123. Palmer, A. C., Smith, G. F., and Turner, S. J.: Cataplexy in a Guernsey bull. Vet. Rec., *106*:421, 1980.

124. Parker, A. J.: Canine epileptic convulsions: Treatment. Illinois Vet., *16*(4):5, 1973.

125. Parker, A. J.: Epilepsy in the dog. Illinois Vet., *16*(3):5, 1973.

126. Parker, A. J.: A preliminary report on a new anti-

epileptic medication for dogs. J. Am. Anim. Hosp. Assoc., *11*:437, 1975.

127. Parker, A. J.: Treatment of feline and canine seizure disorders. *In* Kirk, R. W. (ed.): Current Veterinary Therapy VII. Small Animal Practice. Philadelphia, W. B. Saunders Co., 1980.

128. Parker, A. J., and Cunningham, J. G.: Successful surgical removal of an epileptogenic focus in a dog. J. Small Anim. Pract., *12*:513, 1971.

129. Parker, A. J., O'Brien, D., and Musselman, E. E.: Diazoxide treatment of metastatic insulinoma in a dog. J. Am. Anim. Hosp. Assoc., *18*:315, 1982.

130. Parker, W. A., and Shearer, C. A.: Phenytoin hepatotoxicity: A case report and review. Neurology, *29*:175, 1979.

131. Parry, H. B.: Epileptic states in the dog with special reference to canine hysteria. Vet. Rec., *61*:23, 1949.

132. Pasten, L. J.: Diphenylhydantoin in the canine: Clinical aspects and determination of therapeutic blood levels. J. Am. Anim. Hosp. Assoc., *13*:247, 1977.

133. Pedersoli, W. M., Redding, R. W., and Nachreiner, R. F.: Blood serum concentrations of orally administered diphenylhydantoin in dogs and pharmacokinetic values after an intravenous injection. J. Am. Anim. Hosp. Assoc., *17*:271, 1981.

134. Pellegrini, A., Gloor, P., and Sherwin, A. L.: Effect of valproate sodium on generalized penicillin epilepsy in the cat. Epilepsia, *19*:351, 1978.

135. Penry, J. H., and Porter, R. J.: Epilepsy: Mechanisms and therapy. Med. Clin. North Am., *63*:801, 1979.

136. Plechner, A. J., and Shannon, M.: Food-induced hypersensitivity. Mod. Vet. Pract., *58*:225, 1977.

137. Prince, D. A.: Neurophysiology of epilepsy. Annu. Rev. Neurosci., *1*:395, 1978.

138. Prynn, R. B.: Medical management of the epileptic patient. J. Am. Anim. Hosp. Assoc., *11*:435, 1975.

139. Raskin, N. H., and Fishman, R. H.: Neurologic disorders in renal failure. N. Engl. J. Med., *294*:143, 1976.

140. Redding, R. W., and Prynn, R. B.: Seizures. *In* Kirk, R. W. (ed.): Current Veterinary Therapy. III. Philadelphia, W. B. Saunders Co., 1968.

141. Redenbaugh, J. E., Sato, S., Penry, J. K., Dreifuss, F. E., and Kipferberg, H. J.: Sodium valproate: Pharmacokinetics and effectiveness in treating intractable seizures. Neurology, *30*:1, 1980.

142. Resnick, S.: Hypocalcemia and tetany in the dog. Vet. Med./Sm. Anim. Clin., *67*:637, 1972.

143. Robertson, B. T., and Giles, H.: Complete heart block associated with vegetative endocarditis in a dog. J. Am. Vet. Med. Assoc., *161*:180, 1972.

144. Rogers, W. A., Donovan, E. F., and Kociba, G. J.: Idiopathic hyperlipoproteinemia in dogs. J. Am. Vet. Med. Assoc., *166*:1087, 1975.

145. Rogers, W. A., Donovan, E. F., and Kociba, G. J.: Idiopathic hyperlipoproteinemia in dogs. J. Am. Vet. Med. Assoc., *166*:1087, 1975.

146. Ross, M., Lowe, J. M., Cooper, B. J., Reimers, T., and Froscher, B.: Hypoglycemic seizures in a Shetland pony: A new clinical syndrome. Cornell Vet., in press.

147. Rossdale, P. D.: Modern concepts of neonatal disease in foals. Equine Vet. J., *4*:1, 1972.

148. Rossdale, P. D.: Pulmonary function in the newborn foal. Proc. Am. Assoc. Equine Pract., *18*:69, 1972.

149. Roye, D. B., Serrano, E. E., Hammer, R. H., and Wilder, B. J.: Diphenylhydantoin in dogs and cats. Am. J. Vet. Res., *34*:947, 1973.

150. Russo, M. E.: The pathophysiology of epilepsy. Cornell Vet., *71*:221, 1981.

151. Sakai, K., Sastre, J. P., Salvert, D., Touret, M., Toyhama, M., and Jouvet, M.: Tegmentoreticular projections with special reference to the muscular atonia during paradoxical sleep in the cat: An HRP study. Brain Res., *176*:233, 1979.

152. Sanders, J. E., and Yeary, R. A.: Serum concentrations of orally administered diphenylhydantoin in dogs. J. Am. Vet. Med. Assoc., *172*:153, 1978.

153. Sanders, J. E., Yeary, R. A., Fenner, W. R., and Powers, J. D.: Interaction of phenytoin with chloramphenicol or pentobarbitol in the dog. J. Am. Vet. Med. Assoc., *175*:177, 1979.

154. Sanders, J. E., Yeary, R. A., Powers, J. D., and deWet, P.: Relationship between serum and brain concentrations of phenytoin in the dog. Am. J. Vet. Res., *40*:473, 1979.

155. Schenker, S., Breen, K. J., and Hoyumpa, A. M.: Hepatic encephalopathy: Current status. Gastroenterology, *66*:121, 1974.

156. Sheading, R. G., Meuten, D. J., Chew, D. J., Knaack, K. E., and Houpt, K. H.: Primary hypoparathyroidism in the dog. J. Am. Vet. Med. Assoc., *176*:439, 1980.

157. Sheather, A. L.: Fainting in foals. J. Comp. Pathol. Ther., *37*:106, 1924.

158. Sheather, A. L.: Fainting in foals. J. Comp. Pathol. Ther., *37*:106, 1924.

159. Sherding, R. G.: Hepatic encephalopathy in the dog. Compend. Contin. Ed., *1*:55, 1979.

160. Skinner, S. F., Robertson, L. T., Artero, M., and Gerding, R. K.: Longitudinal study of phenobarbital in serum, cerebrospinal fluid, and saliva in the dog. Am. J. Vet. Res., *141*:600, 1980.

161. Spehlmann, R., and Colley, B.: The effect of diazepam (Valium) on experimental seizures in unanesthetized cats. Neurology, *18*:52, 1968.

162. Starzl, T. E., Porter, K. E., Watanabe, K., and Putnam, C. W.: Effects of insulin, glucagon, and insulin/glucagon infusions on linear morphology and cell division after complete portacaval shunt in dogs. Lancet, *1*:821, 1976.

163. Steinberg, S. H.: Insulin-secreting pancreatic tumors in the dog. J. Am. Anim. Hosp. Assoc., *16*:695, 1980.

164. Strafuss, A. C., Njoku, C. O., Blauch, B., and Anderson, N. V.: Islet cell neoplasm in four dogs. J. Am. Vet. Med. Assoc., *159*:1008, 1971.

165. Strombeck, D. R., and Rogers, Q.: Plasma amino acid concentrations in dogs with hepatic disease. J. Am. Vet. Med. Assoc., *173*:93, 1978.

166. Strombeck, D. R., Breznock, E. M., and McNell, S.: Surgical treatment for portosystemic shunts in two dogs. J. Am. Vet. Med. Assoc., *170*:1317, 1977.

167. Strombeck, D. R., Krums, S., Meyer, D. and Koppesser, R. M.: Hypoglycemia and hypoinsulinemia associated with hepatoma in a dog. J. Am. Vet. Med. Assoc., *169*:811, 1976.

168. Strombeck, D. R., Meyer, D. J., and Freedland, R. A.: Hyperammonemia due to urea cycle enzyme deficiency in two dogs. J. Am. Vet. Med. Assoc., *166*:1109, 1975.

169. Strombeck, D. R., Rogers, Q., Freedland, R., and McEwan, L. C.: Fasting hypoglycemia in a pup. J. Am. Vet. Med. Assoc., *173*:299, 1978.

170. Strombeck, D. R., Weiser, M. G., and Kaneko, J. J.: Hyperammonemia and hepatic encephalopathy in the dog. J. Am. Vet. Med. Assoc., *166*:1105, 1975.
171. Sturtevant, F., Hoffmann, W. E., and Dorner, J. L.: The effect of three anticonvulsant drugs and ACTH on canine serum alkaline phosphatase. J. Am. Anim. Hosp. Assoc., *13*:754, 1977.
172. Suter, P. F.: Portal vein anomalies in the dog: Their angiographic diagnosis. J. Am. Vet. Radiol. Soc., *16*:84, 1975.
173. Tobin, T., Dirdjosudjono, S., and Baskin, S. I.: Pharmacokinetics and distribution of diphenylhydantoin in kittens. Am. J. Vet. Res., *34*:951, 1973.
174. Tobin, T., Dirdjosudjono, S., and Baskin, S. I.: Pharmacokinetics and distribution of diphenylhydantoin in kittens. Am. J. Vet. Res., *34*:951, 1973.
175. Tyler, H. R.: Neurologic disorders in renal failure. Am. J. Med., *44*:734, 1968.
176. Tyler, H. R.: Neurologic disorders in renal failure. Am. J. Med., *44*:734, 1968.
177. Van der Velden, N. A.: Fits in Tervuren shepherd dogs: A presumed hereditary trait. J. Small Anim. Pract., *9*:63, 1968.
178. Vandevelde, M., and Braund, K. G.: Polioencephalomyelitis in cats. Vet. Pathol., *16*:420, 1979.
179. Vitums, A.: Portosystemic communications in animals with hepatic cirrhosis and malignant lymphoma. J. Am. Vet. Med. Assoc., *138*:31, 1961.
180. Vitums, A.: Portosystemic communications in the dog. Acta Anat., *39*:271, 1959.
181. Vulgamott, J. C., Turnwald, G. H., Hong, G. K., Herring, D. S., Hensen, J. F., and Boothe, H. W., Jr.: Congenital portacaval anomalies in the cat: Two case reports. J. Am. Anim. Hosp. Assoc., *16*:915, 1980.
182. Wallace, M. E.: Keeshonds: A genetic study of epilepsy and EEG readings. J. Small Anim. Pract., *16*:1, 1975.
183. Wauquer, A., Ashton, D., and Melis, W.: Behavioral analysis of amygdaloid kindling in beagle dogs and the effects of clonazepam, diazepam, phenobarbital, diphenylhydantoin, and flunarizone on seizure manifestation. Exp. Neurol., *64*:579, 1979.
184. Wilson, J. W., and Caywood, D. D.: Functional tumors of the pancreatic beta cells. Compend. Contin. Ed., *3*:458, 1981.
185. Wilson, J. W., and Hulse, D. A.: Surgical correction of islet cell adenocarcinoma in a dog. J. Am. Vet. Med. Assoc., *164*:603, 1974.
186. Wolf, A. M.: Canine uremic encephalopathy. J. Am. Anim. Hosp. Assoc., *16*:735, 1980.
187. Yeary, R. A.: Serum concentration of primidone and its metabolites phenylethylmalonamide and phenobarbital in the dog. Am. J. Vet. Res., *41*:1643, 1980.
188. Zieve, L.: Pathogenesis of hepatic coma. Arch. Int. Med., *118*:211, 1966.
189. Zook, B. C., Carpenter, J. L., and Leeds, E. B.: Lead poisoning in dogs. J. Am. Vet. Med. Assoc., *155*:1329, 1969.
190. Schwartz-Porsche, D., Löscher, W., and Frey, H.-H.: Treatment of canine epilepsy with primidone. J. Am. Vet. Med. Assoc., *181*:592, 1982.

Chapter

19   DIENCEPHALON

The diencephalon consists of four general regions, bilaterally symmetric on each side of the median third ventricle (Fig. 19–1):[46–48] the epithalamus—including the habenula, the pineal body, and the stria habenularis thalamus; the thalamus (dorsal thalamus)—the main mass of the organ between the epithalamus and the hypothalamus; the hypothalamus—the ventral and lateral walls of the third ventricle, below the interthalamic adhesion; and subthalamus (ventral thalamus)—lateral and caudal to the hypothalamus, continuous with the mesencephalic tegmentum, and includes the subthalamic nucleus, the endopeduncular nucleus, and the zona incerta. This chapter deals primarily with the major components: the thalamus and the hypothalamus. The epithalamus was considered with the limbic system, and the subthalamus with the extrapyramidal system.

THALAMUS

ANATOMY[49, 56]

The thalamus (dorsal thalamus) is related to the hypothalamus ventrally, and to the internal capsule and caudate nucleus laterally and dor-

sally (Fig. 19–1, Plates 14, 15). It is composed of numerous nuclear masses, partly separated by sheets of myelinated axons, called medullary laminae. These nuclei and laminae are represented bilaterally on either side of the third ventricle. In the following discussion, reference will be made to one side. Keep in mind that this is a bilateral structure, similar to the rest of the nervous system, and that there are two thalami and two hypothalami. The internal medullary lamina divides the thalamus on each side into medial and lateral halves, and splits rostrally to enclose a rostral portion, which includes the rostral thalamic nuclei (Fig. 19–2). The lateral half may be subdivided into its nuclei by dividing it into a dorsal and ventral tier by a dorsal plane. The ventral tier produced by this subdivision can be separated further into three nuclear groups from rostral to caudal by two transverse planes. The thin, external medullary lamina forms the external boundary of the lateral half of the thalamus and is separated from the internal capsule by a narrow nuclear mass, the thalamic reticular nucleus. As a result of these divisions, the following nuclear groups and some examples of their specific nuclei may be listed.[10]

1. Rostral thalamic group—rostral thalamic nucleus (limbic system).

2. Medial thalamic group—medial dorsal nucleus.

3. Lateral thalamic group:
    Dorsal tier—dorsolateral nucleus, caudolateral nucleus, pulvinar.
    Ventral tier—ventral rostral nucleus (extrapyramidal), ventral lateral nucleus (cerebellar), ventral caudal group: ventral caudal medial nucleus (cranial nerve sensory relay), ventral caudal lateral nucleus (spinal nerve sensory relay).

4. Caudal thalamic group—medial geniculate nucleus (auditory), lateral geniculate nucleus (vision).

5. Intralaminar—midline thalamic group: central medial nucleus, paraventricular nucleus.

6. Thalamic reticular nucleus (ARAS).

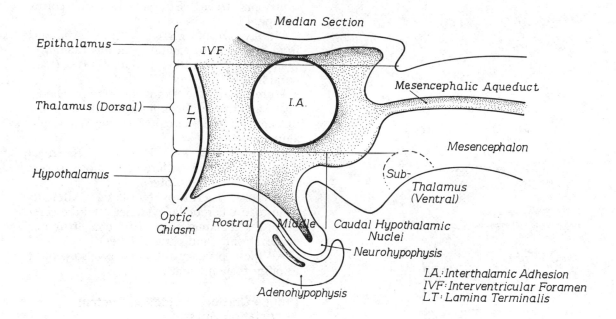

Median Section

Epithalamus

IVF

Thalamus (Dorsal)

L T

I.A.

Mesencephalic Aqueduct

Mesencephalon

Hypothalamus

Sub-
Thalamus
(Ventral)

Optic
Chiasm

Rostral   Middle

Caudal Hypothalamic
Nuclei

Neurohypophysis

Adenohypophysis

I.A.: Interthalamic Adhesion
IVF: Interventricular Foramen
LT: Lamina Terminalis

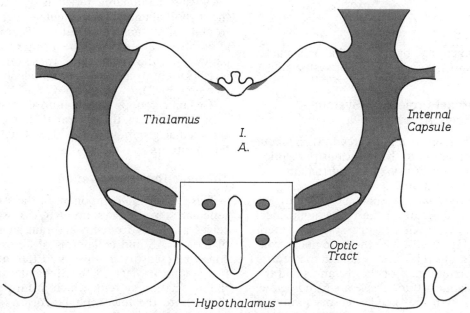

Transverse Section Through Optic Tracts and Internal Capsule

Thalamus

I.
A.

Internal
Capsule

Optic
Tract

Hypothalamus

Figure 19–1. Divisions of the diencephalon.

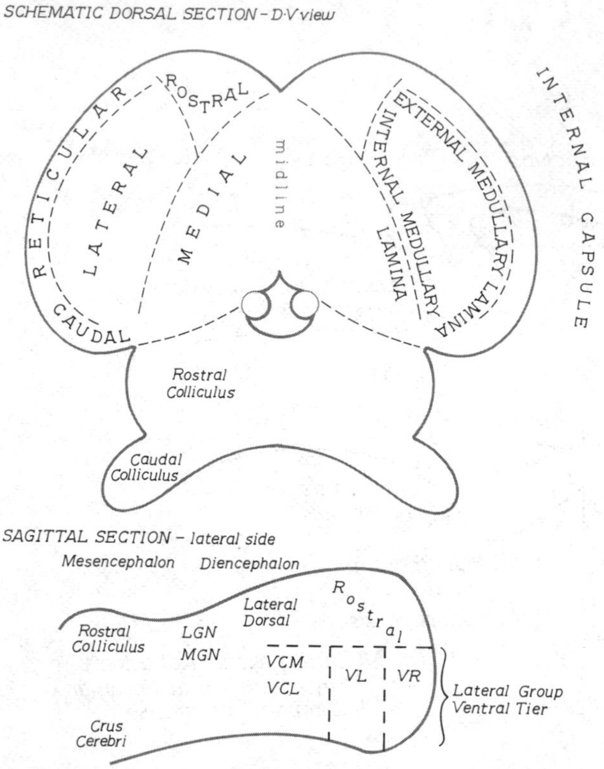

SCHEMATIC DORSAL SECTION – D·V view

SAGITTAL SECTION – lateral side

Figure 19–2. Thalamic nuclear groups. VR, Ventral rostral; VL, ventral lateral; VCM, ventrocaudal medial; VCL, ventrocaudal lateral; LGN, lateral geniculate nucleus; MGN, medial geniculate nucleus.

FUNCTION

On a functional basis, the thalamic nuclei can be grouped into three major systems.

Direct Cortical Projection System— Primary Relay Areas

This system has been referred to throughout the text in relation to the conscious perception pathways of sensory systems and thalamic relays of motor systems.

Sensory System. A thalamic relay to the telencephalon occurs in the conscious projection pathway of all sensory systems except olfaction (Fig. 19–3). The thalamic nuclei concerned with this relay are located in the ventral tier of the lateral half of the thalamus and the caudal thalamic group. These are listed below, with a review of the specific sensory pathways afferent to them and the general area of the telencephalon to which each nucleus projects:

VENTRAL CAUDAL LATERAL NUCLEUS. Afferents from spinothalamic tracts (GSA, GVA), medial lemniscus (GP). Efferents to somesthetic cortex (trunk and limbs).

VENTRAL CAUDAL MEDIAL NUCLEUS.

Afferents from quintothalamic tract (GSA, GP), solitariothalamic tract (GVA, SVA). Efferents to somesthetic cortex (head).

LATERAL GENICULATE NUCLEUS. Afferents from optic tract.[15] Efferents to visual cortex (occipital lobe).

MEDIAL GENICULATE NUCLEUS. Afferents from brachium of caudal colliculus (auditory, vestibular). Efferents to auditory cortex (temporal lobe).

Motor System. Axons of extrapyramidal nuclei and the cerebellum have synapses in the thalamus in their circuitry to the telencephalon.

VENTRAL ROSTRAL NUCLEUS. Afferents from the pallidum. Efferents to motor cortex (frontal and parietal lobes).

VENTRAL LATERAL NUCLEUS. Afferents from rostral cerebellar peduncle and the cerebellorubrothalamic tract. Efferents to motor cortex (frontal and parietal lobes).

All these primary relay nuclei also project to other thalamic nuclei.

Diffuse Cortical Projection System— Association System

These thalamic nuclei receive axons only from other diencephalic and telencephalic sources, such as the primary relay thalamic nuclei and the thalamic reticular system nuclei, the hypothalamus, the cingulate gyrus, the frontal cortex, and the striatum. There are no afferents received from the primary afferent pathways in the brain stem. These nuclei project diffusely to all parts of the telencephalon (see Fig. 19–3).

Thalamic groups that comprise this system include nuclei in the rostral thalamic group, the medial group, and the dorsal tier of the lateral group.

Thalamic Reticular System

This system is a component of the ascending reticular activating system (ARAS), which receives afferents from lower brain stem levels of the ARAS and collaterals of all ascending conscious sensory pathways. Efferents from this system project to the thalamic nuclei of the association system, which in turn projects diffusely to the telencephalic cortex (see Fig. 19–3).

Thalamic groups composing the thalamic reticular system include nuclei in the intralaminar (midline) and reticular groups.

Experimental evidence for the efferent pathways and functions of these systems comes from the following:

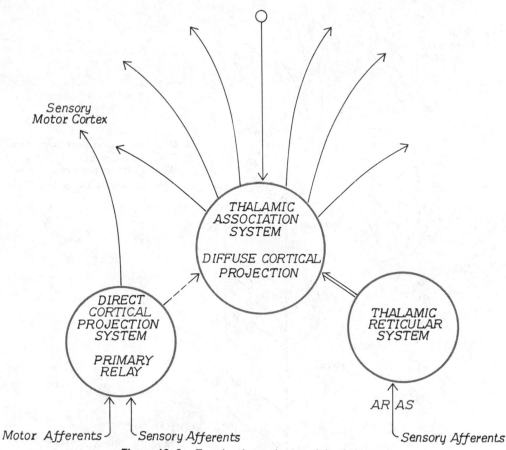

Figure 19–3. Functional organization of the thalamus.

1. If the cortex of the telencephalon is removed, retrograde degeneration occurs in those thalamic nuclei that project to the cortex.[38, 40] Such degeneration occurred in the first two systems described (direct cortical projection, diffuse cortical projection) and not in the third system (thalamic reticular).

2. Mild electrical stimulation of nuclei in the direct cortical projection system produces activity only in specific areas of the telencephalic cortex, those to which these nuclei project. Stimulation of any one of the nuclei in the thalamic reticular system produces a slow, spreading, diffuse activity of the entire telencephalic cortex. This is mediated by the nuclei of the thalamic association system.

ASCENDING RETICULAR ACTIVATING SYSTEM (ARAS)

The ARAS is part of the reticular formation, which consists of a network of neurons in the central portion or core of the brain stem from the medulla, through the pons and midbrain, into the diencephalon.[21, 22, 33]

The ARAS receives afferents from all conscious projection pathways of the sensory systems—exteroception, interoception, and proprioception. As these conscious sensory pathways (spinal and cranial) ascend through the brain stem to the primary relay nuclei in the thalamus, collaterals are given off into the reticular formation (Fig. 19–4).

Most of these collaterals synapse in the reticular formation. Neurons of the ARAS then continue the impulse flow rostrally, in a multisynaptic pattern to one of two areas in the diencephalon: the thalamic reticular or hyposubthalamic reticular system. A few collaterals ascend through the ARAS without synaptic interruption to terminate in one of these two diencephalic areas.

The diencephalic portion of the ARAS stimulates the entire cerebral cortex diffusely. The thalamic reticular system affects the cerebral

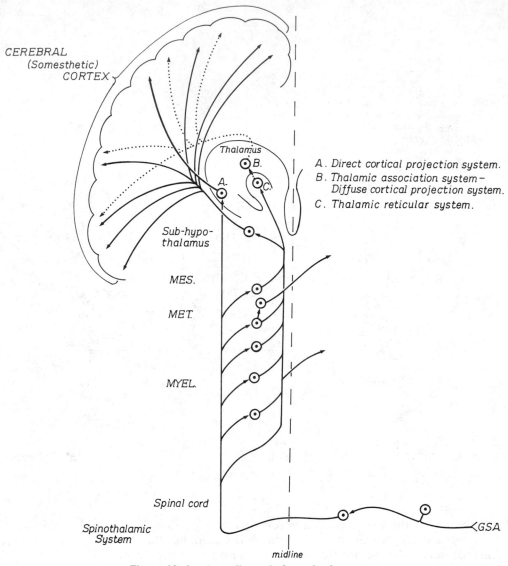

CEREBRAL
(Somesthetic)
CORTEX

Thalamus
B.
A.
C.

A. Direct cortical projection system.
B. Thalamic association system –
   Diffuse cortical projection system.
C. Thalamic reticular system.

Sub-hypo-
thalamus

MES.

MET.

MYEL.

Spinal cord

Spinothalamic
System

GSA

midline

Figure 19–4. Ascending reticular activating system.

cortex by way of the diffuse telencephalic connections of the nuclei of the association system.

The ARAS functions to "arouse" the cerebral cortex, to awaken the brain to consciousness, to prepare the cortex to receive ascending impulses from any sensory modality. It is responsible for maintaining wakefulness. Decreased activity of the ARAS is associated with sleep. Sleep, a highly complex mechanism, is mediated through centers near the midline of the pons and medulla. These centers influence the activity of the ARAS.

Stimulation of dorsal roots, somesthetic tracts, or any part of the ARAS of the sleeping animal arouses it to the awake state. This can

be observed in the animal as well as on its electroencephalogram. This does not occur with stimulation of a primary relay nucleus in the thalamus. In that case, only the specific projection area of the cerebral cortex shows activity. Conversely, lesions that destroy the ARAS cause a comatose state.

The ARAS is thought to be the seat of consciousness. Both central nervous system depressants and stimulants function on the ARAS. The ARAS may be responsible for the ability to focus attention on particular sources of stimuli, rejecting all others. Thus it monitors the myriad of stimuli that ascend to thalamic levels, accepting what is needed for conscious perception and rejecting what is irrelevant.

Disturbances of consciousness can result from lesions that affect the neuronal activity of the ARAS in the brain stem or the neuronal activity of the cerebral cortex. Intracranial injury can produce stupor-semicoma from diffuse cerebral edema or from contusion and hemorrhage in the midbrain and pons of the brain stem. If the semicomatose patient with an intracranial injury has evidence of voluntary limb movements, normal vestibular movements of the eyeballs upon manipulation of the head, no cranial nerve deficits referable to a brain stem lesion, and pupils that may be asymmetric or miotic but respond to light, then the semicoma is probably more due to cerebrocortical dysfunction. The prognosis is guarded, but more favorable than for the patient who is semicomatose with clinical evidence of a brain stem lesion that is interfering with the function of the reticular formation in the ARAS.

Summary of Thalamic Function

1. The thalamus is the chief sensory-integrating system of the neuraxis. It functions in the integration and relay of all types of sensory and motor pathways between lower and higher centers.

2. It may serve as the site of conscious perception of some sensory modalities. This is most evident after a lesion destroys the somesthetic cerebral cortex and the perception of some modalities is preserved.

3. It functions in the ARAS as part of the mechanism for maintaining consciousness, for producing a state of attention, or for producing sleep.

CLINICAL SIGNS

Focal thalamic lesions in domestic animals are rare and would be difficult to localize. Involvement of the direct cortical projection pathways could produce variable degrees of deficits in those systems, such as: lateral geniculate nucleus—contralateral hemianopsia; ventral caudal lateral nucleus—contralateral proprioceptive deficit and hypalgesia; ventral rostral and lateral nuclei—contralateral dysmetria.

Lesions in the limbic system nuclei or tracts result in behavioral changes. Lesions in the thalamic reticular system nuclei result in disturbances of consciousness (depression, semicoma) or seizures. Rostral thalamic lesions may cause leaning, head turning, propulsive

circling, or ocular deviation toward the side of the lesion—the adversive syndrome. Animals with thalamic lesions occasionally act as if they were experiencing pain.

CLINICAL EVALUATION OF THE UNCONSCIOUS ANIMAL

Clinical evaluation of the emergency unconscious patient requires a systematic approach, because the time available for appropriate diagnostic and therapeutic decisions may be brief.[18, 41-43]

Decrease in the level of consciousness can occur from either a diffuse or widespread multifocal lesion of both cerebrums, or a lesion affecting the ARAS of the rostral brain stem. Except for traumatic lesions with bilateral cerebral edema and the various diseases that produce diffuse polioencephalomalacia in animals, acute organic diseases that destroy both cerebral hemispheres are rare.

In both of these conditions, although the primary lesions are cerebrocortical in location, the brain stem will be affected by the brain edema, increased intracranial pressure, or metabolic encephalopathy to contribute to the comatose state. It is unlikely that a lesion confined to the cerebral cortex will produce coma. Most coma results from brain stem lesions.

The pathophysiologic causes of coma can be grouped into four categories: (1) bilateral diffuse, primarily cerebral disease, (2) dorsal tentorial mass lesions that compress or displace the brain stem, (3) ventral tentorial destructive lesions, and (4) metabolic encephalopathy.

Dorsal and ventral tentorial lesions often produce focal neurologic signs. These lesions include neoplasia, abscesses, hemorrhage or contusion or both, localized inflammations, and infarction.

Diffuse brain stem or cerebral destructive lesions may produce symmetric nonlocalizing neurologic signs and coma. These include inflammations, degenerative lesions (polioencephalomalacia, lipodystrophy terminally), injury with or without hemorrhage, and hydrocephalus.

Metabolic encephalopathy, including drug intoxications, usually does not produce focal neurologic signs or alterations of the cerebrospinal fluid.

Be aware of the prolonged postictal coma or stupor that can follow seizures from any cause, including idiopathic epilepsy.

The history of the onset of coma is important. The first fact to establish is whether an injury was observed, or could have happened unobserved. In cases in which an injury could not have occurred, an abrupt onset of coma with structural lesions is more common in ventral tentorial lesions. Space-occupying dorsal tentorial lesions show other evidence of focal signs before the onset of coma. The coma of polioencephalomalacia usually is preceded by ataxia and blindness for at least 6 to 12 hours. Do not overlook drug-induced coma in domestic animals. Drugs used by the owner may have been consumed accidentally in large quantities by the patient.

NEUROLOGIC EXAMINATION

The neurologic examination may be helpful in defining the site and kind of lesion. Six aspects of the examination should be emphasized.

State of Consciousness. This should be documented carefully, especially to allow one to accurately follow the course of the disease and response to therapy. *Depression* or *obtundation* are present when an animal responds slowly or inappropriately to verbal stimuli. Some animals may appear disoriented or even act delirious. *Stupor* or *semicoma* means the patient is generally unresponsive except to vigorous and repeated stimuli that may necessarily be painful. *Coma* means complete unresponsiveness to repeated noxious stimulation.

Vision. Normal response to the menace test generally determines that the central visual pathway to the visual cerebral cortex is intact. In addition, the involvement of the cerebellum in this response is normal. If the menace test is absent but pupillary responses to light and facial muscle function are normal, this usually locates the lesion in the cerebral hemispheres. Severe brain stem lesions interfere with the pupillary responses and may depress the cerebral cortex sufficiently to allow no response to the menace test. This is part of the unconscious state from an ARAS lesion. Intact vision in a semicomatose recumbent patient would indicate a brain stem lesion.

Pupillary Size and Response. Structural disease of the rostral brain stem that is severe enough to cause semicoma or coma usually produces fixed pupils either at midpoint or dilated. Metabolic disease that produces the same degree of unconsciousness usually spares the pupillary light reaction. The pupils may be small but reactive in metabolic disease. In acute diffuse cerebrocortical disease, pupils often are symmetrically small. Severe rostral brain stem compression produces dilated, unresponsive pupils. As a unilateral dorsal tentorial (cerebral) lesion herniates and compresses the brain stem, the pupil on the affected side may first become small but remain reactive to light, followed by dilation of the pupil. This is usually all on the same side as the cerebral space-occupying lesion (neoplasm, abscess) from compression of the oculomotor general visceral efferent neurons. The general visceral efferent neurons are apparently more susceptible to compression than the general somatic efferent neurons. As the compression increases, the pupils become fixed in midposition or dilation and unresponsive to light. This is a poor prognosis. Severe medullary lesions will also result in pupils fixed in mid-position and unresponsive to changes in light.

Extremely small, slit or pinpoint pupils are seen in both metabolic and diffuse cerebrocortical or unilateral dorsal tentorial structural lesions. In the comatose patient reactive pupils imply a metabolic disease, and unreactive pupils strongly suggest structural brain stem disease.

Eye Movements. In animals, testing eye movements in the semicomatose or comatose patient is limited to moving the head rapidly to detect normal vestibular nystagmus. Be cautious in patients with head injury that may also have a cervical vertebral injury. Caloric testing for vestibulo-ocular reflexes is unreliable in the domestic animal. Loss of any eye movement response to moving the head from side to side in a dorsal plane suggests structural brain stem disease with loss of the medial longitudinal fasciculus and is a poor prognosis. Asymmetric or abnormal responses may occur if there is damage to the nuclei or nerves of cranial nerves III, IV, and VI. Bilateral destruction of the labyrinth in the inner ear or the eighth cranial nerve will prevent any response of the eye to head movement. In severe metabolic disease these responses may be absent as well. If abnormal nystagmus is present, this implies that the medial longitudinal fasciculus and other ascending pathways are intact from vestibular nuclei to the nuclei that innervate the extraocular muscles.

Respirations. Irregularities of respiration may occur with serious brain disease. Cheyne-Stokes respiration may occur with severe bilateral cerebral disease, or diencephalic disease, or both. Mesencephalic lesions may cause a regular sustained hyperventilation referred to as central neurogenic hyperventilation. More caudal brain stem lesions produce bizarre, abnormal breathing patterns often referred to as irregular or ataxic breathing. This usually precedes respiratory arrest.

Traumatic lesions that injure the thorax may produce respiratory abnormalities unrelated to a brain stem lesion.

Motor Responses. The pattern of spontaneous motor function or the motor response to painful stimuli may aid in the localization of the lesion. In metabolic disease only symmetric deficits occur. Asymmetric deficits suggest structural disease.

In acute disease with mild asymmetric motor responses, the deficient side may be ipsilateral to a brain stem lesion or contralateral to a cerebral lesion. Shortly after the acute onset of a unilateral cerebral lesion, the animal will be ambulatory and may have a mild contralateral paresis and ataxia. There may be a tendency to turn the head or eyes toward the side of the lesion and to circle in that direction. The obtunded, blind animal with a paretic, ataxic gait is more likely to have a bilateral cerebral lesion than a brain stem lesion. Decerebrate rigidity occurs with midbrain lesions, and is characterized by recumbency accompanied by rigid extension of all the limbs and opisthotonus. Opisthotonos with extensor rigidity of the forelimbs and the hindlimbs flexed forward at the hips with the other joints extended suggests a ventral tentorial lesion with involvement of the rostral cerebellum.

A comatose patient with decerebrate rigidity and normally reactive pupils probably has a metabolic disease, whereas a similar comatose patient with fixed, unreactive pupils has a structural brain stem lesion.

In metabolic disease, obtundation and semicoma usually precede the motor signs, whereas in dorsal tentorial lesions the opposite occurs.

CAUSES. The causes of altered states of consciousness are numerous. The most common cause is trauma. Evaluation of patients with intracranial injury is described in Chapter 20. The metabolic diseases and intoxications that may alter the state of consciousness and produce coma as the main clinical sign or as one of the terminal clinical signs are listed in Tables 19–1 and 19–2.[27] Be aware of hallucinogenic drugs that may be available to the patient in its environment. Other considerations are severe infections, terminal stages of lysosomal storage diseases, congenital hydrocephalus with hemorrhage from mild trauma, neoplasia, and vascular disorders.

DIAGNOSIS AND PROGNOSIS. Ancillary procedures that are used will depend on the information obtained from the history and examination of the patient. Included in the data base may be the CBC, blood electrolytes, glucose, BUN, creatinine, and serum osmolality. Some toxins can be diagnosed from blood or urine examination. Cerebrospinal fluid examination is of value if there has been no head injury.

Prognosis depends on the location and the nature of the lesion and whether it is amenable to therapy. For example, if the patient is comatose following intracranial injury, the lesion may be a hemorrhagic contusion of the mesencephalon, which has a poor prognosis, or the primary lesion may be a cerebral contusion with secondary edema and increased pressure on the brain stem. The latter lesion has a better prognosis for recovery following therapy for cerebral edema.

TABLE 19–1. METABOLIC DISEASES THAT MAY PRODUCE COMA

Pancreatic disease:
    Beta cell neoplasia—hypoglycemia
    Diabetes mellitus—hyperglycemia and ketoacidosis
Liver disease: hyperammonemia, hypoglycemia
Renal disease: uremia, acidosis, hypocalcemia
Myocardial disease: ischemic anoxia
Pulmonary disease: anoxic anoxia, acidosis
Adrenal disease:
    Hypoadrenocortical crisis—hyperkalemia
Anemia: carbon monoxide poisoning, hemorrhage
Osmotic abnormalities:
    Water intoxication—hypo-osmolar state
    Salt poisoning—hyperosmolar state, hypernatremia
Nutritional deficiency: thiamine deficiency
Acidosis, severe
Heat stroke-hyperthermia

TABLE 19–2. POISONS THAT MAY PRODUCE COMA

Hexachlorophene[55]	Lead salts
Cyanide	Dinitrophenol
Barbiturates	Kerosene
Ethylene glycol	Nitrobenzene
Benzene hexachloride, benzene	Turpentine
Amphetamine sulfate	Arsenic
Carbon tetrachloride	Zinc phosphide

HYPOTHALAMUS

ANATOMY

The hypothalamus is that part of the diencephalon that forms the ventral and lateral walls of the ventral portion of the third ventricle. It extends from the lamina terminalis and optic chiasm rostrally through the mamillary bodies caudally (see Fig. 19–1, Plates 14, 15). The ventral surface of the hypothalamus between these areas is the tuber cinereum. A ventral extension of the tuber cinereum is the infundibulum or pituitary stalk. Proximally, the infundibulum widens where it joins the hypothalamus to form the median eminence of the tuber cinereum. Distally, the infundibulum expands to form the distal part of the neurohypophysis, the neural lobe of the hypophysis (pituitary gland).

The hypothalamus may be divided transversely from rostral to caudal into three groups of nuclei.

1. Rostral (chiasmatic) group—preoptic area (part of telencephalon, fuses with rostral hypothalamus), supraoptic nucleus, paraventricular nucleus, rostral hypothalamic area.

2. Intermediate (tuberal) group—infundibular nucleus (arcuate), dorsomedial nucleus, ventromedial nucleus, lateral hypothalamic area.

3. Caudal (mammillary) group—mammillary body, caudal hypothalamic area.

In addition, three longitudinal zones can be recognized throughout each hypothalamus—the periventricular zone, the middle zone, and the lateral zone.

Hypothalamic Connections

Afferent

TELENCEPHALON (rhinencephalon). Fornix—from hippocampus to mammillary bodies; stria terminalis—from amygdaloid body; medial forebrain bundle—from septal area; pallidohypothalamic fibers—from pallidum (extrapyramidal).

DIENCEPHALON. Thalamic—hypothalamic fibers.

MESENCEPHALON. Mammillary peduncle—collaterals of brain stem afferent pathways—GVA, SVA, from visceral modalities. Dorsal longitudinal fasciculus in the periventricular central grey substance—collaterals from the pathways in the solitary tract —GVA, SVA.

Efferent

MAMMILLOTHALAMIC TRACT. To rostral thalamic nucleus.

HYPOTHALAMOTEGMENTAL PATHWAYS. Mammillotegmental tract—to mesencephalic reticular formation to influence brain stem and spinal cord GVE system; periventricular fibers and dorsal longitudinal fasciculus—to brain stem and spinal cord GVE system.

HYPOTHALAMOHYPOPHYSEAL TRACT. The hypothalamohypophyseal tract courses into the neurohypophysis.[60] Neurosecretory products from the supraoptic and paraventricular nuclei (oxytocin, vasopressin or antidiuretic hormone) course through the supraopticohypophyseal and paraventriculohypophyseal tracts to the neural lobe, in which they are elaborated into the capillary bed and ultimately course to the effector organ to exert their activity.[4] The neurosecretory products from the mediobasal hypothalamic nuclei flow through the axons of the tuberohypophyseal tract, and are released terminally into the capillaries of the neurohypophysis and circulate by way of the portal vessels to the sinusoids of the adenohypophysis to influence the endocrine activity of the cells in the pars distalis. These are the adenohypophyseal releasing factors that are produced in hypothalamic nuclei.[52] There is some evidence that endocrines secreted by the adenohypophysis may circulate back to the neurohypophysis, where they can influence the brain.[3]

FUNCTION

The hypothalamus serves as a higher center for regulation of visceral motor activity. Its nuclei act as the upper motor neuron for visceral function; therefore, they are considered the upper motor neuron in the autonomic nervous system. Stimulation of the rostral hypothalamus elicits parasympathetic activity, whereas stimulation of the caudal hypothalamus elicits sympathetic activity throughout the body. The hypothalamus functions without voluntary control. The neocortex does not order hypothalamic activity; nevertheless, the hypothalamus is subject to its influence. As an example, consider the gastrointestinal signs that accompany fear, pain, and emotional states. Visceral motor activity associated with the function of the olfactory and limbic system is mediated through the hypothalamus. In addition, the hypothalamus regulates the activity of a large portion of the body's endocrine system by way of neurosecretory products elaborated from hypothalamic nuclei.

CLINICAL SYNDROMES

Numerous clinical syndromes have been related to lesions that disturb the hypothalamus and adjacent structures.

Abnormal Behavior. Selective ventral hypothalamic lesions in cats produce rage. Cattle with a pituitary gland abscess are often depressed and hold their head and neck extended as if "star gazing."

Diabetes Insipidus.[1, 7-9, 20, 32, 37] Diabetes insipidus is the loss of control of water excretion due to the failure of production or transport and release of antidiuretic hormone (ADH) into the blood stream.[44, 45] This failure to resorb water from the kidney tubules causes polyuria, and secondarily polydipsia. The urine specific gravity is consistently very low (1.002 to 1.005) and does not concentrate when water consumption is stopped, but does show response of the kidney to the intramuscular injection of extracts containing ADH.[5] In a study of 26 dogs with neoplasms of the adenohypophysis, 92 per cent had the clinical diagnosis of diabetes insipidus from direct pressure of the neoplasm on the nuclei in the hypothalamus (supraoptic nuclei).[6, 12, 13, 28, 51]

Abnormal Temperature Regulation.[29] Abnormal temperature control may be manifested as hyperthermia, hypothermia, or poikilothermia. A heat loss center is located in the rostral hypothalamic area which normally responds to elevated body temperatures by initiating sweating, increased respirations, vasodilation, and panting. A heat conservation center is located in the caudal and lateral hypothalamic areas that responds to depressed body temperature by initiating piloerection, shivering, vasoconstriction, and increased basal metabolic rate, thereby increasing feeding. Lesions of these centers inhibit their normal regulatory function: in the case of the heat loss center they cause hyperthermia, while in the heat conservation center they cause hypothermia. Hyperhidrosis (excessive sweating) may accompany hyperthermia with disturbances of these centers. Bilateral destruction of the descending hypothalamotegmental tracts concerned with the conservation and dissipation of the body heat may produce poikilothermia, in which the body temperature varies with the environmental temperature. Poikilothermia occasionally results from intracranial injuries that affect the hypothalamus. Cattle with abscessed pituitary glands and displacement of the hypothalamus may be hypothermic.

Abnormal Appetite.[19, 23, 35] Abnormalities in appetite are expressed as hyperphagia and obesity, or anorexia and cachexia. A satiety center resides in the ventromedial hypothalamic nucleus. If destroyed bilaterally, hyperphagia and obesity result, which may be accompanied by savageness. In the lateral hypothalamic area there is a feeding center responsible for the stimulation of appetite. Lesions in this center cause anorexia that is complete, resulting in cachexia and eventual death. The amygdaloid body is also involved in appetite control.

The adiposogenital syndrome (Froelich's syndrome) results from hypothalamic lesions involving the satiety center and the mediobasal nuclei concerned with gonadal stimulation by way of the hypophysis. Such animals become obese and their genitalia atrophy.[50, 51]

Abnormal Carbohydrate Metabolism. The hypothalamus is involved with the regulation of the blood sugar level of the body. The exact mechanism of this control is unknown. Lesions involving the ventral wall of the third ventricle have been associated with hyperglycemia, glycosuria, and abnormal glucose tolerance curves.

There are reports in the veterinary literature of neoplasms of the pars intermedia in horses associated with hyperglycemia and glycosuria that are unresponsive to insulin.[2, 6, 25, 30, 58, 59] These neoplasms usually exert pressure on the hypothalamus as they grow dorsally out of the hypophyseal fossa. In addition, these animals often exhibit a failure to shed their winter hair coat through the warm months of the year.[2, 16] Hyperthermia and hyperhidrosis also have been reported with these neoplasms, and occasionally diabetes insipidus and a ravenous appetite.

Abnormal Heart Rate. Alterations of cardiovascular function have been observed in cattle with abscesses of the hypophysis and involvement of the hypothalamus. The interference with the role of the hypothalamus in autonomic function results in a marked slowing of the heart, or bradycardia.

Abnormal Sensorium. Hypothalamic lesions that interfere with its role in the ARAS may result in variations in the state of consciousness, occasionally producing semicoma.

Hyperadrenocorticoidism.[34] Hyperadrenocorticoidism often accompanies neoplasms of the adenohypophysis that produce adrenocorticotropic hormone or a similar acting polypeptide hormone.[11, 17] This syndrome has been reported with chromophobe adenomas and pars intermedia neoplasms of the canine pituitary. If the hypothalamus is compromised by the neoplasm, various signs of hypothalamic dysfunction may accompany the signs of hyperactivity of the adrenal cortex.

Signs of hyperadrenocorticoidism include[24, 26, 31, 36, 53, 54, 56] (1) polyuria, polydipsia, polyphagia; (2) bilaterally symmetric alopecia with sparing of the head and distal extremities, thin hypotonic skin, patchy hyperpigmentation, comedones, keratin plugs, petechiae or ecchymoses, and calcinosis cutis; (3) pendulous, flaccid abdomen, enlarged liver; (4) atrophic testicles or prolonged anestrus; (5) lameness (osteoporosis), skeletal muscle atrophy, and weakness; and (6) rarely clinical myotonia. In laboratory tests, the complete blood count shows stress response (lymphopenia, eosinopenia); there are elevated serum cholesterol, glucose, alanine aminotransferase, and alkaline phosphatase levels; urinary specific gravity is from 1.008 to 1.014; and there is evidence of glycosuria.

Diencephalic Syndrome. A diencephalic syndrome is observed in human infants usually less than one year old. It is characterized primarily by an alert, euphoric state and emaciation despite adequate caloric intake. Most have a rostral hypothalamic neoplasm. A similar syndrome was described in a 3-year-old Doberman pinscher with a rostral hypothalamic astrocytoma.[39] Hypothermia, bradycardia, and a failure to drink accompanied the emaciation despite an adequate appetite.

REFERENCES

1. Andersson, B.: Thirst—and brain control of water balance. Am. Sci., 59:408, 1971.
2. Bäckström, G.: Hirsutism associated with pituitary tumors in horses. Nord. Vet. Med., 15:778, 1963.
3. Beigland, R. M., and Page, R. B.: Pituitary-brain vascular relations: A new paradigm. Science, 204:18, 1979.
4. Bisset, G. W., Clark, B. J., and Errington, M. L.: The hypothalamic neurosecretory pathways for the release of oxytocin and vasopressin in the cat. J. Physiol., 217:111, 1971.
5. Bovee, K. C.: Urine osmolality as a definitive indicator of renal concentrating capacity. J. Am. Vet. Med. Assoc., 155:30, 1969.
6. Brandt, A. J.: Über Hypophysenadenom bei Hund und Pferd. Skand. Vet. Tidskr., 30:875, 1940.
7. Breitschwerdt, E. B.: Clinical abnormalities of urine concentration and dilution. Compend. Contin. Ed., 3:414, 1981.
8. Breitschwerdt, E. B., and Root, C. R.: Inappropriate secretion of antidiuretic hormone in a dog. J. Am. Vet. Med. Assoc., 175:181, 1979.
9. Breitschwerdt, E. B., Verlander, J. W., and Hribernik, T. N.: Nephrogenic diabetes insipidus in three dogs. J. Am. Vet. Med. Assoc., 179:235, 1981.
10. Cabral, R. J., and Johnson, J. I.: The organization of mechanoreceptive projections in the ventrobasal thalamus of sheep. J. Comp. Neurol., 141:17, 1971.
11. Capen, C. C., and Koestner, A.: Functional chromophobe adenoma of the canine adenohypophysis. An ultrastructural evaluation of neoplasm of pituitary corticotrophs. Pathol. Vet., 4:326, 1967.
12. Capen, C. C., Martin, S. L., and Koestner, A.: Neoplasms in the adenohypophysis of dogs. Pathol. Vet., 4:301, 1967.
13. Capen, C. C., Martin, S. L., and Koestner, A.: The ultrastructure and histopathology of an acidophil adenoma of the canine adenohypophysis. Pathol. Vet., 4:348, 1967.
14. Cheatham, M. L., and Matzke, H. A.: Descending hypothalamic medullary pathways in the cat. J. Comp. Neurol., 127:369, 1966.
15. Cummings, J. F., and de Lahunta, A.: An experimental study of the retinal projections in the horse and sheep. Ann. N.Y. Acad. Sci., 167:293, 1969.
16. Eriksson, K. S., Dyrendahl, S., and Grunfelt, D.: A case of hirsutism in connection with hypophyseal tumor in a horse. Nord. Vet. Med., 8:807, 1956.
17. Feldman, E. C.: Effect of functional adrenocortical tumors on plasma corticol and corticotropin concentrations in dogs. J. Am. Vet. Med. Assoc., 178:823, 1981.
18. Fisher, C. M.: The neurological examination of the comatose patient. Acta Neurol. Scand. [Suppl.], 36:45, 1979.
19. Fonberg, E.: The effect of hypothalamic and amygdalar lesions on alimentary behavior and thermoregulation. J. Physiol., 63:249, 1971.
20. Grauer, G. F.: The differential diagnosis of polyuric-polydypsic diseases. Compend. Contin. Ed., 3:1079, 1981.
21. Jouvet, M.: Biogenic amines and the states of sleep. Science, 163:32, 1969.
22. Jouvet, M.: Neurophysiology of the states of sleep. Physiol. Rev., 47:117, 1967.
23. Keesey, R. E., and Pawley, T. L.: Hypothalamic regulation of body weight. Am. Sci., 63:558, 1975.

24. Kelly, D. F., Siegel, E. T., and Berg, P.: The adrenal glands in dogs with hyperadrenocorticism: A pathologic study. Vet. Pathol., 8:385, 1971.

25. King, J. M., Kavanaugh, J. F., and Bentinck-Smith, J.: Diabetes mellitus with pituitary neoplasms in a horse and a dog. Cornell Vet., 52:133, 1962.

26. Kirk, G. R., Boyer, S., and Hutcheson, D. P.: Effects of o,p':DDD on plasma cortisol levels and histology of the adrenal gland in the normal dog. J. Am. Anim. Hosp. Assoc., 10:179, 1974.

27. Kirk, R. W., and Bistner, S. I.: Handbook of Veterinary Procedures and Emergency Treatment. 2nd ed. Philadelphia, W. B. Saunders Co., 1975.

28. Koestner, A., and Capen, C. C.: Ultrastructural evaluation of the canine hypothalamic-neurohypophyseal system in diabetes insipidus associated with pituitary neoplasms. Pathol. Vet., 4:513, 1967.

29. Krum, S. H., and Osborne, C. A.: Heat stroke in the dog: A polysystemic disorder. J. Am. Vet. Med. Assoc., 170:531, 1977.

30. Loeb, W. F., Capen, C. C., and Johnson, L. E.: Adenomas of the pars intermedia associated with hyperglycemia and glycosuria in two horses. Cornell Vet., 56:623, 1966.

31. Lorenz, M. D., Scott, D. W., and Pulley, L. T.: Medical treatment of canine hyperadrenocorticoidism with o,p'-DDD. Cornell Vet., 63:646, 1973.

32. Madewell, B. R., Osborne, C. A., Norrdin, R. A., Stevens, J. R., and Hardy, R. M.: Clinicopathologic aspects of diabetes insipidus in the dog. J. Am. Anim. Hosp. Assoc., 11:497, 1975.

33. Magoun, H. W.: The ascending reticular activating system. Res. Publ. Assoc. Res. Nerv. Ment. Dis., 30:480, 1952.

34. Meijer, J. C.: An investigation of the pathogenesis of pituitary-dependent hyperadrenocorticism in the dog. Thesis, University of Utrecht, 1980.

35. Mrosovsky,, N., and Sherry, D. F.: Animal anorexias. Science, 207:837, 1980.

36. Mulnix, J. A.: Adrenal cortical disease in dogs. Scope, 19:12, 1975.

37. Mulnix, J. A., Rijnberk, A., and Hendriks, H. J.: Evaluation of a modified water-deprivation test for diagnosis of polyuric disorders in dogs. J. Am. Vet. Med. Assoc., 169:1327, 1976.

38. Murray, M.: Degeneration of some intralaminar thalamic nuclei after cortical removals in the cat. J. Comp. Neurol., 127:341, 1966.

39. Nelson, R. W., Morrison, W. B., Lurus, A., and Miller, J. B.: Diencephalic syndrome secondary to intracranial astrocytoma in a dog. J. Am. Vet. Med. Assoc., 179:1004, 1981.

40. Peacock, J. H., and Combs, C. M.: Retrograde cell degeneration in adult cat after hemidecortication. J. Comp. Neurol., 125:329, 1965.

41. Plum, F., and Posner, J. B.: The diagnosis of stupor and coma. 2nd ed. Philadelphia, F. A. Davis, 1972.

42. Posner, J. B.: Clinical evaluation of the unconscious patient. Clin. Neurosurg., 22:281, 1975.

43. Posner, J. B.: The comatose patient. J.A.M.A., 233:1313, 1975.

44. Richards, M. A.: Polydipsia in the dog. The differential diagnosis of polyuric syndromes in the dog. J. Small Anim. Pract., 10:651, 1970.

45. Richards, M. A., and Sloper, J. C.: Diabetes insipidus—the complexity of the syndrome. Acta Endocrinol., 62:627, 1969.

46. Rioch, D. M.: Studies on the diencephalon of carnivora. I. Nuclear configuration of the thalamus, epithalamus, and hypothalamus of the dog and cat. J. Comp. Neurol., 49:1, 1929.

47. Rioch, D. M.: II. Nuclear configuration and fiber connections of subthalamus and midbrain of the dog and cat. J. Comp. Neurol., 49:121, 1929.

48. Rioch, D. M.: III. Certain myelinated fiber connections of the diencephalon of the dog and cat. J. Comp. Neurol., 53:319, 1931.

49. Rose, J. E.: The thalamus of the sheep: Cellular and fibrous structure and comparison with pig, rabbit, and cat. J. Comp. Neurol., 77:469, 1942.

50. Saunders, L. Z., and Rickard, C. G.: Craniopharyngioma in a dog with apparent adiposogenital syndrome and diabetes insipidus. Cornell Vet., 42:490, 1952.

51. Saunders, L. Z., Stephenson, H. C., and McEntee, K.: Diabetes insipidus and adiposogenital syndrome in a dog due to an infundibuloma. Cornell Vet., 41:445, 1951.

52. Schally, A. V., Kastin, A. J., and Arinura, A.: Hypothalamic hormones: The link between brain and body. Am. Sci., 65:712, 1977.

53. Schecter, R. D., Stabenfeldt, G. H., Gribble, D. H., and Ling, G. V.: Treatment of Cushing's syndrome in the dog with an adrenocorticolytic agent (o,p'-DDD). J. Am. Vet. Med. Assoc., 162:629, 1973.

54. Scott, D. W.: Cushing's Disease (hyperadrenocorticism). Abstracts, 66th Annual Conference, Ithaca, N.Y., New York State College of Veterinary Medicine, 1974, 36–38.

55. Scott, D. W., Bolton, G. R., and Lorenz, M. D.: Hexachlorophene toxicosis in dogs. J. Am. Vet. Med. Assoc., 162:947, 1973.

56. Siegel, E. T., Kelly, D. F., and Berg, P.: Cushing's syndrome in the dog. J. Am. Vet. Med. Assoc., 157:2081, 1970.

57. Sychowa, B.: The morphology and topography of the thalamic nuclei of the dog. Acta Biol. Exp., 21:101, 1961.

58. Tasker. J. B., Whiteman, C. E., and Martin, B. R.: Diabetes mellitus in the horse. J. Am. Vet. Med. Assoc., 49:393, 1966.

59. Urman, H. K., Ozcan, H. C., and Tekeli, S.: Pituitary neoplasms in two horses. Zentrabl. Veterinaermed., 10:257, 1963.

60. Zambrano, D., and de Robertis, E.: Ultrastructure of the hypothalamic neurosecretory system of the dog. Z. Zellforsch. Mikrosk. Anat., 81:264, 1967.

DIAGNOSIS AND EVALUATION OF TRAUMATIC LESIONS OF THE NERVOUS SYSTEM

CENTRAL NERVOUS SYSTEM [2, 13, 19, 22, 23, 28, 30, 31, 33, 35, 42]

BRAIN

The management of patients who present with intracranial injuries should follow a specific list of priorities which is similar to that for any severe injury.

Establish a Patent Airway. Respiratory hypoxia causes cellular anoxia. Hypercapnia increases the cerebral blood flow in the cranial cavity by vasodilation, and increases cerebral edema, which must be avoided. The unconscious patient should be intubated. If therapy is required in the conscious patient, tracheostomy may be performed. Repeated hyperventilation reduces the partial pressure of carbon dioxide.

Stop Major External Hemorrhage

Treat the Shock.[26] The intracranial injury rarely causes shock. The shock that the patient with intracranial injury often experiences is due to tissue damage and loss of blood from other organs. These should be examined at this time for any life-threatening lesions. The temperature, pulse, and respirations should be recorded for evaluation of the response to

treatment and for signs of deterioration from a brain stem lesion.

Evaluate the Neurologic Status. The assessment of the neurologic status of a patient with intracranial injury does not require exhaustive knowledge of the neuroanatomy and neurophysiology of the brain to arrive at a clinical diagnosis, recommend therapy, and determine a baseline for further evaluation. If possible, an eyewitness account of the accident and a description of the patient immediately following the accident should be obtained and compared with the present evaluation. The most important signs to evaluate are similar to those described under coma in Chapter 19.

STATE OF CONSCIOUSNESS. This is the best evaluation for signs of progressive cerebral hypoxia. The various levels of consciousness may be described as coma (unconscious and no response to painful stimuli), semicoma or stupor (unconscious but responsive to painful stimuli), delirium, confusion, depression, and alertness. The important factor is to describe what response you observe.

PUPIL SIZE AND RESPONSE. Bilateral miotic, bilateral mydriatic, or asymmetric pupils all suggest brain stem contusion of varying degrees. Unresponsive mydriatic pupils bilaterally are usually due to an irreversible midbrain lesion. Miotic pupils that become mydriatic and unresponsive suggest midbrain edema or compression by a progressing cerebral lesion, and an indication for more aggressive therapy. Asymmetric and bilaterally miotic pupils also occur with primarily acute cerebral lesions. These may change remarkably in the first few hours following the injury. A favorable prognosis is indicated by a change from pupillary abnormality to normal. Before concluding that the pupillary abnormality is due to a midbrain lesion, the eyeballs should be examined carefully for lesions. Unilateral lesions in the cerebellar nuclei may also cause anisocoria. Medullary lesions may cause pupils fixed at mid-size.

POSTURE AND MOTOR FUNCTION. In the recumbent animal, determine whether there is any voluntary movement of the limbs in response to painful stimuli. If reflexes are absent, this usually indicates there is an additional spinal cord lesion present. The posture of decerebrate rigidity, extensor rigidity of all four limbs, may occur with severe brain stem lesions that are usually caudal to the red nucleus. Rostral cerebellar lesions may cause opisthotonus and extensor rigidity of the forelimbs. Severe vestibular disturbance peripherally or centrally in the pons and medulla causes head tilt, or neck and body flexion, or both. Lateral neck flexion may occur with unilateral brain stem lesions. If the patient is ambulatory, determine any degree of paresis or ataxia that may be present by careful observation of gait and response to the testing of postural reactions.

VISION. In the absence of lesions in the eyeball or postorbital area, visual deficits in patients with intracranial lesions usually are due to contusion or edema of the visual cerebral cortex. Pupillary response is normal if there are no accompanying rostral brain stem lesions. In the recumbent, conscious animal, vision can only be tested by the palpebral response to menacing gestures toward the eyes. In the severely depressed animal you may not be able to assess visual perception.

OTHER CRANIAL NERVE FUNCTION. Initial loss of cranial nerve function suggests laceration of the cranial nerve along its course from the brain stem, or contusion and hemorrhage in the brain stem involving its fibers or nucleus. Loss of cranial nerve function subsequent to the initial examination suggests compression and hypoxia, and a more guarded prognosis. When this occurs, it is helpful in localizing the lesion.

RESPIRATIONS. Serious brain stem injury may cause irregularities of respiration. Cheyne-Stoke's respiration occurs with diencephalic lesions, hyperventilation with mesencephalic lesions, and irregular or ataxic respirations with medullary lesions. Ataxic respirations usually precede respiratory arrest. Development of these respiratory irregularities and a slowing of the pulse rate are poor prognostic signs.

Signs of vestibular system disturbance (head tilt, truncal torsion, rolling, abnormal nystagmus) can occur with lesions of the vestibular nuclei in the medulla or of the labyrinth in the inner ear. With a nuclear lesion there should be other signs of involvement of adjacent medullary structures. It is important to determine the source of the vestibular system injury, because the prognosis is better for injuries to the inner ear membranous labyrinth. These labyrinthine contusions often are associated with a fracture of the petrosal bone, and hemorrhage often occurs from the external ear canal. If the patient is conscious, with voluntary limb movement, and has no other signs of brain stem involvement, it may recover from the peripheral receptor damage by compensation. This will take from weeks to months, and a residual head tilt and mild ataxia may persist. Vestibular system signs may accompany cerebellar signs with cerebellar lesions. Compensation from cerebellar injury is often remarkable.

Another test of brain stem function is that of vestibular nystagmus. Normally rapid movement of the head from side to side in a dorsal plane elicits a nystagmus, with the quick phase toward the direction of head movement. Lesions that interrupt the medial longitudinal fasciculus or the brain stem portion of neurons in cranial nerves III, IV, or VI prevent this normal vestibular nystagmus in an animal with a normal membranous labyrinth. It may also be absent in a severely depressed animal.

Do not overlook the possibility of multiple injuries. For example, a patient may present as recumbent, semicomatose, and in shock, with pain perceived from the thoracic limbs and with mild voluntary thoracic limb withdrawal attempts, but with complete analgesia and paralysis caudal to the thoracolumbar junction. Such a patient has intracranial injury and a transverse injury of the caudal thoracic spinal cord.

In order to follow the patient's course, a baseline neurologic assessment must be made as soon as possible, and the neurologic status must be reevaluated continually to determine whether the treatment used should be continued or altered.

Cerebral edema is considered to be the usual sequel to intracranial injury, and the primary lesion for which treatment is instituted. The most common gross lesion in the dog and cat with severe intracranial injury is hemorrhage on the median plane in the midbrain tegmentum. This causes semicoma or coma, tetraplegia with or without torticollis, and abnormal pupillary size or response. Subarachnoid hemorrhage, if present, is minimal and often associated with a focal cerebral laceration and hemorrhage. Subdural and extradural hemorrhages are less common. As a rule following an injury, the clinical signs reach their maximum severity within a few hours. Uncontrolled cerebral edema may cause progression of the intracranial signs.

Medical Treatment

The brain edema that occurs following an injury probably results from two mechanisms.[14] Vasogenic edema results from increased permeability of the endothelial cells of brain capillaries associated with contusion and hemorrhage. This is an extracellular edema that predominates in the white matter. Hypoxia may result from injury to the cardiorespiratory system and the cerebral vasculature with decreased perfusion. Hypoxia causes cytotoxic edema with swelling of neurons, glia, and endothelial cells. Corticosteroids are most useful in treating vasogenic edema, and hypertonic solutions are most efficacious in cytotoxic edema. Both drugs will decrease production of cerebrospinal fluid.[43, 44]

Medical treatment is instituted to correct and prevent cerebral edema, and should consist primarily of high levels of corticosteroids, an oxygen-rich atmosphere, and in some instances hypertonic fluids.[3, 16, 20, 24, 29, 42, 45-47] Dexamethasone (Azium) should be administered in a dose of 2 to 4 mg per kg repeated at 6- to 8-hour intervals. This is similar to the treatment used for shock, and may already have been instituted. Some clinicians use lower doses (0.2 mg per kg) if the patient is not in shock.[13] This therapy should be continued for 2 to 3 days, then at decreasing doses for another few days.

There is not complete agreement on the beneficial effects of corticosteroids in experimental brain injury and in some clinical trials in humans.[9, 49] Clinical results in veterinary medicine support its efficacy.

The use of hypertonic fluids is controversial.[24, 37] They should be used only in the stuporous or comatose patient, and precautions are necessary in their use. If there is any reason to believe that hemorrhage in the cranial cavity has not been controlled, this treatment is contraindicated.[36] In the absence of bleeding from the nares or external ear canals, and in the absence of palpable skull fractures that could injure venous sinuses or the middle meningeal artery, it may be safe to assume that continual hemorrhage inside the cranial cavity is not a consideration. It is also contraindicated in dogs that have suffered significant blood loss as a result of their injuries, if the drug is adminis-

tered before this blood loss has been corrected.[38] This is not a problem once the arterial and central venous pressures are normal. Mannitol (Osmitrol, 20 per cent) should be administered intravenously over a 10-minute period at a dose of 2 gm per kg, and repeated once or twice at 3- to 4-hour intervals. Smaller doses of mannitol may be just as effective, but these have not been evaluated clinically in domestic animals. A dose of 0.25 gm per kg of mannitol was as effective as 1.0 gm per kg in persons with head injury.[25] In experimental brain injury it has been shown that the increased cerebrospinal fluid pressure responds to intravenous mannitol in 30 minutes, whereas responses to corticosteroids take about 6 hours.[20] Large doses of hypertonic solutions should not be used without concomitant maintenance of a near normal fluid volume to prevent severe dehydration that can attend the use of these solutions. If hypovolemic shock is present, the blood volume can be reestablished with isotonic lactated Ringer's solution. Hypertonic solutions can be administered simultaneously.[24] It is also important not to overhydrate the patient. This stresses the heart and increases the potential for a rebound effect on the intracranial pressure when the hypertonic fluid therapy is stopped. Monitoring of the central venous pressure and the gum perfusion time should help determine the reestablishment of normal blood volume.

Intravenous dimethylsulfoxide (DMSO) has the effect of reducing the increased intracranial pressure produced by intracranial injury.[10, 11] It is given intravenously at the rate of 2 gm per kg of a 40 per cent solution. Limited clinical use in the horse and dog have shown no obvious untoward side effects. More data are necessary to determine if it is as useful clinically as those therapies already accepted. The experimental data do not support an additive effect of DMSO to that of mannitol or corticosteroids.

Naloxone has been effective experimentally in treating spinal cord injury.[23] Its clinical efficacy has not been determined. Release of endorphins may contribute to the ischemic necrosis at the site of the injury. Naloxone counteracts the effects of endorphins and restores normal vascular perfusion to the spinal cord.

The patient should be placed in an oxygen cage with its head elevated to prevent hypoxia and hypercapnia, which result in cerebral edema.

For a favorable prognosis, a response to

medical therapy should be seen in 6 to 8 hours following treatment. The patient must be reevaluated constantly. If there are signs of improvement, continue the therapy and observation. Any sign of deterioration is an indication for more vigorous medical therapy or possibly surgery.

Having evaluated the patient's neurologic status and instituted medical therapy, skull radiographs may be obtained to determine the presence and severity of fractures of the skull bones that bound the cranial cavity. If there are compound fractures or a depressed fracture that obviously encroaches on the brain, surgery should be performed.

Surgical Treatment[28, 32, 42]

Surgery is considered to repair a fractured skull and to decompress a swollen brain. The latter is a last resort that is rarely performed.

The decision to operate to prevent further compression of nervous tissue from the expanding cerebral edema depends on the results of the neurologic evaluation. A patient who presents as comatose, tetraplegic, and with dilated, unresponsive pupils probably has severe contusion with hemorrhage in the midbrain and pons of the brain stem and is not likely to be helped by surgery. The prognosis is grave. No improvement in the comatose patient with miotic pupils after 24 to 36 hours of medical therapy is an indication for more vigorous medical therapy or possibly surgery.

A patient whose signs deteriorate from those of the initial assessment is a candidate for more vigorous medical therapy or surgical decompression. Such signs include progression from depression or delerium to semicoma, or from semicoma with normal or miotic pupils to semicoma or coma with dilated, unresponsive pupils. A decreasing pulse rate and deep irregular respirations are signs of deterioration. These signs indicate an expanding hematoma or uncontrolled cerebral edema. Surgical decompression is performed by removing a large portion of the calvaria. This is done unilaterally if the side of the hematoma can be identified, and bilaterally if there is diffuse cerebral edema.

If radiographs indicate a fracture involving a venous sinus or the middle meningeal artery, or the signs suggest a unilateral cerebral lesion (contralateral cortical visual deficit, or hemiparesis or both), exploratory surgery may be performed to remove a blood clot. Ultimately, this is the most accurate way to locate extradural hemorrhage.

If the patient slowly returns to consciousness and response to painful stimuli improves, then the medical therapy should be continued but the patient must be reevaluated continually. A patient may go from a few days to a week with minimal signs, and then neurologic signs may slowly deteriorate. This suggests slow extradural or subdural bleeding and cerebral compression.

Occasionally, patients with intracranial injury are presented with seizures or status epilepticus. Diazepam (Valium) in 5-mg doses, intramuscular or intravenous, should be used to stop the seizures. If they persist, barbiturates should be administered. The barbiturate may help reduce cerebral edema.[4] When the seizures have stopped, the patient can be evaluated for further neurologic injury.

Patients that are restless or delerious should be given intravenous diazepam (Valium) in a dose of 5 to 10 mg, provided that a neurologic assessment of the patient is made prior to administering the drug.

Whole body hypothermia has been used to reduce cerebral edema and cellular metabolic demands for oxygen, but the response is too variable to recommend it for routine therapy. However, hyperthermia should be prevented. If the patient is presented hypothermic, attempts should not be made to raise the body temperature, for the hypothermia may be advantageous to the patient.

Therapy Guidelines

1. Ambulatory, confused, depressed: corticosteroids.
2. Delerious: corticosteroids and diazepam.
3. Seizures: diazepam.
4. Recumbent, semicomatose, comatose: mannitol, corticosteroids.
5. *Be patient:* Many dogs and cats will improve to become functional pets after serious intracranial injury. This may take weeks to months to occur. They recover best from cerebral injury and will make remarkable recovery from cerebellar injury. Brain stem injuries carry a much more guarded prognosis.

Adequate nursing care is essential to prevent death from complications. The bladder and rectum should be evacuated regularly. The recumbent patient should be turned as often as possible.

SPINAL CORD[6, 7, 12, 27, 34, 39, 41, 52]

Spinal cord injuries are also described in Chapter 10.

Lumbar, Sacral, and Caudal Segments

The signs that are seen with injury to the lumbar, sacral, and caudal segments of the spinal cord are the same as those that occur with injury of the roots of the spinal nerves of these segments. These include complete analgesia, areflexia, and atonic muscles in the area innervated by these segments. They are described in detail under the peripheral nervous system injuries. In the dog, the caudal segments usually are located over the body of the sixth lumbar vertebra, the sacral segments over the body of the fifth lumbar vertebra, and the last three lumbar segments over the body of the fourth lumbar vertebra. In the cat the sacral segments are often over the body of the sixth lumbar vertebra, and the last three lumbar segments are over the body of the fifth lumbar vertebra. Injury to these segments of the spinal cord is more serious than injury to the roots, and recovery from malacia and hemorrhage should not be expected.

Focal Lesion Between the Third Thoracic and Fourth Lumbar Segments

Focal lesions in one or more of the spinal cord segments from the third thoracic to the fourth lumbar that cause complete dysfunction of the injured tissue from concussion, contusion, or laceration result in paraplegia with intact pelvic limb spinal reflexes, and analgesia of the trunk and limbs caudal to the lesion.

These lesions usually are associated with vertebral fractures and displacements of the vertebral canal. The most common site is the caudal thoracic and cranial lumbar region. Lesions here often result in the Schiff-Sherrington syndrome, which is characterized by rigidly extended hypertonic thoracic limbs and flaccid, hypotonic, paralyzed analgesic pelvic limbs with intact spinal reflexes. The thoracic limbs have normal voluntary motor function despite their marked hypertonia, can perform all the postural reactions and spinal reflexes, and have intact sensation.

If the vertebral canal is displaced at the site of the injury, decompressive laminectomy and realignment should be performed. If there is complete discontinuity of the vertebral canal, nothing can be done for the patient to recover the lost neurologic function. Displacements between 50 and 100 per cent of the vertebral canal have a more guarded prognosis. The smaller the displacement, the more favorable the prognosis. However, this still must be guarded, for at the time of the injury the displacement of the vertebral canal may have

been complete, with the involved vertebrae returning to a position of partial displacement. In addition, the examiner cannot determine clinically whether the damage is contusion or laceration. Functional and organic neurologic deficit cannot be differentiated.

Recovery from concussion occurs spontaneously within a few minutes of the time of the accident. Recovery from contusion caused by compression may be enhanced by laminectomy at the site of the vertebral column injury.[6, 8, 40, 51] Some advocate a midline myelotomy if spinal cord swelling is evident.[28] This should be performed as soon as possible after the diagnosis has been made. The prognosis is more favorable if there are any indications of the functioning of tracts that pass through the site of the lesion, such as voluntary movement of a pelvic limb, tail wagging in response to the examiner, or the perception of pain.

These focal lesions can occur from traumatic rupture of an intervertebral disk, which is diagnosed as a narrow space between adjacent vertebrae. In some instances, there is no lesion in the vertebral column to associate with the focal lesion in the spinal cord. In the absence of localizing vertebral column injury, a myelogram is recommended in order to diagnose if there is significant spinal cord swelling to warrant laminectomy and incision of the dura at the site of the swelling.

Medical therapy for the injured spinal cord should include high doses of corticosteroids and possibly hypertonic fluids, as indicated for the injured brain.[18] These should be administered immediately, followed by surgery if it is indicated. It is essential that following a severe injury surgery be performed at once. The longer the delay the less efficacious is the decompression.

Cervical Spinal Cord

Injuries to the spinal cord from the sixth cervical to the second thoracic segments cause tetraparesis or tetraplegia, with depressed spinal reflexes from the thoracic limbs and hyperactive spinal reflexes from the pelvic limbs. Horner's syndrome (miosis, protruded third eyelid, smaller palpebral fissure, and enophthalmos) occurs with lesions in the first three thoracic segments. Injuries cranial to the sixth cervical segment cause spastic tetraparesis or tetraplegia with hyperactive reflexes in all four limbs. If the injury is severe, Horner's syndrome and respiratory difficulty occur. Death occurs from respiratory failure. The patient should be assessed for respiratory function and this should be supplemented if necessary.

The rationale for medical and surgical therapy is similar to that for the thoracic and lumbar areas. Be aware that significant displacement may accompany fractures of the atlas or axis or both, and the patient may still be ambulatory. These dogs must be handled with extreme care. Neurologic signs can be expected to be worse following anesthesia for radiography or surgery, but this is temporary if the surgeon has been careful.[50]

Penetrating injuries to the spinal cord are uncommon in domestic animals. Gunshot wounds occasionally occur, and cause varying degrees of neurologic deficit. If one side of the spinal cord is injured, paresis or paralysis is found in the limb or limbs on the same side as the lesion. There is no obvious loss of sensation caudal to the lesion because the ascending sensory pathways for pain are located bilaterally. In all patients the foreign material should be removed, and antibiotics should be administered.

In any patient with injury to the nervous system, it is important to ascertain how the animal performed at the site of the accident. The spinal cord and peripheral nerves may be subject to complete transection by injuries. Therefore, it is helpful to know whether the signs of loss of neurologic function occurred immediately or over a period of a few minutes to hours. If a period of time elapsed between the injury and the onset of signs, an anatomic transection did not occur.

When examining an injured dog that is not in shock and has no obvious life-threatening lesions but shows the typical signs of the Schiff-Sherrington syndrome, it is easy to overlook injury to the body cavities in the haste to diagnose the location of the spinal cord lesion. A diaphragmatic hernia may be overlooked and become life-threatening during or following surgery for the spinal cord lesion.

PERIPHERAL NERVOUS SYSTEM

Injuries of peripheral nerves are also described in Chapter 4.

THORACIC LIMB

Radial Nerve

The radial nerve innervates all the extensors of the elbow, carpus, and digits. The elbow extensors (triceps brachii) are innervated at the proximal end of the humerus. These muscles must function for the animal to support its weight normally on the thoracic limb. The carpal and digital extensors are innervated at the proximal end of the radius and ulna. The radial nerve supplies sensory innervation to the cranial and lateral surface of the forearm and dorsal surface of the forepaw.

Injuries to the radial nerve at the level of the elbow usually are associated with fractures of the humerus. The animal cannot extend its carpus and digits, and walks supporting its weight on the dorsal surface of the paw. Hypalgesia or analgesia occurs in the autonomous zone of the sensory distribution of the nerve (Fig. 9–4).

With injuries to the radial nerve medial to the shoulder or more proximally, the patient is unable to support its weight on that limb because of inability to extend the elbow. In addition, the carpus and digits cannot be extended, and hypalgesia or analgesia occurs in the sensory distribution of the nerve. These rarely take place alone at this site. More commonly, the injury is a root avulsion.

Brachial Plexus—Roots of C6–T2[17]

Although the signs that appear following injuries to the brachial plexus or its roots of origin are predominantly those of radial nerve paralysis at the level of the shoulder, there are frequently deficits of other peripheral nerves that leave the brachial plexus. If the musculocutaneous nerve is injured, the limb will be dragged along the floor because of inability to flex the elbow. If the axillary and/or thoracodorsal nerves that innervate the flexors of the shoulder are injured, the elbow will be dropped. Injury to the median and ulnar nerves that innervate the carpal and digital flexors can be determined only by observing failure to flex these joints on testing the flexor reflex, or analgesia in the autonomous zone of their sensory distribution, including the caudal surface of the forearm and the palmar and lateral surfaces of the forepaw. The thoracic limb flexor reflex requires the function of the muscles innervated by the axillary and radial (shoulder flexors), musculocutaneous (elbow flexors), and median and ulnar (carpal and digital flexors) nerves. Careful observation of this reflex may reveal deficits of one or more of its components.

Multiple peripheral nerve involvement is usually caused by contusion or avulsion of the roots of the brachial plexus. This is the most susceptible portion of the peripheral nerve to trauma. The degree of peripheral nerve injury depends on which roots are avulsed. The C8 and T1 roots are affected most commonly, and present as radial, median, and ulnar paralyses. Avulsion of C6 and C7 is reflected as a musculocutaneous, suprascapular, and sometimes axillary nerve paralysis. Usually when most of these roots are avulsed the line of analgesia is at the level of the elbow. Avulsion of ventral roots with sparing of dorsal roots may account for some obvious disparities in motor and sensory deficits. Ipsilateral Horner's syndrome may accompany root avulsions that involve the first two or three thoracic spinal nerves.

Contusion of the brachial plexus medial to the shoulder is rarely by itself the primary site of injury producing the neurologic deficit in the limb.

There is no specific therapy for these avulsions. The torn ends of the rootlets are widely separated and extremely delicate to handle. At least 2 to 3 weeks should be allowed for recovery from contusion without avulsion or laceration. Following this amputation should be considered. Tendon transplantation and arthrodesis of carpus or both carpus and elbow have been recommended in selected cases. The results are not always satisfactory and depend on careful presurgical neurologic evaluation of the patient.[5, 15, 21]

PELVIC LIMB

The sciatic nerve (L6, L7, S1) innervates the caudal thigh muscles (biceps femoris, semimembranosus, and semitendinosus), which are concerned primarily with stifle flexion and extension and hip extension. The tibial nerve from the sciatic innervates the caudal leg muscles (gastrocnemius, and superficial and deep digital flexors), which extend the tarsus and flex the digits. Its sensory distribution is to the caudal surface of the leg and plantar surface of the paw. The peroneal nerve from the sciatic innervates the cranial leg muscles (cranial tibial, long digital extensor, and peroneus longus) that flex the tarsus and extend the digits. Its sensory distribution is to the cranial and lateral surfaces of the leg and the dorsal surface of the paw.

The femoral nerve (L4, L5, L6) innervates part of the iliopsoas muscle, which is a flexor of the hip, and all of the quadriceps muscle, which is an extensor of the stifle and is necessary for the animal to support weight on its pelvic limb. The saphenous branch of the femoral nerve is sensory to the medial side of the thigh, leg, and paw.

The complete flexor reflex in the pelvic limb requires the innervation of the hip flexors (iliopsoas, rectus femoris, sartorius, and tensor fascia lata) by the lumbar spinal nerves 2 to 4, femoral, saphenous, and cranial gluteal nerves; the sciatic nerve innervation of the flexors of the stifle; the peroneal nerve innervation of the tarsal flexors; and the tibial nerve innervation of the digital flexors.

Sciatic Nerve

The sciatic nerve is most commonly injured at the place that it crosses the greater ischiatic notch of the ilium, where it may be involved in a pelvic fracture, and in the caudal thigh, where displaced femoral fractures may affect it. It is also subject to injury by hypodermic injections into the caudal thigh muscles. The prognosis for recovery depends on the nature of the material injected and whether or not it directly entered the nerve.

Sacroiliac luxations may severely contuse the roots that compose the sciatic nerve. The L6 and L7 roots both pass on the ventral surface of the sacrum medial to this articulation, where they are subject to injury.

An animal can have a lacerated sciatic nerve, and still perceive pain from a stimulus to the second digit and withdraw the pelvic limb from the stimulus by flexion of the hip. This occurs because of the saphenous nerve innervation to the medial side of the paw, and the intact innervation to the flexors of the hip. No action is seen in the tarsus and digits. Partial stifle flexion may occur owing to the function of the gracilis (obturator nerve) and caudal part of the sartorius (femoral nerve). Muscle tone should be palpated during this procedure to help evaluate the nerve injury.

When presented with an animal with obvious musculoskeletal injury in an area closely associated with one of the peripheral nerves described, the first responsibility following the treatment of shock, hemorrhage, and other life-threatening injuries is to evaluate the nervous system. The presence of the musculoskeletal injury may prevent evaluation of motor function. Sensory examination determines if the nerve is functioning, and may determine a partial deficit. A failure of response on the part of the peripheral nervous system does not determine if a nerve has been lacerated by the contusion.

If no response is obtained, a number of alternatives remain to determine if the nerve is lacerated. The nerve may be explored simultaneously with the surgical repair of the skeletal injury, or as a separate procedure. Another alternative is to wait 3 to 4 days and stimulate the nerve using an electromyographic unit or an ordinary dry cell battery connected to two hypodermic needles that can be inserted in the vicinity of the nerve.[1, 7] This is done between the site of the injury and one or more of the muscles innervated by the nerve. If the nerve has been lacerated, Wallerian degeneration will have occurred in the distal segment, and the nerve will be unable to conduct an impulse. If the nerve is bruised but anatomically intact, response in the muscles should be seen following the stimulus. Because a nerve may be proved to be functional does not necessarily mean that it will return to complete function once the contusion is reduced. There may be partial laceration or disruption of nerve fibers. Physiologic testing does not readily allow quantitation of partial nerve disruption.

At least 2 to 3 weeks should be allowed for recovery of nerve function in contused nerves. The disrupted ends of lacerated nerves should be apposed and sutured.[27] Regeneration occurs at best at the rate of 1 to 4 mm per day. Measurement from the site of the injury to the site of muscle innervation provides an estimate of the time necessary for regeneration.

Lumbar, Sacral, and Caudal Roots

The lumbar, sacral, and caudal spinal nerves and their roots are injured by fractures of the associated vertebrae. Injury to the roots of the spinal nerves L6, L7, and S1 appears as a sciatic nerve paralysis. Injury to the roots of spinal nerves S1, S2, and S3 causes inability to close the anus, analgesia of the anus and perineal region, and distention of the bladder and rectum. Injury to caudal nerves causes analgesia of and inability to move the tail. The level of the vertebral fracture and displacement determines the degree of neurologic deficit.

In most patients these roots and spinal nerves are not lacerated but are severely contused and often compressed by displacement of the vertebral canal. If the displacement cannot be corrected, a laminectomy should be done to free the involved roots. Spinal nerve roots are part of the peripheral nervous system and are subject to the same principles of healing and regeneration.

REFERENCES

1. Allam, M. W., Nulsen, F. E., and Lewey, F. H.: Electrical intraneural bipolar stimulation of peripheral nerves in the dog. J. Am. Vet. Med. Assoc., *114*:87, 1949.
2. Averill, D. R., Jr.: Intracranial injuries. *In* Kirk, R. W. (ed.): Current Veterinary Therapy. IV. Philadelphia, W. B. Saunders Co., 1971.
3. Ballinger, W. F., Rutherford, R. B., and Zuidema, G. D.: The Management of Trauma. 2nd ed. Philadelphia, W. B. Saunders Co., 1973.
4. Belopavlovic, M., and Buchthal, A.: Barbiturate therapy in the management of cerebral ischemia. Anesthesiology, *35*:271, 1980.
5. Bennett, D., and Vaughan, L. C.: The use of muscle relocation techniques in the treatment of peripheral nerve injuries in dogs and cats. J. Small Anim. Pract., *17*:99, 1976.
6. Brasmer, T. H.: Evaluation and therapy of spinal cord trauma. *In* Kirk, R. W. (ed.): Current Veterinary Therapy V. Philadelphia, W. B. Saunders Co., 1975.
7. Chrisman, C. L., Burt, J. K., Wood, P. K., and Johnson, E. W.: Electromyography in small animal clinical neurology. J. Am. Vet. Med. Assoc., *160*:311, 1972.
8. Committee on Trauma, American College of Surgeons: The Management of Fractures and Soft Tissue Injuries. Philadelphia, W. B. Saunders Co., 1960.
9. Cooper, P. R., Moody, S., Clark, W. K., Kirkpatrick, J., Maravilla, K., Gould, A. L., and Drane, W.: Dexamethasone and severe head injury: A prospective double blind study. J. Neurosurg., *51*:307, 1979.
10. de la Torre, J. C., Johnson, C. M., Goode, D. J., and Mullan, S.: Pharmacologic treatment and evaluation of permanent experimental spinal cord trauma. Neurology, *25*:508, 1975.
11. de la Torre, J. C., Kawanaga, H. M., Rowed, D. W., Johnson, C. M., Goode, D. J., Kajihara, K., and Mullan, S.: Dimethyl sulfoxide in central nervous system trauma. Ann. N.Y. Acad. Sci., *243*:362, 1975.
12. Ducker, T. B., and Hamit, H. F.: Experimental treatments of acute spinal cord injury. J. Neurosurg., *30*:693, 1969.
13. Fenner, W.: Head trauma and nervous system injury. *In* Kirk, R. W. (ed.): Current Veterinary Therapy VIII: Small Animal Practice. Philadelphia, W. B. Saunders Co., in press.
14. Fishman, R. A.: Brain edema. N. Engl. J. Med., *293*:706, 1975.
15. Frost, W. W., and Lumb, W. V.: Radiocarpal arthrodesis: A surgical approach to brachial paralysis. J. Am. Vet. Med. Assoc., *149*:1073, 1966.
16. Greene, G. C.: An experimental model of spinal cord compression simulating intervertebral disk disease in the dog. Master's Thesis, Auburn University, 1976.
17. Griffiths, I. R.: Avulsion of the brachial plexus in the dog. *In* Kirk, R. W. (ed.): Current Veterinary Therapy VI. Philadelphia, W. B. Saunders Co., 1977.

18. Griffiths, I. R.: Vasogenic edema following acute and chronic spinal cord compression in the dog. J. Neurosurg., 42:155, 1975.
19. Hoerlein, B. F.: Canine Neurology. 2nd ed. Philadelphia, W. B. Saunders Co., 1971.
20. Hooshmand, H., Dove, J., Houff, S., and Suter, C.: Effects of diuretics and steroids on CSF pressure. Arch. Neurol., 21:499, 1969.
21. Hussain, S., and Pettit, G. D.: Tendon transplantation to compensate for radial nerve paralysis. Am. J. Vet. Res., 28:336, 1967.
22. Kirk, R. W., and Bistner, S. I.: Handbook of Veterinary Procedures and Emergency Treatment. 2nd ed. Philadelphia, W. B. Saunders Co., 1975.
23. Knecht, C. D.: Considerations for medical treatment of spinal cord injury. In Kirk, R. W. (ed.): Current Veterinary Therapy VIII. Small Animal Practice. Philadelphia, W. B. Saunders Co., in press.
24. Leonard, J. L., and Redding, R. W.: Effects of hypertonic solutions on cerebrospinal fluid pressure in the lateral ventricle of the dog. Am. J. Vet. Res., 34:213, 1973.
25. Marshall, L. F., Smith, R. W., Rauscher, L. A., and Shapiro, H. M.: Mannitol dose requirements in brain-injured patients. J. Neurosurg., 48:169, 1978.
26. Martin, D. B.: Intensive care of the shock patient. Gaines Vet. Symp., 19:27, 1969.
27. Martin, S. H., and Bloedel, J. R.: Evaluation of experimental spinal cord injury using cortical evoked potentials. J. Neurosurg., 39:75, 1973.
28. Mendenhall, H. V., Litwah, P., Hurraspe, D. J., Ingram, J. T., and Lumb, W. V.: Aggressive pharmacologic and surgical treatment of spinal cord injuries in dogs and cats. J. Am. Vet. Med. Assoc., 168:1026, 1976.
29. Miller, J. D., and Leech, P.: Effects of mannitol and steroid therapy on intracranial volume-pressure relationships in patients. J. Neurosurg., 42:274, 1975.
30. Oliver, J. E.: Intracranial injury. In Kirk, R. W. (ed.): Current Veterinary Therapy VII: Small Animal Practice. Philadelphia, W. B. Saunders Co., 1980.
31. Oliver, J. E., Jr.: Management of the patient with acute head injury. Gaines Vet. Symp., 19:22, 1969.
32. Oliver, J. E., Jr.: Surgical approaches to the canine brain. Am. J. Vet. Res., 29:353, 1968.
33. Oliver, J. E., Jr.: Intracranial injury. In Kirk, R. W. (ed.): Current Veterinary Therapy VI. Philadelphia, W. B. Saunders Co., 1977.
34. Osterholm, J. L.: The pathophysiological response to spinal cord injury. J. Neurosurg., 40:5, 1974.
35. Palmer, A. C.: The accident case. IV. The significance and estimation of damage to the central nervous system. J. Small Anim. Pract., 5:25, 1964.
36. Parker, A. J.: Blood pressure changes and lethality of mannitol infusions in dogs. Am. J. Vet. Res., 34:1523, 1973.
37. Parker, A. J.: Some clinical dangers of mannitol therapy. J. Am. Anim. Hosp. Assoc., 10:175, 1974.
38. Parker, A. J., and Smith, C. W.: Lack of functional recovery from spinal cord trauma following dimethylsulphoxide and epsilon amino caproic acid therapy in dogs. Res. Vet. Sci., 27:253, 1979.
39. Parker, A. J., Park, R. D., and Stowater, J. L.: Traumatic occlusion of segmental spinal veins. Am. J. Vet. Res., 35:857, 1974.
40. Parker, A. J., and Smith, C. W.: Functional recovery from spinal cord trauma following incision of spinal meninges in dogs. Res. Vet. Sci., 16:276, 1974.
41. Parker, A. J., Marshall, A. E., and Sharp, J. G.: Study of the use of evoked cortical activity for clinical evaluation of spinal cord sensory transmission. Am. J. Vet. Res., 35:673, 1974.
42. Rucker, N. C., Lumb, W. V., and Scott, R. J.: Combined pharmacologic and surgical treatments for acute spinal cord trauma. Am. J. Vet. Res., 42:1138, 1981.
43. Sahar, A., and Tsipstein, E.: Effects of mannitol and furosemide on the rate of formation of cerebrospinal fluid. Exp. Neurol., 60:584, 1978.
44. Sato, O., Hara, M., Asai, T., Tsugane, R., and Kageyama, N.: The effect of dexamethasone phosphate on the production rate of cerebrospinal fluid in the spinal subarachnoid space of dogs. J. Neurosurg., 39:480, 1973.
45. Shenkin, H. A., and Bouzarth, W. F.: Clinical methods of reducing intracranial pressure. N. Engl. J. Med., 282:1465, 1970.
46. Sims, M. H., and Redding, R. W.: The use of dexamethasone in the prevention of cerebral edema in dogs. J. Am. Anim. Hosp. Assoc., 11:439, 1975.
47. Sims, M. H., and Redding, R. W.: The use of dexamethasone in the prevention of cerebral edema in dogs. J. Am. Anim. Hosp. Assoc., 11:439, 1975.
48. Swaim, S. F.: Peripheral nerve surgery in the dog. J. Am. Vet. Med. Assoc., 161:905. 1972.
49. Tornheim, P. A., and McLaurin, R. L.: Effect of dexamethasone on cerebral edema from cranial impact in the cat. J. Neurosurg., 48:220, 1978.
50. Trotter, E. J.: Surgical repair of fractured atlas in a dog. J. Am. Vet. Med. Assoc., 161:303, 1972.
51. Trotter, E. J.: Canine intervertebral disc disease. In Kirk, R. W. (ed.): Current Veterinary Therapy V. Philadelphia, W. B. Saunders Co., 1975.
52. Vise, W. M., Yaston, D., and Hunt, W. E.: Mechanisms of norepinephrine accumulation within sites of spinal cord injury. J. Neurosurg., 40:76, 1974.

SMALL ANIMAL NEUROLOGIC EXAMINATION AND INDEX OF DISEASES OF THE NERVOUS SYSTEM

SMALL ANIMAL EXAMINATION

Examination of a patient with a complaint of a neurologic disorder should include review of the history, complete general physical examination, neurologic examination, and appropriate ancillary procedures. The neurologic examination should determine the presence of nervous system lesion(s) and establish the location of the lesion(s) in the nervous system. This is the anatomic diagnosis. Utilization of a routine procedure will provide the examiner with the experience and confidence to make an accurate anatomic diagnosis.

The differential diagnosis will be based on the anatomic diagnosis and the evaluation of the signalment and history. The five major kinds of lesions should be considered: malformation, inflammation, neoplasia, degeneration, and injury. Experience with the specific distribution of lesions that occur in certain disease entities will often lead to a presumptive diagnosis. Further evaluation of the patient with ancillary procedures to determine the cause or to confirm the anatomic diagnosis will depend on the differential diagnosis that is established.

Results of the neurologic examination should always be carefully recorded and not left to memory. Subtle changes may alter the prognosis and course of therapy.

SIGNALMENT

The signalment of the patient provides the examiner with the age, sex, breed, and use of the patient. When considered together with the chief complaint, it may help direct the line of questioning in taking the history. For example, patients less than 1 year old that are presented for seizures are more likely to have an inflammatory than a neoplastic disease. Lead poisoning is more common in dogs less than 1 year of age. Toy breeds with functional hypoglycemia usually have seizures when they are less than 6 months old. Hypoglycemic convulsions caused by functional neoplasms of pancreatic beta cells rarely are seen before 4 years of age. Idiopathic epilepsy often begins between 1 and 3 years of age. Neoplastic disease of the nervous system usually occurs in the older patient, except for lymphosarcoma in cats, neurofibromas, and a spinal cord neuroepithelioma in dogs, which are not limited by age.

The sex of the patient is an important consideration because mammary gland adenocarcinomas of the female rank high among the more common neoplasms that metastasize to the brain. Estrus may lower the seizure threshold in some individuals prone to idiopathic epilepsy.

Of the various breeds, the brachycephalic breeds are more prone to primary brain neoplasms. Although any breed of dog including mixed breeds can develop idiopathic epilepsy, it is most common in miniature poodles, followed by a high incidence in German shepherds, Saint Bernards, and beagles. There are probably few if any breeds in which this disease has not been reported. Any list of incidence by breed probably will vary according to the location from which it is reported. Although the incidence is much lower, there is a predilection by breed for the degenerative diseases of the nervous system that have been recognized and may be inherited. These include globoid cell leukodystrophy in Cairn and West Highland white terriers, a lipodystrophy in German short-haired pointers and English setters, and a diffuse neuronal abiotrophy that presents as cerebellar disease in Kerry blue terriers. Cerebellar cortical abiotrophy is inherited in Gordon setters and the rough-coated collie. Hyperkinetic episodes, the so-called "Scotty cramps," occur in Scottish terriers. Congenital deafness may be familial in Old English sheepdogs and dalmatians. Some puppies of toy breeds and breeds that hunt have abnormalities in glucose metabolism that cause episodic weakness, collapse, or convulsions.

Although there are many causes of weakness and ataxia in the pelvic limbs, intervertebral disk protusion rarely occurs before 1 year of age in chondrodystrophic breeds and only occasionally before 5 years in the larger breeds. Young Afghan hounds have an hereditary necrosis of spinal cord white matter. Cervical vertebral malformation occurs in young Basset hounds from C2 to C4 and in young or adult Great Danes and Doberman pinschers from C5 to C7. Older German shepherds have a high incidence of degenerative myelopathy.

HISTORY

The line of questioning followed in taking the history of the patient depends on the chief complaint. In all cases the review should include a summary of the past medical and surgical history unrelated in time to the present complaint.

If the chief complaint is an injury, the questioning will focus on the authenticity of the trauma, when it occurred, when the signs first appeared, and how they have changed to the present time. By 24 hours after an injury the signs usually remain static or improve. Progressive neurologic signs usually are not due to a single episode of trauma.

When a dog presents with seizures, it is necessary to obtain as thorough a description of the seizure as possible in order to be certain of its authenticity and to attempt to determine the kind of seizure. The majority of seizures seen in veterinary medicine are generalized (grand mal) seizures. This is the type that occurs with idiopathic epilepsy, intoxications, and many diseases of the prosencephalon with structural lesions. Psychomotor seizures are more common in cases of lead poisoning and diseases of the limbic system. Descriptions of these seizures often include activities of the patient that could be described as bizarre behavior or hysteria prior to the generalized seizure. Partial motor seizures may occur with or without confusion but with no loss of consciousness. These may be characterized by episodic muscular activity limited to a small group of muscles such as the eyelids, lips, all facial muscles, muscles of mastication, or part or all of the musculature of one limb or both limbs on one side of the body. The consistent onset of partial seizures in one muscle area may be associated with a focal brain lesion in the contralateral motor cortex. Only rarely do these partial seizures in dogs slowly spread from the initial muscle group to a wider area of the body in a specific pattern (Jacksonian seizure). Partial seizures involving more of a behavioral abnormality occur with limbic system seizure foci. A careful description of a dog that is "collapsing" may help distinguish a seizure disorder from narcolepsy–cataplexy, or syncope from a cardiac lesion.

The history of patients presented with signs of progressive neurologic disease should include careful documentation of each sign the patient has shown, in order to help determine whether the lesion is focal or disseminated in the nervous system. For example, a patient that first showed paresis (weakness) and ataxia of the pelvic limbs that progressed to complete paraplegia and then developed a head tremor, head tilt, and abnormal nystagmus necessarily has lesions in more than one location to explain the signs. A progressive thoracolumbar spinal cord lesion and a lesion in the cerebellomedullary region of the brain would account for these signs. Such a multifocal distribution of lesions is characteristic of an inflammatory lesion such as the encephalomyelitis caused by the canine distemper virus or toxoplasmosis, or cryptococcosis in dogs and cats. The signs of inflammatory disease usually progress faster than those of the familial degenerative diseases. A neurofibroma of a spinal nerve of the brachial plexus that invades the vertebral canal through an intervertebral foramen and compresses the spinal cord often first causes an undiagnosed lameness in the affected thoracic limb, followed by lower motor neuron paresis of that limb with neurogenic muscular atrophy. Following invasion of the vertebral canal by the neoplasm and compression of the spinal cord, a spastic paresis and ataxia appear in the ipsilateral pelvic limb. This is followed by tetraparesis and tetraplegia with hyperreflexia, and spasticity of the pelvic limbs and depressed reflexes in the thoracic limbs. In some instances of what seems to be a sudden onset of disease, thorough questioning of the owner may elicit previous signs that indicate a progressive disorder. As a rule signs that are precipitous in onset and not progressive are due to injury or loss of vascular integrity. The latter is exemplified by the ischemic or hemorrhagic myelopathy associated with fibrocartilaginous emboli. Be aware that neoplastic disease may produce rapidly progressive signs with a fairly sudden onset.

In the young animal, malformation or diseases acquired in utero must be considered, and the patient's history should document whether the signs were present from birth or as soon as the patient was ambulatory enough for the signs to be recognized. This is particularly important in patients with signs of cerebellar disease. In the cat, the panleukopenia virus induces a cerebellar degeneration in the fetus or neonate. The signs when the patient is ambulatory are nonprogressive. A nonprogressive cellular degeneration or malformation of unknown cause may occur in utero in the dog. Herpesvirus may cause cerebellar degeneration in the first 2 weeks of life in the dog. Progressive cerebellar signs commencing around 3 months of age may be the onset of a diffuse inflammatory disease such as canine distemper encephalitis or a progressive cerebellar degeneration. In Kerry blue terriers a diffuse neuronal abiotrophy begins in the Purkinje cells of the cerebellum and causes a cerebellar ataxia, usually around 10 to 12 weeks of age. There is evidence for an hereditary basis for this disease. The signs of globoid cell leukodystropy in Cairn and West Highland white terriers usually begin between 3 and 6 months of age. These often include cerebellar in addition to spinal cord signs.

If intoxication is suspected, a thorough search should be carried out to find a possible source of the intoxicant. Lead may be considered from lead-based paints, linoleum, tarpaper, and batteries. Many insecticides contain chlorinated hydrocarbons that can cause generalized myoclonus or generalized seizures. Others contain organic phosphates that can cause myoclonic activity, or seizures, or both, in addition to salivation, vomiting, diarrhea, and initially miosis. Dial soap contains hexachlorophene, which can produce seizures, stupor, or coma. Ethylene glycol (antifreeze) may produce similar signs following a brief period of ataxia.

A history of progressive seizures with increasingly shorter interictal periods is typical of neoplasia of the prosencephalon. The review should include a previous history of the diagnosis of neoplasia in other systems of the body.

GENERAL PHYSICAL EXAMINATION

In all patients in which a neurologic examination is indicated, it should be preceded by a thorough general physical examination of all other body systems. Some inflammatory diseases of the nervous system also affect other organ systems. Seizures may occur in patients with extensive liver or kidney disease or functional pancreatic islet neoplasms. Primary disease of other systems may be manifested by episodes of weakness or collapse. Examples include hypoglycemia, cardiorespiratory diseases, and hypoadrenocorticoidism. Musculoskeletal diseases often are confused with neurologic disease.

NEUROLOGIC EXAMINATION[7, 16-18]

The neurologic examination can be divided into five parts: mental attitude-behavior, gait, postural reactions, spinal nerves, and cranial nerves. In this description an intact reflex only requires the function of the peripheral nerves being tested and the segments of the spinal cord or brain stem in which the afferent axon enters and the cell bodies and axons of the efferent neurons are located. A reaction depends on the same components as the reflex, plus the ascending pathways through the white matter of the spinal cord and brain stem to the cerebellum and sensorimotor cortex of the cerebrum, and the descending pathways that return from the cerebrum by way of its internal capsule, and the white matter of the brain stem and spinal cord. The lower motor neuron has its cell body and dendritic zone in the ventral grey column of the spinal cord or specific cranial nerve nucleus in the brain stem. Its axon leaves the central nervous system and courses through peripheral nerves to its telodendron in the group of muscle fibers it innervates. The upper motor neurons have cell bodies and dendritic zones in collections of grey matter in the cerebrum (motor cerebral cortex) or brain stem (red nucleus, reticular nuclei). Their axons descend in tracts through the white matter in the brain and spinal cord to end in telodendria in the vicinity of the lower motor neuron that they ultimately influence.

The precise order in which the parts of a neurologic examination are performed varies with the preference of the examiner and the attitude of the patient. An initial assessment should be made of the patient's mental attitude and behavior. If the patient is resting quietly in a cage at the time of examination, the cranial nerve examination may be done first. If the patient is excited or apprehensive, it may be more convenient to perform the cranial nerve examination after the patient has been handled during the examinations of gait, postural reactions, and reflexes.

Mental Attitude-Behavior

An assessment should be made of the patient's mental attitude, sensorium, or behavior. The owner is usually the best judge of the subtle changes in the patient's behavior and should be questioned about this. Is the patient bright, alert, and responsive on your first approach and throughout the examination? The various terms that characterize alterations of this attitude and behavior are depression, lethargy, unresponsiveness, stupor, coma, anxiety, disorientation, hyperactivity, hysteria, propulsion, and aggression.

As a rule, these alterations in the animal's normal sensorium reflect disturbances in the diencephalon and telencephalon and often implicate some portion of the limbic system. It is especially important to evaluate these carefully in the recumbent patient. Cervical spinal cord disease that produces recumbency will not alter the patient's mental attitude except that some animals may become frantic and hyperexcitable if they are unable to get up. The same degree of tetraplegia can occur with a brain stem lesion that severely alters the patient's responsiveness to its environment.

Gait

Examination of the gait should be done in a place where the patient may be allowed to move freely, unleashed, and the ground surface is not slippery. The floor of many examining rooms is too slippery for adequate evaluation of the patient's gait. In some patients with vertebral column injury with spinal cord contusion resulting in paresis and ataxia, moving the patient on a slippery floor may cause a fall, and further injury may result. A carpeted room is ideal.

The degree of functional deficit dictates the necessity for further examination of strength and coordination. A patient that is tetraplegic—unable to support its weight or move its limbs when the weight is borne on them—need not have further tests performed for the postural reactions. A grade 0 paraplegic patient need not be examined for postural reactions in the pelvic limbs, but the thoracic limbs should be examined carefully. Occasionally, a patient with progressive myelitis may present as paraplegic because of an extensive thoracolumbar spinal cord location of the lesion but also have an asymmetric thoracic limb gait because of a less severe focus of the lesion in the cervical spinal cord. An early sign in dogs with ascending myelomalacia associated with an acute intervertebral disk extrusion may be a hesitant, stumbling, awkward gait in the thoracic limbs. The severity of advanced pelvic limb weakness is evaluated best by holding the patient suspended at the base of the tail and observing its gait. The degree of pelvic limb strength and coordination present following a thoracolumbar spinal cord lesion may be graded according to the following scheme:

  5—Normal strength and coordination
  4—Can stand to support; *minimal paraparesis and ataxia*
  3—Can stand to support but frequently stumbles and falls; *mild paraparesis and ataxia*
  2—Unable to stand to support; when assisted, moves limbs readily but stumbles and falls frequently; *moderate paraparesis and ataxia*
  1—Unable to stand to support; slight movement when supported by the tail; *severe paraparesis*
  0—Absence of purposeful movement; *paraplegia*

Postural Reactions

Following observation of the gait for strength and coordination, the postural reactions can be tested especially to determine if there are less obvious deficits in strength and coordination when the gait appears to be normal. Each of these requires that all major components of the peripheral and central nervous systems be intact. They are not of localizing value by themselves.

Wheelbarrowing. The thoracic limbs may be tested by supporting the patient under the abdomen so that the pelvic limbs are off the ground surface and forcing the patient to walk on its thoracic limbs. The normal animal walks with symmetric movements of both thoracic limbs and the head extended in normal position. Patients with lesions of the peripheral nerves of the thoracic limbs, cervical spinal cord, or brain stem may have asymmetric movements, with stumbling or knuckling over on the dorsum of the paw of the affected limb. Hypermetria occasionally is observed. With more severe lesions in this area, there is a tendency to carry the head flexed with the nose close to and occasionally reaching the ground surface for support. If no deficit is observed, extend the neck while the animal is wheelbarrowed. This sometimes reveals a mild deficit, a tendency to knuckle over on the dorsum of the paw, which was not observed before. This may be helpful to confirm a cervical spinal cord lesion in Great Danes or Doberman pinschers that have a cervical vertebral malformation and show mild pelvic limb paresis and ataxia, but no overt thoracic limb signs.

Hopping—Thoracic Limb. While still supporting the pelvic limbs, hop the animal on one thoracic limb while holding the other off the ground surface so that the entire weight of the body is supported by the limb to be tested. Move the dog forward and to each side but especially laterally, and observe the strength and coordination of the limb. Repeat this on the other thoracic limb and compare the response. Asymmetry occurs with paresis or ataxia. Hypermetria may be seen with general proprioceptive or cerebellar deficits. This is an effective way of determining minor deficits when the gait appears to be normal, as occurs with contralateral cerebral sensorimotor cortex lesions.

Extensor Postural Thrust. The same sequence of tests can be done on the pelvic limbs. The extensor postural thrust reaction is performed by holding the patient off the ground surface by supporting it caudal to the scapulae, lowering it to the ground surface, and observing the patient extend its pelvic limbs to support its weight. Moving the patient forward and backward in this position tests the symmetry of pelvic limb function, strength, and coordination.

Hopping—Pelvic Limb. Continuing to support the patient by the thorax so that the thoracic limbs are not in contact with the ground surface, one pelvic limb can be held up and the patient forced to hop laterally or forward on the supporting limb. Both pelvic limbs should be tested this way and the responses compared. It is important to compare the pelvic limb hopping responses with each other and not the ipsilateral thoracic limb. Normally the hopping response of the pelvic limb seems more stiff or hypertonic, with a slightly larger excursion than that of the thoracic limb.

Hemistanding and Hemiwalking. The patient's ability to stand and walk with the thoracic and pelvic limbs on one side can be tested by holding the opposite thoracic and pelvic limbs off the ground surface and forcing the patient to walk forward or to the side. These are referred to as the hemistanding and hemiwalking reactions. With a large dog or uncooperative patient that resists hopping, you may be able to evaluate the hopping responses by observing the responses of the limbs during hemiwalking.

A patient with a unilateral lesion of the sensorimotor cortex or internal capsule may have a normal gait but show deficits in its postural reactions on the side opposite the lesion. Attempts to hemiwalk on the contralateral side are delayed and/or exaggerated (hypermetric) and spastic, and stumbling may occur. With unilateral cervical spinal cord lesions, the limbs on the same side as the lesion show a deficiency in the gait and are unresponsive on postural reaction testing, including inability to support the animal in the hemiwalking reaction.

Placing. Other postural reactions that can be tested include placing with the thoracic limbs. The patient is supported off the ground surface and its thoracic limbs are brought to the edge of a table or similar surface so that the dorsal surface of the paws makes contact. This test should be performed on both thoracic limbs simultaneously and individually, with and without blindfolding the patient. Vision can compensate for the sense of position when the general proprioceptive system is abnormal.

Tonic Neck Reaction. The tonic neck reaction involves extension of the head and neck so that the nose is directed dorsally. The normal patient responds by extension of all the joints of both thoracic limbs. A patient with disease of the general proprioceptive system in the cervical spinal nerves, cervical spinal cord, or medulla fails to extend its carpus or digits or both, and these joints passively flex so that the weight is borne on the dorsal surface of the paw. The same response may occur if a patient is paretic either as a result of disease of the motor neurons that innervate the thoracic limb, or in the white matter of the spinal cord that influences these motor neurons.

Proprioceptive Positioning. Proprioceptive positioning tests this afferent system by determining the patient's ability to recognize when the paw has been flexed so that the weight is borne on its dorsal surface. The normal animal returns the paw to its usual position. In patients with severe paresis, this test may also be deficient.

Spinal Nerves

Spinal nerve evaluation includes assessment of muscle tone and size, spinal reflexes, and cutaneous sensation. Muscle tone and spinal reflexes are evaluated best when the patient is in lateral recumbency and as relaxed as possible. It is important to test muscle tone, tendon reflexes, and the flexor reflex to noxious stimuli, in that order, to maintain the cooperation of the patient.

Muscle Tone. Muscle tone is evaluated by passive manipulation of the limbs individually. The degree of resistance is determined to be less than normal (hypotonic), normal, or more than normal (hypertonic). The latter may be referred to as spasticity. The degree of spasticity varies from a mild increased resistance to passive manipulation, to a marked increase that may be "clasp knife" in character. It is referred to as "clasp knife" because as attempts are made to flex a limb, the degree of extension of the limb increases, until suddenly it gives way to complete flexion without resistance.

Hypotonia usually occurs with lower motor neuron disease, whereas upper motor neuron disease is characterized by hypertonia or spasticity. The functional integrity of the lower motor neuron is necessary to cause muscle cell contraction in order to maintain muscle tone. It is also necessary to maintain the normal health of the muscle cell it innervates. When

denervated, these cells degenerate. This is observed clinically as neurogenic atrophy and can be detected electromyographically by the production of abnormal potentials in resting muscle. The upper motor neuron influences the activity of the lower motor neuron to produce voluntary motor activity and to maintain muscle tone for support of the body against gravity. Although the upper motor neuron includes both facilitatory and inhibitory functions on the activity of the lower motor neuron, when the upper motor neuron is diseased the result usually observed is a release of the lower motor neuron from inhibition and overactivity of the facilitatory mechanism. This release is seen as hypertonia or spasticity.

Dogs that are tetraplegic should be held in a supporting position to observe the muscle tone in the limbs and any voluntary responses. Usually dogs with cervical spinal cord disease will have rigidly extended limbs, and the entire trunk and limbs will feel stiff when you hold the dog up and move the limbs along the ground surface. The hypertonia may be severe enough to permit the patient to stand unsupported. Tetraplegic dogs with diffuse neuromuscular diseases such as polyradiculoneuritis are hypotonic or atonic and appear and feel limp when you attempt to hold them in a supporting position. There is no reflex extension of the limb and no support elicited by placing the paws on the ground. Instead the limbs buckle under the weight of the body.

Patellar Reflexes. The most reliable tendon reflex is the patellar reflex. It is the only tendon reflex that is present in all normal animals. It is obtained by lightly tapping the patellar tendon with the patient in lateral recumbency and as relaxed as possible for proper evaluation. A pediatric neurologic hammer is the most useful instrument, but any hard object such as scissor handles can be used. The reflex can be elicited in all normal dogs and is mediated by the femoral nerve through the fourth to sixth lumbar spinal cord segments. The degree of normal response varies with the breed. Large breeds of dogs have a brisker reflex than the short-limbed breeds like the dachshund. The response should be evaluated as absent (0), hyporeflexic (+1), normal (+2), hyperreflexic (+3), or clonic (+4). This reflex should be tested with the patient lying on each side. An absent reflex or hyporeflexia occurs when there is disease of a portion of the reflex arc. Hyperreflexia or clonus is often present in upper motor neuron disease.

Biceps and Triceps Reflex. In the thoracic

limb, the biceps and triceps reflexes can be elicited in many dogs that are relaxed and in lateral recumbency. Lightly tapping the tendon of insertion of the triceps proximal to the olecranon elicits a slight extension of the elbow. The reflex is mediated by the radial nerve through the seventh and eighth cervical and first and second thoracic spinal cord segments. The biceps reflex is elicited by placing a finger on the distal ends of the biceps and brachialis muscles at the level of the elbow. Tapping this finger with the hammer elicits a slight flexion of the elbow. The muscle contraction can be palpated in some instances when no movement of the joint is seen. The musculocutaneous nerve mediates this reflex through the sixth, seventh, and eighth cervical spinal cord segments. The normal patient has a mild reflex response to these stimuli. In a few normal patients they are difficult to elicit. They are absent when there is disease of some portion of the reflex arc. They may be hyperactive in some patients with disease of the upper motor neuron.

See Chapter 10 for a discussion of other tendon reflexes.

Flexor Reflex—Pelvic Limb. The flexor reflexes to painful stimuli determine the integrity of the reflex arc as well as the pathway in the central nervous system that is concerned with the patient's response to painful stimuli. The most reliable stimulus is pressure exerted on the base of the toenail with hemostats. Many normal animals do not respond to the stimulus of a pin. In the pelvic limb, the flexor reflex is mediated by the sciatic nerve through the sixth and seventh lumbar spinal cord segments and the first sacral segment. Abnormality of the motor portion of the sciatic nerve distal to the pelvis causes paralysis, hypotonia, and atrophy of the flexors of the stifle, tarsus, and digits as well as of the extensors of the hip, tarsus and digits. There is no resistance to flexion or extension of the tarsus. On walking with a sciatic nerve paralysis, the tarsus is lower on the affected side and the paw may be placed on its dorsal surface; however, the limb is able to support weight as long as the femoral nerve is intact.

Sensory branches of the peroneal nerves supply the dorsal surface of the paw. The plantar surface is supplied by tibial nerve sensory branches. The medial side of the paw is supplied by the saphenous nerve, a branch of the femoral nerve at the femoral triangle. This enters the spinal cord through the fourth to sixth lumbar segments. A patient may have a contused sciatic nerve from a pelvic fracture and have no function of the muscles innervated by this nerve and analgesia of the lateral, dorsal, and plantar surfaces of the paw. However, the intact saphenous nerve provides sensation to the medial surface of the paw. If this area is stimulated the patient will flex the hip with the intact innervation of the iliopsoas muscle, but the stifle, tarsus, and digits fail to flex. For this reason both the medial and lateral surfaces of the paw should be tested for reflex responses as well as pain perception.

Pain Perception. The patient shows signs of pain when the impulses generated by a noxious stimulus have entered the spinal cord over the peripheral nerves and dorsal roots and are relayed to tracts in the lateral funiculi of the spinal cord bilaterally. These tracts ascend the spinal cord in the lateral funiculi, and continue through the medulla, pons, and mesencephalon to specific nuclei in the thalamus for relay to the somatic sensory cerebral cortex. Pain may be evidenced when the impulses reach the thalamus or cerebrum.

Flexor Reflex—Thoracic Limb. In the thoracic limb the thoracodorsal, axillary, musculocutaneous, median, ulnar, and radial nerves are responsible for flexion of the shoulder, elbow, carpus, and digits when a painful stimulus is applied to the paw. These arise from the sixth cervical to the second thoracic spinal cord segments. The specific sensory nerve stimulated depends on the location of the stimulus. The median and ulnar nerves innervate the skin of the palmar surface of the paw; the radial nerve supplies the dorsal surface. In the forearm the radial nerve supplies the skin on the cranial and lateral surfaces. The ulnar nerve supplies the caudal surface and the musculocutaneous nerve the medial surface. Be aware of the amount of overlap of the cutaneous innervation by these nerves (Fig. 9–4).

Crossed Extensor Reflex. In patients with upper motor neuron disease and release of the lower motor neuron, a crossed extensor reflex may be elicited in the recumbent animal when the flexor reflex is stimulated. This occurs in the limb opposite the one being tested for a flexor reflex. To avoid voluntary extension of the contralateral limb as a response to pain, the flexor reflex first should be elicited with as mild a stimulus as is necessary and the opposite limb observed for extension. When elicited in a patient in lateral recumbency this is an abnormal reflex, indicative of upper motor neuron disease.

Perineal Reflex. The perineal reflex is elicited by stimulating the anus with a noxious stimulus and observing contraction of the anal sphincter and flexion of the tail. It is mediated by branches of the sacral and caudal nerves through the sacral and caudal segments of the spinal cord.

Cutaneous Reflex. The cutaneous reflex is the contraction of the cutaneous trunci in response to mild stimulation of the skin of the trunk. It can be elicited from the thoracic and most of the lumbar region. The regional segmental spinal nerves contain the sensory neurons that are stimulated. The impulses are carried into the related spinal cord segments and then relayed through the white matter of the spinal cord cranially to the eighth cervical spinal cord segment. Here synapse occurs on lower motor neurons of the lateral thoracic nerve that innervate the cutaneous trunci. This reflex may require multiple stimulation to elicit, and occasionally normal dogs resist this stimulation and show no reflex. This reflex may be useful in diagnosing the level of a complete transverse thoracolumbar spinal cord lesion.

Cranial Nerves

The cranial nerve examination should be performed at the time that the patient is in the most cooperative attitude. The procedure for examining the cranial nerves is described here, with the specific cranial nerves being examined indicated in parentheses.

Observe the head for any evidence of a head tilt (vestibular VIII), facial muscle asymmetry from weakness or contracture-hemifacial spasm (VII), or atrophy of the muscles of mastication (motor V). Palpate these muscles for tone and atrophy. With one eye of the patient covered, menace the opposite eye with threatening gestures of the hand, being careful to avoid striking the patient or stimulating the hair with air currents (II-VII). Repeat this on the opposite side. If the response is absent, check the eyelids for ability to close (VII). Observe the symmetry of the pupils and their reaction to light in either eyeball (II–III). Observe the eyes for evidence of abnormal position, strabismus (III, IV, VI, vestibular VIII), or abnormal nystagmus (vestibular VIII). Move the head from side to side to generate normal vestibular nystagmus. This stimulates the vestibular nerve (VIII), and impulses pass through the vestibular nuclei (medulla) and medial longitudinal fasciculus (medulla-pons-midbrain) to abducent neurons

in the medulla for abduction and oculomotor neurons in the midbrain for adduction. Test the corneal and palpebral reflexes (sensory V–VII), ear movement (VII), and the position of the philtrum (VII). Examine the commissure of the lips for hypotonia that exposes mucosa and allows saliva to escape (VII). Check the skin sensation to blunt forceps from the corners of the eyelids (lateral angle-maxillary nerve V; medial angle-ophthalmic nerve V) and the mucosa of the nasal septum (ophthalmic nerve V). If further evaluation is necessary a pin can be used over the entire surface of the head. If evaluation is difficult and a deficit is suspected, the most sensitive area to test with a blunt object is the mucosa of the nasal septum inside each naris. Observe the jaws for normal closure (motor V). Open the mouth and observe whether resistance is normal (motor V). Observe the position of the tongue, its movements and size (atrophy), and pull on it to test its strength (XII). Check the gag reflex by probing the pharynx with a finger (IX, X).

Additional Tests: Visual. Additional tests may be performed for certain of the cranial nerves if an abnormality is suspected. If a visual deficit is suspected from the menace test, the patient should be walked through a maze once with the lights on and again with the lights off. After observing the patient without a blindfold, cover one eye and repeat the maneuver through the maze. Observe this for each eye. These tests for vision test not only the eyeball and second cranial nerve, but also the central visual pathway to the visual cerebral cortex. Because approximately 65 per cent (cat) to 75 per cent (dog) of the optic nerve axons cross in the optic chiasm, clinically a patient will show a unilateral blindness with an ipsilateral optic nerve lesion or a contralateral lesion in the optic tract, lateral geniculate nucleus, optic radiation, or visual cerebral cortex. The deficit is more complete with optic nerve lesions, and the pupil on the affected side may be more dilated than the pupil in the normal eyeball and unresponsive to light directed to the affected eyeball. The pupil in the blind eyeball will respond to light directed to the normal eyeball as long as the oculomotor nerve (III) is intact. With unilateral lesions in the central visual pathway from the optic tract to the visual cerebral cortex, pupillary function is normal. This occurs because some of the optic nerve axons concerned with pupillary control cross in the optic chiasm as well as in the pretectal area, so that impulses stimulated by light in one retina reach both oculomotor nuclei. Lesions in the central visual pathway from the optic tract caudally may only produce a deficient menace response in the eye on the opposite side and may not be detected when the patient walks around objects in a room, even with the normal eye covered. This is because there are optic nerve axons from the eyeball with the menace deficit that do not cross in the optic chiasm.

Disease of one optic nerve causes blindness in that eye with a normal or slightly dilated pupil and no response to light directed into that eye. Both pupils constrict to light placed in the opposite eye.

Disease of one oculomotor nerve causes a widely dilated pupil on that side that is unresponsive to light directed into either eyeball.

Cerebellar lesions may cause a failure of the menace response, but visual function and facial muscle function are normal in all other tests. These patients will have significant evidence of cerebellar disease in their posture and gait.

Additional Tests: Vestibular. For further examination of the vestibular system (vestibular VIII), the head should be held laterally over each shoulder with the exposed eyeball covered except for the limbus. Observe the eyeball for the development of a positional nystagmus. Make a similar observation with the head and neck extended and both eyeballs covered with the lower eyelids except for the limbus at the superior portion of the eyeball. In the normal patient no nystagmus develops and the corneas remain in the center of the palpebral fissure. In patients with unilateral disease of the vestibular system, the eye on the affected side is depressed and does not elevate into the center of the fissure, and nystagmus may be observed. The head should be moved from side to side and the normal vestibular nystagmus elicited should be observed. In bilateral peripheral vestibular disease or severe lesions in the brain stem, this response may be absent. This lack of normal eye movement offers a poor prognosis in animals with intracranial injury. In unilateral vestibular lesions the rapidity of the response may not be equal in both directions of head movement.

The nystagmus elicited by spinning the patient should be observed, and the rapidity and duration compared following spinning both to the left and the right. An assistant is needed to hold the patient in a normal standing position and spin it rapidly six or seven times. The postrotatory nystagmus elicited is observed immediately upon stopping the spin.

The presence of a spontaneous or positional nystagmus or a postrotatory nystag[mus] markedly different on each side is [a] disturbance of the vestibular system [with a] turbance of the peripheral portion of this system (the eighth cranial nerve), the abnormal spontaneous or positional nystagmus is either horizontal or rotatory, with the quick phase directed toward the side opposite the lesion. The postrotatory nystagmus developed after spinning the patient to the opposite side from the lesion is depressed when compared with the response observed on spinning the patient toward the side of the lesion. With extensive bilateral peripheral vestibular disease the examiner may not be able to elicit nystagmus.

A horizontal, rotatory, or vertical spontaneous or positional nystagmus occurs with disturbance of the central portion of the vestibular system. In addition, with central vestibular lesions the direction of the nystagmus may vary with changes in the position of the head. A rapid pendular congenital nystagmus may occur in puppies with or without abnormalities of the visual system.

Vestibular system disease is characterized by loss of balance. Disease on one side produces ipsilateral head tilt, and the patient will lean, fall, or roll toward the side of the lesion. Strength and postural reactions are normal. Abnormal nystagmus may occur and may be spontaneous or positional. Peripheral vestibular system lesions cause a jerk nystagmus directed away from the side of the lesion (quick phase).

Peripheral Vestibular System Disease
Seldom roll
Nystagmus: quick phase always to opposite side
Other signs: facial paresis-paralysis
Horner's syndrome (cat, dog)

Central Vestibular System Disease
More tendency to roll
Nystagmus: quick phase may change directions
with different head positions
vertical
Other signs: ipsilateral hemiparesis-ataxia
slow postural reactions
depression
head tremor, hypermetria
dysphagia
medial strabismus
weak jaw, atrophy of masticatory
muscles
facial hypalgesia

The sense of smell (I) and hearing (cochlear VIII) are difficult to evaluate unless the deficit is complete. Usually the owner's observations of the patient in its natural environment are more reliable for determination of these sensations.

A copy of the neurologic examination form routinely used at the New York State College of Veterinary Medicine follows at the bottom of this page.

SUMMARY OF SIGNS WITH LESIONS AT SPECIFIC LOCATIONS (TABLE 21–1)

SPINAL CORD

Lumbosacral: Fourth Lumbar to Fifth Caudal Segments

With *complete destruction* from the fourth lumbar through the fifth caudal segments, there is flaccid paraplegia—no support, gait, or movement of pelvic limbs and tail (except for slight hip flexion), no postural reactions in the pelvic limbs, areflexia of the flexor, patellar, and perineal reflexes, atonia or soft muscles, with no resistance to manipulation of pelvic limbs or tail, neurogenic atrophy in chronic lesions, a dilated anus, and analgesia from the pelvic limbs, tail, and perineum.

With *partial destruction* of grey and white matter between the fourth lumbar and fifth caudal segments, there is flaccid paraparesis and ataxia of pelvic limbs with normal thoracic limbs; postural reactions of pelvic limbs are attempted but poorly accomplished; hyporeflexia or areflexia of flexor, perineal, and patellar reflexes; hypotonia—normal or weak resistance to manipulation of pelvic limbs, and hypotonic anus; slight neurogenic atrophy in chronic lesions; and normal or depressed pain perception (hypalgesia) from pelvic limbs, tail, and perineum.

Neurologic Examination

Signalment:
History:

Mental Status:
Gait and Posture:

Cranial Nerves:
  II Menace   OS   OD
     Pupils
     Ophthalmoscopic
 III Pupils   Strabismus
  V Motor: Mand.
     Sensory: Ophth. Max. Mand.

  VI Strabismus

VII
VIII Cochlear
     Vestibular: Head tilt
        Nystagmus: Resting
                   Positional
                   Postrotatory
                   Vestibular

Muscle Tone-Size

Spinal Reflexes:

Patellar	LH	RH
Biceps	L	R
Triceps	L	R
Perineal		Tail
Flexor	LF	RF Crossed
	LH	RH Extensor
Pain Perception		

IX, X *Postural Reactions:*
XII

Wheelbarrowing	LF	RF
Hopping	LH	RH
Extensor postural thrust	LH	RH
Hemistand	L	R
Hemiwalk	L	R
Proprioceptive positioning	LF	RF
	LH	RH
Tonic neck and eye	Tactile	
Placing: Optic		

Anatomic diagnosis:

Differential diagnosis:

Plan:

Thoracolumbar: Third Thoracic to Third Lumbar Segments

With *complete destruction* or *dysfunction,* when the focal site is between the third thoracic and third lumbar segments, there occurs spastic paraplegia, with no voluntary support, gait, or movement of pelvic limbs, no postural reactions in the pelvic limbs, and normal or hyperactive flexor and patellar reflexes. Crossed extensor reflex may occur, muscle tone is normal or hypertonic, but occasionally

TABLE 21–1. RELATIONSHIP OF CLINICAL SIGNS TO ANATOMIC SITE OF LESION

Clinical Signs	Functional System	Anatomic Location
Inability to prehend	Masticatory and tongue muscles	Cranial nerves V, XII, pons-medulla
Dysphagia	Tongue, palatal, pharyngeal, and esophageal muscles	Cranial nerves IX, X, XI, XII, medulla
Drooling	Facial paralysis, dysphagia	Cranial nerve VII, middle ear, medulla Cranial nerves IX, X, medulla
Head tilt Nystagmus Loss of balance	Vestibular system	Inner ear, medulla, cerebellum
Rolling	Vestibular system	Medulla, cerebellum (inner ear)
Strabismus	Cranial nerves to extraocular muscles, vestibular system	Cranial nerves III, IV, VI, midbrain-medulla Inner ear-medulla-cerebellum

Circling
  With loss of balance
  Without loss of balance
	Vestibular system
	Limbic system(?)
		Inner ear, medulla, cerebellum
		Frontal lobe, rostral thalamus

Head and eye deviation-turning to one side	Limbic system(?)	Frontal lobe, rostral thalamus
Pacing, head pressing	Limbic system	Frontal lobe, rostral thalamus
Opisthotonos	Upper motor neuron	Rostral cerebellum, midbrain

Blindness	Visual System
	  Dilated, unresponsive pupils
	  Normal pupils
		Eyeball, optic nerves
		Visual cortex-cerebrum, (midbrain)

Depression, semicoma, coma	Ascending reticular activating system	Pons to thalamus-cerebral cortex
Seizures		Cerebrum, thalamus-hypothalamus
Hyperesthesia, hyperactivity to external stimuli	Ascending reticular activating system	Thalamus, cerebrum
Aggressive behavior, mania-hysteria, odontoprisis	Limbic system	Thalamus, cerebrum
Tremor Associated with movements, head and neck	Cerebellar system	Cerebellum
Associated with movements, head, trunk, limbs	Multiple systems	Diffuse CNS
Episodic, not associated with movements, head, trunk, limbs		Thalamus, cerebrum
Bradycardia, hypothermia, hyperthermia	UMN for general visceral efferent system	Hypothalamus
Irregular-ataxic respirations	UMN for respiratory muscle LMN	Pons-medulla

hypotonic, and there is analgesia from the area caudal to the lesion.

With *partial destruction* or *dysfunction,* when the focal site is between the third thoracic and third lumbar segments, there is spastic paraparesis and ataxia of pelvic limbs with normal thoracic limbs. All postural reactions are poorly performed in the pelvic limbs, flexor and patellar reflexes are normal or hyperactive, crossed extensor reflex may occur, muscle tone is normal or hypertonic, and pain perception is normal or depressed from the area caudal to the lesion. The same signs may be observed with lesions from L4 to L6 if they are confined to the white matter.

Caudal Cervical: Fifth Cervical to Second Thoracic Segments

With *partial destruction* of grey matter between the fifth cervical and the second thoracic segments, tetraparesis and ataxia of all four limbs are found, with the thoracic limb deficit worse than that of the pelvic limb, or there is tetraplegia with the patient in lateral recumbency. Thoracic limbs are hyporeflexic or areflexic, have normal tone or are hypotonic, and neurogenic atrophy occurs if there is a chronic lesion. The pelvic limbs show normal reflexes or are hyperreflexic, have normal tone or are hypertonic, and there is no atrophy. Pain perception is normal or depressed from all four limbs, or depressed from thoracic limbs only. All postural reactions are performed poorly, with the thoracic limb function worse than that of the pelvic limb. There is miosis, protruded third eyelid, ptosis, and enophthalmos with T1–T3 lesions.

Cranial Cervical: First Cervical to Fifth Cervical Segments

With *partial destruction* or *dysfunction,* when the focal site is between the first and fifth cervical segments, spastic tetraplegia may be observed if the lesion is severe with the patient in lateral recumbency. No postural reactions are present, reflexes are normal or hyperactive in all four limbs, crossed extensor reflexes may occur, muscle tone is normal or hypertonic; and there may be hypalgesia from the area caudal to the lesion. With less severe lesions there may be spastic tetraparesis and ataxia of all four limbs. The deficit in the pelvic limbs is usually worse than that in the thoracic limbs.

Postural reactions are performed poorly, reflexes are normal or hyperactive, crossed extensor reflexes may occur, muscle tone is normal or hypertonic, and pain perception is normal or depressed from the area caudal to the lesion. The same signs may be observed with lesions from C5 to C7 that are confined to the white matter. Occasionally the deficit in the thoracic limbs is worse than that in pelvic limbs if the lesion is a midline compression of the cervical spinal cord or is at the cervical intumescence.

MEDULLA AND PONS

Lesions in the medulla and pons result in spastic tetraparesis and ataxia of all four limbs or tetraplegia, ipsilateral spastic hemiparesis and ataxia (unilateral lesions), central vestibular signs, depression and irregular respirations, and hypalgesia of the trunk and limbs.

Signs of cranial nerve deficit are as follows: facial hypalgesia or analgesia (sensory V), paresis or paralysis of masticatory muscles (motor V), medial strabismus (VI), facial paresis or paralysis (VII), pharyngeal paresis (IX, X), and tongue paresis (XII).

CEREBELLUM

With diffuse lesions the signs are symmetric ataxia with preservation of strength, dysmetric gait (hypometria or hypermetria), truncal ataxia, head tremor, muscle hypertonia, occasional abnormal nystagmus, and bilateral menace deficit.

With unilateral lesions the signs are usually ipsilateral, occasionally contralateral. The body and the head tilt toward the side of the lesion, occasionally away from side of lesion, and there may be ipsilateral menace deficit.

With severe rostral lesions there may be opisthotonos and rigidly extended forelimbs, and the pelvic limbs will be extended forward by hip flexion.

MESENCEPHALON (Midbrain)

With lesions in this area, the following signs occur: opisthotonus with rigid extension of all limbs (decerebration), spastic tetraparesis and ataxia of all four limbs, spastic hemiparesis if the lesion is unilateral (usually contralateral), depression, stupor (semicoma), or coma, and hypalgesia of the head, trunk, and limbs. Signs of cranial nerve deficit are ventrolateral strabismus (III) and mydriasis and nonreactive pupil (III). There is deviation of the eyeballs in certain positions of the head, and the head and neck are flexed laterally, with the nose directed toward the shoulder with severe midline or unilateral lesions in the tegmentum. Visual deficits may be observed in acute lesions.

DIENCEPHALON (Thalamus and Hypothalamus)

Bilateral lesions of the diencephalon produce the following signs: slow postural reactions bilaterally, mild ataxia, bilateral visual deficit with dilated unresponsive pupils (optic tracts), and bilateral hypalgesia (ventral caudal lateral and medial nuclei).

Unilateral lesions are indicated by contralateral deficient postural reactions, contralateral visual deficit with normal pupils, contralateral hypalgesia (most noticeable in the head), and the adversive syndrome—propulsive circling, and head and eye deviation toward the side of lesion.

With lesions which are either bilateral or unilateral the manifestations are: depression, stupor (semicoma), or coma, behavioral changes, seizures, and the following hypothalamo-hypophyseal disorders: body temperature, glucose metabolism, appetite control, autonomic nervous system, water balance, gonadal function, and thyroid and adrenal function.

TELENCEPHALON (Cerebrum)

Lesions in this area are evidenced by changes in a number of ways. Changes in behavior or temperament include depression (lethargy, obtundation), stupor (semicoma), lack of recognition of owner or environment and bewilderment, loss of trained habits, and irritable, hysterical, maniacal, or aggressive behavior. In propulsion the animal often paces and circles in one direction, and turns the head and eyes in one direction; this direction is usually toward a unilateral lesion, called the "adversive" syndrome (turn to). This may require a rostral thalamic involvement in the

lesion. Seizures are partial (contralateral face or limbs or both) or generalized (grand mal, psychomotor). The gait usually is normal, but contralateral postural reactions are deficient. Bilateral lesions produce blindness. Unilateral lesions produce contralateral visual deficit with normal pupil responses to light. Occasionally contralateral facial hypalgesia occurs. Rarely the hypalgesia is observed in the contralateral trunk and limbs. Acute diffuse lesions may produce bilateral miosis. Pseudobulbar paresis rarely may be observed on voluntary movement: contralateral lower facial paralysis (lip and nose), pharyngeal paresis, and tongue paresis.

ANCILLARY EXAMINATION

Following determination of the anatomic diagnosis from the neurologic examination, a differential diagnosis will be made based on the lesion location, history, and signalment of the patient. The ancillary examinations that are performed will be determined by the differential diagnosis. Cerebrospinal fluid examination is often one of the most useful procedures and is described in Chapter 3. Radiography and myelography are included in that discussion. More sophisticated procedures will depend on what is available to the clinician.

INDEX OF THE DISEASES OF THE NERVOUS SYSTEM OF DOGS AND CATS

The diseases of the nervous system of dogs and cats that have been referred to in this book are organized here anatomically and according to the five basic kinds of lesions these diseases produce in the nervous system. These include the following:

Malformation of the nervous tissue

Injury—from external trauma and from internal compression by adjacent structures such as a neoplasm, abscess, or vertebral malformation

Inflammation—usually caused by an infectious agent

Neoplasia—primary neoplasm of nervous tissue

Degeneration—from metabolic diseases, nutritional causes, intoxications, or vascular impairment.

A final category are those diseases primarily considered to be idiopathic. Following each disease is its location in the book.

MALFORMATION
    Cranial Nerve—Ocular
      Collie eye syndrome, 292
      Persistent hyaloid vasculature, 282
      Optic nerve hypoplasia, 293
      Microphthalmia, 293
      Congenital deafness, 308
      Congenital vestibular syndrome, 246
      Congenital nystagmus, 252
    Spinal Cord—Neuromuscular
      Meningomyelocele, 26
      Spinal dysraphism, 26, 194
      Myelodysplasia, 26, 184, 194
      Hydromyelia, 49, 208
      Hypomyelinogenesis-dysmyelinogenesis, 149
      Swimmer syndrome, 208
    Brain
      Exencephaly, 24
      Duplication of prosencephalon, 24
      Craniofacial malformation, 24
      Hydranencephaly, 24
      Lissencephaly, 25, 265, 331
      Congenital hydrocephalus, 47, 208, 295, 330
      Hypomyelinogenesis-dysmyelinogenesis, 149
      Cerebellar malformation, 263, 265
      Griseofulvin-induced malformation, 293

INJURY
    Peripheral Nerve
      External, 70, 361
        Brachial plexus avulsion, 73, 361
        Sacrocaudal fracture, 73, 363
        Petrosal bone injury, 110, 249
      Internal
        Lumbosacral stenosis, cauda equina syndrome, 74
        Dysphagia (neoplasia), 109
        Facial paralysis (neoplasia), 109
        Brachial plexus neurofibroma, 197
    Spinal Cord
      External, 81,182, 184, 196, 359
      Internal, 81
        Intervertebral disk extrusion, 81, 183, 186, 196
        Neoplasia, 183, 189, 197, 417
        Lymphosarcoma (cats), 189, 197
        Neuroepithelioma (dogs), 189, 423
        Multiple cartilaginous exostosis, 189
        Thoracic vertebral malformation, 190
        Atlantoaxial malformation, 199
        Caudal cervical malformation-malarticulation, 200
        Cervical malformation (Bassett hounds), 204
        Vertebral osteomyelitis-diskospondylitis, 190, 204

        Spondylosis deformans, 191
        Dural ossification, 191
        Vertebral exostosis-hypervitaminosis A, 204
    Brain
      Brain injury, 295, 331
      Cerebellar injury, 272
      Extramedullary neoplasm, 411

INFLAMMATION
    Peripheral Nerve—Muscle
      Polyradiculoneuritis, 74
      Acute idiopathic polyneuropathy, 77
      Experimental allergic neuritis, 76
      Brachial plexus neuritis-neuropathy, 77
      Chronic polyneuritis-polyneuropathy, 78
      Postrabies vaccine polyneuritis, 77
      Toxoplasma neuritis, 74, 383
      Feline chronic relapsing polyneuritis, 173
      Myositis
        Infectious, 84
        Idiopathic immune-mediated, 84
        Masticatory, 85
        Polymyositis, 85
        Feline polymyositis-polymyopathy, 86
      Otitis media-interna, 109, 248
      Hemifacial spasm, 109
      Trigeminal neuritis, 110
      Optic neuritis, 293
    Spinal cord
      Canine distemper myelitis, 146, 191, 204, 381
      Toxoplasma myelitis, 83, 191, 383
      Cryptococcal myelitis, 191, 384
      Feline infectious peritonitis-myelitis, 192, 385
      Feline polioencephalomyelitis, 83
      Canine myoclonus, 146, 381
      Suppurative meningitis-myelitis, 204
      Cerebrospinal nematodiasis, 205
    Brain
      Acquired hydrocephalus, 47
      Feline polioencephalomyelitis, 83, 330
      Rabies encephalomyelitis, 112, 383
      Canine distemper encephalitis, 250, 272, 293, 294, 296, 330, 381
      Toxoplasma encephalitis, 250, 272, 293, 295, 330, 383
      Cryptococcal meningoencephalitis, 272, 293, 330, 384
      Canine infectious hepatitis-encephalitis, 383
      Feline infectious peritonitis-encephalitis, 250, 330, 385
      Granulomatous encephalitis (reticulosis), 250, 272, 293, 382, 419
      Chronic encephalitis of Pug dogs, 384
      Cuterebra myiasis, 251, 272
      Optic neuritis, 293
    Diffuse
      Rabies encephalomyelitis, 112, 383
      Canine distemper encephalomyelitis, 146, 191, 204, 250, 272, 293, 330, 381

The neurologic examination provides the basis for localizing the lesion in the nervous system. The following is a listing of the diseases, previously classified by kind of lesion, arranged on the basis of the primary anatomic area that may be affected and show clinical signs.

CEREBRAL
Hydrocephalus
Exencephaly
Duplication of prosencephalon
Hydranencephaly
Lissencephaly
Rabics encephalitis
Canine distemper encephalitis

Toxoplasma encephalitis
Cryptococcal encephalitis
Feline infectious peritonitis-encephalitis
Granulomatous encephalitis (reticulosis)
Chronic encephalitis of Pug dogs
Feline ischemic encephalopathy
Cerebrovascular accident
Poisons
Cuterebra myiasis
Thiamin deficiency
Neoplasia
Storage disease
Lead poisoning
Idiopathic epilepsy
Cerebral anoxia-hypoxia
Hepatic encephalopathy
Behavior abnormalities
Springer spaniel "rage" syndrome
Feline polioencephalomyelitis
Injury
Diencephalic syndrome

BRAIN STEM
Rabies encephalitis
Canine distemper encephalitis
Toxoplasma encephalitis
Cryptococcal encephalitis
Canine infectious hepatitis-encephalitis
Feline infectious peritonitis-encephalitis
Cuterebra myiasis
Granulomatous encephalitis (reticulosis)
Chronic encephalitis of Pug dogs
Neoplasia
Thiamin deficiency encephalopathy
Pituitary neoplasia
Injury

CEREBELLUM
Malformation
Neuronal abiotrophy
Canine distemper encephalitis
Toxoplasma encephalitis
Cryptococcal encephalitis
Granulomatous encephalitis (reticulosis)
Feline infectious peritonitis-encephalitis
Injury
Infarction
Neoplasia
Storage disease

SPINAL CORD
Meningomyelocele
Spinal dysraphism
Myelodysplasia
Hydromyelia
Fibrocartilaginous embolic myelopathy
Degenerative myelopathy
Hereditary neuronal abiotrophy (Swedish Lap-
land dog)
Hereditary spinal muscular atrophy (Brittany
spaniels)
Stockard's paralysis
Canine distemper myelitis

Toxoplasma myelitis
Cryptococcal meningomyelitis
Granulomatous myelitis (reticulosis)
Diffuse myelomalacia
Feline polioencephalomyelitis
Canine myoclonus
Tetanus
Strychnine poisoning
Scotty cramps-hyperkinesis
External Injury
Internal Injury
Neoplasia
Lymphosarcoma
Neuroepithelioma
Neurofibroma
Intervertebral disk extrusion
Multiple cartilaginous exostosis
Vertebral malformation
Thoracic
Cervical malformation-malarticulation
Occipitoatlantoaxial
Bassett hound
Osteomyelitis-diskospondylitis
Spondylosis deformans
Dural ossification
Vertebral exostosis-hypervitaminosis A
Feline infectious peritonitis-myelitis
Suppurative meningitis-myelitis
Hereditary myelopathy with myelinolysis (Af-
ghan hound)
Demyelinating myelopathy (miniature poodles)
Intramedullary neoplasia
Progressive axonopathy (boxer)
Spinocerebellar tract degeneration

NEUROMUSCULAR- SPINAL NERVES
Botulism
Tick paralysis
Polyradiculoneuritis
Acute idiopathic polyneuropathy
Experimental allergic neuritis
Brachial plexus neuritis-neuropathy
Lumbosacral stenosis
Injury
Brachial plexus avulsion
Toxoplasma neuritis
Aortic thrombosis–ischemic neuromyopathy
Myasthenia gravis
Chronic polyneuritis-polyneuropathy
Postrabies vaccine polyneuritis
Distal denervating disease
Inherited hypertrophic neuropathy (Tibetan
mastiff)
Giant axonal neuropathy
Distal symmetric polyneuropathy
Metabolic neuropathy
Myositis
Infectious
Idiopathic immune-mediated
Masticatory
Polymyositis
Feline polymyositis-polymyopathy
Congenital myotonia

Exertional myopathy
Nutritional myopathy
Neuromuscular esophageal defect
Tetanus
Strychnine poisoning
Scotty cramps-hyperkinesis
Canine sensory neuropathy
Feline chronic relapsing polyneuritis
Trigeminal sensory neuropathy
Swimmer syndrome

CRANIAL NERVES
Laryngeal paresis (Bouviers)
    Congenital
    Hypothyroid
Otitis media-interna (VII, VIII, sympathetics)
Dysphagia—neoplasia
Facial paralysis—neoplasia, hypothyroid, idiopathic
Hemifacial spasm—idiopathic, inflammatory
Trigeminal neuritis
Neuromuscular esophageal defect
Trigeminal sensory neuropathy
Progressive retinal atrophy
Collie eye syndrome
Persistent hyaloid vasculature
Microphthalmia
Optic nerve hypoplasia
Retinal dysplasias
Optic neuritis
Congenital nystagmus
Congenital deafness
Congenital vestibular syndrome
Feline vestibular syndrome
Canine vestibular syndrome
Petrosal bone injury
Antibiotic degeneration of vestibulocochlear neurons

DIFFUSE
Griseofulvin-induced malformations in cats
Rabies encephalomyelitis
Canine distemper encephalomyelitis
Toxoplasma encephalomyelitis
Cryptococcal encephalomyelitis
Granulomatous encephalomyelitis (reticulosis)
Canine infectious hepatitis-encephalitis
Feline infectious peritonitis-encephalomyelitis
Feline polioencephalomyelitis
Narcolepsy-cataplexy
Hypomyelinogenesis-dysmyelinogenesis
Poisons
"Shaker dogs," nonsuppurative encephalomyelitis
Cerebrospinal nematodiasis
Storage diseases

The following diseases of small animals are summarized here owing to lack of or an incomplete coverage elsewhere in the textbook.

Canine Distemper Encephalitis. Canine distemper is a multisystemic disease of dogs caused by a morbillivirus in the family Para-myxoviridae. The lesions and clinical signs of the disease in the nervous system are extremely variable and depend on the age of the dog, its immune status, the strain of the virus, and the location of the lesions.

The grey matter is primarily involved in most susceptible young puppies and in older dogs with specific viral strains. This is a mild nonsuppurative inflammatory lesion with variable neuronal degeneration. The rare case that follows live virus vaccination by 5 to 7 days has an extensive grey matter lesion predominantly in the pons and adjacent brain stem.

The acute neuronal grey matter form in young dogs is usually associated with acute death or extensive seizures, propulsion, stupor or hysteria, and ataxia. In older adult dogs, the grey matter form may be a chronic lesion and produce mild clinical signs related mainly to cerebral disturbance: dullness, propulsion, and seizures.

The white matter lesion initially consists of demyelination without inflammation that may or may not be associated with clinical signs, depending on how extensive the lesion is and where it is located. The nonsuppurative inflammation that follows this demyelination may produce extensive necrosis and result in clinical signs. This is the usual lesion in the subacute or more chronic form of canine distemper at any age. The demyelination and nonsuppurative inflammation with necrosis are usually multifocal and scattered through the spinal cord and brain, predominantly in white matter. Lesions are often most profound in the white matter of the spinal cord, cerebellum, and optic tracts. Clinical signs, therefore, reflect this multifocal distribution. Clinical signs of spinal cord disease and cerebellovestibular disease are most commonly observed in various combinations.

Seizures can occur in any form of this disease but most often occur in the acute grey matter form. Rarely, this disease produces a chronic sclerosing lesion in the cerebral white matter that may be associated with visual deficit and seizures.

Myoclonus can occur with any form of this disease but most often is the primary clinical sign associated with a very mild nonsuppurative inflammation in the vicinity of the grey matter, the cell bodies of which innervate the muscles involved in the myoclonus.

CSF occasionally is normal, usually contains a mild elevation of protein, and sometimes a mild pleocytosis with lymphocytes and mononuclear cells. Approximately 50 per cent of dogs with canine distemper encephalomyelitis will have canine distemper antibodies detectable in the CSF.

As a rule, the disease is progressive but occasionally this progression stops spontaneously and improvement may occur. There is no specific therapy.

Granulomatous Meningoencephalomyelitis. Granulomatous meningoencephalomyelitis is an idiopathic inflammatory disease of the central nervous system of dogs. It has been described previously as inflammatory reticulosis, granulomatous reticulosis, and histiocytic encephalitis.[4, 6, 22, 32, 33] Primary reticulosis of the central nervous system is the general term for massive accumulation of histiocyte-like cells around blood vessels. If these perivascular cells consist only of histiocytic cells, it is considered to be a neoplasm. More commonly these perivascular accumulations of cells are a mixture of lymphocytes, plasma cells, and histiocytes which more closely resembles an inflammatory lesion. These lesions have been called the inflammatory form of reticulosis. More recently this disease has been referred to as granulomatous meningoencephalomyelitis.[6]

The lesion consists of a large perivascular concentric proliferation of lymphocytes, plasma cells, and histiocytes. These massive accumulations of cells compress and invade the adjacent parenchyma. The lesion predominates in white matter, although grey matter and meninges may be affected.

Three forms of this disease occur: focal, disseminated, and ocular. The focal form is a mass lesion that results from the involvement of a large number of blood vessels in one site. The accumulation of these cells in whorls around adjacent blood vessels results in a mass or space-occupying lesion. These occur more commonly in the cerebellar white matter (peduncles) or cerebral white matter and less commonly in the brain stem or spinal cord. In the disseminated form many widely scattered blood-vessel–related lesions occur throughout the white matter of the entire central nervous system. The ocular form, consisting of an extensive lesion throughout the optic nerves, is referred to as optic neuritis. Occasionally it is accompanied by a focal or disseminated lesion elsewhere in the central nervous system.

The cause of this disease is unknown; no etiologic agent has been identified with any consistency. Most viral isolation procedures have been unrewarding. Some forms of the disease may resemble lymphosarcoma.[39] The lesion also resembles experimental allergic encephalitis, which supports a possible immunologic basis for the disease.

The disease is most common in dogs and occurs primarily in young adults, but patients have been observed from six months to ten years of age. Poodles and other small breeds are commonly affected.[33] The onset of the disease is variable from acute to chronic, and progression of signs can be rapid or slow or may stop progressing after a short period of time. Occasionally fever may accompany the clinical neurologic signs.

The clinical signs reflect the location of the lesion in the nervous system. If the lesion is focal in the cerebellomedullary region, the neurologic signs will reflect involvement of the cerebellum, vestibular system, upper motor neuron, general proprioceptive system, and occasionally the cranial nerve neurons. If the focal lesion is in the cerebrum, the clinical signs may include seizures, behavioral changes, visual and postural reaction deficits, and propulsion-adversive syndrome.

In the disseminated form of the disease the signs may reflect a diffuse or multifocal location. This will often include involvement of the cerebellomedullary region.[4]

In the ocular form of the disease there will be blindness with dilated unresponsive pupils.[14, 36] In some patients the optic disc may be involved, with edema and hemorrhage that can be observed with the ophthalmoscope. In a few patients, other clinical signs will reflect the disseminated or focal extension of this lesion elsewhere in the central nervous system.

Cerebrospinal fluid usually is abnormal with mild elevations of leukocytes consisting of lymphocytes and large mononuclear cells; protein is usually mildly elevated. Occasionally protein is increased without pleocytosis; sometimes the pleocytosis is severe. Neutrophils in the cerebrospinal fluid are uncommon.

There is no treatment for the primary disease, but some patients will improve on corticosteroid therapy for a variable period of time.[32, 33] The initial treatment should consist of oral prednisolone at 1 to 2 mg per kg per day. Improvement is often seen in a few days if therapy is started early in the course of the disease. The dose should be slowly decreased and continued on an alternate-day basis. Most patients will require continued therapy to prevent recurrence of the signs. Improvement may last for several months in some dogs, although most will ultimately succumb to the progression of this disease. The ocular form of this disease may be treated initially with the retrobulbar injection of corticosteroids.

The prognosis for permanent recovery is poor, but for temporary improvement for weeks or months it is fair to good. Better results are obtained when therapy is started early in the course of the disease.

Canine Infectious Hepatitis-Encephalitis. The canine infectious hepatitis adenovirus attacks endothelial cells of blood vessels throughout the body, including those in the nervous system. Many dogs with severe hepatitis caused by the virus may have involvement of the nervous system vessels but to an extent that is insufficient to produce neurologic signs. Occasionally these nervous system vessels are severely involved and vasculitis and hemorrhage develop rapidly in the brain stem, producing a rapidly progressive tetraparesis-ataxia, semicoma, coma, seizures, and death. These signs may be accompanied by fever, vomiting, and diarrhea.

Rabies. Rabies is an encephalomyelitis caused by a neurotropic virus that affects all species of warm-blooded animals. It is a fatal disease that usually causes death by 10 days after the onset of clinical signs. The incubation period from exposure to clinical signs is extremely variable.

The clinical signs are also quite variable. It has been said that the most typical clinical description of rabies is how atypical the signs can be.[15] Cattle often begin with a pelvic limb paresis and ataxia and a paralyzed hypalgesic tail. Horses often present with signs of spinal cord disease.

In dogs and cats the behavioral abnormality is variable.[26] Some will show a marked disturbance with hyperirritability and destructive or vicious biting of animate or inanimate objects. These signs may be episodic. They may eat dirt, sticks, and stones. Dysphagia causes profuse salivation. Seizures, paralysis, and death may follow. Others will show more depression associated with a progressive paresis and ataxia of the gait and medullary signs of facial, pharyngeal, and jaw paralysis. Intense conjunctival congestion is often present.

Cats are highly susceptible and often show a pronounced excitatory stage of the disease before progressive paralysis occurs. Cats that develop rabies following vaccination with modified live virus usually begin with lameness-paresis of the pelvic limb that was injected.[10] This progresses to paraparesis and rigidly extended pelvic limbs, followed by tetraparesis and recumbency. Signs of ascending spinal cord disease prevail. Medullary signs are uncommon, and these cats often survive longer than those with the natural form of the disease. The same ascending paralysis occurs in dogs following rabies vaccination.[28, 38] This form of the disease may not be fatal.

Pseudorabies. Pseudorabies is a diffuse nonsuppurative encephalomyelitis and ganglioneuritis caused by the *Herpesvirus suis*. Pseudorabies is endemic in swine and also affects cattle, sheep, dogs, and cats. In most species other than swine, it produces a rapidly fatal disease. Most affected dogs and cats die within 24 to 48 hours of the onset of clinical signs.[8, 20, 34] There is often severe pruritus, with self-mutilation at the site at which the virus gained entrance into the peripheral nerves and migrated to the central nervous system; this is usually around the head region.

Initially, along with the pruritus there may be signs of restlessness, profuse salivation, ataxia, vocalization, and tremors. This may be accompanied by fever, vomition, and dyspnea. These signs rapidly progress to profound depression, head pressing, seizures, coma, and death. Occasionally pruritus does not occur.[41] The source of the virus to carnivores is the consumption of virus-contaminated tissues of swine, cattle, rats, or mice.

In swine the disease is most severe in the baby pig, and the clinical signs decrease in severity with age. The disease is rapidly fatal in baby pigs and may be very mild and transient in adult pigs.

Toxoplasmosis. *Toxoplasma gondii* is a protozoan that causes disease in a wide variety of animal species. As an acquired neurologic disease toxoplasmosis is most common in dogs and cats, but the incidence in these species is low in my experience. The organism most commonly causes lesions in the lung, liver, intestine, muscle, and nervous system. Not all organs are always affected in any one patient. Immunosuppressed animals or those with immunologic disorders are more susceptible to this disease.

Any portion of the central nervous system and the roots of spinal nerves can be affected.[1] The organism produces a varying degree of necrosis and mostly nonsuppurative encephalomyelitis of both grey and white matter. Mild lesions consist of numerous focal areas of degeneration, gliosis, and lymphoid perivascular cuffs; severely necrotic areas will contain neutrophils in the inflammation and hemorrhage. These lesions are either scattered throughout the central nervous system, organized into one focal lesion with characteristics of a granuloma, or diffusely distributed in a periventricular location. Organisms are found free in the tissues or in macrophages, or are encysted. Encysted organisms may be found unassociated with any inflammation.

Clinical signs will be determined by the location and extent of the lesion. The rapidly progressive periventricular lesion produces diffuse signs of brain disease and early death. A focal thoracolumbar granuloma will affect only the pelvic limbs. Young dogs affected in the lumbosacral intumescence may develop a remarkable rigidity and muscle atrophy in the paretic pelvic limb(s). Myositis may accompany this spinal cord lesion. Multifocal neurologic signs are suggestive of this diagnosis. Patients have been observed with signs that predominantly reflect disease in the cerebrum, or cerebellum, or cervical or thoracolumbar spinal cord.

Chorioretinitis is often observed in these patients and is due to the same protozoal agent. CSF is usually abnormal with elevation of protein and pleocytosis with variable cell type occasionally including neutrophils; CSF is xanthochromic if hemorrhage has occurred.

Cryptococcosis. *Cryptococcus neoformans* causes a systemic mycosis that produces a diffuse leptomeningitis in all domestic animals. It is more commonly observed in cats than dogs, but the overall incidence is low in my experience.[42] Immune deficiency or immunosuppression may be involved in the pathogenesis of the infection. The lesion is diffuse throughout the meninges and sometimes throughout the ventricular system, with involvement of the adjacent parenchyma. The meningeal lesion often extends into the parenchyma along the penetrating blood vessels. This may be grossly visible on transverse sections as gelatinous cysts.

The degree of inflammation associated with the massive accumulation of organisms is variable. The lack of inflammatory reaction is often remarkable. Mild inflammation involves lymphocytes and monocytes. More extensive inflammation may include neutrophils and occasionally eosinophils. Granulomatous lesions may occur with macrophages, giant cells, and fibroblastic scarring. The organisms are free in the tissues or in macrophages.

The CSF usually contains many organisms that are readily identified as fungal agents. Specific identification of *Cryptococcus neoformans* requires special procedures. A similar infection has been seen in humans caused by a closely related fungus of the *Rhodotorula* genus.

Clinical signs are variable but usually reflect a diffuse or multifocal distribution and are progressive. Cerebellomedullary signs are often apparent and may be combined with spinal cord and/or cerebral signs. Generalized seizures may occur in cats and can be elicited by extending the neck.

Ocular involvement with chorioretinitis and optic neuritis is common.[3, 5, 9, 13, 19] This may be due to extension of the meningeal lesion from the meninges at the base of the brain along the optic nerve to the eyeball. Other sites of infection include the nasal cavity, frontal sinus, lymph nodes, lungs, skin and subcutis, kidney, spleen, muscle, gastrointestinal tract, and tympanic bullae.

A latex agglutination cryptococcal antigen test is now available for the clinical diagnosis of this disease in humans and domestic animals.

Although cryptococcal infection in some non–nervous tissues have been successfully treated with amphotericin B and 5-fluorocytosine,[29] there are no reports of its efficacy against infection of the nervous system in animals.

Chronic Encephalitis of Pug Dogs. A chronic granulomatous meningoencephalomyelitis has been recognized in young Pug dogs in California and the northeastern United States. The onset of the disease has ranged from 9 months to 4 years of age and has affected both males and females. In most individuals the clinical signs have been present from 1 to 6 months before death or euthanasia. A few have died after only a few days of clinical signs.

The signs predominantly reflect lesions in the cerebrum, with generalized seizures being the most commonly reported sign. Owners will also report varying degrees of ataxia, paresis, circling, and depression. Besides generalized seizures, these dogs may also exhibit partial motor seizures with muscle spasms of the face or the limbs on one side of the body. Neurologic examination will usually reveal unilateral or occasionally bilateral postural reaction deficits, visual deficits with normal pupil responses to light, and occasionally a tendency to turn the head or circle to one side propulsively. These reflect the major cerebral location of the lesion. Some dogs will have signs of central vestibular system involvement and, more rarely, cerebellar lesions. Spinal cord signs are less frequent or are masked by the signs of brain lesions. Occasionally these dogs will scream as if in pain, but no extracranial source can be localized. Death is usually preceded by coma or status epilepticus.

Cerebrospinal fluid is usually abnormal with moderate elevations in lymphocytes and other mononuclear cells and total protein.

The lesion consists of a diffuse degeneration of white matter and less often grey matter associated with large perivascular cuffs of lymphocytes and histiocytes. The parenchymal necrosis is severe in some parts of the lesion and may be visible on gross examination of transverse sections of the preserved cerebrum. Astrocytosis with proliferation of glial processes is often widespread in the areas of degenerate white matter. In some dogs there is significant involvement of grey matter with this inflammatory lesion or with a laminar type of necrosis of the cerebral cortex. The latter lesion may be secondary and reflect anoxic changes associated with persistent generalized seizures. Areas of lymphocytic meningitis are common.

This disease has been recognized but not reported previously in California,[44] where a large number of affected dogs all came from one kennel in the Sacramento area. It has been observed in Massachusetts,[43] and I have studied this disease in three littermates from Connecticut with onset of clinical signs at 9, 18, and 19 months of age, and in three unrelated Pug dogs from New York State. Viral isolation studies were unsuccessful in two of these dogs. The etiology remains unknown. A possible familial predisposition warrants investigation.

There is no specific therapy. The generalized seizures are often refractory to anticonvulsant drugs. Corticosteroid therapy has not been rewarding to date.

Feline Infectious Peritonitis. Feline infectious peritonitis is a disease that affects multiple systems in cats and is caused by a coronavirus. The granulomatous form affects the nervous system and the lesion usually consists of an extensive ependymitis, choroid plexitis, and adjacent encephalitis and myelitis throughout the central nervous system.[23, 24, 27, 35, 40] In some there is also an extensive leptomeningitis. An immune complex–mediated vasculitis is thought to be responsible for the nervous system lesion. There is usually an extensive accumulation of lymphoid and mononuclear inflammatory cells and occasionally neutrophils in this lesion. In some this is accompanied by an extensive exudation of protein into the lesion and CSF. Analysis of the CSF reflects this inflammatory response and usually contains high levels of protein and extensive pleocytosis. Rarely this disease produces a focal granulomatous lesion in the spinal cord or brain.

This is usually a chronic slowly progressive disease, and clinical signs are often diffuse and nonspecific. Common neurologic signs include paraparesis, abnormal nystagmus, and seizures. Involvement of the cerebellomedullary region is common and causes tremor, ataxia with loss of balance, and tetraparesis. Hyperesthesia often occurs and may reflect the leptomeningitis. These signs are frequently accompanied by a fever, depression, weight loss, and occasionally other signs of a chronic systemic illness. Ocular lesions of uveitis often accompany the neurologic disease. Hypergammaglobulinemia and a significantly elevated feline infectious peritonitis antibody titer are usually present.

Cats with this disease have a poor prognosis. Occasionally vigorous therapy with corticosteroids and immunosuppressive-cytotoxic drugs may stop the disease process and result in improvement if the signs are mild.

Thiamin Deficiency Encephalopathy. Thiamin deficiency produces nervous system lesions and clinical signs more commonly in cats than dogs. It occurs in cats fed a fish diet high in thiaminase, a diet inadequate in thiamin, or food that is cooked, which destroys thiamin.[2, 25] Prolonged anorexia may lead to thiamin deficiency. In cats stressed with a clinical illness, the period of anorexia necessary to produce this is shortened. In dogs, this disease is most commonly associated with feeding cooked food.

Lesions consist of a bilaterally symmetric degeneration of brain stem nuclei.[21] This degeneration is most evident in vestibular nuclei, caudal colliculi, oculomotor nuclei, red nuclei, lateral geniculate nuclei, and habenular nuclei. Basal nuclei and the cerebral cortex occasionally are involved.

Clinical signs in cats begin with anorexia and a sudden onset of cerebellovestibular ataxia, followed by dilation of pupils that respond poorly to light.[11, 21] Seizures, head ventroflexion, coma, and death follow. The seizures can often be elicited on handling the cat and include a severe tonic flexion of the entire vertebral column and head. These cats act as if they were trying to roll into a ball.

Dogs with thiamin deficiency usually show an initial depression and spastic paraparesis that progresses to ataxia, torticollis, circling, and finally an inability to stand.[30, 31] Generalized seizures usually occur after the dog is recumbent. Menace responses may be absent, suggesting a cerebrocortical visual deficit.

Treatment with a few milligrams of thiamin early in the course of the disease will usually result in complete recovery.[11]

REFERENCES

1. Averill, D. R., and de Lahunta, A.: Toxoplasmosis of the canine nervous system: Clinicopathologic findings in four cases. J. Am. Vet. Med. Assoc., 159:1134, 1971.
2. Baggs, R. B., de Lahunta, A., and Averill, D. R.: Thiamin deficiency encephalopathy in a specific pathogen free cat colony. Lab. Anim. Sci., 28:323, 1978.
3. Bistner, S., de Lahunta, A., and Lorenz, M.: Generalized cryptococcosis in a dog. Cornell Vet., 61:440, 1971.
4. Braund, K. G., Vandevelde, M., Walker, T. L., and Redding, R. W.: Granulomatous meningoencephalomyelitis in six dogs. J. Am. Vet. Med. Assoc., 172:1195, 1978.
5. Carlton, W. W., Feeney, D. A., and Zimmerman, J. L.: Disseminated cryptococcosis with ocular involvement in a dog. J. Am. Anim. Hosp. Assoc., 12:53, 1976.
6. Cordy, D. R.: Canine granulomatous meningoencephalomyelitis. Vet. Pathol., 16:325, 1979.
7. de Lahunta, A.: Feline neurology. Vet. Clin. North Am., 6:433, 1976.
8. Dow, C., and McFerran, J. B.: Aujeszky's disease in the dog and cat. Vet. Rec., 75:1099, 1963.
9. Edwards, N. J., and Rebhun, W. C.: Generalized cryptococcosis: A case report. J. Am. Anim. Hosp. Assoc., 15:439, 1979.
10. Esh, J. B., Cunningham, J. G., and Wiktor, T. J.: Vaccine induced rabies in four cats. J. Am. Vet. Med. Assoc., 180:1336, 1982.
11. Everett, G. M.: Observations on the behavior and neurophysiology of acute thiamin-deficient cats. Am. J. Physiol., 141:439, 1944.
12. Fankhauser, R., Fatzer, R., Luginbuhl, H., and McGrath, J. T.: Primary reticulosis of the CNS in animals. Adv. Vet. Sci. Comp. Med., 16:40, 1972.
13. Fischer, C. A.: Intraocular cryptococcosis in two cats. J. Am. Vet. Med. Assoc., 158:191, 1971.
14. Fischer, C. A., and Liu, S.-K: Neuro-ophthalmologic manifestations of primary reticulosis of the central nervous system in a dog. J. Am. Vet. Med. Assoc., 158:1240, 1971.
15. Fox, F. H.: Personal communication, 1982.
16. Fox, M. W.: Conditioned reflexes and innate behavior of the neonate dog. J. Small Anim. Pract., 4:85, 1963.
17. Fox, M. W.: The clinical behavior of the neonatal dog. J. Am. Vet. Med. Assoc., 143:1331, 1963.
18. Fox, M. W.: The development and clinical significance of superficial reflexes in the dog. Vet. Rec., 75:378, 1963.
19. Gelatt, K. N., McGill, L., and Perman, V.: Ocular and systemic cryptococcosis in a dog. J. Am. Vet. Med. Assoc., 162:370, 1973.
20. Gore, R., Osborne, A. D., Darke, P. G. G., and Todd, J. N.: Aujeszky's disease in a pack of hounds. Vet. Rec., 101:93, 1977.
21. Jubb, K. V., Saunders, L. Z., and Coates, H. V.: Thiamine deficiency encephalopathy in cats. J. Comp. Pathol. Bacteriol., 66:217, 1956.
22. Koestner, A., and Zeaman, W.: Primary reticulosis of the central nervous system in dogs. Am. J. Vet. Res., 23:381, 1962.
23. Kornegay, J. N.: Feline infectious peritonitis: The central nervous system form. J. Am. Anim. Hosp. Assoc., 14:580, 1978.
24. Legendre, A. M., and Whitenack, D. L.: Feline infectious peritonitis with spinal cord involvement in two cats. J. Am. Vet. Med. Assoc., 167:931, 1975.
25. Loew, F. M., Martin, C. L., Dunlop, R. H., Maplehof, R. J., and Smith, S. I.: Naturally-occurring and experimental thiamin deficiency in cats receiving commercial cat food. Can. Vet. J., 11:109, 1970.
26. Minor, R.: Rabies in the dog. Vet. Rec., 101:516, 1977.
27. Montali, R. J., and Strandberg, J. D.: Extraperitoneal lesions in feline infectious peritonitis. Vet. Pathol., 9:109, 1972.
28. Pedersen, N. C., Emmons, R. W., Selcer, R., Woodie, J. D., Holliday, T. A., and Weiss, M.: Rabies vaccine virus infection in three dogs. J. Am. Vet. Med. Assoc., 172:1092, 1978.
29. Pierost, E., McKee, J. M., and Crawford, P.: Successful medical management of severe feline cryptococcosis. J. Am. Anim. Hosp. Assoc., 18:111, 1982.
30. Read, D. H., and Harrington, D. D.: Experimentally induced thiamine deficiency in Beagle dogs: Clinical observations. Am. J. Vet. Res., 42:989, 1981.
31. Read, D. H., Jolly, R. D., and Alley, M. R.: Polioencephalomalacia in dogs with thiamine deficiency. Vet. Pathol., 14:103, 1977.
32. Russo, M. E.: Primary reticulosis of the central nervous system in dogs. In Kirk, R. W. (ed.): Current Veterinary Therapy: Small Animal Medicine VIII. Philadelphia, W. B. Saunders Co., in press.
33. Russo, M. E.: Primary reticulosis of the central nervous system in dogs. J. Am. Vet. Med. Assoc., 174:492, 1979.
34. Shell, L. G., Ely, R. W., and Crandell, R. A.: Pseudorabies in a dog. J. Am. Vet. Med. Assoc., 178:1159, 1981.
35. Slauson, D. O., and Finn, J. P.: Meningoencephalitis and panophthalmitis in feline infectious peritonitis. J. Am. Vet. Med. Assoc., 160:729, 1972.
36. Smith, J. S., de Lahunta, A., and Riis, R. C.: Reticulosis of the visual system in a dog. J. Small Anim. Pract., 18:643, 1977.
37. Vandevelde, M.: Primary reticulosis of the central nervous system. Vet. Clin. North Am., 10:57, 1980.
38. Vandevelde, M., and Fatzer, R.: Neurological complications in three dogs after vaccination with a

tissue culture rabies vaccine. Vlaams Diergen. Tijds., *43*:253, 1974.

39. Vandevelde, M., Fatzer, R., and Fankhauser, R.: Immunohistologic studies in primary reticulosis of the canine brain. Vet. Pathol., *18*:577, 1981.

40. Weiss, R. C., and Scott, F. W.: Feline infectious peritonitis. *In* Kirk, R. W. (ed.): Current Veterinary Therapy: Small Animal Practice VII. Philadelphia, W.B. Saunders Co., 1977.

41. Whitley, R. D., and Nelson, S. L.: Pseudorabies (Aujeszky's disease) in the canine. Two atypical cases. J. Am. Anim. Hosp. Assoc., *16*:69, 1980.

42. Wilkinson, G. T.: Feline cryptococcosis: A review and seven case reports. J. Small Anim. Pract., *20*:749, 1979.

43. Averill, D. A., Jr.: Personal communication, 1982.

44. Holiday, T., and Cordy, D. R.: Personal communication, 1982.

EQUINE NEUROLOGIC EXAMINATION AND INDEX OF DISEASES OF THE NERVOUS SYSTEM

EQUINE NEUROLOGIC EXAMINATION

Examination of a horse with a neurologic disorder should include review of the history, complete general physical examination, neurologic examination, and appropriate ancillary procedures. The neurologic examination should determine the presence of a nervous system lesion(s) and establish the location of the lesion(s) in the nervous system. This is the anatomic diagnosis. Utilization of a routine procedure will provide the examiner with the experience and confidence to make an accurate anatomic diagnosis.

The differential diagnosis will be based on the anatomic diagnosis and the evaluation of the signalment and history. The five major kinds of lesions should be considered: malformation, inflammation, neoplasia, degeneration, and injury. Experience with the specific distribution of lesions that occur in certain disease entities will often lead to a presumptive diagnosis. Further evaluation of the patient

with ancillary procedures to determine the cause or confirm the anatomic diagnosis will depend on the differential diagnosis that is established.

Results of the neurologic examination should always be carefully recorded and not left to memory. Subtle changes may alter the prognosis and course of therapy.

SIGNALMENT

The signalment should include a description of the breed, sex, age, color, and use of the patient. A few neurologic diseases are specific to particular breeds. The young Arabian foal has a presumed hereditary cerebellar cortical abiotrophy. A similar condition exists in the Gotland pony breed. Signs are present at birth or usually occur prior to 4 to 6 months of age. Seizures have been observed in Arabian foals at a few months of age. These may be inherited and usually resolve spontaneously in a few months. An atlanto-occipital malformation has been seen only in Arabians or Arabian-cross foals. Some are born showing severe spasticity of the limbs and tetraparesis, while others do not show signs, according to the owners, until several months of age. Narcolepsy has been observed in Shetland ponies and may begin prior to 6 months of age. Night blindness (stumbling and falling while being ridden during and after dusk) has been seen in the Appaloosa breed. Neurologic signs due to congenital malformation of the nervous system usually are present at birth and are nonprogressive. Cervical stenotic myelopathy is a vertebral malformation with spinal cord compression. It is not breed-specific but is more common in the younger animal from 6 months to about 2 years of age. It is more common in the rapidly growing male thoroughbred, where it may be familial. A diffuse spinal cord degeneration of unknown pathogenesis is seen in all breeds and usually causes signs prior to 6 months of age. A similar disease has been described as familial in zebras. Acute hepatoencephalopathy (Theiler's disease) is not usually seen in foals less than 1 year old. Melanomas are common in the grey horse. More cases of myelitis syndrome associated with a protozoal agent have been seen in mature standardbred horses.

HISTORY

In addition to the data applicable to the present illness, the history should include a summary of all past medical and surgical events. The line of questioning referable to the chief complaint depends on the nature of the complaint.

Careful documentation of the onset and course of a neurologic disorder is important in order to distinguish between a traumatic or acute vascular disorder and a disorder of a progressive nature such as inflammation, degeneration, or neoplasia. As a rule, 24 hours after an injury the neurologic signs are static or improved. Progressive neurologic signs are not usually caused by a single episode of trauma. It is common for an owner to blame a neurologic disorder on an injury from a fall when in fact the underlying progressive neurologic disorder caused the fall. Be aware that neoplastic involvement of the nervous system occasionally may occur suddenly and progress rapidly. Cervical stenotic myelopathy may have a slow insidious onset and progress, or occur suddenly without obvious evidence of progression. Thus any neurologic signs caused by a space-occupying or compressive type of lesion may appear suddenly even though the primary lesion is slowly progressive. Equine degenerative myeloencephalopathy always has a slow insidious onset and progresses slowly.

If the neurologic disorder has been progressive, the examiner should carefully document the occurrence of each sign to determine if the lesion is focal or diffuse in the nervous system. A patient with progressive paresis and ataxia of the pelvic limbs with normal thoracic limb function that subsequently develops a facial paresis and hemiatrophy of the tongue must have more than one lesion to explain the signs. Such a multifocal distribution of lesions is characteristic of an inflammatory lesion such as protozoal encephalomyelitis in horses. By careful questioning of an owner concerning the onset of neurologic signs, it may become apparent that there were previous signs, suggesting a progressive problem.

The history of previous or concurrent diseases affecting other body systems should be investigated in the patient as well as in the rest of the herd. Upper respiratory disease, abortions, or minor illness with fever may have occurred in a herd in which one or more horses have neurologic signs caused by equine herpesvirus I (rhinopneumonitis). In this disease, a history of other horses affected with a mild transient ataxia may be found on examination of a patient that became recumbent in a 24- to 48-hour period. A history of strangles infection in the patient or in the herd may accompany the signs of a brain abscess due to *Streptococcus equi*. Determine if there is a present or past history of a problem similar to that shown by the patient in other related or unrelated animals. Evidence of a family history may help document an hereditary disease.

The environment should be examined directly or indirectly for a source of toxins or possible poisonous vegetation. A *Fusarium* species of mold infecting corn has been implicated in equine leukoencephalomalacia, a rare disease today.

Centaurea species (yellow star thistle and Russian knapweed) are involved in the pathogenesis of nigropallidal encephalomalacia. The pyrrolizidine alkaloids from species of *Senecio* (ragwort and common groundsel), *Amsinckia* (fiddle-neck), or *Crotalaria* (wild pea) produce a chronic hepatic cirrhosis that may result in hepatic encephalopathy. A syndrome of episodic ataxia and muscle spasms—"staggers"—may occur in horses consuming rye grass, or paspallum grasses infected with ergot *(Claviceps paspali)*. Ataxia and cystitis have been associated with feeding on *Sorghum* grasses (sorghum, sudan, Johnson grass). Locoweed poisoning has been reported in horses grazing on *Oxytropis* and *Astragalus* herbs. They showed wasting, abnormal gait, and hypersensitivity during handling.

Horses grazing in fields in which lead fallout has occurred from industrial wastes have been poisoned. A source of growth of *Clostridium botulinum* is often difficult to document. External wounds or internal lesions infected with this organism should be considered as a source of toxin in cases of suspected botulism.

The vaccination history of the animal is important in evaluating differential diagnosis for the various viral encephalitides, equine infectious anemia, and strangles infection. Rhinopneumonitis titers apparently are not necessarily protective against the neurologic form of this disease. Biologics of equine origin such as tetanus antitoxin may be implicated as the source of an agent causing acute hepatic necrosis and encephalopathy.

GENERAL PHYSICAL EXAMINATION

The complete general examination of all body systems other than the nervous system should precede the neurologic examination. Primary disease of other systems may be manifested by neurologic signs. The severe cerebral disorder of hepatic encephalopathy is a common example of this in the horse. Other extracranial encephalopathies include neonatal septicemia and maladjustment syndrome (respiratory distress syndrome, cerebral hypoxia), neonatal hypoglycemia, transit tetany, and hypomagnesemia. In such cases the signs are often intermittent. Patients with cardiac malformations may present with episodes of weakness or collapse (syncope). The same can occur with hypoadrenocorticoidism. Musculoskeletal disorders most frequently are confused with signs of neurologic disease. Palpation of limbs and joints sometimes aided by simultaneous auscultation may reveal fractures that are the cause of the clinical signs. A rectal examination should be included and can assist in defining sublumbar muscle tenderness (myositis). A grossly distended bladder can be expected in most recumbent horses, but in a standing horse usually is suggestive of paralysis of the bladder. Palpable crepitus associated with the pelvic cavity and hip area in a horse with a severe lameness, muscle atrophy, or pelvic limb paresis should be studied carefully. Often these apparently abnormal findings are not associated with a bony lesion. Palpation may reveal firm muscles and cold skin in aortic-iliac thrombosis. Neuritis of the cauda equina may present because of dysuria or obstipation. Epistaxis often accompanies cranial nerve deficits caused by guttural pouch mycosis. Surface wounds should be looked for in consideration of tetanus, botulism, or rabies. Ticks may be implicated in producing a flaccid paralysis of foals.

NEUROLOGIC EXAMINATION

The neurologic examination should include evaluation of the mental status, gait and posture, postural reactions, spinal nerves, and cranial nerves. The order in which the parts of a neurologic examination are performed is unimportant; however, those procedures that will upset the patient the least should be performed first. Complete spinal reflex examination cannot be assessed in most horses that are ambulatory; however, in such cases it is reasonable to assume that they are present even if they possibly are exaggerated.

Mental Status and Behavior

The owner should be questioned regarding the behavior of the patient. He or she can best judge if it has changed and can inform you of how the patient normally responds. The breed and age may influence the behavior. It is especially important to judge the mental status carefully in the recumbent patient. Cervical spinal cord disease may produce recumbency without altering the animal's behavior.

If its behavior is unchanged, the animal will remain alert and responsive. Horses with suspected botulism may be recumbent and too weak to move but usually respond to the examiner. Occasionally, some depression is observed. A recumbent animal that is obtunded, semicomatose, having seizures, or is delirious has a brain lesion. Sometimes a horse that is down due to spinal cord disease, aortic thrombosis, myositis, or acute vestibular disease will act delirious in its frantic struggle to get up. The most remarkable alterations in behavior usually occur with hepatic encephalopathy.

Gait and Posture

Neurologic abnormalities that affect the tracts that ascend from or descend to the spinal cord produce varying degrees of spasticity, ataxia, and paresis that can be observed in the gait. With spinal cord disease, the earliest signs are usually spasticity and ataxia. With more severe lesions, paresis becomes apparent. These will result from lesions of the tracts in the white matter as occurs regularly in cervical stenotic myelopathy and equine degenerative myeloencephalopathy. The spasticity and paresis result from upper motor neuron tract lesions, with spasticity being the earliest sign. The ataxia results from a general proprioceptive tract lesion.

Spasticity may be manifested as a stiff, short-strided gait. The limbs will often strike the ground sharply with a slapping sound. The thoracic limbs may delay slightly at the end of protraction before striking the ground. This makes them appear to float before landing, and there may be a mild hypermetria from general proprioceptive system deficits. The general proprioceptive ataxia may cause the hindquarters to sway, a prolonged pelvic limb stride associated with a delay in the onset of protraction, an abduction of the pelvic limb on protraction or adduction, with the limb crossing under the body and sometimes stepping on the opposite limb. Severe swaying and delays in protraction or pivoting and sinking on a limb may also be due to the paresis of voluntary movement from upper motor neuron lesions.

The horse should be moved at the walk and trot in a straight line, walked in large and small circles in both directions, and backed. It may help to observe subtle deficits if this is also done on a gentle slope. Blindfolding may exacerbate an ataxia if it is vestibular in origin. It has little effect on the ataxia caused by spinal cord lesions. Slight asymmetry in length of strides may be detected by walking next to the horse stride for stride. Allowing the horse to move freely without a lead in a paddock also may be helpful. The horse with mild general proprioceptive ataxia from spinal cord disease may gait fairly well in a straight path but show ataxia on quickly turning at the end of a paddock.

The patient's gait should be observed for spasticity, ataxia, and paresis while the examiner stands off to the side of the horse as it is walked. First, concentrate on the pelvic limbs, then the thoracic limbs. Observe the animal as it turns to reverse its direction. Observe the thoracic limb gait as the horse is walked with the head and neck extended. This may cause a thoracic limb to scuff the ground or float excessively on protraction when there is mild cervical spinal cord disease.

Sway: Signs of weakness, or ataxia, or both may be elicited by gently pushing the hindquarters or pulling the patient by the tail to one side as it is standing and walking (the sway response). The normal horse resists these movements, or steps briskly to the side as it is pushed or pulled. The weak horse can be pulled easily to the side and may stumble or fall. The ataxic horse may easily be thrown off stride and stumble. The weak horse also may tend to buckle or collapse when strong pressure is applied with the fingers to the withers and loin region.

Circle: Turn the horse at a walk in a fairly small circle and observe the initiation of protraction and degree of limb excursion as it turns. Circle the horse in both directions. The ataxic horse may sway to one side, be slow to protract a limb, cross its limbs, or step on its opposite limb. The ataxic animal may abduct the outside pelvic limb too far as it is pushed or moved in a small circle. This may appear as a hypermetric movement similar to the stringhalt action, and is assumed to be a sign of a general proprioceptive tract lesion. The animal that is circled may keep a clinically affected pelvic limb fixed in one position on the ground and pivot around it without moving it. The same failure to protract the limb may be seen on backing. It may even force the horse into a "dog-sitting" posture. This is assumed to be caused by a lesion in the general proprioceptive tracts, or the upper motor neuron tracts, or both. It usually occurs in the more severely affected patient. It is often difficult to distinguish paresis from ataxia, but in most instances it is unimportant because of the close anatomic relationship of the ascending general proprioceptive and descending upper motor neuron tracts in the white matter of the spinal cord.

Occasionally, with general proprioceptive tract lesions the animal may hold an affected limb longer in an abnormal position (crossed or abducted) when placed there by the examiner.

As a rule mild lesions of the tracts in the cervical spinal cord cause a more obvious deficit in the pelvic limbs but usually some thoracic limb deficit can be detected. If no thoracic limb deficit is observed and the pelvic limb signs are mild, the lesion either could be in the thoracolumbar spinal cord or in the cervical spinal cord. If the pelvic limb signs are moderate or severe with normal thoracic limbs, the lesion causing the signs is limited to the thoracolumbar spinal cord. When the pelvic limb signs are very severe but the thoracic limb signs are very subtle, then the possibility of a thoracolumbar lesion *and* a mild cervical lesion, or a diffuse spinal cord lesion, should be considered. Similarly, a moderate thoracic limb deficit with mild pelvic limb signs may be due to multifocal or diffuse lesions and is unlikely to be caused by a focal cervical spinal cord contusion. Most multifocal myelopathies in horses are inflammatory (myelitis) and most diffuse diseases are equine degenerative myeloencephalopathy.

A hypertonic, spastic, short-strided gait may occur with cerebellar disease with a mild degree of hypermetria. This gait, which is seen in Arabians with cerebellar cortical abiotrophy, can best be described as an apparent delay in the onset of the voluntary movement followed by an exaggerated response. The exaggerated response may produce a quick, short stride with limited joint movement (hypermetria). In the disease in Arabians these signs are symmetric in all four limbs but may be more obvious in the thoracic limbs. Strength is normal and there is no general proprioceptive ataxia in cerebellar disease. A head tremor and an abnormal menace response consistently accompany the gait abnormality. In unilateral cerebellar disease the abnormal gait usually is observed in the ipsilateral limbs.

Unilateral cerebral lesions generally do not interfere with the gait unless accompanied by increased intracranial pressure. Extensive manipulations that require extra coordinated efforts (hopping, righting, standing up) may elicit some minimal abnormalities in the contralateral limbs. If circling occurs, it is usually toward the side of the cerebral lesion. These lesions may be localized best by a visual deficit in the contralateral eyeball with normal pupillary response bilaterally. If increased intracranial pressure also is present, however, the pupillary responses also may be deficient. A dilated, unresponsive pupil may occur on the same side as a cerebral space-occupying lesion from oculomotor nerve compression.

When lesions affect the vestibular system peripherally (otitis media), or centrally in the vestibular nuclei or vestibular portions of the cerebellum, there is usually a head and body tilt toward the side of the lesion. If the lesion is peripheral, strength and general proprioception are normal and the animal drifts or lurches toward the affected side. Although such an animal shows no weakness or lack of knowledge as to where its limbs are located, it may show a slightly wide base stance, presumably for better balance. Blindfolding accentuates this loss of balance and may cause the animal to fall to the affected side. Further examination of the eyeballs may elicit other abnormalities due to lesions in this system (see section on cranial nerve examination).

Spinal Nerves

It should be remembered that an intact reflex only requires the muscles, their peripheral nerves, and the segments of brain stem or spinal cord from which the afferent neurons enter and the efferent neurons leave the CNS. A pain response on the part of the patient requires the afferent peripheral nerve and the white matter of the spinal cord and brain stem to the grey matter of the sensory cortex. Such a response usually is seen as a reaction on the part of the patient that also requires an intact pathway from the sensory motor cortex of the cerebrum through the white matter of the brain and spinal cord to efferent neurons and their axons in peripheral nerves. These efferent neurons of such reflex arcs and reactions, along with their terminal neuromuscular junctions, are the final common pathway of all motor function and are termed the lower motor neuron. All descending connections of neurons that help regulate the function of these LMNs are termed upper motor neurons. Thus the UMN includes the grey matter of the cerebral motor cortex, cerebellum, and brain stem nuclei (red nucleus, substantia nigra, reticular formation) and their descending tracts.

The upper motor neuron contains tracts that are both facilitatory and inhibitory to the function of the lower motor neuron; however, when upper motor neuron lesions exist there is usually a resulting "release" of the lower motor neuron from inhibition. Thus upper motor neuron signs are classically those of hypertonia of muscles and hyperreflexia of reflex arcs. If the lower motor neuron is affected, passive manipulation of the appropriate limb will reveal decreased or absent tone (flaccidity). Muscle tone cannot be assessed in a limb that the horse is lying on. Such lower motor neuron lesions also affect the local reflex arcs and thus cause depressed or absent reflexes. The last characteristic of lower motor neuron lesions is rapid muscle atrophy that results from denervation of peripheral muscles. Myelitis (i.e., protozoal) that affects the grey matter as well as the white matter produces observable atrophy of pelvic limb muscles if the lesion involves segments L4 through S1, and of the thoracic limb muscles if it is in segments C6 through T2. This is often asymmetric. In tetanus, the remarkable hypertonia results from neurotoxin interference with interneurons in the spinal cord that normally inhibit lower motor neuron reflex function.

The tendon reflexes should be examined first because they do not elicit a pain response. As a rule, these require a recumbent animal and can only be tested adequately in the limbs the animal is not lying on. Lower motor neuron lesions or lesions anywhere in the reflex arc cause hyporeflexia or areflexia, whereas upper motor neuron lesions result in reflexes that at least are present and may be hyperreflexic.

Patellar Reflex. This is elicited by holding the limb relaxed in a partially flexed position and striking the intermediate patellar ligament. This normally produces stifle extension. Striking the ligament with the edge of the hand will usually elicit the reflex. This reflex is mediated through the femoral nerve and primarily the L4 and L5 segments of the spinal cord. The femoral nerve is also sensory to the medial side of the limb through its saphenous nerve branch.

Triceps Reflex. Hold the relaxed limb in partial flexion, tap the triceps tendon at the olecranon, and observe for a mild elbow extension. This is mediated through the radial nerve and the cervical intumescence (C7, C8, T1). This nerve is also sensory to the midlateral surface of the arm and forearm. If this nerve is injured proximal to the triceps innervations the animal will drag or stand on the dorsum of the hoof and cannot support weight on the limb. This would also occur if the cell bodies in the cervical intumescence were affected. If the nerve is injured in the arm distal to the triceps innervation, weight can be supported but the digit cannot be extended; therefore the patient stands on the dorsum of the hoof.

Flexor Reflex—Pelvic Limb. Use fingers, forceps, or an electric prod on the coronary band or heel bulb, depending on the severity of the neurologic deficit. Use whatever is necessary to determine the reflex as well as the response to pain without upsetting the patient any more than is necessary.

The flexor reflex response requires the sciatic nerve and spinal cord segments L6, S1, and S2. If the sensory stimulation is restricted to the dorsal metatarsal region, the peroneal nerve will be stimulated. The plantar metatarsal region is innervated by the tibial nerve branch of the sciatic nerve. The coronary band receives both tibial and peroneal nerve innervation. Flexion of the stifle, hock, and digit is mediated by the sciatic nerve and its peroneal and tibial branches. Hip flexion is mediated by the entire lumbar spinal cord and the segmental innervation of the psoas major muscle.

When this reflex is performed, *two* observations should be made: first, the amount of reflex initiated, and second, the animal's cerebral response to the painful stimulus. The reflex only requires the sciatic nerve and the sixth lumbar and first and second sacral spinal cord segments. The cerebral response to pain requires that the sensory portion of these components *plus* the ascending spinal cord tracts that transmit sensory information to the rostral

brain stem and cerebral cortex be intact. The cerebral response to pain may be manifested by one or more of the following: pupillary dilation, altered respirations, head, ear, eyeball, and trunk movements, or kicking if the limb stimulated is not paralyzed. Lesions in the peripheral nerve being tested produce hypalgesia or analgesia and a depressed or absent reflex response. Lesions in the ascending spinal cord tracts for the sensory modalities perceived as pain produce hypalgesia or analgesia without any loss of the reflex function. Transverse spinal cord lesions that produce paresis or paralysis caudal to the lesion may be localized by finding a line of hypalgesia or analgesia along the body wall.

The cutaneous reflex also may be helpful in localizing a thoracolumbar spinal cord lesion. Gentle pin pricking of the skin along the dorsal and lateral aspects of the body wall elicits a quivering of the skin of the trunk from contraction of the cutaneous trunci muscle. The sensory stimulation is carried to the spinal cord segments by the dorsal branches of the segmental spinal nerves at the level of the stimulation. The sensory information is relayed cranially from that point through the spinal cord white matter to the first thoracic and eighth cervical segments, where it initiates action in the lower motor neuron cell bodies of the lateral thoracic nerve which innervates the cutaneous trunci. A lesion anywhere along this pathway may interfere with this reflex.

Flexor Reflex—Thoracic Limb. Stimulation of the coronary band or heel bulb stimulates the dendritic zone of neurons in the median nerve (and ulnar nerve laterally). The response of flexion of the digit, carpus, elbow, and shoulder requires the function of the last three cervical and first two thoracic spinal cord segments and the axillary, musculocutaneous, median, ulnar, and radial nerves.

A lesion that involves the spinal cord at the level of the cervical intumescence produces tetraparesis with lower motor neuron signs in the thoracic limbs (atonia, areflexia, atrophy) owing to the disturbance of the grey matter from C6 to T2, and upper motor neuron signs in the pelvic limbs (normal or exaggerated reflexes, and hypertonia without atrophy) due to the disturbance to the upper motor neuron tracts in the spinal cord white matter at C6 to T2.

A local cervical reflex similar to the cutaneous reflex of the trunk can be elicited by gently pricking the skin of the lateral neck and observing flicking of the skin of the neck due to contractions of the cutaneus colli and brachiocephalicus muscles. Some severe cervical lesions involving grey matter (myelitis) can result in a depressed or absent local cervical reflex.

Perineal Reflex. Mild stimulation of the skin of the perineum elicits reflex closure of the anus and tail flexion if the pudendal, caudal rectal and caudal nerves and the last three sacral and caudal segments of the spinal cord are intact. In horses with rabies the tail and anus may be hypotonic and hypalgesic.

Be sure to observe and differentiate both the reflex response and the cerebral response or reaction to the painful stimuli used. Occasionally, a severe spinal cord lesion has been found to result in hypalgesia confined to the ipsilateral limb or including a portion of the trunk if the grey matter lesion is diffuse. However, this is not common and the other findings in neurologic evaluation best define the site.

The axial musculature and the vertebrae should be palpated for deformities, or focal pain, or both. The few cases of equine myotonia that have been seen were easily detected by palpation of tense hypertrophied muscles that were hypersensitive to mechanical stimulus. Percussion resulted in a prolonged tight muscle "knotting" called a myotonic dimple that lasted less than 2 minutes. These foals do have a stiff, choppy gait in the pelvic and occasionally the thoracic limbs, especially after a period of rest. Acute extensive midcervical myelitis may result in a visual and palpable deformity (scoliosis) of the cervical vertebral column that mimics vertebral fracture or luxation.

SUMMARY OF SIGNS WITH LESIONS AT SPECIFIC AREAS OF THE SPINAL CORD

Lumbosacral Intumescence (L4 through Caudal Segments)

1. Thoracic limbs normal.
2. Ataxic and paretic pelvic limbs, with decreased ability to support weight to paraplegia (total pelvic limb paralysis).
3. Decreased or absent tail, anus, and pelvic limb tone and reflexes. Atrophy of pelvic limb muscles.
4. Hypalgesia or analgesia of the same areas with a line just caudal to the cranial edge of the lesion.
5. Urinary incontinence and obstipation.

Thoracolumbar (T3–L3)

1. Thoracic limbs normal.
2. Pelvic limb spasticity, ataxia, and paresis to paraplegia.
3. Normal tail and anal tone and reflexes and normal or exaggerated pelvic limb reflexes with normal tone or hypertonia. No neurogenic atrophy.
4. Hypalgesia or analgesia caudal to the lesion.
5. Focal area of sweating.
6. Urinary incontinence.

The same signs occur with lesions from L4 to L6 if they are confined to the white matter.

Cervical Intumescence (C6–T2)

1. Paresis (tetraparesis) and ataxia of all four limbs to tetraplegia.
2. Depressed or absent thoracic limb reflexes and tone with atrophy.
3. Normal or exaggerated pelvic limb reflexes and tone.
4. Hypalgesia or analgesia caudal to the cranial edge of the lesion. Hypalgesia may be more pronounced in the thoracic limbs.
5. Sweating of entire side of head and body and Horner's syndrome with severe lesions.

Cervical Spinal Cord Cranial to the Intumescence (C1–C5)

1. Spasticity, ataxia, and paresis (tetraparesis) of all four limbs to tetraplegia. Ataxia and paresis may be more obvious in the pelvic limbs.
2. Normal or exaggerated reflexes and tone in all four limbs.
3. Hypalgesia caudal to the lesion.
4. Sweating of entire side of head and body and Horner's syndrome with severe lesions.

The same signs may occur with lesions at C6 or C7 if they are confined to the white matter.

Cranial Nerves

I. Olfactory Nerve. Clinical deficit in smell rarely is encountered in the horse. Normal function may be observed by the patient's ability to smell the hand of the examiner or its feed.

II. Optic Nerve. Visual deficits may be seen as the animal maneuvers in its environment or through a maze. In the normal animal a sudden gesture of the hand toward the eye elicits immediate closure of the palpebral fissure and the head may jerk away from the movement. It is imperative to perform this maneuver far enough from the animal that contact is not made and air currents cannot be felt. The afferent component of this pathway includes the ipsilateral refractive media of the eyeball, the retina, optic nerve, and chiasm and primarily the contralateral optic tract, lateral geniculate nucleus (thalamus), and the optic radiation and occipital cortex of the cerebrum. The latter structures are contralateral to the eyeball being tested because 80 to 90 per cent of the optic nerve axons cross in the optic chiasm in the horse. The lower motor neuron involved is the facial nucleus in the medulla and facial nerve to the orbicularis oculi. There is indirect evidence that the pathway between the visual cerebral cortex and the facial nucleus involves the cerebellum or is influenced by the cerebellum. Young Arabians with cerebellar cortical abiotrophy do not respond to the menace gesture with eyelid closure, yet they have no facial palsy or visual deficit. Very young foals also may not respond, or become refractory during repeated testing. Thus, in horses with a poor or absent menace response it is important to determine whether they can see by other means.

Space-occupying or necrotic lesions in one cerebrum produce a contralateral visual deficit which can be observed by the failure to respond to the menace gesture, and by walking the patient through a maze, especially with the normal eye blindfolded. Bilateral lesions of the optic radiation (leukoencephalomalacia) or visual cortex (hepatic encephalopathy, viral encephalitides) produce a bilateral visual deficit. Pupillary responses to light are normal. Only if the lesion is in the eyeball or optic nerve or chiasm are pupillary light responses abnormal. Bilateral optic tract lesions also interfere with this but unilateral lesions may not. The afferent pathway to light directed into the eyeball is the same as for the menace gesture to the level of the lateral geniculate nucleus. The axons for this function pass by the neurons in this thalamic nucleus and synapse in the pretectal region of the brain stem. These second neurons in the afferent pathway in turn synapse on neurons in both oculomotor nuclei. Crossing can occur at the optic chiasm, as well as at the pretectal and oculomotor nuclear levels. Therefore, shining the light in one eyeball produces reflex pupillary constriction in both eyeballs. The efferent lower motor neuron is the parasympathetic preganglionic neuron in the oculomotor nucleus and its axon

in cranial nerve III (oculomotor nerve). Synapse occurs in the ciliary ganglion just caudal to the eyeball and postganglionic axons innervate the constrictor muscle of the pupil in the iris. This pupillary constriction pathway is limited to the brain stem and is spared by lesions affecting the visual pathways in the cerebrum.

In severely depressed animals the amount of pupil closure to light may be minimal, but the pupil usually is not mydriatic. An excited animal may have very widely dilated pupils that respond poorly to light. Prior to directing the light through the pupil for this reflex, pupillary apertures should be checked for size and symmetry. A widely dilated pupil in a normal eyeball suggests an oculomotor nerve deficit. It is unresponsive to light directed into either eyeball. The normal pupil responds when light is directed into the mydriatic pupil only if the optic nerve of the affected eyeball is intact. A partially dilated pupil may occur in severe unilateral retinal or optic nerve lesions and only responds to light directed into the normal eyeball. Bilateral severe miosis may occur with acute diffuse cerebral lesions. Severe brain stem contusions can produce a range of pupillary abnormalities that may change rapidly in the first few hours after the injury. Progressive bilateral dilation is a grave sign and suggests progressive edema in the mesencephalon.

Although a partially miotic pupil that contracts well to light is an easily recognized part of Horner's syndrome in other species, it can be difficult to detect in the horse. The most striking features of Horner's syndrome in the horse are ipsilateral hyperhidrosis, hyperthermia of the head, and cranial neck and ipsilateral ptosis of the upper eyelid. Other findings include mild miosis, congestion of nasal and conjunctival membranes, and increased lacrimation. This syndrome is seen in guttural pouch mycosis and surgery (postganglionic), deep cervical injections, space-occupying cervical lesions, and experimental section of the cervical sympathetic trunk (preganglionic). This is because the sympathetic supply for the eye and blood vessels of the head is carried in the cervical sympathetic trunk adjacent to the cervical vagus nerve. These fibers pass up the neck to the cranial cervical ganglion on the wall of the guttural pouch adjacent to the internal carotid artery, and the postganglionic fibers follow other vessels and nerves to all parts of the head.

The optic nerve should be observed with the ophthalmoscope as part of the neurologic examination. It occasionally may reflect increased intracranial pressure by the appearance of swelling at the optic disk.

III. Oculomotor Nerve (to Dorsal, Ventral and Medial Recti, Ventral Oblique, and Levator Palpebrae). The parasympathetic component of the oculomotor nerve is tested along with the optic nerve and visual pathway examination.

IV. Trochlear Nerve (to Dorsal Oblique).

VI. Abducent Nerve (to Lateral Rectus and Retractor Bulbi). The function of the extraocular muscles and their innervation by cranial nerves III, IV, and VI are tested simultaneously by observing the position of the eyeballs in the orbits and their movements. An abnormal position (strabismus) occurs if there is interference with the innervation of these muscles.

Without experimental or direct clinicopathologic correlation, the specific position of the strabismus in the horse for paralysis of each of these three cranial nerves is unknown. Comparing with other species and with humans, an oculomotor palsy should produce a lateral and ventral strabismus. Ptosis and mydriasis may accompany this due to paralysis of the levator palpebrae and pupillary constrictor muscles, respectively. A trochlear nerve palsy should cause the medial aspect of the pupil to rotate dorsally.

An abducent nerve palsy should cause a medial strabismus and possible lack of eyeball retraction (with protrusion of the third eyelid) when the corneal reflex is tested. These forms of strabismus should be present in all positions of the head because of the muscle paralysis.

Be aware of the strabismus associated with disturbances of the vestibular system. There is a direct anatomic connection between the vestibular system (cranial nerve VIII, vestibular nuclei, and vestibular part of cerebellum) and these extraocular muscle neurons by way of the medial longitudinal fasciculus (MLF) in the brain stem. Vestibular abnormalities may interfere with the normal tonic mechanism controlling eyeball position relative to head position and a strabismus may result. This is usually ventral and sometimes medial and may correct itself in certain positions of the head. The affected eyeball will abduct and adduct (normal vestibular nystagmus) if the head is moved from side to side. With unilateral vestibular disorders this vestibular strabismus occurs on the ipsilateral side.

If there is bilateral disturbance of the vestibular system or the MLF, then moving the head from side to side does not induce a normal eyeball movement (vestibular nystagmus). This is a grave sign in intracranial injuries, because it indicates that a brain stem lesion has occurred to interfere with the MLF.

V. Trigeminal (to Muscles of Mastication and Sensation to Most of Head). Lesions that affect the mandibular nerve innervation of the muscles of mastication bilaterally cause a dropped jaw and inability to close it. Unilateral lesions can be detected best by the atrophy of the temporal and masseter muscles that can be palpated.

The sensory function of this cranial nerve can be tested by gentle palpation of the eyelids medially (ophthalmic nerve) and laterally (ophthalmic and maxillary nerves), which causes the palpebral fissure to be closed (facial nerve). This is the palpebral reflex. Gentle palpation of the cornea with the lids held open tests the sensory function of the ophthalmic nerve and the extraocular muscle innervation that causes the eyeballs to be retracted (oculomotor and abducent nerves) and the third eyelid to protrude passively. This is the corneal reflex. Gentle palpation or light pin pricking of the upper lip and nostrils tests the maxillary nerve, and of the lower lip, tongue, and cheek tests the mandibular nerve response. In a depressed animal palpation of the nasal septum with a blunt probe may be required to elicit a hypalgesia (ophthalmic nerve).

Idiopathic hyperesthesia, referred to as trigeminal neuralgia, has been assumed in horses that continually rub one side of their faces.

Lesions that involve the spinal tract of the trigeminal nerve on the side of the medulla can produce a sensory deficit without paresis of the masticatory muscle (Fig. 12–4).

Cerebral lesions that interfere with the somesthetic cortex of the parietal lobe can produce a mild contralateral hypalgesia, most evident in the sensitive nasal septum.

VII. Facial Nerve (to Muscles of Facial Expression). This is the lower motor neuron of many of the reflexes that have been tested that produce closure of the palpebral fissure (menace, corneal, palpebral). Paresis or paralysis of these facial muscles causes the ear, upper eyelid, and the lower lip to droop, and the upper lip and nose to be pulled toward the normal side. A mild paresis may be detected by careful observation of the use of the lips on prehension and the lack of action of the nostrils on inspiration.

Injury to the buccal branches on the side of the face (recumbency, facial trauma) causes signs of paresis in the lips and nostrils only.

The facial nucleus can be affected by lesions in the medulla. The nerve can be involved in meningitis, otitis media, guttural pouch mycosis, or presumably by a selective transient neuritis (idiopathic facial paralysis). The diffuse neuropathy that primarily affects the cauda equina (neuritis of the cauda equina) also may affect other spinal and cranial nerves, including the facial nerve.

VIII. Vestibulocochlear Nerve

1. The cochlear division mediates the sensory modality interpreted as sound. Deafness most often is due to lesions of this nerve or the receptor in the cochlear duct. Congenital deafness is caused by aplasia or degeneration of this receptor end organ. Bilateral otitis media and otitis interna cause deafness. Unilateral deafness associated with otitis media and otitis interna may be difficult to detect.

2. The vestibular division innervates the receptor end organs in the semicircular ducts, macula, and utricle that function in the orientation of the head with the body, limbs, and the eyes. Vestibular system abnormalities can occur with lesions in the eighth cranial nerve, vestibular nuclei in the medulla, or vestibular components of the cerebellum. The abnormal posture of head, body, and eyes and the abnormal gait have been described. In addition, abnormal nystagmus may be observed. With peripheral nerve disorders (injury, otitis media or interna), the quick phase of the nystagmus always is directed to the opposite side from the lesion (head tilt), and may be horizontal or rotatory. In the first few days after the onset of the signs the nystagmus may be spontaneous—visible at all times. After this it may be elicited only by holding the head in different positions—positional nystagmus. With lesions in the central components of the vestibular system, the positional nystagmus may change direction with different positions of the head.

Remember that in pure vestibular system abnormalities there is no loss of strength. With unilateral vestibular disorders (otitis media-interna) the ataxia is asymmetric with tilting of the head and leaning, falling, or rolling of the body toward the side of the lesion. With diffuse cerebellar cortical disease (e.g., as occurs in Arabian foals), strength is normal and the remarkable hypertonic dysmetria is symmetric.

Patients with otitis media or interna may present with a sudden onset of clinical signs, and a frantic attitude.

IX, X, XI. Glossopharyngeal, Vagus, and Spinal Accessory Nerves. The most important clinical deficits of one or more components

of these nerves are laryngeal and pharyngeal paralysis. The cell bodies of the neurons that innervate these muscles are in the nucleus ambiguus of the medulla. The peripheral nerves are associated closely with the portion of the guttural pouch often affected by mycotic infections, and dysphagia often occurs with this disease.

Pharyngeal paralysis can be detected by observing the appearance of food and water at the nostrils, inability to swallow food or water, and inadequate swallowing of a stomach tube. The degree of difficulty depends on whether the lesion is unilateral or bilateral. Dysphagia is a common sign in rabies, probably due to lesions in the medulla. Be aware that severe diffuse cerebral disease may cause swallowing difficulties even though there is no primary lesion in the nucleus ambiguus. Also remember that myositis of the pharyngeal and lingual muscles may interfere with the swallowing function. Dysphagia is also one of the most prominent signs of the diffuse lower motor neuron paralysis in suspected botulism.

Laryngeal paralysis can be detected by the characteristic inspiratory dyspnea (roaring) that is audible on respiration. Neuropathy of these cranial nerves associated with chronic lead poisoning may cause pharyngeal and laryngeal paralysis.

XII. Hypoglossal Nerve (Motor to Tongue Muscles). Paralysis of one nerve produces atrophy of the ipsilateral half of the tongue but does not interfere much with its function. Bilateral palsy interferes with swallowing. The normal tongue resists attempts to pull it from the mouth. The paretic tongue can be pulled from the mouth easily and is slow to return. In a severely depressed horse the tongue may be pulled from the mouth easily, and it will hang out for a while before being returned to the mouth. Occasionally the tip may be chewed on. This can occur without a hypoglossal neuron lesion. The upper motor neuron (extrapyramidal nuclear) lesions in yellow star thistle poisoning may cause sudden dystonia of the masticatory (V), facial (VII), and tongue (XII) muscles that interferes with prehension and swallowing functions, occasionally accompanied by behavior changes and leaning and/or circling tendencies.

Palpate the skull for any deformities.

INTERPRETATION OF CSF ANALYSIS

Normal values for equine CSF analysis are as follows: cisternal pressure, 161 to 456 mm

H_2O; protein, 0 to 92 (mean 37) mg per dl; RBC, 0; WBC, 0 to 5 mm³; creatine kinase, 0 to 7 (mean 1) IU; glutamic-oxalacetic transaminase, 18 to 43 (mean 30) Sigma-Frankel units; and lactic dehydrogenase, 0 to 5 (mean 1.5) IU. There is no significant difference in cytology or protein and enzyme levels between fluid from the cerebellomedullary cistern and the lumbosacral subarachnoid space. It should be clear and colorless.[10]

As a general rule injury to the CNS results in a xanthochromic (yellow) CSF with slightly elevated protein (80 to 150 mg per dl) or occasionally a definitely bloody sample. However, large hemorrhages may be present epidurally with very little change in CSF. This can depend partly on the site of collection. If a brain or cranial cervical lesion is suspected, then an atlanto-occipital sample should be taken. A lumbosacral sample should be taken for all spinal cord problems caudal to this. Other diseases that can result in xanthochromic CSF with elevated protein and a few mononuclear cells (10 to 30 per mm³) are intracarotid injections of drugs such as promazine, deep cerebral abscess (*Streptococcus equi*), vertebral osteomyelitis, and acute wobbler syndrome. Classically equine herpesvirus I (rhinopneumonitis) vasculitis/myelopathy results in a xanthochromic fluid with elevated protein (80 to 200 mg per dl) and little or no cellular response. The CSF changes with protozoal myelitis are variable. Although a moderately elevated protein (100 to 200 mg per dl) and mononuclear pleocytosis (50 to 100 per mm³) can be expected, the CSF is often normal. The arboviral encephalitides produce a pleocytosis that can vary in nature. In Venezuelan equine encephalomyelitis and eastern equine encephalomyelitis during the acute phase, a high neutrophil count (<100 to 500+ per mm³) can be expected that will change to a predominantly small mononuclear pleocytosis over several days. Western equine encephalomyelitis produces a less marked pleocytosis (50 to 200 per mm³) that is predominantly (>50 per cent) small mononuclear cells. In all cases the protein content also is elevated to about 100 to 300 mg per dl. Rabies virus encephalomyelitis alters the CSF results in a manner similar to that in western equine encephalomyelitis. The most common diffuse cerebral disease, hepatoencephalopathy, does not effectively alter the CSF findings, although a slight yellow discoloration may be apparent as a result of the profound dehydration and icterus.

INDEX OF DISEASES OF THE NERVOUS SYSTEM OF HORSES

The diseases of the nervous system of the horse that have been referred to in this book are organized here according to the five basic kinds of lesions that these diseases produce in the nervous system. These include the following:

Malformation of the nervous tissue

Injury—from external trauma and from internal compression by adjacent structures such as a neoplasm, abscess, or vertebral malformation

Inflammation—usually caused by an infectious agent

Neoplasia—primary neoplasm of nervous tissue

Degeneration—from metabolic diseases, nutritional causes, intoxications, or vascular impairment.

A final category are those diseases primarily considered to be idiopathic. Following each disease is its location in the book.

The neurologic examination provides the basis for localizing the lesion in the nervous system. The following is a listing of the diseases, previously classified by kind of lesion, arranged on the basis of the primary anatomic area that may be affected and show clinical signs:

CEREBRAL
Congenital hydrocephalus
Injury
Protozoal encephalitis
Rabies

Viral encephalomyelitis
Herpesvirus I encephalitis (rare)
Leukoencephalomalacia, mycotoxic
Abscess
Hepatic encephalopathy
Epilepsy

BRAIN STEM
Injury
Protozoal encephalitis
Herpesvirus I encephalitis
Parasitic encephalitis
Abscess
Nigropallidal encephalomalacia
Pituitary neoplasm

CEREBELLUM
Protozoal encephalitis
Parasitic encephalitis
Abscess
Injury
Neuronal abiotrophy
Paspalum staggers
Rye grass poisoning

SPINAL CORD
Hamartoma
External injury
Internal injury
Vertebral malformation
Occipitoatlantoaxial
Cervical: cervical stenotic myelopathy
Thoracolumbar
Synovial cyst
Neoplasia
Protozoal myelitis
Herpesvirus I myelitis
Nonsuppurative myelitis
Parasitic myelitis
Degenerative myelopathy
Fibrocartilaginous embolic myelopathy
Tetanus
Shivering

NEUROMUSCULAR—SPINAL NERVE
Injury
Botulism
Aortic thrombosis—ischemic neuromyopathy
Polyneuritis-neuritis of cauda equina
Nutritional myopathy
Exertional myopathy
Myotonia
Tetanus
Shivering

CRANIAL NERVES
Injury
Laryngeal hemiplegia
Guttural pouch mycosis
Otitis media-interna
Protozoal encephalitis

Optic nerve hypoplasia
Optic neuropathy
Night blindness

DIFFUSE
Rabies encephalomyelitis
Leukoencephalomalacia, mycotoxic
Paspalum staggers
Rye grass poisoning
Miscellaneous poisons

The following diseases of horses are summarized here owing to lack of or incomplete coverage elsewhere in the textbook.

Rabies.   Rabies, an encephalomyelitis caused by a neurotropic virus, is usually fatal by 10 days after the onset of clinical signs. The clinical signs are variable.[9]

A common initial clinical sign is ataxia that is usually diagnosed as due to focal spinal cord disease. The presence or progression to hyperesthesia should indicate a more diffuse problem. Paresis and ataxia will progress to recumbency and seizures often occur near the terminal stage of the disease. Medullary signs of cranial nerve deficit are not common. Other signs observed in the course of the disease may include visual deficit, behavioral changes, odontoprisis, incontinence, anal and tail paresis and hypalgesia, muscle spasms, roaring, sweating, and fever.

Viral Encephalomyelitis.   The equine viral encephalitides are the inflammations of the central nervous system of horses caused by a group of togaviruses that usually reside in birds and are transmitted to the horse by a biting insect. In the United States these include Eastern, Western, and Venezuelan equine encephalomyelitis. The lesion is a diffuse nonsuppurative meningoencephalomyelitis that varies in intensity with the virus involved. Most clinical signs reflect the involvement of the cerebral hemispheres: lethargy, unresponsiveness, aimless walking along a fence or in circles, and blindness. With involvement of the brain stem and spinal cord, ataxia and paresis occur and may progress to recumbency. The Eastern and Venezuelan viruses produce a more progressive lesion and more clinical signs than does the Western variety. Fever and anorexia usually accompany the neurologic signs.

REFERENCES

1. Adams, L. G., Dollahite, J. W., Romane, W. M., Bullard, T. L., and Bridges, C. H.: Cystitis and ataxia associated with sorghum ingestion by horses. J. Am. Vet. Med. Assoc., *155*:518, 1969.
2. de Lahunta, A.: Neurological problems of the horse. Proc. Am. Assoc. Equine Pract. *19*:25, 1973.
3. de Lahunta, A.: Diagnosis of equine neurologic problems. Cornell Vet., *68*:122, 1978.
4. Ferris, D. H., and Beamer, P. D.: Comparative studies of equine encephalomyelitis caused by nematodes, viruses, and mycotoxins. Proc. Am. Assoc. Equine Pract., *17*:173, 1971.
5. Gabel, A. A., and Koestner, A.: The effects of intracarotid artery injection of drugs in domestic animals. J. Am. Vet. Med. Assoc., *162*:1397, 1963.
6. Harries, W. N., Baker, F. P., and Johnston, A.: An outbreak of locoweed poisoning in horses in southwestern Alberta. Can. Vet. J., *13*:141, 1972.
7. Harrington, D. D.: Pathologic features of magnesium deficiency in young horses fed purified rations. Am. J. Vet. Res., *35*:503, 1974.
8. Holliday, T. A.: The nervous system–examination. *In* Catcott, E. J., and Smithcors, J. F. (eds.): Equine Medicine and Surgery. 2nd ed. Wheaton, Ill., American Veterinary Publications, Inc., 1972.
9. Joyce, J. R., and Russell, L. H.: Clinical signs of rabies in horses. Compend. Contin. Ed., *3*:S56, 1981.
10. Mayhew, I. G., Whitlock, R. H., and Tasker, J. B.: Equine cerebrospinal fluid: Reference values of normal horses. Am. J. Vet. Res., *38*:1271, 1977.
11. Mayhew, I. G., and Ingram, J. T.: Neurologic evaluation of the horse. Proc. Am. Assoc. Equine Pract., *24*:525, 1978.
12. Woods, J. R.: Neurologic examination of the horse. Okla. Vet., *24*:11, 1972.

FOOD ANIMAL NEUROLOGIC EXAMINATION AND INDEX OF DISEASES OF THE NERVOUS SYSTEM

**FOOD ANIMAL NEUROLOGIC
    EXAMINATION
INDEX OF DISEASES OF THE NERVOUS
    SYSTEM OF FOOD ANIMALS**

The neurologic evaluation of any species of animal follows the physical examination and is for the purpose of observing abnormalities that reflect a disturbance of the nervous system and locating where this disturbance has affected the nervous system. This assessment is the anatomic diagnosis. A differential diagnosis is then established for a disease at the site of the anatomic diagnosis. This differential diagnosis will reflect the clinician's knowledge of the signalment, and history of the onset and course of the disease. Appropriate ancillary studies are then planned based on the diseases under consideration in the initial differential diagnosis. Evaluation of these results and further evaluation of the patient and the disease course will result in a presumptive diagnosis. A prognosis is then considered and therapy planned for this presumptive diagnosis.

The purpose of the neurologic examination is to establish where the lesion or disturbance is located in the nervous system. Five major anatomic sites may be considered: neuromuscular, spinal cord, brain stem, cerebellum, and cerebral.

Neuromuscular diseases usually cause profound weakness with loss of tone, reflexes, and atrophy. Involvement of only one limb usually implicates a peripheral nerve problem. Bilateral gait abnormalities in an alert, responsive animal usually incriminate a spinal cord lesion. Gait deficits and cranial nerve abnormalities occur with brain stem lesions. Circling with a head tilt and other signs of imbalance occur with vestibular system disturbance. Propulsive circling without signs of vestibular disturbance reflects a frontal lobe or rostral thalamic lesion. Spastic ataxia, dysmetria, and head tremor occur with cerebellar lesions. A disturbed sensorium or abnormal behavior implicates a brain stem and/or cerebral lesion. Blindness with normal pupils incriminates the cerebrum. Seizures occur primarily with cerebral lesions.

FOOD ANIMAL NEUROLOGIC EXAMINATION[3, 4]

The description of the neurologic examination in small animals (Chapter 21) is generally applicable to the small or young food animals: goats, sheep, young pigs, calves, and foals. The equine neurologic examination (Chapter 22) is generally applicable to the bovine animal.

Evaluate the animal's sensorium and behavior by watching its response to its environment and to you. Abnormalities suggest brain disease, especially of the cerebrum.

Evaluate its ability to stand and walk. Observe the gait while walking, turning corners, walking with the neck extended, walking in a small circle in both directions, and backing. Observe the animal walking and running loose in an enclosed area. With a cooperative animal and difficult problem it may help to observe these on a sloped surface. Observe the animal's response when it is being pulled to the side by the tail (swaying) as it is walked. Small food animals can be observed while being hopped on each limb in a lateral direction, and while standing and walking on the limbs on one side only (hemistanding, hemiwalking). The gait will be abnormal with neuromuscular, spinal cord, caudal brain stem, and cerebellar lesions but not with lesions confined to the cerebrum. Neurologic gait abnormalities include paresis, ataxia, spasticity, and dysmetria.

In the recumbent animal, evaluate the tone

in the limbs, anus, and tail, the patellar and all flexor reflexes, the perineal reflex, and pain perception from the limbs, anus, and tail. The patellar and flexor reflexes should be done on the nonrecumbent side. Test the cutaneous reflex. Palpate for muscle atrophy and palpate the vertebral column for shape and for pain. Except for the patellar reflex, most of these can be determined in the standing animal.

If the animal is recumbent but can readily stand up on its forelimbs and sit like a dog, its lesion is at least caudal to T2. If it cannot reach this position, the lesion is usually in the cervical spinal cord or brain stem. With caudal cervical spinal cord lesions, the animal may be able to flex its neck laterally and raise the head and neck off the ground. With severe cranial cervical lesions, only the head can be moved.

Evaluate vision (during walking; menace response—II, central visual pathway—VII), pupillary size and response to light (II, III), eyeball position (III, IV, VI, and vestibular), normal and abnormal nystagmus (vestibular), facial muscle strength (VII), masticatory muscle size and strength (V), facial sensation (V), ability to swallow (IX, X, XI), tongue strength (XII), facial temperature, and nasal sweating (sympathetic).

Based on this examination, the anatomic diagnosis should be determined. Is the lesion neuromuscular, spinal cord, brain stem, cerebellum, cerebral, multifocal, or diffuse? Only then should the kind of lesion be considered. In establishing the differential diagnosis, consider five categories of lesions: malformation, injury, inflammation, neoplasia, degeneration (vascular, toxic, metabolic, nutritional). Ancillary studies will be determined from the diseases selected for the differential diagnosis.

INDEX OF DISEASES OF THE NERVOUS SYSTEM OF FOOD ANIMALS

The diseases of the nervous system of food animals that have been referred to in this book are organized here according to the five basic kinds of lesions that these diseases produce in the nervous system. These include the following:

Malformation of the nervous tissue
Injury—from external trauma and from internal compression by adjacent structures such as a neoplasm, abscess, or vertebral malformation
Inflammation—usually caused by an infectious agent
Neoplasia—primary neoplasm of nervous tissue
Degeneration—from metabolic diseases, nutritional causes, intoxication, or vascular impairment.

A final category are those diseases primarily considered to be idiopathic. Following each disease is its location in the book.

The neurologic examination provides the basis for localizing the lesion in the nervous system. The following is a listing of the diseases, previously classified by kind of lesion, arranged on the basis of the primary anatomic area that may be affected and show clinical signs.

CEREBRAL
Prosencephalic hypoplasia
Meningoencephalocele
Hydranencephaly (Akabane, blue-tongue viruses)
Prosencephalic duplication
Hereford encephalomyopathy
Congenital hydrocephalus
Vitamin A deficiency-seizures
Rabies encephalitis
Brain abscess
Injury
Thrombotic meningoencephalitis *(H. somnus)*
Caprine viral leukoencephalitis (CAE)
Parelaphostrongylus tenuis encephalitis
Arsanilic acid poisoning (pig)
Mercury poisoning
Lead poisoning
Salt poisoning
Water intoxication
Storage disease
Coccidiosis-seizures
Hepatic encephalopathy
Polioencephalomalacia

BRAIN STEM
Polioencephalomyelitis (pig)
Rabies encephalitis
Listeriosis
Caprine leukoencephalitis (CAE)
Parelaphostrongylus tenuis encephalitis
Thrombotic meningoencephalitis *(H. somnus)*
Abscess
Injury
Leptomeningitis

CEREBELLUM
In utero bovine virus diarrhea infection
In utero hog cholera virus infection
Neuronal abiotrophy
Abscess
Listeriosis
Injury
Paspalum staggers
Phalaris staggers
Rye grass staggers

SPINAL CORD
Meningomyelocele
Myelodysplasia
Diplomyelia
Diastematomyelia
External injury
Internal injury
    Atlantoaxial malformation
    Abscess
    Lymphosarcoma
    Neurofibroma
Polioencephalomyelitis (pig)
Rabies encephalomyelitis
Fibrocartilaginous embolic myelopathy
Poliomyelomalacia (pig)
Arsanilic acid poisoning (pig)
Caprine viral leukomyelitis (CAE)
Parelaphostrongylus tenuis myelitis
Haloxon intoxication (sheep)
Nutritional myelopathy (pig)
Swayback—nutritional myelopathy
Myelin disorder of Charolais
Tetanus
Spastic paresis
Spastic syndrome

NEUROMUSCULAR—SPINAL NERVE
Injury
Botulism
Triorthocresylphosphate poisoning
Neurofibroma
Polyneuritis
Myotonia (goat)
Nutritional myopathy
Tetanus
Spastic paresis
Spastic syndrome

CRANIAL NERVE
Optic neuropathy–Vitamin A deficiency
Cyclopia
Ocular malformations
Otitis media-interna (VII, VIII)
Congenital nystagmus

DIFFUSE
Rabies encephalomyelitis
Polioencephalomyelitis (pig)
Caprine leukoencephalomyelitis (CAE)
Parelaphostrongylus tenuis encephalomyelitis
Thrombotic meningoencephalomyelitis
  (*H. somnus*)
Paspalum staggers
Phalaris staggers
Rye grass staggers
Snakeroot poisoning
Hereditary neuraxial edema
Hypomyelinogenesis-dysmyelinogenesis
Myelin disorder of Charolais
Arsanilic acid poisoning (pig)
Storage disease
Malignant catarrhal fever
Sporadic bovine encephalomyelitis

For the following bovine diseases, either they have not been described in this textbook or their descriptions have been limited.

Listeriosis. Listeriosis is a bacterial meningoencephalitis caused by *Listeria monocytogenes*.[5] It affects ruminants of all ages but more commonly young adults over 1 year old. Occasionally outbreaks occur associated with a silage diet. The organism grows well in an environmental pH of greater than 5.4. The organism enters the brain via the blood or over the trigeminal nerve, and lesions are most profound in the pons and medulla.

Signs may be acute in onset and include depression, vestibular disturbance (loss of balance, head tilt, abnormal nystagmus, circling), facial paresis to paralysis, tetraparesis and ataxia, medial strabismus, dysphagia, weak jaw and tongue, and occasionally cerebellar signs (head tremor, hypermetria), and sialosis. The latter may cause significant acidosis. Seizures and blindness usually do not occur.

Fever may occur only early in the disease. CSF usually has a mild lymphoid-mononuclear pleocytosis and elevated protein.

The prognosis for response to antibiotic therapy is better if the patient is still able to stand and walk. Treat with 40,000 units of penicillin per kg bid for 7 to 14 days. Decrease the dose to one half for next 7 days. Treat the acidosis with bicarbonate.

Leptomeningitis. Suppurative leptomeningitis is caused by a number of bacteria in young calves. *Escherichia coli, Pasteurella* sp., and *Pneumococcus* sp. are often cultured. Clinical signs reflect diffuse brain disease, but the caudal brain stem and cerebellar deficits predominate.

Tetraparesis and ataxia progress to recumbency. Head tilt, head tremor, abnormal nystagmus may be accompanied by depression to semicoma and occasionally opisthotonos. These calves are usually not blind, not hyperesthetic, and do not seizure. Hypopyon and fever may be present.

CSF contains a marked neutrophilic pleocytosis and moderate protein elevation. If an organism is cultured, the antibiotic to which it is most sensitive should be administered.

Polioencephalomalacia - Cerebrocortical Necrosis. Polioencephalomalacia is a disease of all ruminants.[6] It is most common in young cattle 3 to 18 months old. It is more common in cattle on a heavy grain ration and often follows a dietary change to less roughage by 3 to 4 weeks. It affects individual dairy cattle or occurs in outbreaks in grain-fed feedlot cattle.

Typically the onset is acute with a mild generalized ataxia rapidly followed by blindness with normal pupillary responses, depression, head pressing, and dorsomedial strabismus. Miosis may be severe. Recumbency follows in a few hours, with semicoma and opisthotonos, rigidly extended limbs, and abnormal nystagmus. Seizures are seen only occasionally.

This is a metabolic encephalopathy due to a deficiency of thiamin. This may be due to excessive growth of thiaminase-producing organisms in the rumen or formation of analogs that compete with thiamin as a coenzyme. The metabolic defect results in a degeneration most profound in the cerebral cortex.

CSF may be normal or may contain mild increases in leukocytes and protein.

The sooner the treatment is started with thiamin, the better the prognosis. Treat with intravenous thiamin at 10 mg per kg every 3 hours. Most show signs of improvement by the third treatment if recovery is to occur. Treat seriously affected cattle with mannitol (20 per cent, 1 to 2 gm per kg) for the cytotoxic edema.

Many of the herd may have marginal thiamin adequacy and should be treated with oral or intramuscular thiamin. Roughage should be increased to 50 per cent of the diet and Brewer's yeast can be added.

Lead Poisoning.   Lead poisoning occurs in all ages of cattle including young calves that have access to lead paint, batteries, or crank case oil.

An acute form occurs in calves or adults. Generalized seizures are common. Other signs of hyperactivity include excessive chewing, facial twitches, bellowing, charging, mania, hyperesthesia, odontoprisis, and head pressing. Recumbency with opisthotonos and extensor rigidity may follow. They are usually blind with normal pupil responses to light. Death often occurs in 24 hours.

A subacute form occurs in adults and consists of blindness with normal pupil responses, depression to stupor, ataxia, head pressing, circling, grinding of the teeth, and a head bob. There are usually no ruminal contractions, and constipation is common.

CSF can be normal or have mild elevation in protein and mononuclear cells.

Treatment is often effective if administered early. It consists of calcium EDTA in a continuous flow at 110 to 220 mg per kg, followed by 2 rapid doses of 110 mg per kg each at a 6-hour interval. Pentobarbital may be needed to control seizures.

Salt-Water Imbalance.   Cytotoxic edema will occur if the osmolality of the central nervous system is upset by either excessive amounts of sodium ion in the diet or a diet with water deprivation or the animal suddenly consumes a large quantity of water. Signs mostly reflect a cerebral disturbance: dullness to hyperesthesia, tremors, muscle spasms, seizures, and blindness. Ataxia, paresis, nystagmus, opisthotonos, and coma follow brain stem involvement in severe cases. Death can occur suddenly.

Hypernatremia has been observed in veal calves that are raised in confinement and fed solely on milk replacement containing whey that has excessive salt; these calves have no access to water.

Cerebrocortical necrosis has been observed in cattle with water deprivation.

With direct or indirect (water deprivation) salt poisoning, serum and CSF sodium and chloride levels are elevated and the osmolality is increased. Water-intoxicated calves have depressed osmolality and electrolyte levels, intramuscular hemolysis, and hemoglobinuria.

Thrombotic Meningoencephalitis.   Thrombotic meningoencephalitis is a bacterial disease of cattle caused by *Hemophilus somnus*. It is most common in feedlot cattle 8 to 12 months old but also is observed in dairy cattle. It is often associated with stress and may affect several animals over a few days.

Septic vasculitis and thrombosis occur in blood vessels throughout the brain and spinal cord. Clinical signs reflect the parenchymal lesions that result from the vascular impairment and inflammation. Ataxia and paresis progress to recumbency and severe depression. Occasionally death occurs suddenly. Blindness is not common and more often is unilateral. Seizures occur occasionally and there is usually more depression than instability. Mania and hyperesthesia are uncommon.

There may also be fundic lesions of chorioretinitis, synovitis, myositis, laryngitis, pleuritis, or pneumonia. Fever and leukocytosis with neutrophilia are common. CSF contains excessive neutrophils and protein, and the organism may be cultured from the CSF, blood, joints, or pleural cavity.

Some cattle respond to early treatment with tetracyclines, penicillin, or sulfonamides. Administer oxytetracycline intravenously at 10 mg per kg every 12 hours for 3 treatments.

Malignant Catarrhal Fever.   This is a presumed viral disease of cattle with a reservoir of the infectious agent in sheep. It affects multiple organs with a primary lesion of fibrinoid necrotizing vasculitis. The nervous system is involved in the head and eye form. The lesion of vasculitis and associated meningitis and encephalomyelitis is diffuse through the central nervous system. Clinical signs are nonspecific and include depression, ataxia, and paresis. Blindness and seizures are rare. Ocular lesions primarily affect the cornea and conjunctiva. In addition to diarrhea, clinical signs of respiratory system disease may occur. Fever is persistent, and leukopenia may occur.

Sporadic Encephalomyelitis (Buss disease). This is a diffuse nonsuppurative meningoencephalitis and serositis (pleuritis, pericarditis, peritonitis) caused by *Chlamydia pecoris* or a paramyxovirus. Calves less than 6 months old are most susceptible, and the disease is more acute with recumbency or opisthotonos but not blindness. In older cattle the signs are more vague and include depression and mild paresis and ataxia. Fever and leukopenia usually occur. Some respond to early treatment with tetracyclines.

Rabies. Cattle of all ages that are exposed to wildlife or dogs are susceptible. The signs are extremely variable. In general two forms are observed. The acute, maniacal, furious form is accompanied by hyperesthesia, bellowing, ataxia, charging of animate or inanimate objects, and sexual excitement. Blindness and seizures are rare. These cattle may collapse and die in 1 to 2 days. In the milder, dull, paralytic form, there is an ascending paralysis. Initially there is pelvic limb paresis and ataxia, a flaccid tail that is hypalgesic or analgesic, and anal atonia with tenesmus and sucking and blowing of air in the rectum. The pelvic limbs become hypalgesic as the paresis and ataxia occur in the thoracic limbs. Sialosis, yawning, and occasionally weak bellowing occur. Recumbency and death usually occur in 6 to 7 days.

Hepatic Encephalopathy. Hepatic encephalopathy follows the liver lesion and dysfunction associated with the consumption of plants containing pyrrolizidine alkaloids *(Senecio, Crotolaria,* and *Amsinckia* spp.).[2] Clinical signs, which include dullness, propulsive walking, circling, and head pressing, predominantly reflect a cerebral disturbance. Aggressive behavior may occur with charging and persistent bellowing. Blindness and seizures may follow. In addition, some calves may be icteric and have a photodermatitis.

High-producing dairy cows that consume large amounts of high-energy feed during the dry period may develop an extensively fatty liver.[1] Encephalopathy may follow with vague signs of cerebral dysfunction: staring into space, elevated head, and tremors. Mild ataxia and paresis may occur and progress to recumbency.

REFERENCES

1. Deem, D. A.: Bovine fatty liver syndrome. Compend. Contin. Ed., *2*:S185, 1980.
2. Finn, J. P., and Tennant, B.: Hepatic encephalopathy in cattle. Cornell Vet., *64*:136, 1974.
3. Hofmeyer, C. F. B.: Evaluation of neurologic examination of sheep. J. S. Afr. Vet. Assoc., *49*:45, 1978.
4. Leighton, R. L.: Neurologic examination of cattle. Vet. Scope, *8*:2, 1968.
5. Rebhun, W. C., and de Lahunta, A.: Diagnosis and treatment of bovine listeriosis. J. Am. Vet. Med. Assoc., *180*:395, 1982.
6. Smith, M. C.: Polioencephalomalacia in goats. J. Am. Vet. Med. Assoc., *174*:1328, 1979.

CASE DESCRIPTIONS

Each case description has three parts: the first part is the description of the neurologic disorder; the second part includes the neuroanatomic diagnosis and how this was determined, the differential diagnosis, and the ancillary data available in the case; and the third part includes the course of the disease, the final clinical or necropsy diagnosis, and a brief discussion of the syndrome.

Case 1: Case Description

Signalment. A 4-year-old female Great Dane-cross.

Chief Complaint. Weakness and ataxia.

History. Starting 5 months prior to examination, this dog had episodes of coughing and gasping. Numerous examinations during this time did not result in a definite diagnosis. The owner commented that the dog's eyes looked different during this period of time. One month prior to examination, a veterinarian observed anisocoria from a small left pupil. About 10 days prior to examination, the dog began to lose coordination in the pelvic limbs and a head tilt was apparent. The ataxia progressed to the thoracic limbs.

Examination. The dog was alert and responsive but seemed disoriented in space. Its head was tilted to the left. It was reluctant to stand but could do so unassisted, and it continually leaned against the wall on its left side. When excited, the dog nearly tipped over toward its left side. Its strength seemed to be normal.

Postural reactions were difficult to test because of the animal's disorientation. It frantically grasped for support when picked up to perform postural tests. There was a suggestion that the left pelvic limb hopped poorly.

Hypertonia was marked in the thoracic limbs and mild in the pelvic limbs. There was no atrophy. Patellar reflexes were hyperactive (plus 3) bilaterally. Biceps and triceps reflexes were present. Flexor reflexes and the perineal reflex were all normal and pain perception was normal.

On cranial nerve examination there was observed in the left eye a small pupil, protruded third eyelid, and smaller palpebral fissure. The head was tilted to the left (left ear more ventral). On holding the head and neck in extension the left eyeball did not elevate normally in the fissure. A positional abnormal nystagmus occurred that was mostly rotatory to

the right. There was a moderate atrophy of the tongue muscles on the left side. The gag reflex was normal.

Diagnosis

Neuroanatomic Diagnosis. These signs indicated a caudal brain stem lesion on the left side. The vestibular signs (head tilt, tipping of the body to the left, strabismus, and abnormal nystagmus) were severe. The degree of severity suggested central vestibular involvement. The tongue atrophy indicated hypoglossal nucleus or nerve involvement, which could not occur with otitis media or other middle and inner ear disease. The signs of Horner's syndrome (miosis, protruded third eyelid, and smaller palpebral fissure) were due to sympathetic nerve paralysis to the orbital structures. This can occur with middle ear disease. Horner's syndrome would be unlikely with medullary disease without more evidence of medullary involvement accompanied by ipsilateral severe hemiparesis. The history of gagging and coughing suggested paresis of pharyngeal muscles and could occur with disease of the pharyngeal branches of the ninth and tenth cranial nerves on one side. This also would not accompany an otitis media.

If the earliest observations of gagging and anisocoria were reliable, they suggest involvement of these nerves long before any vestibular signs or other signs of brain stem involvement. The latter occurred later and would be best explained by an extramedullary or extracranial mass involving the pharyngeal branches of the ninth and tenth cranial nerves and the sympathetic trunk or the cranial cervical ganglion, which later grew into the cranial cavity and compressed the left side of the medulla. The failure to observe any facial paresis indicated that the lesion should be caudal to the internal acoustic meatus. Within the medulla the vestibular nuclei extend farther caudal than the facial nucleus and could be affected by a compressing mass at that point.

Differential Diagnosis. As suggested, an extramedullary mass lesion would best explain the development of this syndrome. An inflammatory lesion of the middle ear was excluded on anatomic grounds. Inflammations of the medulla in the dog rarely produce such specific cranial nerve deficits. An exception could be an extramedullary abscess, but these are rare in the dog. In most animals they are associated with otitis media and petrosal bone abscesses. The progression of signs, with vestibular signs coming late in onset, did not suggest this pathogenesis. A chronic meningitis or diffuse meningeal neoplastic process possibly could produce these signs if it was concentrated on the left side of the medulla. However, this would not explain the Horner's syndrome. The signs were too progressive for any traumatic or ischemic degenerative lesion. Most other degenerations would not be this focal in nature. Progression and age ruled out malformation.

Ancillary Studies. Cerebrospinal fluid had an opening pressure of 140 mm H_2O. After removing 2 cc of clear, colorless fluid the closing pressure was 60 mm H_2O. It contained 3 RBC and no WBC per cmm, and 71 mg of protein per dl.

Plain radiographs were normal. Scintigraphy only slightly suggested increased uptake of radioisotope on the left side of the caudal fossa.

Outcome

The ancillary studies supported the diagnosis of an extramedullary mass. The brain-CSF barrier had been disturbed and the protein was moderately elevated. There was no indication of a primary suppurative inflammatory lesion. Following anesthesia for the ancillary studies the vestibular signs were remarkably exacerbated, and the dog continually attempted to roll to the left side.

In the dog this form of vestibular disturbance is usually only seen with vestibular nuclear lesions or lesions of the vestibular components of the cerebellum.

The dog was still difficult to evaluate for postural reactions but did show evidence of more difficulty manipulating the paws on the left side, which was further indication of involvement of the left side of the medulla.

Prognosis for recovery was poor without surgical intervention and was guarded with it. It was difficult to keep the dog from injuring itself when it rolled. The owner elected to have euthanasia performed.

Necropsy Findings. Four days after these studies necropsy revealed massive enlargement of the vagosympathetic trunk in the cranial cervical region. It included the distal ganglion of the vagus and extended into the cranial cavity through the tympano-occipital fissure and jugular foramen. Within the cranial cavity this mass measured 14 mm in diameter and compressed the medulla caudal to the trapezoid body and seventh and eighth cranial nerves (Fig. 24–1). The intracranial portion of the hypoglossal neurons was distended with neoplastic tissue, as was the spinal portion of the eleventh cranial nerve. The glossopharyngeal and vagal neurons were directly involved in the large intracranial mass. Although the mass spared the cranial cervical ganglion, the adjacent sympathetic trunk was involved. On microscopic examination this neoplasm was diagnosed as a neurofibroma.

The course of the disease, with sympathetic and

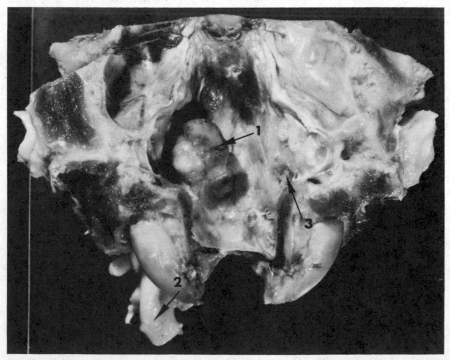

Figure 24–1. Case 1: Dorsoventral view of ventral aspect of caudal fossa of cranial cavity with the brain removed. The mass on the left (*1*) is continuous through the jugular foramen and tympano-occipital fissure with a similar mass in the vagosympathetic trunk (*2*). The normal right jugular foramen is indicated (*3*).

pharyngeal areas being the first presumed to be involved, is highly suggestive that the mass began outside the cranial cavity in the region of the tympano-occipital fissure. This is further supported by the late onset of the vestibular signs. There is no indication of when the hypoglossal involvement began, since this would have required visualization of the hemiatrophy of the tongue.

Remember that Horner's syndrome can be produced by lesions in a wide range of anatomic locations. The presence of other signs of neurologic disturbance usually determines the site of the lesion in the sympathetic nervous system. Dogs with persistent choking, gagging, or coughing for which no explanation can be found in the pharynx should be evaluated for a possible partial paralysis of the pharyngeal muscles.

Case 2: Case Description

Signalment. A 5-year-old male Great Dane.

Chief Complaint. Inability to use the pelvic limbs.

History. Two days prior to examination the dog had been out walking with its owner and on returning to the house developed difficulty using its pelvic limbs. Within a few minutes it collapsed on these limbs and could not get up.

Examination by a veterinarian the next morning revealed paraplegia with a normal patellar reflex, absent flexor reflex, and depressed perineal reflex. There was also urinary incontinence.

Examination. On examination two days after the onset of signs the dog was alert and responsive, but had no voluntary use of the pelvic limbs—grade 0 paraplegia. Occasionally a mild degree of hip flexion occurred on walking the dog on its thoracic limbs with the pelvic limbs held up by the tail. Thoracic limb and trunk function were normal.

The pelvic limbs were hypotonic to manipulate. Both patellar reflexes were brisk (plus 3). Pelvic limb flexor reflexes were both absent. No pain was perceived from digits three through five or the dorsal, lateral, or plantar aspects of the paws. Stimulation of the medial side of the paw elicited pain and excited mild hip flexion. The anus was dilated, atonic, and areflexic. The tail was atonic and unresponsive to the perineal reflex. Pain was absent from the tail, perineum, caudal thigh, and skin distal to the stifle, except on the medial side of the leg and paw. Sensation was normal from the cranial thigh region. There was a line of analgesia at about the L6 vertebra. No pain was elicited on manipulation of the caudal lumbar and sacral vertebrae.

The bladder was distended and urine often was dribbled involuntarily.

Diagnosis

Neuroanatomic Diagnosis. These clinical signs indicated that there had been complete destruction of the caudal, sacral, and last two lumbar segments or spinal nerves. The preserved patellar reflex and pain on the medial side of the leg and paw indicated that segments L4 and L5 and the femoral and saphenous nerves were intact. Normal sensation in the cranial thigh region indicated that the L4 segment and lateral cutaneous femoral nerve were intact. The dorsal branches of the emerging spinal nerves course caudally to supply the skin one to two vertebral lengths caudal to their site of origin from the vertebral canal. Therefore the line of analgesia is often one to two vertebrae caudal to the spinal nerve that emerges from the intervertebral foramen and supplies the skin up to the line of analgesia. When the stimulus from the medial side of the paw entered the spinal cord over the L4 and L5 dorsal rootlets, the reflex disseminated to the L5 through L1 segments to initiate contraction of the psoas major and iliacus muscles and hip flexion was observed. Destruction of the L6, L7, and S1 segments prevented stimulation of alpha motoneurons of the sciatic nerves. Therefore no flexion of the stifle, tarsus, or digits occurred. Bladder paralysis was due to the lesion of the sacral segments.

Differential Diagnosis. The acute onset without recognized signs of progression suggested an acute traumatic lesion or sudden vascular compromise. There was no history to support external trauma. A severe acute intervertebral disk extrusion at L4-L5 or L5-L6 could produce these signs. This is reasonable in a 5-year-old Great Dane. There was no associated pain on manipulation of the caudal lumbar vertebrae. Such pain may occur with intervertebral disk extrusions but is uncommon with vascular lesions causing myelopathy. Sudden infarction of these spinal cord segments from fibrocartilaginous emboli would produce this sort of onset and clinical signs. The acute onset and total sudden destruction are not compatible with either intra- or extramedullary neoplasms, or inflammatory lesions or malformations.

Ancillary Studies. Plain radiographs were normal. A myelogram indicated a slight intramedullary swelling from the middle of the fourth lumbar vertebra to the L5–L6 articulation.

Cisternal cerebrospinal fluid was clear and colorless and contained normal cells and 68 mg of protein per dl.

Outcome

The ancillary studies supported an ischemic myelopathy of the involved spinal cord segments. Hemorrhage, or edema, or both may occur in this lesion and could account for the intramedullary swelling that was observed on the myelogram. Elevated CSF protein levels often occur from the tissue destruction that accompanies this lesion. It may be much more apparent if the CSF is sampled closer to the lesion. An intramedullary neoplasm would not produce such a sudden onset of signs.

No change occurred over 1 week's observation and the owner elected to have euthanasia performed on the dog.

Necropsy Findings. At necropsy the lumbosacral intumescence appeared slightly swollen, and on opening the dura there was a brownish-yellow discoloration on the surface of the caudal lumbar and sacral segments, along with small hemorrhages. On transverse sections there was a gross lesion from the fifth lumbar segment caudally. In the caudal part of the L5 segment there was a mild brown discoloration of the grey matter. The L6, L7, sacral, and caudal segments were soft and most of the grey matter and a variable amount of the adjacent white matter were distinctly hemorrhagic or discolored grey. On microscopic examination this was a severe hemorrhagic necrotizing myelopathy—a hemorrhagic infarct (Fig. 24–2). Fibrocartilaginous embolic material was present in arteries and veins. There was no apparent degeneration of associated intervertebral disks.

The final diagnosis was fibrocartilaginous embolic ischemic and hemorrhagic myelopathy bilaterally from the caudal portion of the L5 segment through the caudal segments.

I have observed this disease in many different breeds at all levels of the spinal cord.[5, 18] Spontaneous recovery, compensation, or both occurred in many of these patients. The prognosis for recovery is better if the paresis is incomplete and the lesion spares the grey matter of the cervical or lumbar intumescences. If recovery is going to occur there usually will be some evidence of this within 1 week after the onset of the neurologic signs. Although

degenerate intervertebral disks that rupture into vertebral bodies are presumed to be the source of this fibrocartilaginous embolic material in the leptomeningeal and parenchymal vessels in humans, there is no evidence yet to support this in the dog. Intervertebral disk material has been observed herniated into the ventral internal vertebral venous plexus and this has been proposed as the source of the emboli.[8, 19]

Case 3: Case Description

Signalment. An 11-year-old female collie.

Chief Complaint. Unable to use the pelvic limbs.

History. Ten days prior to examination this dog became lame in the left thoracic limb. One week later the dog began to drag the left pelvic limb, and within 3 days it went down in the pelvic limbs and could not get up.

Examination. The dog had been recumbent for 1 day when it was examined. It lay in lateral recumbency and could not assume a sternal position. If picked up and supported by the trunk and tail, it would walk on the thoracic limbs with short, stiff strides. The pelvic limbs were paraplegic, grade 0. The trunk had to be supported or it would swing to the side, causing the dog to fall.

There were no postural reactions present in the pelvic limbs. The right thoracic limb was stiff but responded normally to hopping. The left thoracic limb was slow in hopping. Both pelvic limbs and the right thoracic limb were hypertonic on passive manipulation. The left thoracic limb was hypotonic

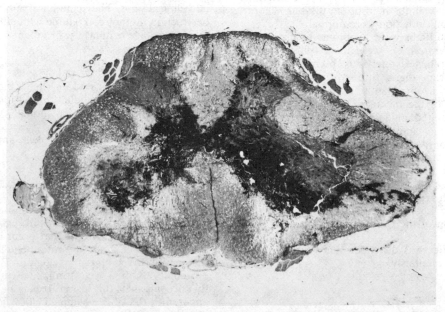

Figure 24–2. Case 2: Transverse section of L7 spinal cord segment with extensive hemorrhagic necrosis of grey matter and ischemic necrosis of white matter. Hematoxylin and eosin.

and mild atrophy was apparent in most muscles of that limb. No pain was elicited on neck manipulation.

Patellar reflexes were both brisk (plus 3). Both triceps reflexes were brisk, as was the right biceps reflex. No biceps reflex was elicited on the left. Flexor reflexes were normal in all four limbs. There was normal pain perception from the thoracic limbs but distinct hypalgesia in the pelvic limbs. A line of hypalgesia was detected in the cranial thoracic region.

Cranial nerve examination was normal. However, the left pupil was consistently smaller than the right. The left third eyelid protruded and the eyeball seemed depressed in the orbit. The left palpebral fissure was smaller than the right.

Diagnosis

Neuroanatomic Diagnosis. These signs indicated that there was a focal spinal cord lesion in the cranial thoracic region. A transverse lesion at the third thoracic segment would cause a spastic paraplegia and loss of trunk strength. Partial involvement of T2 and T1 on the left along with T3 would cause a complete left Horner's syndrome if the grey matter or ventral roots were affected. Partial involvement of T1 and C8 grey matter or roots on the left would account for the mild left thoracic limb signs and atrophy that were observed. The asymmetry suggested by the course described in the history, the left thoracic limb signs, and Horner's syndrome would indicate that a progressive lesion had grown on the left side, compressing the spinal cord from left to right.

Differential Diagnosis. The localizing signs, signs of asymmetry, progressive course, and age of the dog all indicated a diagnosis of a neoplasm compressing the spinal cord. Extramedullary neoplasms are more common and cause more evidence of asymmetry than intramedullary lesions. Neurofibromas are common in the dog. They occasionally occur in the sympathetic trunk and invade the vertebral canal via the rami communicantes, spinal nerves, and roots. If the trunk was involved at the level of the cervicothoracic ganglion, the Horner's syndrome would have preceded the spinal cord signs. An epidural metastasis at this site could also explain these signs. Extramedullary neoplasms may grow slowly to substantial size with concomitant spinal cord compression without obvious neurologic signs if the displacement is slow. However, it seems that when a critical point in the ability of the compressed vasculature to supply the spinal cord is passed, then ischemia occurs and clinical signs are rapidly progressive even over a few days, as observed in this patient. Anesthesia for ancillary studies of these patients may precipitate further ischemia if it decreases cardiac outflow and normal blood flow with proper oxygenation to this compromised section of the spinal cord.

The lack of history and the presence of progressive signs excluded external trauma. Intervertebral disk extrusion could not be excluded, but this is an unusual site for it to occur. The rate of speed of progression and localizing signs were unusual for an inflammatory lesion. Ischemic degeneration would be unlikely to take this long to develop if the initial onset of left thoracic limb lameness is considered pertinent.

Ancillary Studies. Plain radiographs were normal. The dye column on the lumbar myelogram stopped abruptly over the caudal aspect of the body of T2, and, in fact, a small amount of dye escaped from the vertebral canal and was seen dorsally adjacent to the spine of T3 and ventrally along the ventral aspect of the vertebral body of T2 (Fig. 24–3).

Cisternal CSF was clear, colorless, and contained no cells and 31 mg of protein per dl. The pressure was normal.

Outcome

The ancillary studies supported the clinical diagnosis of an extramedullary cranial thoracic space-occupying lesion. Exploratory surgery was recommended but because of the age of the dog and severity of the signs, the owner elected to have euthanasia performed.

Necropsy Findings. At necropsy a large, firm nodular mass was found located in the thorax on the left longus colli muscle involving the cranial aspect of the left thoracic sympathetic trunk and left cervicothoracic ganglion. This mass extended dorsally between the first two ribs and entered the vertebral canal through the intervertebral foramen between T1 and T2. It compressed the left first thoracic spinal nerve and expanded into the epidural space, where it compressed the spinal cord to the right (Fig. 24–4). The second and especially the third spinal cord segments were the most compressed. The third thoracic segment was reduced to less than one-half its normal width. The mass was diagnosed as a neurofibroma.

This case emphasizes the value of Horner's syndrome in the localization and interpretation of lesions. This syndrome probably occurred before the gait deficit if it can be assumed that the sympathetic trunk and cervicothoracic ganglion were affected initially before the mass expanded into the vertebral canal. Most spinal cord neoplasms are extramedullary and therefore are amenable to surgical removal if they can be diagnosed before the spinal cord compromise and the associated clinical deficit are marked.

Case 4: Case Description

Signalment. An 8-year-old male coonhound.

Chief Complaint. Weakness and ataxia.

History. About 4 weeks prior to examination this dog was noticed to be slow on treeing a raccoon.

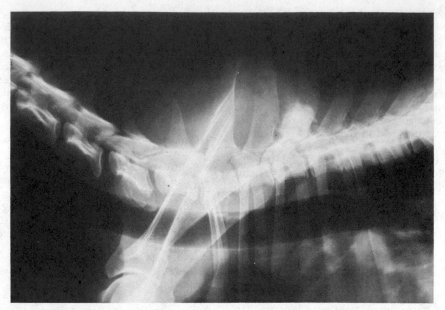

Figure 24–3.   Case 3: Lumbar Skiodan myelogram demonstrating a block to normal flow at the T2–T3 articulation and leakage of dye into the epaxial area beside the spine of T3.

This occurred 1 month after the dog had been bitten by a raccoon. The dog continued to "slow down" when hunting. Six days prior to examination it could not stand unassisted. The pelvic limbs seemed more affected than the thoracic limbs.

Examination. The dog was reasonably alert and responsive. It could not stand unassisted. If supported it veered off to the right and walked slowly with stiff, awkward movements, tipping to the right. The limbs appeared markedly hypertonic. The animal's strength seemed good but it was very disoriented. The head was tilted to the right and the neck was curved to the right (concave right). Along with this posture the head and neck were extended more than normal. The trunk often weaved from side to side and a head tremor was evident.

On postural reaction testing there was greater deficit on the left than on the right side. Postural reactions were difficult to test because of the dog's disorientation. The deficit was especially evident in the hopping responses. The dog would fall on attempting to hemiwalk on the left side. Proprioceptive positioning was absent on the left side.

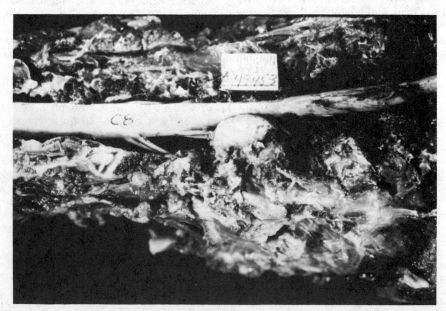

Figure 24–4.   Case 3: Necropsy exposure of neurofibroma in the epidural space compressing the left first thoracic spinal roots and the second thoracic spinal cord segment.

The dog preferred left lateral recumbency and with little stimulation would assume a position of opisthotonos. The thoracic limbs would extend rigidly. The pelvic limbs often were flexed.

There was marked hypertonia in the limbs. This was more apparent in the left limbs when the dog was in right lateral recumbency. No atrophy was evident. Patellar reflexes were both brisk (plus 3). Of the thoracic limb tendon reflexes only the left triceps reflex was apparent. Perineal and flexor reflexes were all present. Pain was intact and no significant hypalgesia could be detected.

On cranial nerve examination the only abnormalities were referable to the vestibular system. The head was tilted to the right. On neck extension a positional nystagmus was induced that was rotatory to the right side. On the same maneuver the right eye was noted to drift ventrally and laterally. However, in some positions of the head it was in a normal position, and both eyes abducted and adducted well on moving the head from side to side.

Diagnosis

Neuroanatomic Diagnosis. The signs of vestibular disturbance were prominent in this case—the right head tilt, leaning and falling to the right, vestibular strabismus of the right eye, and abnormal nystagmus. With disturbance of the peripheral nerve or receptor portions of the vestibular system the abnormal nystagmus would be directed away from the side of the disturbance, which is denoted by the direction of the head and body tilt. In this case the abnormal nystagmus was directed to the same side as the head tilt, which indicates disturbance of the central portions of the vestibular system.

Even more obvious were the signs of other systems being affected that only occur in the brain stem. The marked degree of bilateral thoracic limb hypertonia, the truncal ataxia and tendency to opisthotonic posture would only be expected with central involvement of the descending upper motor neuron portion of the reticular formation, or possibly the rostral vermal portion of the cerebellum, or both. These signs suggested a tendency toward decerebration. Experimental rostral cerebellar lesions may produce opisthotonos with flexion instead of extension of the pelvic limbs. The deficit in postural reactions which was most pronounced on the left in the hopping, hemiwalking, and proprioceptive positioning responses implicated lesion of the upper motor neuron and general proprioception tracts in the brain stem.

Cerebellar, vestibular, and UMN-GP deficits could well be explained by a caudal fossa lesion. The predominantly left-sided postural reaction deficit should be explained by a predominantly left-sided pontine or medullary lesion. This reflected damage to the left rubrospinal and reticulospinal tracts which mostly cross at their origin in brain stem nuclei rostral to the lesion, and damage to the left spinocerebellar and cuneocerebellar tracts that project mostly to the cerebellum from the trunk and limbs on the same side.

The predominance of right-sided central vestibular signs may reflect a multifocal lesion in the cerebellum or medulla with disturbance of these structures on the right side, or these may be paradoxical vestibular signs from a left-sided cerebellar medullary lesion.

The remarkable preservation in strength and sensorium in the face of severe cerebellar-vestibular

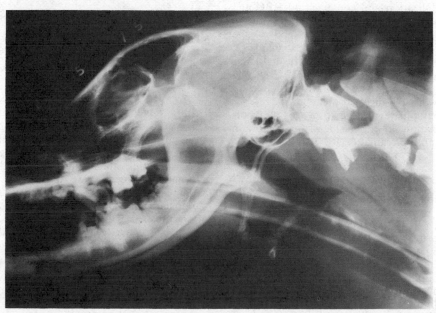

Figure 24–5. Case 4: Lateral radiograph of skull showing an oval area of opacity in the position of the tentorium cerebelli.

disturbance suggested that the lesion might be extramedullary and compressing these structures rather than intramedullary, unless it was predominantly in the cerebellar medulla.

Although the history implicated a raccoon bite 1 month prior to the onset of neurologic signs, all the signs observed were the antithesis of coonhound paralysis, which produces profound paresis with loss of tone and reflexes, and muscle atrophy. Further, the onset of this disease usually follows the incriminating bite by 7 to 10 days.

Differential Diagnosis. The signs of a progressive focal lesion in the caudal fossa of an aged dog are suggestive of a neoplastic disease.

A focal inflammatory lesion that was proliferative and space-occupying could produce these signs. Granulomatous encephalitis (reticulosis) would be the most common lesion of this type. Toxoplasmosis occasionally may produce a focal granulomatous lesion. A bacterial abscess, although rare in the dog, also should be considered. These are most commonly associated with the extension of a suppurative lesion in the middle and inner ear to the meninges and occur more commonly in pigs and cats. Such a focal lesion with space-occupying signs would not be compatible with canine distemper encephalitis. Cryptococcal leptomeningitis usually produces more diffuse signs, although cerebellar-vestibular signs are common.

Traumatic lesions would be excluded by the history and progressive course. Degenerative lesions are more diffuse except for vascular accidents. The latter are not associated with a progressive course. Malformations were excluded by the age of the patient.

Ancillary Studies. Two cisternal cerebrospinal fluid samples were obtained. The first was on the second day of hospitalization and contained 40 RBC and 14 mononuclear cells per cmm, and 98 mg of protein per dl. The second sample was obtained on the fourth day. The opening pressure was 265 mm H_2O; closing pressure was 120 mm H_2O. The fluid was clear and colorless but contained 8 RBC and 40 WBC per cmm. The latter were mostly mononuclear cells. There were 176 mg of protein per dl.

Plain radiographs revealed an oval area of abnormal mineralization on either side of the tentorium cerebelli within the cranial cavity (Fig. 24–5).

Outcome

On the second day of hospitalization all the signs were slightly worse. In addition, the left pupil was slightly larger than the right, although both still responded to light. On the third day the signs of decerebration seemed more profound. The dog could make no effort to get up. When held in a standing position the thoracic limbs extended caudally and the neck extended in an opisthotonic posture. Voluntary limb movement could still be induced. The dog would struggle to maintain some semblance of balance but to no avail.

The cerebrospinal fluid abnormality confirmed the central location of a lesion and helped to substantiate a neoplasm as the cause, as indicated by the increased intracranial pressure, the mild elevation in cells, and moderate elevation of protein. Radiography further substantiated the extramedullary neoplastic nature of the lesion. The degree of mineralization suggested an osseous neoplasm and not a meningioma.

With a poor prognosis for survival more than a few days and a guarded prognosis for surgical recovery, the owner elected euthanasia.

Necropsy Findings. A large, firm nodular mass completely enveloped the tentorium cerebelli and projected ventrally, severely compressing the middle and rostral portions of the cerebellar vermis and paravermal lobules (Fig. 24–6). At the most compressed portion of the cerebellum it measured only 7 mm thick (Fig. 24–7). The caudal vermis projected caudally into the foramen magnum. The entire pons and medulla were compressed by the mass growing into the cerebellum. Dorsal to the tentorium the mass compressed the medial side of each occipital lobe.

On microscopic examination the mass was an osteogenic sarcoma.

The kind of lesion and its location clearly explain the clinical signs and results of the ancillary studies. It was not possible to determine if the predominance of right-sided vestibular signs resulted from a left- or right-sided lesion. There was bilateral involvement of the vestibular portions of the cerebellum as well as the vestibular nuclei. There was no clinical evidence of visual disturbance from the mild compression of each occipital lobe.

Case 5: Case Description

Signalment. A 6-year-old spayed female Boston terrier.

Chief Complaint. Seizures.

History. Seven weeks prior to examination the first seizure was observed. Three seizures occurred over a 2-hour period, each lasting 1 to 2 minutes. It was reported that these began with the dog shaking all over, salivating, then falling on its side, and they alternated between severe rigidity and shaking. The animal appeared to lose consciousness. A veterinarian had prescribed primidone therapy. A number of seizures occurred over the 7-week period, but their exact occurrence was not well documented. Seizures did occur the day before admission.

Examination. On initial examination the dog appeared to be blind. The pupils were dilated and unresponsive to light. The dog stumbled from side to side on walking.

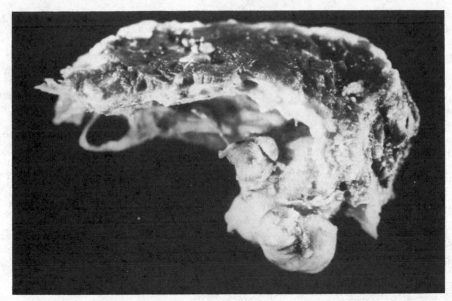

Figure 24–6. Case 4: Lateral view of the calvaria removed at necropsy with the mass at the site of the tentorium cerebelli.

Thorough neurologic examination the following day revealed a reasonably alert and responsive dog. The gait was essentially normal. Occasionally the right forepaw was slow to protract on turning left and would almost turn over onto its dorsal surface.

On wheelbarrowing the right thoracic limb occasionally stumbled. The hopping response was slow in the right limbs, especially the right pelvic limb. The right pelvic limb was slower to respond on walking backward with the pelvic limbs. Hemistanding was normal. Hemiwalking was slow and awkward on the right side. The proprioceptive positioning response was slow in both right limbs. Placing was normal. On extending the neck, the right tho-

racic limb occasionally flexed distally so that the dorsal surface was on the ground.

Muscle tone was normal. No atrophy was observed. Both patellar reflexes were brisk. Biceps and triceps reflexes were absent. Perineal and flexor reflexes were normal, as was pain perception.

On cranial nerve examination the menace response appeared to be slightly slower from the right lateral field. On walking the dog through a maze to the left no object was bumped but on walking to the right occasionally an object was hit. Pupils were normal in size and responsive to light. There was a suggestion that there was less response to mild stimulation of the nasal mucosa with a blunt instru-

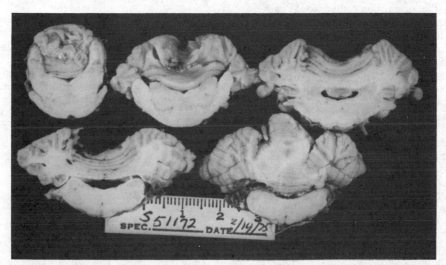

Figure 24–7. Case 4: Transverse sections at the level of the pons and medulla, showing the compression of the cerebellum and brain stem caused by the tentorial mass.

ment on the right side. The rest of the cranial nerves were normal.

Diagnosis

Neuroanatomic Diagnosis. The clinical signs observed on the day following hospital admission all suggested a left cerebral lesion. A lesion in the centrum semiovale would interfere with ascending conscious proprioceptive neurons from the thalamus and descending upper motor neuron projections from the motor cortex, explaining the essentially normal gait but deficient contralateral postural reactions. If the lesion was confined to the sensorimotor cortex, the same systems would be affected and cause the same signs. The slight right facial hypalgesia could result from a lesion in the same location affecting the general somatic afferent neuronal projection from the thalamus. Although pain perception pathways ascend bilaterally from the limbs, trunk, and face on one side, the predominance of the contralateral projection is usually only detected for the face with unilateral thalamic or cerebral lesions. Involvement of the optic radiation in the left centrum semiovale would account for the observed visual deficit on the right side.

Similarly, the same systems could be affected on the left side of the diencephalon in a fairly small area. The GP and UMN systems are together in the internal capsule or could be affected separately in the ventrocaudolateral thalamic nucleus and crus cerebri, respectively. The left optic tract and left ventrocaudomedial thalamic nucleus involvement would explain the visual deficit and facial hypalgesia, respectively.

Why did the initial examination indicate blindness with dilated unresponsive pupils and a paretic-ataxic gait that were absent on the following day? These signs can be explained by a bilateral optic nerve or chiasm lesion such as occurs most commonly with optic neuritis, plus a more diffuse mild lesion, probably in the brain stem, that would cause the generalized paresis and ataxia. These lesions would be unlikely to appear suddenly and resolve in a 36- to 48-hour period. The blindness with paresis and ataxia could be a prolonged postictal depression. The dog was observed to seizure the day before admission and had been blind and ataxic since then. These signs commonly are seen for a short period of time, (usually less than 3 hours) following a seizure, and then they completely disappear. However, occasionally they last for 1 to 2 days after a seizure. The presence of dilated unresponsive pupils is unusual as a sign of postictal depression.

A third explanation is that these signs were the result of fairly severe intracranial pressure elevation associated with a mass lesion. The blindness reflected bilateral cerebral compression or edema. The dilated unresponsive pupils were due to the cerebral mass compressing the mesencephalon and ventrally located oculomotor neurons. Such lesions frequently cause pupillary dilation (general visceral efferent deficiency) without strabismus (general somatic efferent deficiency). The same brain stem compression could cause the paresis and ataxia. This is probably the best explanation in view of the results of the neurologic examination performed after these signs resolved, which indicated a primary left cerebral lesion. However, the more typical sign that results from an expanding cerebral mass is ipsilateral pupillary dilation from the asymmetric ipsilateral cerebral herniation and compression of the midbrain.

There is no obvious answer to this dilemma, except that an organic lesion involving these other structures is not compatible with the signs observed. Postictal depression or increased intracranial pressure or both may be involved.

Differential Diagnosis. Progressive seizures in an aged dog associated with interictal signs of a focal cerebral lesion are highly suggestive of a neoplasm. Brachycephalic breeds are thought to be especially prone to gliomas, which further adds to this diagnosis.[3] A focal inflammatory lesion such as a toxoplasma granuloma, bacterial abscess, or granulomatous encephalitis (reticulosis) could produce these signs. Canine cerebral abscesses are rare. All three of these should produce abnormalities in the cerebrospinal fluid.

With no immediate or past history of trauma and the presence of progressive signs this would be unlikely. Posttraumatic seizures occasionally occur but require a history of injury associated with signs of significant intracranial injury.

Malformation at this age would be unlikely. Most degenerative disorders are diffuse and do not produce focal signs. Vascular injuries are the exception, but the signs should be sudden in onset and not progressive. Extracranial metabolic diseases are excluded because of the presence of a focal neurologic deficit. Idiopathic epilepsy would be excluded by the age of onset and the interictal neurologic abnormality.

Ancillary Studies. The CBC, BUN, serum glucose, and electrolytes were normal. The cisternal cerebrospinal fluid opening pressure was 160 mm H_2O; 3 cc of a clear colorless fluid were withdrawn. The closing pressure was less than 30 mm H_2O. The fluid contained 4 RBC and 2 WBC per cmm, and 39 mg of protein per dl.

Plain radiographs of the skull and thorax were normal.

Outcome

Elevated CSF protein levels with normal color and cells commonly occur with intracranial neoplastic disease. Although the opening pressure was in the high normal range, the drop to below 30 after the sampling (the lowest number that can be recorded) suggested a decreased total size of the CSF-containing space. This would be more significant if only 2 cc—the standard amount—were removed and would not cause such a large drop in pressure. Ordinarily on removal of 2 cc from the cerebellomedullary cistern the closing pressure is not less than one-half of the opening pressure. If it is, this suggests a smaller total volume of CSF from a subarachnoid space compromised by a space-occupying lesion.

Plain radiographs are helpful only if a neoplastic lesion is adjacent to the skull and has eroded it, or if the neoplasm is of cartilage or bone that has mineralized. Primary and most metastatic brain neoplasms cannot be visualized. Even meningiomas that may be mineralized usually are not visualized.

For the next week of hospitalization, no seizures were observed in the animal. The dog's neurologic status remained unchanged except that the right menace deficit and facial hypalgesia no longer could be detected. All signs were referable to a left frontal lobe location.

Because of the poor prognosis for recovery and guarded prognosis if the suspected mass could be localized further by scintigraphy and operated on, the owner elected euthanasia.

Necropsy Findings. The rostral pole of the left frontal lobe was distended. The cortical surface was thin and fluctuated on palpation. The affected gyri included the prorean, precruciate, rostral suprasylvian, and rostral compositus. On transverse section there was a well-demarcated mass in the center of the left frontal lobe. It was soft, grey, gelatinous, and contained numerous fluid-filled cystic spaces (Fig. 24–8). The white matter of the left parietal lobe caudal to the mass was swollen. No other lesions were observed. On microscopic examination this mass was an astrocytoma.

The necropsy confirmed a left cerebral astrocytoma as the cause of the focal neurologic signs and presumably the cause of the progressive seizures in this aged Boston terrier. This does not solve the

dilemma of an exact explanation for the presenting signs that had resolved by the following day. There was no evidence at the time of necropsy of cerebral herniation, or direct compression of the optic nerves or chiasm. Postictal depression with atypical pupillary dilation remains the best explanation.

This case exemplifies the value of careful neurologic examination of the patient with seizures. Observation of interictal deficits strongly supports an organic brain lesion and would not occur in idiopathic epilepsy or most extracranial and metabolic disease.

Case 6: Case Description

Signalment. A 3-year-old female mongrel setter.

Chief Complaint. Abnormal pelvic limb function.

History. Five days prior to examination this dog left its home. Four days later it was found lying alongside a road unable to get up.

Examination. On initial examination the dog was alert and responsive. It sat in sternal recumbency but refused to get up on its pelvic limbs. If assisted, thoracic limb function was normal. The right pelvic limb seemed to have normal neurologic function but the dog was reluctant to bear weight on the limb. The left pelvic limb was less functional and stood with the dorsal aspect of the paw turned over on the ground.

Tone, reflexes, and pain perception were normal in the right pelvic limb. Voluntary motion was readily induced. The left pelvic limb would flex slightly at the hip when handled, but even on noxious stimulation there was no flexion of the stifle or tarsus and no pain was perceived from the paw, leg, or caudal thigh except along the medial aspect. The patellar reflex was normal.

The tail was atonic, areflexic, and analgesic. The

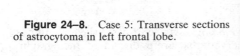

Figure 24–8. Case 5: Transverse sections of astrocytoma in left frontal lobe.

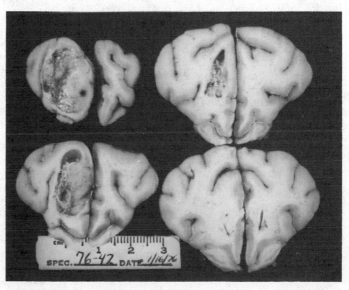

anus was partly dilated. Slight response to perineal stimulation occurred on the right side. Pain was perceived from the right side of the perineum and not the left. The left proximal caudal thigh region was also analgesic. The bladder was distended and had to be expressed manually.

Diagnosis

Neuroanatomic Diagnosis. Neurologic deficit was limited to the left sciatic nerve or its roots of origin, the left sacral nerves or roots, and the caudal nerves bilaterally. The L4 and L5 roots and spinal nerves were preserved on the left because of the intact patellar reflex (femoral nerve) and intact pain sensation on the medial aspect of the limb (saphenous nerve). Hip flexion was normal because of the intact L1-L5 roots and spinal nerves to the psoas major muscle. Sensation was normal over the cranial thigh region because of the intact L4 roots and spinal nerve (lateral cutaneous femoral nerve). The deficit of the left sacral roots or nerves was reflected in the atonic, areflexic, analgesic left anus and perineum (pudendal nerve) and analgesic proximal caudal thigh area (caudal cutaneous femoral nerve). The bladder paralysis was due to bilateral pelvic nerve paralysis or bilateral sacral nerve paralysis. The total tail deficit reflected a bilateral caudal nerve lesion. The lesion must explain a left L6 through S3 spinal nerve lesion and bilateral pelvic and caudal nerve lesion.

Differential Diagnosis. The presumed acute onset, along with the history of finding this dog beside the road, and the pain and abnormality palpated in the skeletal structures of the pelvic region, were highly presumptive of a traumatic lesion of external origin. The signs of neurologic deficit can be explained readily by contusion of roots and spinal branches of peripheral nerves.

A sacrocaudal fracture and luxation could account for the total dysfunction of the caudal nerves. The left sciatic palsy could have occurred from fracture of the ischium with medial displacement of the cranial portion and hip, which contused the nerve as it passed distally medial to the greater trochanter of the femur. Fracture of the body of the ilium at the greater ischiatic notch with displacement of the bone fragments may have contused the sciatic nerve as it passed over this notch. Sacral fractures with sacroiliac luxation will contuse the ventral branches of L6 and L7 spinal nerves that must course caudally on the ventromedial aspect of this joint to form the sciatic nerve. The same traumatic lesion can easily contuse the sacral nerve ventral branches as they emerge from the pelvic sacral foramina.

Ancillary Studies. Radiography revealed a craniodorsal dislocation of the right hip, a sacrocaudal fracture with ventral displacement of the caudal vertebrae, and a fracture of the sacrum at the left sacroiliac joint which was subluxed (Figs. 24–9, 24–10).

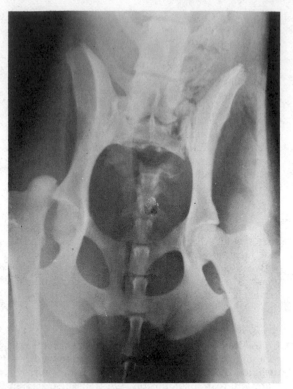

Figure 24–9. Case 6: Ventrodorsal radiograph showing right coxofemoral luxation and left fracture of sacrum with sacroiliac subluxation.

Outcome

Within a few days the dog recovered sensation in the distribution of the left sciatic nerve but motor function remained absent. Within the next 10 days the dog began to get up and walk. Neurologic function of the right pelvic limb was normal. The left pelvic limb could support weight normally (femoral nerve). The limb was advanced by hip flexion (iliopsoas muscle–lumbar nerves), but the animal walked with the stifle extended and the paw placed with its dorsal surface on the ground due to the persistent sciatic palsy. Incontinence persisted from the pelvic nerve injury. The tail remained paralyzed and analgesic.

After 1 month with no improvement, euthanasia was performed.

Necropsy Findings. At necropsy the skeletal injuries were observed that were diagnosed radiographically. The caudal nerves were torn and fibrosed at the sacrocaudal fracture. The left L7 spinal nerve ventral branch was discolored and entirely embedded in fibrous tissue ventromedial to the sacroiliac joint. A portion of the left L6 spinal nerve ventral branch was involved in the same fibrous adhesion. The ventral branches of the sacral nerves were embedded in hemorrhage and fibrous tissue. No spinal cord lesions were observed.

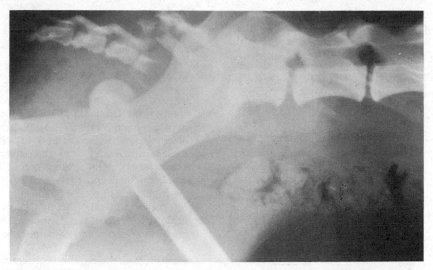

Figure 24–10. Case 6: Lateral radiograph showing sacrocaudal fracture and separation.

Case 7: Case Description

Signalment. An 8-year-old small female mongrel.

Chief Complaint. Head tilt.

History. Six weeks prior to examination this dog fairly suddenly developed a mild right head tilt. This sign slowly became worse, although some days it seemed better. For the preceding week or two some difficulty in the dog's gait had been observed.

Examination. The dog was alert and responsive. Its head was constantly tipped to the right to a marked degree. Occasionally the dog drifted to the right as it walked. Strength and general proprioception seemed normal in the gait.

On postural reaction testing there was a slight asymmetry with a slower response with the right limbs, especially the right pelvic limb. This was only observed in the hopping response. Muscle tone and all spinal reflexes were normal. No atrophy was evident. Pain perception was normal.

On cranial nerve examination there was anisocoria, with the right pupil slightly larger than the left. The pupillary light reflex responses were intact, but the right pupil never contracted as much as the left. Frequently the right eyeball assumed a ventrolateral position. However, this was not constant in all positions of the head. When the head was moved from side to side to observe vestibular nystagmus, both eyeballs were able to fully adduct and abduct. There was no spontaneous nystagmus at rest. With the head held flexed to the left a vertical to slightly rotatory left nystagmus occurred. This rotatory left nystagmus was exacerbated after the dog was rolled over once. The normal nystagmus induced by moving the head from side to side was slower than normal, especially on moving the head to the left. No other cranial nerve deficits were observed.

Diagnosis

Neuroanatomic Diagnosis. These signs, which are predominantly vestibular, indicated a lesion in the right side of the brain in the caudal fossa. The reason for locating the lesion in the central and not peripheral portion of the vestibular system is because of the postural reaction deficit. Nothing about the vestibular signs indicated a central lesion. All were compatible with a disturbance of the peripheral receptor. The only possible exception was the occasional vertical component of the abnormal nystagmus. If this were consistently only vertical, it should indicate a central lesion. A variation from vertical to rotatory has been seen in peripheral diseases. However, in peripheral disease the direction of the rotation is away from the side of the head tilt. This is determined by the direction of movement of the 12 o'clock point on the limbus of the eyeball in relation to the dog's left or right side.

Peripheral vestibular disturbances may accompany otitis media or otitis interna. The only additional neuroanatomic structures that can be affected by this disease in the dog are the facial nerve (facial paralysis), cochlear nerve (deafness), and postganglionic sympathetic nerves (Horner's syndrome). Postural reactions are not directly interfered with by vestibular system disorders. Lesions in the medulla that interfere with the upper motor neuron, or general proprioceptive system, or both cause a slowing of the postural reaction responses. A severe lesion in these tracts in the medulla causes an ipsilateral spastic hemiparesis and ataxia. A mild lesion may produce only a postural reaction deficit. A lesion in the cerebellar peduncles that disturbs the general proprioceptive system in the spinocerebellar and cuneocerebellar tracts produces an ipsilateral hemiataxia if severe or only a deficit in ipsilateral postural reactions.

The ventrolateral strabismus that was inconstant and easily elicited by head and neck extension is a common finding in the eye on the same side as the other signs of a vestibular disturbance. It results from the disturbance in normal tonic input from the vestibular system to the nuclei of the cranial nerves that innervate the extraocular muscles. To differentiate this from the strabismus of an oculomotor nerve paralysis, in the latter the strabismus is constant and the ability to adduct the eyeball is impaired.

The larger right pupil was not explained by ocular examination. It could have reflected mild oculomotor nerve compression on the floor of the cranial cavity. However, there were no associated clinical signs of increased intracranial pressure. Lesions in cerebellar nuclei occasionally are associated with pupillary asymmetry.

Differential Diagnosis. Progressive signs of a focal right cerebellomedullary lesion in an aged dog are most suggestive of a mass lesion. Neoplasia, granulomatous encephalitis (reticulosis), or abscess must be considered. This is a common clinical presentation in a dog with a papilloma or carcinoma of the choroid plexus of the fourth ventricle. The white matter of the cerebellar medulla and peduncles is a common site affected by granulomatous encephalitis (the inflammatory form of the reticulosis lesion).[7, 9] An abscess of the right cerebellomedullary angle from a similar lesion in the petrosal bone usually produces a facial paresis or paralysis along with the central vestibular signs. These are rare in dogs. The inflammatory disease caused by canine distemper, toxoplasmosis, or cryptococcosis usually produces multifocal or diffuse lesions and signs. Injury and ischemic lesions produce sudden onset of signs and nonprogression.

Ancillary studies. Plain radiographs of the skull, including the tympanic bullae, were normal.

Cerebrospinal fluid had an opening pressure of 90 mm H_2O. It was clear and colorless and contained 166 RBC and 103 WBC per cmm. All the latter were mononuclear cells. There were 286 mg of protein per dl and the closing pressure was 80 mm H_2O.

Outcome

The ancillary studies supported a focal granulomatous inflammation as the cause of the clinical signs. Space-occupying lesions in the caudal fossa often do not elevate CSF pressure. If the meninges are involved in the granulomatous encephalitis lesion it is common for the protein and leukocytes to be moderately increased, as in this patient.

This is a lesion that occurs within the parenchyma and would not be amenable to surgery. It usually continues to progress in its development, although the rate may be slow. In some instances corticosteroid therapy has been thought to slow its progression, but only temporarily. The owner elected to have euthanasia performed.

Necropsy Findings. At necropsy the area of the right choroid plexus was enlarged and a grey-brown color. On transverse section three lesions were observed. At the right cerebellomedullary angle there was a large area of brown discoloration with a whorled appearance that blended with the adjacent parenchyma (Fig. 24–11). It involved all the right cerebellar peduncles and adjacent cerebellar medulla. It extended into the adjacent medulla, where it involved the caudal cerebellar peduncle, vestibular nuclei, and the spinal tract and nucleus of the trigeminal nerve. No signs of facial hypalgesia were observed to relate to the involvement of the central projections of the trigeminal nerve. The rest of the lesion distribution explained the clinical signs observed.

Two additional smaller focal whorled brown lesions were observed. One occupied a portion of the ventral septal nuclei, caudate nucleus, rostral commissure, column of the fornix, and adjacent rostral diencephalon, all on the left side. The other was smaller and located in the right parahippocampal gyrus and adjacent hippocampus. No signs were related to these areas. The only signs that could be predicted to occur from the areas disturbed by these lesions are changes in behavior and attitude, or seizures, or both.

On microscopic examination all these lesions were diagnosed as granulomatous encephalitis. No organism was identified.

Case 8: Case Description

Signalment. A 5-year-old gelded Thoroughbred.

Chief Complaint. Muscle atrophy and weak pelvic limbs.

History. Two months prior to initial examination atrophy occurred in the horse's left masseter muscle. The onset was rapid, over a one-week period. The horse continued to race well. One week prior to examination, while the animal was being rested for a sesamoid problem, atrophy was observed in the right gluteal region and an altered gait occurred.

Examination. The gelding was alert and responsive. The pelvic limb gait was abnormal. There was a slight delay in the onset of the protraction phase of the right pelvic limb. On the horse's turning to the left the hind quarters swayed left, and it had difficulty coordinating the right pelvic limb with the left. When the hindquarters were pushed to the right the right pelvic limb was slow to abduct. On backing, it was slow to retract from the supporting position. There was distinct atrophy of the right middle gluteal and tensor fascia lata muscles. Tail and anal tone and the perineal reflex were normal. No hypalgesia was detected.

The left masseter muscle was severely atrophied. The left temporal muscle was mildly atrophied. There was no lack of jaw tone or strength and no

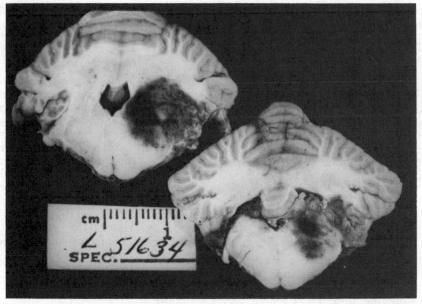

Figure 24–11. Case 7: Transverse sections of granuloma in the right side of the cerebellum and medulla.

deviation was observed. The remainder of the cranial nerve examination was normal.

Diagnosis

Neuroanatomic Diagnosis. These clinical signs suggested a primary lesion of the muscles that were atrophied, a peripheral neuropathy of the left mandibular and right cranial gluteal nerves, or a multifocal lesion of the central nervous system with lesions in the left trigeminal motor nucleus in the pons and right side of the spinal cord segments L5, L6, and S1 primarily affecting the ventral grey column.

Although the right pelvic limb gait was the most abnormal, the left was not normal and the overall pelvic limb disturbance seemed greater than would be expected if the lesion was confined to the right cranial gluteal nerve or the muscles it innervates. A similar delay in the onset of protraction with forward gait and retraction with backing is seen with spinal cord lesions affecting the white matter cranial to the lumbosacral intumescence. It is not clear whether this is a sign of motor or proprioceptive deficiency. For this reason a spinal cord lesion with white matter and ventral grey column involvement from L5 to S1 was most suspect.

Peripheral neuropathy or primary myopathy with such a distribution as this has not been reported in the horse. A myopathy of the masseter muscles has been reported in debilitated young horses but the involvement is bilateral.

Differential Diagnosis. An inflammatory disease would best explain the multifocal, asymmetric, and progressive nervous system signs. The progressive signs would be untoward for a single episode of trauma, as would the lesion distribution. The repeated contusions that may occur with the cervical malarticulation in the wobbler syndrome may give progressive signs but they are fairly symmetric and reflect a cervical spinal cord location. Degenerative myeloencephalopathy produces symmetric signs of white matter disease in all four limbs and occurs in the young horse. These two spinal cord diseases could not account for the muscle atrophy. Multifocal metastatic neoplasia is rare but conceivably could explain the asymmetry and progression of signs.

The possible inflammatory lesions that should be considered include protozoal encephalomyelitis, parasitic encephalomyelitis, multifocal bacterial encephalomyelitis, and equine polyneuritis (neuritis of the cauda equina). Although cranial nerve signs do occur in some cases of equine polyneuritis, the signs of neuritis of the cauda equina are most profound at that time, with symmetric paralysis and analgesia of the tail, anus, perineum, bladder, and rectum. Similarly, when pelvic limb gait abnormality accompanies the neuritis of the cauda equina there is usually complete loss of function of the caudal and sacral nerves, as just described. *Streptococcus equi* abscesses may occur in the central nervous system of horses and may be multiple, but usually are in the brain. The lesion distribution seen in this case would be unusual for embolic bacterial disease. Migrating larvae of *Strongylus vulgaris* may affect any part of the central nervous system. If this was the cause of the lesion in the motor nucleus of the trigeminal nerve, it would be unusual not to have more signs of damage to adjacent structures in the pons and medulla. The same could be said for embolic bacterial disease or the lesion produced by protozoa. Nevertheless, multifocal grey matter lesions such as these in the horse are most commonly caused by an unidentified protozoan.

Although the viral-induced equine encephalitides produce an encephalomyelitis, the signs are mostly of diffuse brain disease, and focal cranial nerve nuclear signs or asymmetric lumbosacral spinal cord signs would be most unusual.

Ancillary Studies. Repeated studies of the complete blood count, electrolytes, and serum enzymes revealed no significant abnormality. Lumbosacral cerebrospinal fluid was slightly xanthochromic but contained no cells and 70 mg of protein per dl.

Muscle biopsy of the atrophied left masseter muscle revealed neurogenic atrophy. Radiographs of the temporomandibular joints were normal.

Outcome

After 3 weeks of hospitalization and treatment with corticosteroids, the pelvic limb gait abnormality was slightly worse. The horse was discharged but the rapid deterioration of pelvic limb function required rehospitalization 1 week later.

On reexamination the horse was recumbent and could not get up unassisted. It would sit like a dog on its paretic pelvic limbs when it attempted to stand. The hair was worn off the skin over the thigh muscles, where there was severe bruising from struggling to get up. When assisted its thoracic limbs functioned normally. The pelvic limbs were both paretic and ataxic and took short, weak strides. The right limb was worse and would cross under the body or overflex in an exaggerated protraction phase.

There was severe atrophy of the right middle gluteal and tensor fascia lata muscles. There was mild atrophy of the right biceps femoris, semitendinosus, semimembranosus, and gastrocnemius muscles. The right patellar reflex was brisk. The tail and anal tone were reduced, although the perineal reflex was still intact and no hypalgesia could be detected.

On cranial nerve examination the only abnormalities observed were atrophy. There was severe atrophy of the left masseter and temporal muscles and the entire right half of the tongue. Prehension and swallowing were normal except that occasionally a bolus of hay fell out of the mouth.

The neuroanatomic and differential diagnosis remained essentially the same, only now the disease involved the right hypoglossal nucleus or nerve, or both, and more of the lumbosacral intumescence. A protozoan-induced encephalomyelitis remained the most likely disease producing these signs.

Ancillary Studies. A CBC performed on two occasions revealed a leukocytosis with an absolute neutrophilia. Cisternal cerebrospinal fluid was slightly xanthochromic and contained 29 RBC and no WBC per cmm, 29 mg of protein per dl, 55 SF units of aspartate aminotransferase (normal, <30), and no creatine kinase. Lumbosacral CSF was xanthochromic and contained 24 RBC and 31 mononuclear cells per cmm and 166 mg of protein per dl, 87 SF units of aspartate aminotransferase, and

2 international units of creatine kinase (normal, <2).

Because of the progressive signs, and the horse's inability to get up, the owner elected euthanasia.

Necropsy Findings. At necropsy, lesions were confined to the nervous system. On transverse section of the lumbosacral intumescence there were bilateral discolorations and softening from L5 through S2 (Fig. 24–12). The softening was more prominent on the left side. These lesions involved the lateral funiculi and adjacent ventral grey columns. The associated ventral rootlets from L5 and S2 showed a brown discoloration. On microscopic examination this consisted of a severe necrotizing nonsuppurative inflammation of grey and white matter with some hemorrhage. Protozoal organisms were present in the lesion (Fig. 24–13). The lesion in the right ventral grey column was more chronic and correlated with the chronic atrophy of the right middle gluteal and tensor fascia lata muscles. In this lesion the neuronal cell bodies were absent and were replaced by numerous hypertrophied astrocytes.

The right hypoglossal nerve was discolored grey. On transverse sections there was a reddish-brown discoloration in the medulla limited to the site of the right hypoglossal nucleus. On microscopic examination there was degeneration of myelin and axons in the right hypoglossal nerve and the nucleus was entirely devoid of neurons and filled with numerous hypertrophied astrocytes. The same microscopic lesion was found in the pons limited to the motor nucleus of the left trigeminal nerve. A group of protozoal organisms was found adjacent to the hypoglossal nuclear lesion. No other lesions were present in the brain.

The cranial nerve nuclear lesion was presumed to be related to the protozoal agent. In other patients the same lesion has been accompanied by inflammation. Possibly the protozoa gain entry to the central nervous system from muscle over its motoneurons and destroy the cell bodies of these motoneurons.

The active inflammatory lesion in the spinal cord that was presumed to be related to the protozoal organisms that were present previously has been seen confined to the medulla, cerebellum, or cerebrum of horses with signs directly related to the extensive area of destruction that occurs in this disease.

Even with the lack of cranial nerve signs, the signs that related to the spinal cord involvement in this patient are characteristic of this protozoal disease in the horse. The progressive course, asymmetric signs, signs of grey matter involvement, and abnormal cerebrospinal fluid suggest this diagnosis over the others discussed.[6, 12] Electron microscopic studies have shown that this protozoan belongs in the subphylum, Apicomplexa and in the genus *Sarcocystis*.[16]

In a retrospective study of equine spinal cord disease at the New York State College of Veterinary Medicine, it was found that this disease predominated in standardbreds from 1 to 3 years of age. It

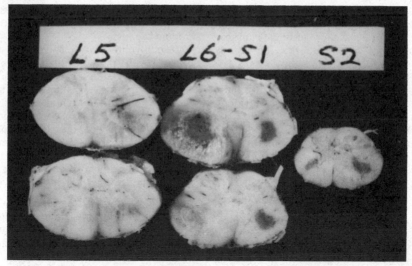

Figure 24–12. Case 8: Transverse sections of the necrotizing inflammatory spinal cord lesion in the lumbosacral intumescence.

has been observed in most all breeds from 1 to 10 years of age and at all times of the year, but especially in the warmer months. The exact identity and life cycle of this protozoan remain to be determined.

Case 9: Case Description

Signalment. A 10-month-old female German shepherd.

Chief Complaint. Weak, incoordinated pelvic limbs.

History. The signs of pelvic limb abnormality began fairly suddenly 1 week prior to examination. There was no opportunity for external injury. The signs of pelvic limb weakness and incoordination progressed during the week before examination.

The only other previous medical illness occurred two months before when the dog had diarrhea for a few days. This responded to antibacterial therapy.

The dog had received canine distemper vaccine as a puppy. The age of the dog when vaccinated and the number of vaccinations had not been recorded.

Examination. The dog was alert and responsive and showed a grade 1 paraparesis and ataxia. It was unable to get up on its pelvic limbs unassisted. If helped by holding the base of the tail both limbs moved voluntarily, but with litttle effect on support

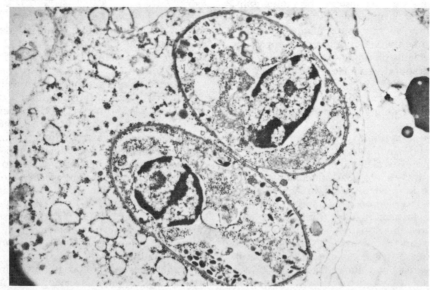

Figure 24–13. Case 8: Electron photomicrograph of two protozoa in cytoplasm of a macrophage in the spinal cord lesion.

or locomotion. The right pelvic limb moved slightly more than the left. There were no responses of either limb to postural reaction testing. Thoracic limb gait and response to postural reaction testing were normal.

Pelvic limb tone was normal. Both patellar reflexes were slightly brisk. Perineal and pelvic limb flexor reflexes were normal. Hypalgesia was evident in both pelvic limbs, perineum, tail, and trunk caudal to the thoracolumbar junction.

Cranial nerve examination was normal.

Diagnosis

Neuroanatomic Diagnosis. These signs of severe UMN paresis and GP ataxia of the pelvic limbs could be caused by a focal or diffuse white matter lesion caudal to T3. The normal or hyperactive pelvic limb reflexes suggested that the lesion was cranial to the L4 segment. The stability of the trunk shown when the dog was walked supported by the tail suggested a lesion caudal to the midthoracic segments. The line of hypalgesia suggested a lesion near the thoracolumbar junction. There were no signs that could not be explained by a focal lesion at this site.

Differential Diagnosis. Progressive spinal cord disease in young dogs of less than 1 year most commonly is caused by canine distemper myelitis. Usually there is some evidence of the multifocal nature of that disease, such as mild thoracic limb signs, or cerebellar-vestibular signs, or both, in addition to the severe paraparesis. Cerebrospinal fluid is often abnormal with a mild elevation of protein and occasionally a pleocytosis.

Thoracolumbar vertebral malformations often produce signs similar to these in dogs less than 1 year of age. Usually the malformation can be palpated but it can always be observed on radiographs.

Although spinal cord neoplasms usually are considered less often in the young animal, a neuroepithelioma is one that has a predilection for young dogs and especially German shepherds.[15, 17] These occur in an intradural extramedullary position at a site between the T10 and L1 spinal cord segments. Myelography is required to confirm this diagnosis.[10, 14] Lymphosarcoma should also be considered at this age.

Occasionally a multiple cartilaginous exostosis that involves a vertebra grows into the vertebral canal and compresses the spinal cord. This occurs in young dogs less than 1 year, but readily can be palpated in the long bones and ribs. The vertebral lesions can be observed on radiographs.

Similar signs are seen in older German shepherds with degenerative myelopathy. This rarely is seen before 4 or 5 years of age and is a slow, insidiously progressive disease that takes months to reach the stage of paraparesis and ataxia manifested by this dog.

Intervertebral disk extrusions produce similar signs; however, they are rarely seen before 4 or 5 years of age in breeds such as the German shepherd and are rare before 18 months in the chondrodystrophic breeds.

Osteomyelitis with spinal cord compression causes severe pain and usually a leukocytosis and fever. It also can be observed on radiographs.

Although paraparesis and ataxia may reflect the onset of an inherited metabolic degeneration of white or grey matter in young dogs, as the lesion progresses the signs reflect the diffuse involvement of the spinal cord and brain. There has been no such lesion reported in German shepherds.

There was no history of trauma, and the progression of signs did not agree with this diagnosis.

Ancillary Studies. The complete blood count was normal. Cerebrospinal fluid pressure was 110 mm H_2O and contained 0 RBC and 1 WBC per cmm, and 18 mg of protein per dl. Plain radiographs were normal.

Outcome

The dog was treated with corticosteroids for a 6-day period. At the end of this period the dog was much improved and walked unassisted with a grade 3 to 4 paraparesis and ataxia. The pelvic limbs were partly flexed on standing and walking, and the left hind paw was frequently dragged on protraction.

The dog was discharged. Three weeks later it returned because the signs had regressed to those observed at the initial examination: a severe grade 1 paraparesis and pelvic limb ataxia. There was still a line of hypalgesia at the thoracolumbar junction. The degree of hypalgesia was worse.

A second cerebrospinal fluid examination revealed 8 RBC and 0 WBC per cmm, and 13 mg of protein per dl.

Because of the severity of the signs and poor prognosis, euthanasia was requested.

Necropsy Findings. At gross necropsy a red-colored swelling was present in an intradural location, mostly on the left side of the T12 spinal cord segment (Fig. 24–14). It measured 15 mm long × 6 mm wide. At its widest point it compressed the spinal cord to a 1 mm-thick band of tissue curved over the right side of the intradural, extramedullary mass (Fig. 24–15). Nerve rootlets coursed through the mass and it was not attached to the dura.

On microscopic examination the mass was extremely cellular, with minimal supporting tissue. The neoplastic cells mostly appeared to be epithelial cells arranged at random, in sheets or around an oval or elongate lumen. It was diagnosed as a neuroepithelioma.

This was one of the first of these neoplasms observed. In retrospect a myelogram should have been done to confirm the diagnosis and locate the lesion for surgical removal.

During the course of progressive spinal cord signs from compression by a neoplasm, intervertebral disk, or malformed vertebrae it is common for brief periods of clinical improvement to occur. These

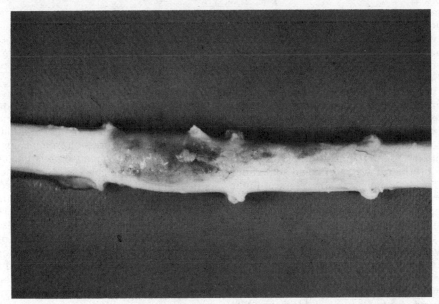

Figure 24–14. Case 9: Intradural spinal cord neoplasm located between the spinal roots of segments T12 and T13 on the left side.

often follow corticosteroid therapy, as was observed in this patient in this report.

Case 10: Case Description

Signalment. A 10-month-old female Arabian horse.

Chief Complaint. Incoordination.

History. At 3 to 4 weeks of age this filly was noticed to stumble occasionally and even fall when running in a paddock. The pelvic limbs splayed out at times. There was no history of any difficulty at birth. These signs of a gait abnormality slowly worsened. They were more noticeable in the pelvic limbs, the hooves of which sometimes were dragged on their dorsal surface.

Examination. This filly was alert and responsive but had a remarkably abnormal gait with spasticity, paresis and ataxia in all four limbs. The abnormal signs were symmetric in the thoracic and pelvic limbs but were worse in the pelvic limbs.

The filly walked with basewide pelvic limbs that had a longer stride than normal, causing the animal to sway from one side to the other. Occasionally the hooves were dragged on their dorsal surface at the onset of the protraction phase of the stride. On turns the hindquarters swayed to the side. The outside pelvic limb often was abducted excessively

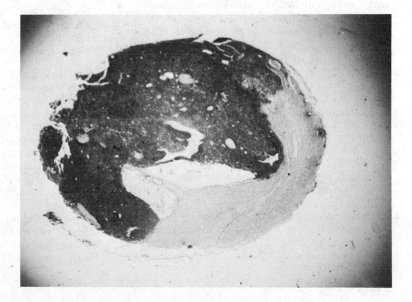

Figure 24–15. Case 9: Transverse section of intradural-extramedullary spinal cord neoplasm at the T12 segment. Hematoxylin and eosin.

during protraction. The thoracic limbs appeared to be hypertonic and spastic, as manifested by a short-strided gait with limited motion of the joints. Occasionally the dorsal surface of the hooves scuffed at the onset of protraction.

Turning the filly in a tight circle exaggerated the ataxia. The pelvic limb on the outside of the turn overflexed or abducted excessively during protraction. The pelvic limb on the inside of the circle occasionally was slow to begin protraction and would remain in one position on the ground, being used as a support for the animal to pivot around. When it did protract it was ataxic and sometimes stepped on the opposite hoof. The thoracic limbs only occasionally were slow to begin protraction or stepped on each other as the animal turned.

Gentle pulling of the filly by the tail to the side as it walked, the sway response, caused it to stumble. There was much less resistance than normal to this tail pressure. Finger pressure applied to the withers or loin caused the filly to sink and almost collapse on the ground.

When allowed to run free in a paddock, the filly showed less gait deficit as it ran in a straight line but remarkable ataxia and some paresis when forced to turn quickly at the end of the paddock.

Muscle tone and size appeared to be normal. The perineal and tail tone and reflexes were normal. No hypalgesia could be detected. Cervical vertebral palpation and manipulation were normal. No abnormal pain was elicited.

Cranial nerve examination was normal.

Diagnosis

Neuroanatomic Diagnosis. The clinical signs of spastic paresis and ataxia reflect a deficit in function of the upper motor neuron and general proprioceptive systems, respectively. The symmetry of signs and abnormality of all four limbs indicate a focal cervical or diffuse spinal cord white matter lesion.

Differential Diagnosis. A diffuse degenerative myeloencephalopathy occurs in young horses of many breeds and causes slowly progressive signs.[11, 12] The onset is prior to 2 years and often prior to 6 months. The signs reflect the diffuse degeneration of neurons in all funiculi. It predominates in the thoracic spinal cord and in the spinocerebellar tracts. This was considered the most likely presumptive diagnosis for this patient.

An atlanto-occipital malformation occurs in Arabian horses and causes cranial cervical spinal cord compression that produces signs at birth or usually by a few months of age. The signs are often quite severe. This malformation can be detected by the abnormal posture of the neck with limited flexion of the atlanto-occipital joint. This immobility, as well as the abnormal vertebra, can be palpated. Radiography will confirm the diagnosis.

Cervical stenotic myelopathy can produce these signs. This is the cervical vertebral malarticulation-malformation that is the cause of cervical spinal

cord compression referred to as the wobbler syndrome. It usually does not produce signs before 6 months of age and would not be expected to produce signs before 1 month of age, as in this patient. Physical and neurologic examination cannot differentiate this disease from degenerative myeloencephalopathy. Radiographic study with careful measurement of the cranial and caudal orifices of each vertebral foramen may reveal stenosis associated with a malformation or malarticulation.

Spinal cord compression from an epidural abscess with or without osteomyelitis is uncommon in the horse. The prolonged course and the absence of other signs of infection and pain on cervical vertebral manipulation would not suggest this diagnosis.

The early age of onset and the long, slowly progressive course would not be expected from the various equine spinal cord inflammatory diseases. Protozoal myelitis is the most common cause of a focal, segmental, cervical spinal cord lesion of an inflammatory nature. It is rare in horses under 1 year of age and usually produces more rapidly progressive signs, although some have been observed to remain unchanged over fairly long periods of time. There was no asymmetry of signs or focal areas of hypalgesia, reflex loss, or atrophy to suggest this diagnosis. Equine herpesvirus type I (rhinopneumonitis), encephalomyelopathy, and vasculitis can produce similar signs owing to the diffuse nature of the spinal cord ischemic leukomyelopathy. However, the signs are always sudden in onset and not progressive, as in this case. *Streptococcus equi* produces parenchymal abscesses in the brain of horses but rarely in the spinal cord. Such a lesion in the spinal cord would most likely produce more severe or asymmetric signs. Similarly, parasitic myelitis would be expected to produce more asymmetric signs and either no progression following one excursion through the parenchyma or more rapid progression from subsequent migration than was observed here.

The slow onset and progression of signs would not be compatible with a traumatic lesion of external origin. The short period of normal posture and gait and the slowly progressive signs would not occur with a spinal cord malformation.

Ancillary Studies. Plain radiographs of the cervical vertebrae from full extension to full flexion were normal. A cisternal myelogram was performed. Although with the neck in full flexion there was interruption but not obstruction to the flow in the ventral aspect of the subarachnoid space over the craniodorsal aspects of each vertebral body, normal flow occurred along the dorsal aspect of the spinal cord. This is a normal phenomenon in the horse. A cervical venogram following the introduction of radiopaque dye into the marrow of the body of the axis revealed no obstruction to flow in the vertebral ventral internal venous plexus.

Lumbosacral and cisternal cerebrospinal fluids were normal.

Outcome

Because of the slowly progressive signs and poor prognosis for normal use of this animal, the owner requested euthanasia.

Necropsy Findings. No gross lesions were apparent in the central nervous system. When the cervical vertebrae were disarticulated no compression of the spinal cord was apparent when it was observed through the interarcuate space as each vertebral articulation was flexed and extended. There were no significant abnormalities in the disarticulated cervical vertebrae.

On microscopic examination there was a diffuse degenerative lesion in the central nervous system that was most apparent in the spinal cord white matter. Myelin degeneration was apparent in all spinal cord segments. This lesion predominated in the lateral and ventral funiculi of the thoracic spinal cord. The spinocerebellar tracts were the most completely involved (Fig. 24–16). Astrocytosis accompanied this lesion. There was axonal degeneration scattered through the white and grey matter of almost all segments, but it was especially pronounced in the nuclei of the dorsal spinocerebellar tracts. It also occurred in various nuclear areas in the brain stem, especially the caudal medullary prorioceptive nuclei.

These lesions are compatible with the diagnosis of degenerative myeloencephalopathy. This disease has been reported in horses and zebras.[11-13] One study of a closely related group of zebras suggested a genetic basis for this disease. Most breeds of horses have been affected, including crossbreeds. No hereditary basis has been established. The mean onset of signs is 6 months, with a range of from near birth to 24 months. There is a chronic progression of signs from the time of onset in most horses. They may eventually stabilize and not progress. Affected horses rarely become recumbent. Recovery does not occur. The disease is presumed to be a form of progressive neuronal degeneration. A nutritional pathogenesis is being investigated.

Case 11: Case Description

Signalment. A 7-year-old female domestic cat.

Chief Complaint. Seizures, behavioral change.

History. The cat experienced a sudden onset of depression, lack of normal responsiveness to its owners, and episodes of jerky movements in the face and left thoracic limb. The following day it was presented to a veterinarian who observed two of the episodes and described the cat as turning its head with jerky shaking movements to the left, and extending the left thoracic limb caudally along the trunk in a series of clonic movements. Similar clonic movements occurred in the left pelvic limb. These were accompanied by facial muscle twitching, excessive salivation, and pupillary dilation. They each lasted about 1 minute, after which the cat seemed to act normally except for expressing resentment at being handled.

The seizures were treated with phenobarbital and thiamine. No more occurred over the next 2 days, and the cat was discharged.

Two weeks later the cat was returned because of a persistent aggressive behavior that made it unmanageable and no longer compatible as a pet.

Examination. The cat was alert and responsive and well oriented to its environment. It resented prolonged handling and would growl and strike

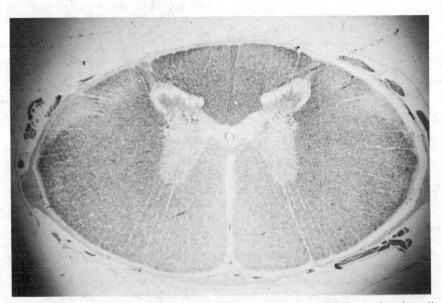

Figure 24–16. Case 10: Transverse section of spinal cord at the T15 segment. Note severity of myelin degeneration in spinocerebellar tracts (dorsolateral funiculi) and in ventral funiculi. Luxol fast blue and cresyl echt violet.

without provocation. No seizure or circling was observed.

The gait was normal, but a mild postural reaction deficit occurred on the left side. The left pelvic limb did not respond as readily as the right with flexion when the cat was backed up in the extensor thrust position. Hopping was also slower in the left pelvic limb. Hopping on each thoracic limb showed only an equivocal deficit in the left thoracic limb, but when the animal was walked forward only on the thoracic limbs (wheelbarrowing) with the neck extended, the left thoracic limb was slower and often adducted and brushed the medial side of the right limb. Normal tone and mass were determined on passive manipulation and palpation of the limb. Patellar and flexor reflexes were normal, as was pain perception. No asymmetry was detected.

There was a persistent menace deficit in the lateral visual field of the left eyeball. Pupillary responses to light were normal. The remaining cranial nerve functions were normal.

Diagnosis

Neuroanatomic Diagnosis. These signs are compatible with a right cerebral lesion. The partial seizure described consistently on the left side of the trunk and left limbs reflects a seizure focus in the contralateral motor cortex. Disturbance of the function of this right sensorimotor cortex or its afferent and efferent processes in the internal capsule does not affect the gait but interferes with the contralateral postural reactions, as seen in this patient. The menace deficit in the left side of the visual field of the left eye with normal pupillary responses to light can be explained by a lesion in the right optic tract, lateral geniculate nucleus, optic radiation, or visual cortex. The latter two would be affected by a right cerebral lesion.

Differential Diagnosis. The most common cause of an acute onset of predominantly unilateral cerebral signs in a cat, followed by partial resolution and often leaving a persistent change in behavior, is an ischemic encephalopathy—cerebral infarction—due to vascular compromise of unknown origin.[4]

External injury could produce similar signs. Accurate documentation of the history should contribute to this diagnosis. Careful observation and palpation of the surface of the head, including the conjunctival surfaces, may show evidence of external injury. Usually following external trauma the cat initially has more severe signs of cerebral disturbance and is slower to resolve than following the cerebral infarction syndrome. Radiography may reveal evidence of an external injury.

One of the most common causes of seizures in cats is thiamine deficiency secondary to prolonged anorexia or all-fish diets with significant thiaminase content. Seizures usually are generalized. Ataxia and pupillary dilation may be observed on interictal

examination, but not the entirely unilateral deficits observed in this patient. The lesion is a diffuse metabolic encephalopathy that ultimately results in a bilateral degenerative lesion in the brain stem. The lack of appropriate history and the presence of focal, lateralizing cerebral signs in this cat would not warrant this diagnosis.

Of the various inflammatory diseases that affect the brain of the cat, a toxoplasma granuloma or bacterial abscess in one cerebrum would best comply with the focal signs observed. In either case the acute onset followed by partial resolution of signs would be unlikely. The agent of feline infectious peritonitis and *Cryptococcus neoformans* produce diffuse meningitis or ependymitis, or both, and diffuse, less localizing signs. Usually if the signs of these diseases reflect a focal area of the involvement, it is referable to the caudal fossa and cerebellomedullary regions, and not the cerebrum. Cerebrospinal fluid should reflect the nature of these inflammatory diseases.

Meningiomas and gliomas occasionally occur in older cats and could produce these focal signs, but the sudden onset and nonprogression of the clinical disorder would be unlikely.

Similarly, the acute onset and lack of progression, as well as the age of onset, would eliminate brain malformation or the degenerative diseases caused by the inborn errors of metabolism. Signs of a unilateral cerebral malformation would be present at birth, or if seizures were the first indication of this lesion they would be expected to occur before a year of age. The feline leukodystrophies and lipodystrophies that have been described have produced signs in young cats less than 6 months old. Although toxic encephalopathy from such chemicals as lead, ethylene glycol, organophosphates, or chlorinated hydrocarbons may produce a sudden onset of seizures, residual signs of a unilateral cerebral lesion or the spontaneous resolution of signs would not be expected.

Ancillary Studies. Radiographs of the skull were normal. Cisternal cerebrospinal fluid contained 1634 RBC per cmm without crenation or xanthochromia, 9 mononuclear cells per cmm, and 18 mg per dl of protein. Tests for feline leukemia virus were negative.

Outcome

The cerebrospinal fluid abnormality was consistent with an ischemic lesion and the inflammatory response to the tissue damage. The red blood cells presumably resulted from the procedure for obtaining the fluid. Erythrocytes from previous hemorrhage usually are crenated and the fluid may be xanthochromic after the cells are removed by centrifugation. Usually the protein also is mildly elevated following the parenchymal destruction that occurs in cerebral infarction.

Because this cat's change in behavior made it incompatible as a pet, euthanasia was requested.

Necropsy Findings. The only gross lesion observed on removal of the brain was a yellow discoloration and softness of the right temporal lobe. On palpation of the transverse sections of the formalin-fixed brain there was softening evident in both pyriform lobes and the adjacent parahippocampal gyri.

Microscopic examination revealed an extensive encephalopathy bilaterally in the parahippocampal gyri and the hippocampus. On the right side the lesion extended into the cerebral cortex of the gyri of the frontal and parietal lobes located laterally. The lesion consisted of parenchymal degeneration with extensive astrocyte proliferation and hypertrophy. These hyperplastic gemistocytes completely filled areas of cortex, with varying degrees of neuron loss and degeneration. Occasionally small areas of cavitation occurred in the hippocampus and parahippocampal gyrus. Small blood vessels were prominent in these areas. A few vessels in the lesion and in the leptomeninges were surrounded by lymphocytes. No primary vessel lesion was observed. These lesions are compatible with an ischemic pathogenesis. The degenerate areas mostly are supplied by branches of the middle cerebral arteries.

These lesions confirmed the diagnosis of feline ischemic encephalopathy or cerebral infarction. The disease has been observed in adult cats of all breeds and ages at all times of the year but primarily in the late summer. Although the cerebral lesion is ischemic in nature, the cause of the ischemia is not known. Vascular lesions have only been observed in a few patients. Viral isolation procedures on tissue culture and electron microscopy on brain tissue have not revealed any agent. No relationship to cardiomyopathy has been observed.

Although the lesion is usually most profound in the distribution of one middle cerebral artery (Fig. 24–17), it is not limited to the area of brain supplied by that vessel. Although the signs reflect a unilateral cerebral lesion, the lesions are often bilateral but worse in one cerebrum. In addition, occasionally lesions occur in the brain stem but to a lesser extent and usually without associated clinical signs.

The prognosis for life in these cats is usually good. Only one death has been observed associated with this lesion, and that occurred within the first 24 hours of recognized signs. Residual signs that may affect the animal's compatibility as a companion include propulsive pacing or circling, seizures, or a change in behavior to aggressiveness.

Case 12: Case Description

Signalment. An 8-month-old female Cairn terrier.

Chief Complaint. Depression and ataxia.

History. At 6 months of age this dog was presented to a veterinarian for lethargy, frequent urination, increased water consumption, and carrying the tail flexed between the pelvic limbs. A granular yellow discharge was noted at the vulva. The dog was treated for cystitis and these signs resolved after 4 days of hospitalization. The vaccination status was considered adequate.

At 8 months old the animal was reexamined for depression, circling, standing with its head pressed against the wall, and abnormal use of the pelvic limbs that had been present for 24 hours. The owner recalled that there were other brief periods when the dog stood quietly staring off into space, seemingly oblivious of the environment.

After 24 hours of hospitalization and treatment with fluids, antibiotics, and steroids the dog's behavior was normal.

Laboratory tests performed at this time revealed a leukocytosis (23,800 per cmm) and neutrophilia (19,278 per cmm). The total plasma protein was low at 4.5 gm per dl (normal: 6.0–7.8). The blood urea nitrogen was slightly low at 9 mg per dl (normal: 10–20). The serum alanine aminotransferase was significantly elevated at 192 Sigma-Frankel units (normal: <50), as was the serum alkaline

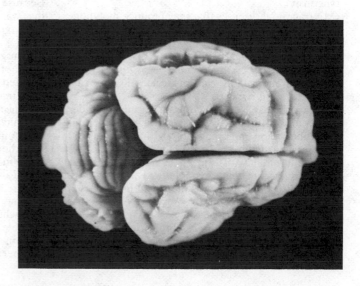

Figure 24–17. Case 11: Dorsoventral view of right cerebral atrophy secondary to cerebral infarction, mostly in the distribution of the right middle cerebral artery. This is another cat with signs similar to those of case 11.

phosphatase at 263 international units (normal: <30). Subsequently, during similar episodes of depression the animal responded to removal of food.

Examination. The dog was small for its breed and age. No physical or neurologic abnormalities were observed.

Diagnosis

Neuroanatomic Diagnosis. Although no signs were observed during the examination, the signs described in the history were suggestive of a diffuse neurologic disorder with cerebral involvement. The depression and change in behavior reflected decreased cerebrocortical or ascending reticular activating system function and limbic system disturbance. The pelvic limb ataxia may reflect mild diffuse brain stem dysfunction, or spinal cord dysfunction, or both.

Differential Diagnosis. Neurologic abnormalities that consist of a transient disturbance of brain function that ceases spontaneously but has a tendency to recur are suggestive of a metabolic abnormality.

Major structural brain lesions rarely produce the signs described with periods of complete recovery. For this reason it would be unlikely that these signs were due to lesions caused by inflammation, injury, malformation, or neoplasia. Minor structural lesions in an area of the brain that does not produce signs of neurologic deficit may initiate seizures, but examination in the interictal period is normal.

Lead poisoning, which is more common in the young dog and may produce signs of gastrointestinal disturbance along with neurologic signs, usually causes seizures. If the encephalopathy is severe, persistent signs of structural disease may occur and produce lethargy, visual deficits, and ataxia. However, these would not be expected to resolve spontaneously.

Extracranial diseases that may produce metabolic encephalopathy include pancreatic beta cell neoplasms or metabolic abnormalities in glycogenolysis that produce hypoglycemia, hepatic disease leading to significant hyperammonemia, renal disease with chronic uremia, and cardiovascular disease that causes cerebral hypoxia.

Beta cell pancreatic neoplasms occur in older dogs and would be unlikely at this age. The metabolic aberration in glycogenolysis that is found in toy breeds usually occurs around 3 months of age. Chronic uremia with encephalopathy at this age could result from renal hypoplasia. The most common cardiovascular diseases that result in decreased cardiac output and cerebral hypoxia are arrhythmias such as ventricular tachycardia and atrial fibrillation, severe heart block, or rarely, dirofilariasis. Hepatic encephalopathy at this age is most commonly due to an abnormal portacaval anastomosis.[2]

Ancillary Studies. Clinical laboratory studies revealed a mild leukocytosis (18,500 per cmm) with neutrophilia (13,300 per cmm), monocytosis (2,600 per cmm), and band cells (600 per cmm). A mild anemia was present (PCV 33; 1.1 per cent reticulocytes). Total serum protein was reduced to 3.2 gm per dl (normal: 5.0–6.7) with both albumin and globulin less than normal: albumin 1.7 gm per dl (normal: 2.6–3.4); globulin 1.5 gm per dl (normal: 2.0–3.9). Liver enzymes were elevated in the serum: alkaline phosphatase 98 international units (<30); alanine aminotransferase 220 Sigma-Frankel units (<50). Bromsulphalein was retained longer than normal—19.5 per cent at 30 minutes (<5). Blood urea nitrogen was normal (13 mg per dl) on one occasion and below normal (5 mg per dl) on another (normal: 10–20 mg per dl). Blood glucose levels varied excessively. On three occasions levels were determined at 201, 56, and 53 mg per dl (normal: 70–110). Urate crystals were found in the urine on one of five urinalyses. Fasting and 2-hour postprandial serum ammonia values were significantly elevated. The patient's levels were 0.27 and 0.24 micromole per L respectively, while in the control animal they were .02 and .02 micromole per L.

Plain radiographs revealed a small liver shadow. This was confirmed at laparotomy when a catheter was placed in an intestinal vein of the jejunum. A portogram showed simultaneous opacification of the caudal vena cava and portal vein and liver (Fig. 24–18). A single vessel looped ventrally and then dorsally as it coursed from the portal vein to the caudal vena cava caudal to the diaphragm. This anastomosis left the portal vein just caudal to its right hepatic branch. This represents a reversal of flow through the splenic and left gastric veins, entering the caudal vena cava at the diaphragm.

Outcome

The ancillary studies confirmed the diagnosis of hepatic encephalopathy due to portacaval shunt. Because the anastomosis consisted of a single vessel that was accessible to ligation, it is a consideration for surgery if there is not excessive portal hypertension.

Conservative therapy was instituted, which consisted of a low protein, high carbohydrate diet that was fed in small amounts at short intervals.[1] An intestinal antibiotic (neomycin sulfate) also was administered for varying periods of time. This dog was alive at 2 years of age, functioning well as a pet 15 months after this diagnosis.

Although this disease more commonly is seen in the young dog, occasionally it has not been diagnosed in a dog until 6 years of age. Although the disease has been reported in numerous breeds, there is some indication that it may be familial in miniature schnauzers. The clinical signs can be extremely variable and reflect involvement of one or more systems including hepatic, gastrointestinal, renal, and nervous systems. Stunting and weight loss are

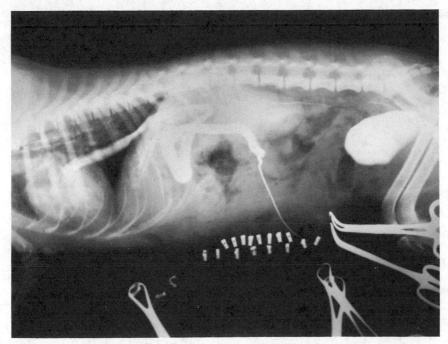

Figure 24–18. Case 12: Portogram following celiotomy and cannulation of a jejunal vein. Two seconds following injection, dye is apparent in the portal vein, its branches in the atrophic liver, a large single portacaval shunt caudal to the liver, and the caudal vena cava. Dye in the kidneys, ureters, and bladder is from a previous injection.

common. Clinical complaints often include anorexia, vomiting, ascites, polyuria, polydypsia, depression, weakness, ataxia, seizures, pacing, disorientation and staring, head pressing, blindness, stupor, and coma.

Hepatic encephalopathy also has been reported associated with urea cycle enzyme deficiencies and advanced liver disease that includes chronic cirrhosis and diffuse neoplastic infiltration.

REFERENCES

1. Barrett, R. E.: Canine hepatic encephalopathy. *In* Kirk, R. W. (ed.): Current Veterinary Therapy VI. W. B. Saunders, Philadelphia, 1977.
2. Barrett, R. E., de Lahunta, A., Roenigk, W. J., Hoffer, R. E., and Coons, F. H.: Four cases of congenital portacaval shunt in the dog. J. Small Anim. Pract., *17*:71, 1976.
3. Berryman, F. C., and de Lahunta, A.: Astrocytoma in a dog causing convulsions. Cornell Vet., *65*:212, 1975.
4. de Lahunta, A.: Feline ischemic encephalopathy—a cerebral infarction syndrome. *In* Kirk, R. W. (ed.): Current Veterinary Therapy VI. W. B. Saunders, Philadelphia, 1977.
5. de Lahunta, A., and Alexander, J. W.: Ischemic myelopathy secondary to presumed fibrocartilaginous embolism in nine dogs. J. Am. Anim. Hosp. Assoc., *12*:37, 1976.
6. Dubey, J. P., Davis, G. W., Koestner, A., and Kiryu, K.: Equine encephalomyelitis due to a protozoan parasite resembling *Toxoplasma gondii*. J. Am. Vet. Med. Assoc., *165*:249, 1974.
7. Fankhauser, R., Fatzer, R., Luginbühl, H., and McGrath, J. T. III: Primary reticulosis of the CNS in animals. Adv. Vet. Sci. Comp. Med., *16*:40, 1972.
8. Hayes, M. A., Creighton, S. R., Boysen, B. A., and Holfeld, N.: Acute necrotizing myelopathy from nucleus pulposus embolism in dogs with intervertebral disk degeneration. J. Am. Vet. Med. Assoc., *173*:289, 1978.
9. Koestner, A., and Zeman, W.: Primary reticuloses of the central nervous system in dogs. Am. J. Vet. Res., *23*:381, 1962.
10. Luttgen, P. J., Braund, K. G., Brawner, W. R., and Vandevelde, M.: A retrospective study of 29 spinal tumors in the dog and cat. J. Small Anim. Pract., *21*:213, 1980.
11. Mayhew, I. G., de Lahunta, A., Whitlock, R. H., and Geary, J. C.: Equine degenerative myeloencephalopathy. J. Am. Vet. Med. Assoc., *170*:195, 1977.
12. Mayhew, I. G., de Lahunta, A., Whitlock, R. A., Krook, L., and Tasker, J. B.: Spinal cord disease in the horse. Cornell Vet. [Suppl. 6], *68*:1, 1978.
13. Montali, R. J., Bush, M., Sauer, R. M., Gray, C. W., and Xanten, W. A.: Spinal ataxia in zebras. Vet. Pathol., *11*:68, 1974.
14. Northington, J. W.: Metrizamide myelography in five dogs and two cats with suspected spinal cord neoplasms. J. Am. Vet. Radiol. Soc., *21*:149, 1980.
15. Schiefer, B., and Dahme, E.: Primäre Geschwülste des ZNS bei Tieren. Acta Neuropathol., *2*:202, 1962.
16. Simpson, C. F., and Mayhew, I. G.: Evidence for

Sarcocystis as the etiologic agent of equine protozoal myeloencephalitis. J. Protozool., *27*:288, 1980.

17. Teuscher, E., and Cherrstrom, E. C.: Ependymoma
of the spinal cord in a young dog. Schweiz. Arch.
Tierheilk., *116*:461, 1974.

18. Zaki, F. A., Prata, R. G., and Kay, W. J.: Necrotizing

myelopathy in five Great Danes. J. Am. Vet. Med.
Assoc., *165*:1080, 1974.

19. Zaki, F. A., and Prata, R. G.: Necrotizing myelopathy
secondary to embolization of herniated intervertebral disk material in the dog. J. Am. Vet. Med.
Assoc., *169*:222, 1976.

APPENDIX

TRANSVERSE BRAIN SECTIONS

Approximate Levels of 16 Plates of Dog Brain

The following transverse sections are arranged from caudal to rostral through the brain. The white matter is stained and appears black, whereas the grey matter is relatively unstained.

Dorsal view of brain stem.

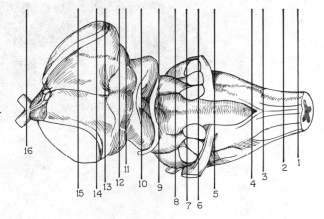

Left lateral surface of the brain stem. (After Evans, H. E., and de Lahunta, Λ.: Miller's Guide to the Dissection of the Dog. Philadelphia, W. B. Saunders Co., 1971.)

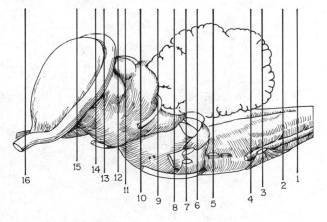

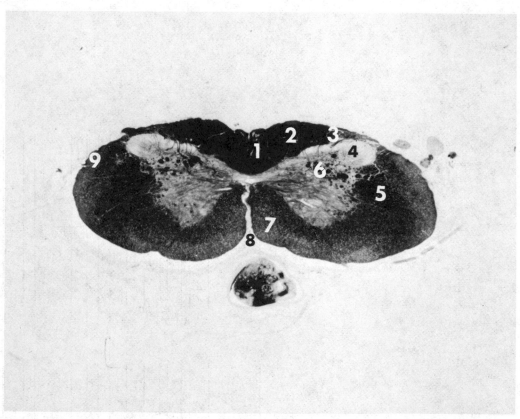

PLATE 1

1. Fasciculus gracilis
2. Fasciculus cuneatus
3. Spinal tract of trigeminal nerve
4. Nucleus of spinal tract of trigeminal nerve–dorsal grey column, first cervical segment
5. Rubrospinal tract
6. Lateral pyramidal (corticospinal) tract
7. Vestibulospinal tract
8. Ventral median fissure
9. Spinocerebellar tracts

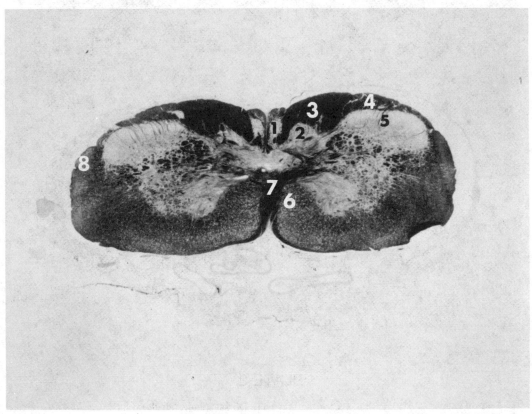

PLATE 2

1. Nucleus gracilis
2. Medial cuneate nucleus
3. Fasciculus cuneatus
4. Spinal tract of trigeminal nerve
5. Nucleus of spinal tract of trigeminal nerve
6. Medial longitudinal fasciculus—tectospinal part
7. Pyramidal decussation
8. Spinocerebellar tracts

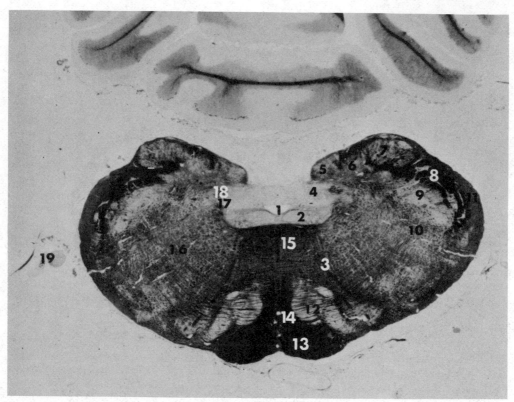

PLATE 3

1. Central canal
2. Hypoglossal motor nucleus
3. Radix of hypoglossal nerve
4. Parasympathetic nucleus of vagus nerve
5. Nucleus gracilis
6. Medial cuneate nucleus
7. Lateral cuneate nucleus
8. Spinal tract of trigeminal nerve
9. Nucleus of spinal tract of trigeminal nerve
10. Nucleus ambiguus

11. Dorsal spinocerebellar tract
12. Olivary nucleus
13. Pyramidal tract
14. Medial lemniscus
15. Medial longitudinal fasciculus—tectospinal part
16. Reticular formation
17. Nucleus of solitary tract
18. Solitary tract
19. Accessory nerve

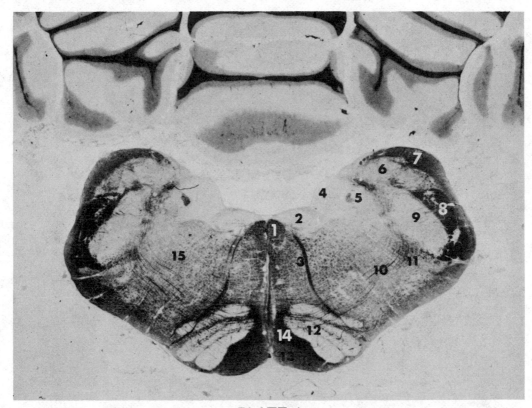

PLATE 4

1. Medial longitudinal fasciculus
2. Hypoglossal motor nucleus
3. Radix of hypoglossal nerve
4. Parasympathetic nucleus of vagus nerve
5. Nucleus of solitary tract
6. Lateral cuneate nucleus
7. Caudal cerebellar peduncle
8. Spinal tract of trigeminal nerve

9. Nucleus of spinal tract of trigeminal nerve
10. Deep arcuate fibers
11. Nucleus ambiguus
12. Olivary nucleus
13. Pyramidal tract
14. Medial lemniscus
15. Reticular formation

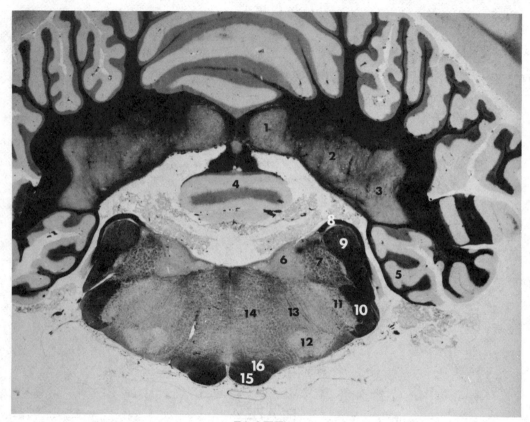

PLATE 5

1. Fastigial cerebellar nucleus
2. Interpositial cerebellar nucleus
3. Lateral cerebellar nucleus
4. Nodulus
5. Flocculus
6. Medial vestibular nucleus
7. Caudal (descending) vestibular nucleus
8. Acoustic stria
9. Caudal cerebellar peduncle
10. Spinal tract of trigeminal nerve
11. Nucleus of spinal tract of trigeminal nerve
12. Facial motor nucleus
13. Ascending facial nerve fibers
14. Reticular formation
15. Pyramidal tract
16. Medial lemniscus

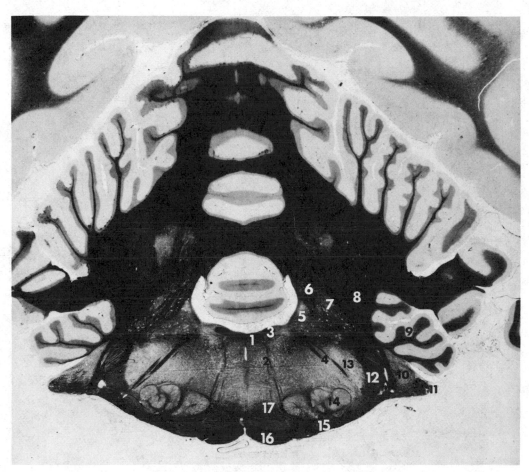

PLATE 6

1. Medial longitudinal fasciculus
2. Abducent nerve fibers
3. Genu of facial nerve
4. Descending facial nerve fibers
5. Medial vestibular nucleus
6. Vestibulocerebellar fibers
7. Lateral vestibular nucleus
8. Caudal cerebellar peduncle
9. Flocculus

10. Cochlear nuclei
11. Vestibulocochlear nerve
12. Spinal tract of trigeminal nerve
13. Nucleus of spinal tract of trigeminal nerve
14. Dorsal nucleus of trapezoid body
15. Trapezoid body
16. Pyramidal tract
17. Medial lemniscus

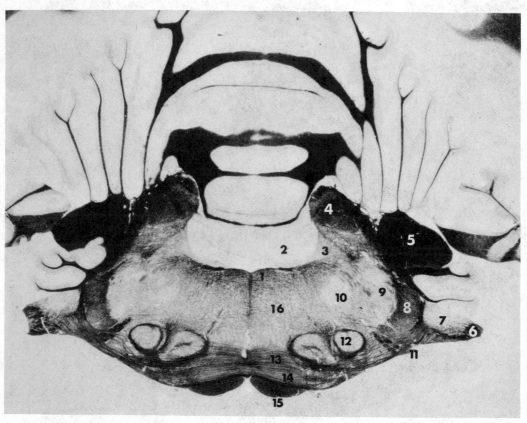

PLATE 7

1. Medial longitudinal fasciculus
2. Rostral medullary velum
3. Rostral vestibular nucleus
4. Rostral cerebellar peduncle
5. Middle cerebellar peduncle
6. Vestibulocochlear nerve
7. Cochlear nuclei
8. Trigeminal nerve
9. Nucleus of spinal tract of trigeminal nerve, rostral part (pontine sensory)
10. Motor nucleus of trigeminal nerve
11. Facial nerve
12. Dorsal nucleus of trapezoid body
13. Medial lemniscus
14. Trapezoid body
15. Pyramid
16. Reticular formation

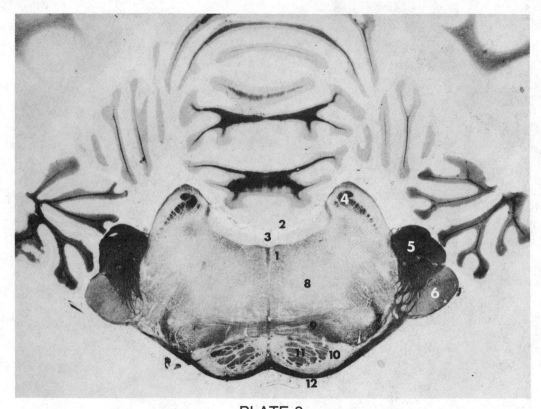

PLATE 8

1. Medial longitudinal fasciculus
2. Rostral medullary velum
3. Fourth ventricle
4. Rostral cerebellar peduncle
5. Middle cerebellar peduncle
6. Trigeminal nerve
7. Lateral lemniscus
8. Reticular formation
9. Medial lemniscus
10. Pontine nuclei
11. Longitudinal fibers of pons
12. Transverse fibers of pons

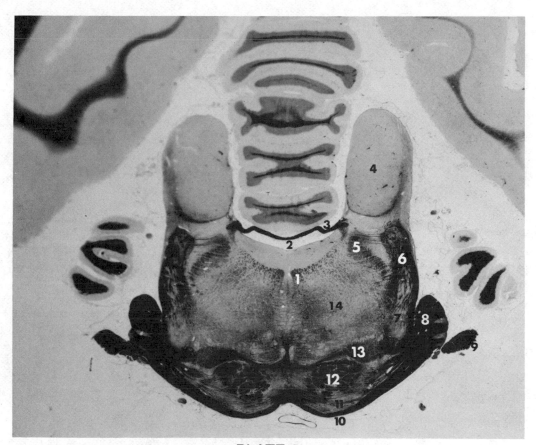

PLATE 9

1. Medial longitudinal fasciculus
2. Fourth ventricle
3. Trochlear nerve
4. Caudal colliculus
5. Rostral cerebellar peduncle
6. Lateral lemniscus
7. Nucleus of lateral lemniscus

8. Middle cerebellar peduncle
9. Trigeminal nerve
10. Transverse fibers of pons
11. Pontine nuclei
12. Longitudinal fibers of pons
13. Medial lemniscus
14. Reticular formation

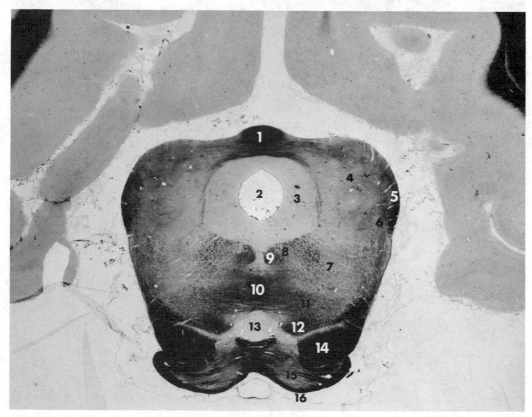

PLATE 10

1. Commissure of caudal colliculus
2. Mesencephalic aqueduct
3. Central grey substance
4. Caudal colliculus
5. Brachium of caudal colliculus
6. Lateral lemniscus
7. Reticular formation
8. Motor nucleus of trochlear nerve
9. Medial longitudinal fasciculus
10. Decussation of rostral cerebellar peduncle
11. Rubrospinal tract
12. Medial lemniscus
13. Intercrural nucleus
14. Crus cerebri
15. Pontine nuclei
16. Transverse fibers of pons

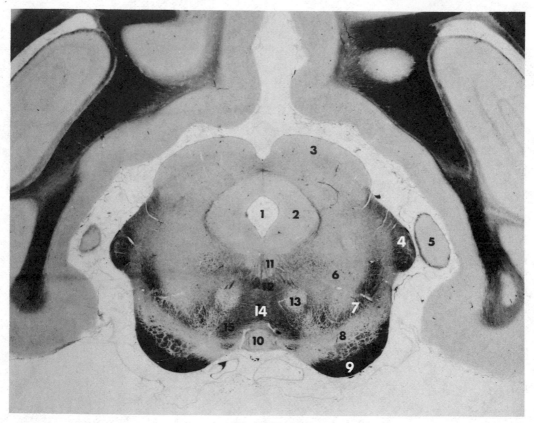

PLATE 11

1. Mesencephalic aqueduct
2. Central grey substance
3. Rostral colliculus
4. Brachium of caudal colliculus
5. Medial geniculate nucleus
6. Reticular formation (deep mesencephalic nucleus)
7. Medial lemniscus
8. Substantia nigra
9. Crus cerebri
10. Intercrural nucleus
11. Oculomotor motor nucleus
12. Medial longitudinal fasciculus
13. Red nucleus
14. Ventral tegmental decussation (rubrospinal neurons)
15. Rubrospinal tract

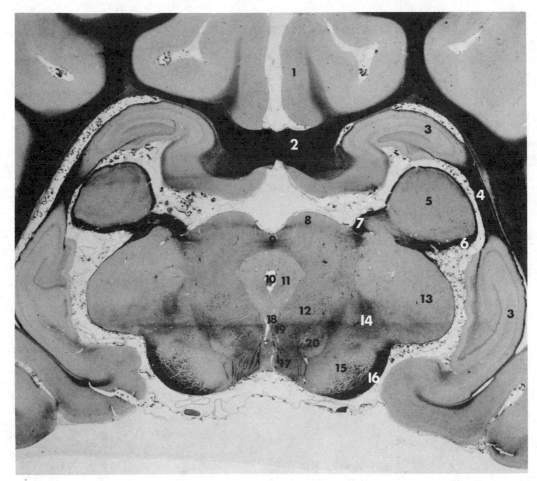

PLATE 12

1. Cingulate gyrus
2. Splenium of corpus callosum
3. Hippocampus
4. Crus of fornix
5. Thalamic nucleus—lateral geniculate
6. Optic tract
7. Brachium of rostral colliculus
8. Rostral colliculus
9. Commissure of rostral colliculus
10. Mesencephalic aqueduct
11. Central grey substance
12. Reticular formation (deep mesencephalic nucleus)
13. Thalamic nucleus—medial geniculate
14. Medial lemniscus
15. Substantia nigra
16. Crus cerebri
17. Oculomotor nerve fibers
18. Parasympathetic nucleus of oculomotor nerve
19. Medial longitudinal fasciculus
20. Red nucleus

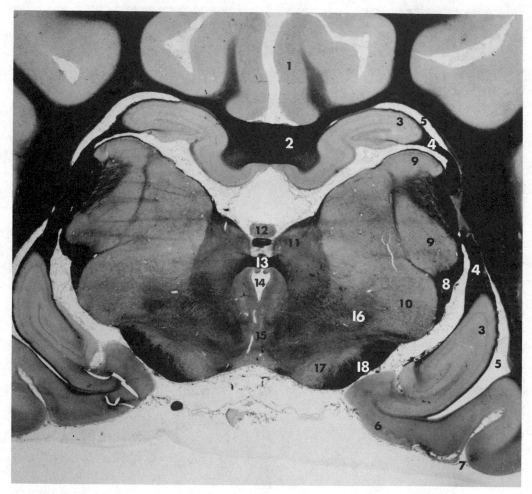

PLATE 13

1. Cingulate gyrus
2. Splenium of corpus callosum
3. Hippocampus
4. Crus of fornix
5. Lateral ventricle
6. Parahippocampal gyrus
7. Lateral rhinal sulcus—caudal part
8. Optic tract
9. Thalamic nucleus—lateral geniculate

10. Thalamic nucleus—medial geniculate
11. Pretectal nuclei
12. Pineal body
13. Caudal commissure
14. Mesencephalic aqueduct
15. Parasympathetic nucleus of oculomotor nerve
16. Medial lemniscus
17. Substantia nigra
18. Crus cerebri

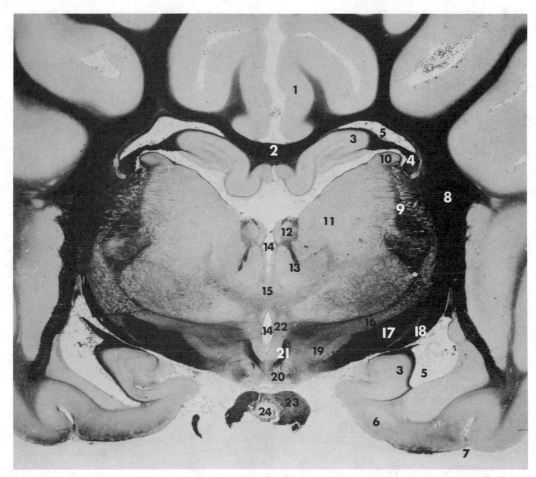

PLATE 14

1. Cingulate gyrus
2. Corpus callosum
3. Hippocampus
4. Crus of fornix
5. Lateral ventricle
6. Parahippocampal gyrus
7. Lateral rhinal sulcus—caudal part
8. Internal capsule
9. Thalamocortical projection fibers
10. Thalamic nucleus—lateral geniculate
11. Thalamic nuclei
12. Habenular nucleus
13. Fasciculus retroflexus (habenulointercrural tract)
14. Third ventricle
15. Interthalamic adhesion
16. Zona incerta
17. Crus cerebri
18. Optic tract
19. Subthalamic nucleus
20. Mammillary nucleus
21. Mammillothalamic tract
22. Caudal hypothalamic region
23. Adenohypophysis
24. Neurohypophysis

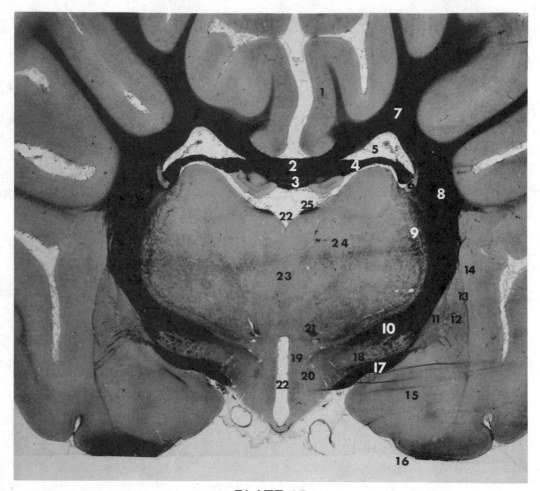

PLATE 15

1. Cingulate gyrus
2. Corpus callosum
3. Body of fornix
4. Crus of fornix
5. Lateral ventricle
6. Caudal caudate nucleus
7. Corona radiata (centrum semiovale)
8. Internal capsule
9. Thalamocortical projection fibers
10. Corticopontine—nuclear—spinal projection fibers
11. Pallidum ⎫
12. Putamen ⎬ Lentiform nucleus

13. External capsule
14. Claustrum
15. Amygdaloid body
16. Pyriform lobe
17. Optic tract
18. Endopeduncular nucleus
19. Hypothalamic nuclei
20. Column of fornix
21. Mammillothalamic tract
22. Third ventricle
23. Interthalamic adhesion
24. Thalamic nuclei
25. Stria habenularis thalami

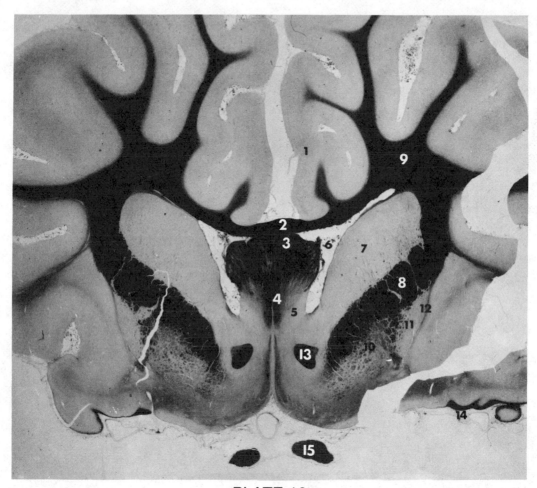

PLATE 16

1. Cingulate gyrus
2. Corpus callosum
3. Body of fornix
4. Column of fornix
5. Telencephalic septum—cellular part (septal nuclei)
6. Lateral ventricle
7. Rostral caudate nucleus

8. Internal capsule
9. Corona radiata (centrum semiovale)
10. Pallidum ⎫ Lentiform nucleus
11. Putamen ⎭
12. External capsule
13. Rostral commissure
14. Lateral olfactory tract
15. Optic nerve

INDEX

Note: Page numbers in *italics* refer to illustrations; those followed by "t" indicate tables.

Malformation *(Continued)*
  cervical vertebrae, in basset hounds, 204
    in Doberman pinschers, 200
    in Great Danes, 200
    in small animals, 199
  definition of, 2
  hereditary, brain-ocular, in Herefords, 27
  index of diseases of, for small animals, 378
  lumbosacral spinal cord, in small animals, 184
  mesencephalic aqueduct, 47
  pathogenesis of, 27
  spinal cord, 26
    in foals, 233
    in large animals, 233
  thoracolumbar spinal cord, 194
  thoracolumbar vertebrae, in small animals, 190
Malformation-malarticulation, of cervical vertebrae,
    in dogs, 200
  in horses, 219
Malignant catarrhal fever, 405
Mammillary body, 319t, *320, 321*
Mammillary peduncle, *320, 321*
Mamillotegmental tract, 319t, *320,* 321
Mammillothalamic tract, 319t, *320,* 321
Mania, 375t
Mannitol, 32
  in brain injury, 358
Mannosidosis, 296t
Mantle layer, 9, *10, 11*
Manx cat, meningomyelocele of, 26
Marginal layer, 9, *10, 11*
Medial forebrain bundle, 319t, 320, *320*
Medial geniculate nucleus, of thalamus, 306, *306*
Medial lemniscus, *160,* 161, *162*
Medial longitudinal fasciculus, 241, *242*
Medulla, 14, 95, 96, *97, 103,* 104, *105*
  clinical signs in, 375t, 376
Medullary reticulospinal tract, 137
Megaesophagus, 69, 107
  neuromuscular defect and, 111
Melanoblasts, 11, *13,* 14
Membrane
  basilar, 304, *305*
  external limiting, of retina, *283,* 285
  internal limiting, of retina, *283,* 286
  vestibular, 304, *305*
Membranous labyrinth, vestibular, 238, *240*
  auditory, 304, *305*
Menace response, in cerebellar disease, 262
Menace test, 289, *290*
Meningitis, suppurative, 204
Meningocele, cerebral, 24
Meningoencephalocele, 24
  in Burmese kittens, 24
Meningomyelocele, 26
  in English bulldogs, 26
  in large animals, 233
  in Manx cats, 26
  in small animals, 184
Mesencephalon, 6, *8,* 17, *17, 18, 19,* 96, *98*
  caudal colliculus of, *306,* 307
  clinical signs in, 375t, 376
  rostral colliculus of, 289
  trigeminal nucleus of, 162
  trigeminal tract of, 162
Mestinon, 70
Metencephalon, 6, *8,* 16
Methiodal sodium, 35
Methylphenidate, 339
Metrizamide, 35
  with seizures, 332

Microphthalmia, 293
Microsmatic species, 316
Micturition
  control of, 123, 124
  neurologic disorders of, 125
Minimum flexion diameter, of equine cervical
    vertebrae, 222
Minimum sagittal diameter, of equine cervical
    vertebrae, 222
Miosis, 116, 122, 291t
Mitral cells, 315
Modiolus, 304
Moldy corn poisoning, in horses, 112
Motor area, of cerebrum, 131, *131*
Motor end plate, 54, *55*
Motor neuron, general visceral efferent, 115
Motor neuron disease, 84
Motor responses, of unconscious animal, 351
Motor systems, 4, 9
Multiple cartilaginous exostosis, 189
Muscle atrophy, examination of, in large animals,
    216
Muscle tone, 177
  examination of, in small animals, 370
Mutilation, self, 173
Myasthenia gravis, 69, 89
  acquired, 69
  congenital, 69
  dysphagia and, 106
Mycotoxicosis, 150
Mydriasis, 121, 122, 291, 291t
Myelencephalon, 6, *8,* 14
Myelin
  disorders of, 149
    in Charolais cattle, 232
Myelinolysis, hereditary, in Afghan hounds, 193
Myelitis
  canine distemper and, 191
  cerebrospinal nematodiasis and, 229
  cryptococcosis and, 191
  equine herpes virus I, 227
  equine nonsuppurative, 228
  equine protozoal, 222t, 225
  feline infectious peritonitis and, 191
  in large animals, 225
  parasitic, in small animals, 205, 229
  Pareluphostrongylus tenuis, 229
  Strongylus vulgaris, in horses, 230
  suppurative, 204
  toxoplasmosis and, 191
  viral, of goats, 228
Myelodysplasia, 26
  in calves, 233
  in small animals, 184
  thoracolumbar spinal cord, in small animals, 194
Myeloencephalopathy, in horses, 222t, 230
Myeloencephalopathy-vasculitis, equine herpes virus
    I, 227
Myelography, 35, *35, 36,* 412
Myelomalacia, diffuse, 82
Myelopathy
  compressive, 81
  degenerative, in German shepherds, 192
    in horses, case study of, 425
  demyelinating, in miniature poodles, 193
  embolic, 81
    fibrocartilaginous, in horses, 232
      in pigs, 232
    of spinal cord, 194, 205
  hereditary myelinolysis and, in Afghan hounds,
    193